Pathology of the
Stomach and Duodenum

Heidrun Rotterdam
Horatio T. Enterline

Pathology
of the
Stomach and
Duodenum

With a Contribution by
Sheldon C. Sommers

With 220 Illustrations

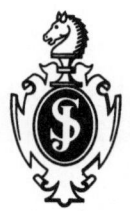

Springer-Verlag
New York Berlin Heidelberg
London Paris Tokyo

Heidrun Rotterdam, M.D. Associate Professor of Surgical Pathology, Department of Pathology, Attending Pathologist, University Hospital, New York University Medical Center, New York, NY 10016, USA

Horatio T. Enterline, M.D. Professor Emeritus of Surgical Pathology, Hospital of the University of Pennsylvania Medical School, Philadelphia, PA 19104, USA

Sheldon C. Sommers, M.D. Clinical Professor of Pathology, Columbia University College of Physicians & Surgeons, New York, NY 10032, USA, Clinical Professor of Pathology, University of Southern California School of Medicine, Los Angeles, CA 90033, USA

Library of Congress Cataloging-in-Publication Data
Rotterdam, Heidrun.
    Pathology of the stomach and duodenum / Heidrun Rotterdam, Horatio
  T. Enterline; with a contribution by Sheldon C. Sommers.
      p.   cm.
    Includes bibliographies and index.
    ISBN-13:978-1-4612-8153-5
    1. Stomach—Diseases. 2. Duodenum—Diseases. I. Enterline,
  Horatio. II. Sommers, Sheldon C. III. Title
    [DNLM: 1. Duodenal Diseases—pathology. 2. Stomach Diseases—
    pathology. WI 300 R851p]
    RC802.9.R67 1988
    616.3′3—dc19
    DNLM/DLC   88-29446

Printed on acid-free paper.

© 1989 by Springer-Verlag New York Inc.
Softcover reprint of the hardcover 1st edition 1989

Typeset by Caliber Design Planning, Inc., New York, New York.

9 8 7 6 5 4 3 2 1

ISBN-13:978-1-4612-8153-5   e-ISBN-13:978-1-4612-3550-7
DOI: 10.1007/978-1-4612-3550-7

Preface

Pathology of the Stomach and Duodenum offers information on all aspects of gastric and duodenal disease including historical, epidemiologic, clinical, and pathophysiologic data with the emphasis on diagnostic gross and microscopic pathology. In an age of ever-increasing subspecialization, we want to stress the importance of evaluating new information in relation to old knowledge, and pathologic features in relation to clinical findings.

We decided to discuss the duodenum in conjunction with the stomach because of the common pathophysiology of some gastric and duodenal diseases, such as peptic ulcer disease. Primary small intestinal diseases, which may also affect the duodenum, however, are excluded here.

We have deliberately cited references of historical interest to offer the reader a perspective on the development of gastroduodenal pathology. The inclusion of chapters on embryology, anatomy, and physiology serves the same purpose of a holistic approach toward the study of disease that must take into account the normal background from which it develops.

The final chapter on miscellaneous lesions deals with rare conditions, many of which reflect the participation of the gastroduodenum in systemic or abdominal disease at large.

Creating a volume of this dimension requires the collaboration of many. We thank Sheldon C. Sommers, M.D., for contributing the chapter on stromal tumors; our families for their patient support; Linda Paul, of the University of Pennsylvania, and Rosemary Gandolfo, of New York University Medical Center, for expert secretarial work; and Pat Kuharic, of Lenox Hill Hospital in New York, and Virginia Meyer, of New York University Medical Center, for illustrations and photographic work.

HEIDRUN ROTTERDAM, M.D.
HORATIO T. ENTERLINE, M.D.

Contents

CHAPTER 1

The Normal Stomach and Duodenum

Embryology

The gastrointestinal tract is derived from the entodermal germ layer, which can be distinguished as a sheet of flat epithelial cells between the ectodermal disc and the blastocyst cavity when the embryo is 8 days old.[1] During the subsequent week, the entodermal cells extend along the wall of the blastocyst cavity until, by the 15th day, they form its entire lining.[2] The formation of head and tail folds results in a division of the entoderm-lined cavity into an intraembryonic portion, the primitive gut, and two extraembryonic portions, the yolk sac and the allantois.

The primitive gut, on the basis of differences in embryonic growth patterns, is divided into three portions: the blind-ending foregut; the midgut, which is temporarily connected with the yolk sac by means of the omphalomesenteric duct; and the blind-ending hindgut. The stomach and proximal, or right, portion of the duodenum are derived from the caudal part of the foregut. The distal portion of the duodenum represents the cephalic part of the midgut. This difference in embryonic derivation is reflected in differences of vascular supply: The stomach and foregut-derived proximal duodenal loop are supplied by the coeliac artery, and the midgut-derived distal portion of the duodenum by the superior mesenteric artery.[3]

In the fourth week of embryonic life the simple straight alimentary tube undergoes its first change in the form of a slight dorsal bulge near the head end, the earliest beginning of the future stomach.[4] The stomach rudiment is initially on a level with the heart rudiment.[3] In the fifth week the gastric part of the foregut is a fusiform dilatation located in the septum transversum, the primitive diaphragm. Its subsequent caudal migration is mainly due to the great enlargement of the thorax by the developing lungs. The stomach, however, like the diaphragm and the lungs, is primarily a cervical structure, as is shown by its innervation.

During the following weeks the appearance of the stomach and duodenum change greatly due to different rates of growth in various regions of the gut and due to rotations. While the growth rate of the intestine increases continually and much more quickly than that of the total body during prenatal life, the growth rate of the stomach decreases by a constant amount over time.[5] In the third month the stomach first rotates about a longitudinal axis, whereby the left side becomes the anterior surface and the right side the posterior surface (Fig. 1-1A). The left vagus nerve comes to innervate the anterior wall, the right vagus nerve the posterior wall. The formation of the greater and lesser curvatures is the result of the relative faster growth of the original posterior part of the stomach as compared with the anterior part.[1] The stomach then rotates about an antero-posterior axis, whereby the pyloric end moves upward and to the right and the cardiac end moves downward and to the left (Fig. 1-1B).

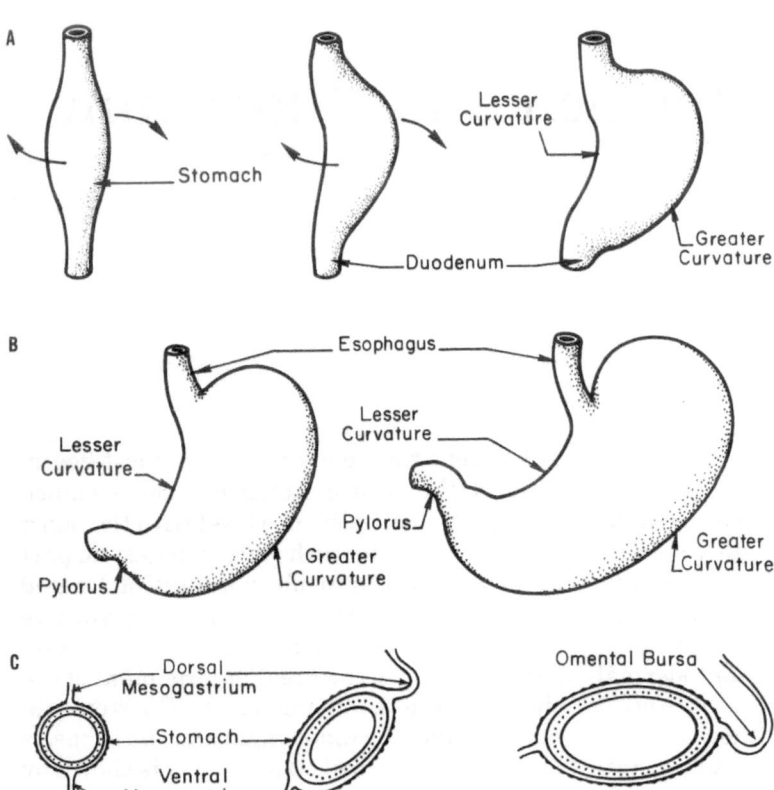

Figure 1-1. Development of the stomach in the third month of embryonic life. **A.** Rotation about a longitudinal axis (*left*) is followed by the relatively faster growth of the original posterior part of the stomach (*center*), resulting in the formation of the lesser and greater curvatures (*right*). **B.** A second rotation of the stomach about an anteroposterior axis results in the upward and right movement of the pylorus and the downward and left movement of the cardia. **C.** Formation of the omental bursa during the process of rotation.

By this double rotation the stomach assumes approximately its adult position. As the stomach rotates, the duodenum takes on the form of a U-shaped loop, rotates to the right, and finally comes to lie retroperitoneally.

Before the rotations the stomach is attached to the dorsal and ventral body walls by peritoneal folds, the dorsal and ventral mesogastrium. At the very beginning of the process of rotation, the dorsal mesogastrium becomes redundant and sags increasingly to the left until a pouch is formed behind the stomach, the omental bursa, with its opening to the right (Fig. 1-1C). Subsequently, in the third and fourth month, the same, originally posterior, mesogastrium lengthens more and more and, with the rotation of the stomach, comes to form the greater omentum.[4]

The ventral mesogastrium undergoes a double change as well. With the development of the liver in its midportion it is divided into a part connecting the anterior abdominal wall with the liver, the falciform ligament, and a part connecting the liver with the lesser curvature of the stomach, the lesser omentum. Following the rotations of the stomach, the ventral mesogastrium becomes a transverse fold and the lesser omentum the ventral boundary of the orifice of the omental bursa.

The histologic development of the gut comprises the differentiation of the two constituent elements of its wall, the entoderm and the visceral mesoderm.[4] The glands are the product of the entoderm, the entire connective tissue and muscle the product of the mesoderm. By the fourth or fifth week the embryonic stomach has a small lumen and a relatively thick multilayered lining.[6] As the organ grows the mucosa becomes thinner and pitted on the surface by primary gastric pits. The glands of the stomach are formed by multiplication and aggregation of entodermal cells, which first form solid cylindric cell masses and then become hollowed out and branch in the 10th week. Initially the peptic glands contain only one cell type. In the fourth month certain cells gradually accumulate cytoplasmic granules and differentiate into parietal cells (Fig. 1-2). Although pepsin is present at 16 weeks, acid production develops much later.

Much of the duodenal differentiation occurs in the second gestational month. When the embryo measures 8.5 mm, there is no duodenal lumen between the outlets of the pancreatic and common bile ducts. In the 15-mm embryo these ducts end in closed cavities. When the embryo measures 15 to 20 mm, vacuoles begin to form in the center and gradually coalesce to form a lumen. By the time the embryo is 23 to 38 mm long, the process of recanalization is completed.[5]

Glands and villi of the duodenum are fairly well formed by the 10th week. Branching of the hollowed cylindric masses of entodermal cells into the underlying mesoderm gives rise to Brunner's glands of the duodenum. Unbranched, simple tubular depressions become the glands of Lieberkühn. In vitro recombination experiments have shown that epithelial morphogenesis and cytodifferentiation are influenced by the mesenchyme. It is of particular interest that duodenal-epithelial morphogenesis is affected by the presence of gastric mesenchyme. The proportion of goblet cells is higher on recombination with gastric mesenchyme than with duodenal mesenchyme.[7]

The visceral mesoderm differentiates into a narrow, loose inner zone, which develops into the lamina propria and submucosa, and a thicker outer zone, which develops into the muscularis propria. The outer surface cells of the mesoderm become the mesothelium. The stomach exhibits a distinct inner circular and outer longitudinal muscle layer by the fourth month.[4]

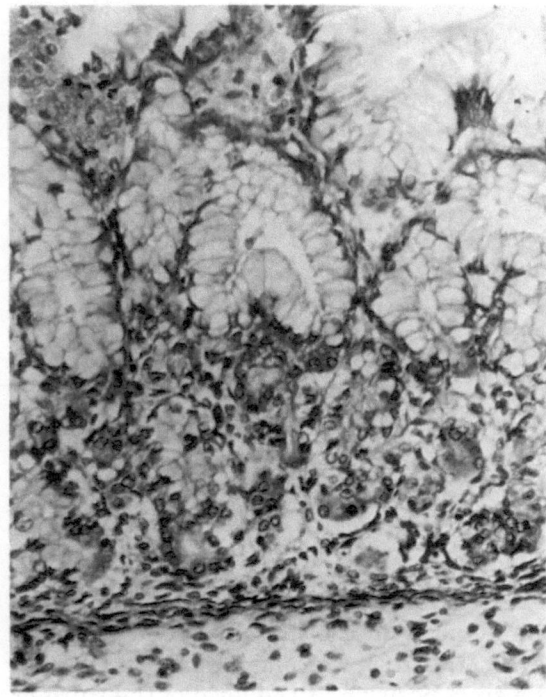

Figure 1-2. Gastric body mucosa in a 4-month-old fetus. Foveolae (*top*) and gastric glands (*bottom*) are recognizable. Within the gastric glands, parietal cells (darker cells) can be distinguished from chief cells (paler cells). HPS, X250, reproduced at 75%.

Anatomy

Stomach

The stomach, also called the *ventriculus* (derived from the Latin *venter* = belly) or *gaster* (Greek), lies in the upper abdomen in the epigastric, umbilical, and left hypochondriac regions. Most of it lies left to the midline. The stomach is surrounded by a number of vital organs that may be secondarily affected by diseases originating in the stomach or, conversely, may secondarily affect the stomach itself. Superiorly the stomach is adjacent to the diaphragm. Inferiorly it is connected to the transverse colon by the gastrocolic ligament, which consists of anterior and poster-

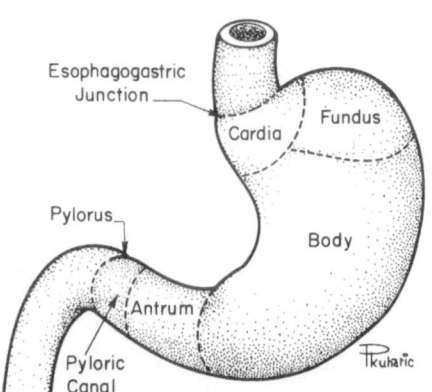

Esophagogastric
Junction

Cardia   Fundus

Pylorus

Body

Antrum

Pyloric
Canal

Pkukaric

Figure 1-3. Normal adult stomach and its different anatomic regions. The greater curvature is on the right of the diagram, the lesser curvature on the left.

ior reflections of the greater omentum. In the supine position the inferior border is at the level of the first or second lumbar vertebra, in the erect position at the level of the third or fourth lumbar vertebra. In senescence the inferior border is 4 to 6 cm lower than in midadulthood. Anteriorly the stomach is partially covered by the left lobe of the liver and partially by the anterior abdominal wall. Posteriorly the body and tail of the pancreas and the splenic and superior mesenteric vessels are found. The lesser sac occupies the potential space between the stomach and these structures. Laterally the stomach is suspended by peritoneal folds, the hepatogastric ligament of the lesser omentum on the left side and the gastrophrenic, gastrosplenic, and gastrocolic ligaments, all parts of the greater omentum, on the right side. The spleen is interposed between the left side of the diaphragm and the left upper posterior surface of the stomach.

The shape and position of the stomach are variable and depend on body build, race, and stomach contents. Japanese have longer and more mobile stomachs than Americans, allowing for easier esophagogastric anastomosis after esophageal resections.[8] The greatest length measured vertically is about 25 cm, the greatest breadth 10 to 12 cm. The

mean capacity varies with age and is approximately 30 cc at birth, 1000 cc at puberty, and an average of 1200 cc in adulthood.[9]

The cardiac orifice communicates with the esophagus and is situated on the left behind the seventh costal cartilage, 10 cm from the anterior abdominal wall and 40 cm from the incisor teeth. The pyloric orifice joins the stomach with the duodenum and is situated 1.2 cm to the right of the midline at the level of the lower border of the first lumbar vertebra, when the body is in the supine position and the stomach is empty. The stomach thus has an oblique axis that slants from the upper left to the lower right and slightly forward. The lesser curvature connects the two orifices on the right and the greater curvature on the left (Fig. 1-3). The cardia (Greek: *heart*) is the rather ill-defined area around the cardiac orifice. The fundus is the dome-shaped bulge to the left above the level of the gastroesophageal junction. At times the term is used to include the entire body, an unfortunate confusion of terminology.[10] The body or corpus is the most capacious central portion between the fundus and the pyloric antrum. The pyloric part represents the distal third of the stomach and is composed of the wider pyloric antrum and the narrow 2.5-cm-long pyloric canal, which opens into the duodenum. The antral area in cadavers with no obvious gastric disease was found to vary from 8 to 17.7% of the total stomach area.[9] The lesser curvature together with the pyloric antrum is the gastric canal or *Magenstrasse* (German: *stomach street*). It is relatively fixed in position, in contrast to the more mobile region of the larger curvature. Many pathologic changes, such as gastritis, peptic ulcer, and carcinoma, are most frequently found along the course of the gastric canal. The pylorus (Greek: *gatekeeper*) is the muscular sphincter at the gastroduodenal junction.

The wall of the stomach is composed of mucosa, submucosa, muscularis propria, and serosa. The mucosa of the empty stomach presents many mostly longitudinal folds, *rugae*, which flatten with increasing gastric distension. Rugae are most prominent in the fundus and body and relatively small in the antrum and adjacent lesser curvature. Variations in the morphology of rugae are important clues for diagnosing certain diseases, such as gastritis, carcinoma, and lymphoma.

The submucosa is composed of loose connective tissue that allows the mucosa to move freely on the muscular layer. It contains blood vessels, lymphatics, and the nerve plexus of Meissner. The muscularis propria is composed of three layers[11]: the incomplete longitudinal layer, which forms mainly two bands along the two curvatures; the almost complete circular layer, which spares only the paraesophageal part of the fundus and forms the pyloric sphincter; and the innermost oblique layer, which invests the fundus and extends down on the anterior and posterior surfaces in two broad sheets that fuse with the circular layer of the incisura angularis, i.e., the lowest point on the lesser curvature. The muscle of the proximal gastric body and fundus is electrically silent.

The gastric slow wave, the pacemaker potential for antral peristalsis, is thought to originate in the longitudinal muscle layer in the midgreater curvature.[11,12] It occurs at regular intervals of about 20 seconds, lasts about 4 seconds, and migrates rapidly around the stomach and more slowly toward the pylorus. This activity is remarkably little affected by disease, drugs, or physiologic influences.[12] Vagotomy produces temporary disorganization.[11]

Antral peristalsis is produced by localized contractions of the circular muscular layer. Contractions arise as shallow indentations approximately 2 cm wide about the middle of the gastric body and accelerate and increase in depth as they move toward the pylorus. At their maximal frequency they occur regularly every 20 seconds or at intervals of some integral multiple of 20 seconds.

The function of the gastric muscle of the fundus and proximal body is not contraction, but receptive relaxation.[11] Receptive relaxation is an active process that occurs as a reflex response to pharyngoesophageal move-

ment and allows for gastric filling by means of a sustained drop in intraluminal pressure. The gastric serosa is part of the visceral peritoneum and is closely attached to the muscular layer.

Arteries of the stomach are derived from the celiac trunk and form two arches along the two curvatures. The left gastric artery, a direct branch of the celiac trunk, reaches the lesser curvature and divides into two branches that run along the front and the back and join with branches of the right gastric artery derived from the hepatic artery. The right and left gastroepiploic arteries, branches of the gastroduodenal and the splenic arteries, respectively, supply the larger curvature. Gastric branches of the splenic artery, so-called *short gastric arteries*, supply as much blood to the stomach as to the spleen.[13] They form a network of vessels in the fundus and, to a lesser extent, in the corpus. An accessory left gastric artery, also called the *posterior gastric artery*, originates from the splenic artery in 48 to 68% of cases and supplies the superior portion of the posterior gastric wall. Inadvertent transection during gastrectomy may cause postoperative bleeding or necrosis of the residual gastric stump.[13]

Veins of the stomach include the right epiploic vein, which joins the superior mesenteric vein; the left gastroepiploic, pyloric, and several short gastric veins, which join the splenic vein; and the left gastric or coronary vein, which runs along the lesser curvature and joins the portal vein. Its communication with the esophageal vein provides the basis for potential shunting of blood from the portal to the systemic venous circulation.

Lymphatics are numerous in the stomach. The major drainage follows the arteries and may be divided into three main areas, each corresponding to both anterior and posterior walls of the stomach (see Fig. 7-45).

1. The medial two-thirds of the vertical portion of the stomach is supplied by lymphatic trunks along the left gastric artery, ending in lymph nodes at the upper ex-

treme of the lesser curvature and sometimes in juxtacardiac nodes.

2. The area from the fundus to the midportion of the greater curvature, exclusive of the region discussed above, is supplied by lymphatic trunks along the splenic and gastroepiploic vessels, ending in the hilar splenic nodes.

3. The lower one-half of the greater curvature and the pyloric and gastroepiploic areas are supplied by lymphatic trunks along the hepatic artery, ending in lymph nodes along the larger curvature and pylorus (i.e., gastroepiploic, peripyloric, pancreatic, duodenal, and superior mesenteric nodes).

Isolated metastases situated on the curvature opposite the neoplasm may occur because of the absence or presence of valvules in subserous lymphatics orienting the flow in a particular direction.[14] Along the left gastric artery long lymph collectors may bypass nodes. Lymphatics along the posterior gastric artery connect with the splenic chain.[14]

The nerve supply to the stomach is provided by the terminal branches of the left and right vagus nerves and by sympathetic branches from the celiac plexus. The excitatory vagal effect is counteracted by the inhibitory action of the sympathetic nerve. Both contain sensory and motor fibers.[11] As the vagus enters the esophageal hiatus, the left or anterior trunk bifurcates into the hepatic branch and the anterior gastric nerve and the right or posterior trunk into the celiac branch and the posterior gastric nerve.[15,16] The anterior gastric nerve descends along the lesser curvature, usually at a distance of 0.5 to 1.0 cm from the serosa, sends off 2 to 12 anterior gastric branches, and terminates in the gastric antrum near the incisura angularis. In some cases, it reaches the pylorus and even the first part of the duodenum.[16] In most cases, the pylorus is innervated by a single descending branch of the hepatic division of the anterior vagus. The posterior gastric nerve follows the left gastric artery, sends off an average of four branches to the posterior

wall of the stomach, and, as a rule, terminates slightly higher on the lesser curvature than does the anterior gastric nerve. Rarely it may reach the pylorus.[15] More commonly the celiac division of the posterior vagus supplies nerves to the posterior wall of the antrum. Considerable individual variation exists as to the exact site of the major vagal divisions, the number of anterior and posterior trunks (double anterior trunks in 19%, double posterior trunks in 17%, multiple trunks in 14%), the size of anterior and posterior trunks (anterior trunk 0.5 to 4.5 mm, posterior 0.5 to 4.7 mm), and the number of anterior and posterior gastric branches.[15] Furthermore, separate gastric nerves often arise from the vagal trunks above the formation of the anterior and posterior gastric nerves. These anatomic variations explain why selective vagotomy may be ineffective if only the major anterior and posterior gastric divisions are sectioned.[16]

In the gastric wall, nerves form four interconnected plexuses: the subserosal, myenteric, submucosal, and mucosal. In contrast to the esophagus, the myenteric plexus of the stomach is particularly dense.[11]

Duodenum

The duodenum derives its name from the Latin *duodeni*, meaning 12 times and referring to its length of about 12 fingerbreadths. It is the most proximal segment of the small bowel and is approximately 26 cm long.[9] In the relaxed and empty state it forms an almost perfect ring, suspended between the duodenohepatic ligament (which represents the free border of the lesser omentum containing the portal vein, the hepatic artery, and the bile duct) proximally and the ligament of Treitz at the duodenojejunal flexure distally. The latter ligament, originally termed "suspensory muscle of the duodenum" by Treitz in 1853, has been shown to represent an expansion of the circular and longitudinal muscle layers of the duodenum and to serve as a sphincter whose function is coordinated with that of the pylorus.[17]

Except for the mobile portion of the duodenum proximal to the duodenohepatic ligament, the remainder is relatively fixed and retroperitonal in location.

When distended, the duodenum shows four distinct parts (Fig. 1-4). The first or ascending part is approximately 5 cm long, movable, and runs backward and slightly upward and to the right from the pylorus. It rests against the liver and the gallbladder on the right and above, the common bile duct on the left and the back, and the loops of the small intestine below. The second or descending part of the duodenum is approximately 8 cm long, has the largest circumference of all parts, and forms an acute angle with the first part. It runs along the right side of the spine to the fourth lumbar vertebra, slightly lower in women than in men.[9] It is in contact with the vena cava, the right kidney, the ascending colon, and the pancreas. The common duct passes obliquely through its left wall about 10 cm from the pylorus. The third or transverse part of the duodenum is approximately 6 cm long and crosses the spine and vena cava and, in almost one-quarter of cases, the aorta. Together with the first and second parts, the third part forms a loop around the head of the pancreas. The fourth part of the duodenum is approximately 7 cm long, begins at an obtuse angle with the third, and ascends on the front of the spine to the top of the second lumbar vertebra, usually overlapping the aorta. Rarely it may reach the left kidney. The tail of the pancreas is behind it, and the mesentery of the small intestine arises on its front.

The duodenal wall has the same basic organization as the remainder of the small intestine. Specific duodenal differences include the absence of circular folds (valves of Kerckring) in the proximal 5 cm and the presence of the largest folds in the fourth part of the duodenum.[18] Circular folds reach a height of 8 to 10 mm and a thickness of 3 to 4 mm, extending one-half to two-thirds around the lumen. They are composed of submucosa and mucosa.

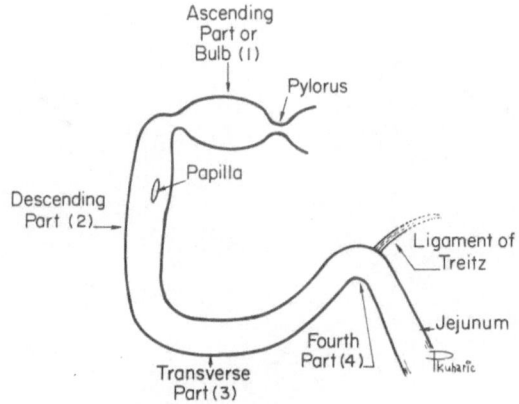

Figure 1-4. Normal adult duodenum and its different anatomic parts.

Arteries of the duodenum are derived from the hepatic and the superior mesenteric arteries. The gastroduodenal artery, a branch of the hepatic artery, runs on the left of the first part and sends off the superior pancreaticoduodenal artery, which provides the chief vascular supply for the front of the duodenum. The second major supply is provided by the inferior pancreaticoduodenal artery, which arises from the superior mesenteric artery. Additional small branches of the pyloric artery and the superior mesenteric artery supply the proximal and distal ends of the duodenum, respectively.[9]

Two venous outflow areas can be distinguished in the duodenum: the larger inferior–anterior area, which drains through the upper anterior, lower anterior, and lower posterior pancreaticoduodenal veins into the upper mesenteric vein; and the smaller superior–posterior area, which drains through the right gastric and upper posterior pancreaticoduodenal veins directly into the portal vein.[12] Individual differences exist as to the number of pancreaticoduodenal veins, the exact areas from which blood is drained, the anastomoses, and places of opening.

Lymphatic drainage occurs via the preaortic lymph nodes.

Nerves of the duodenum are derived from the solar plexus.

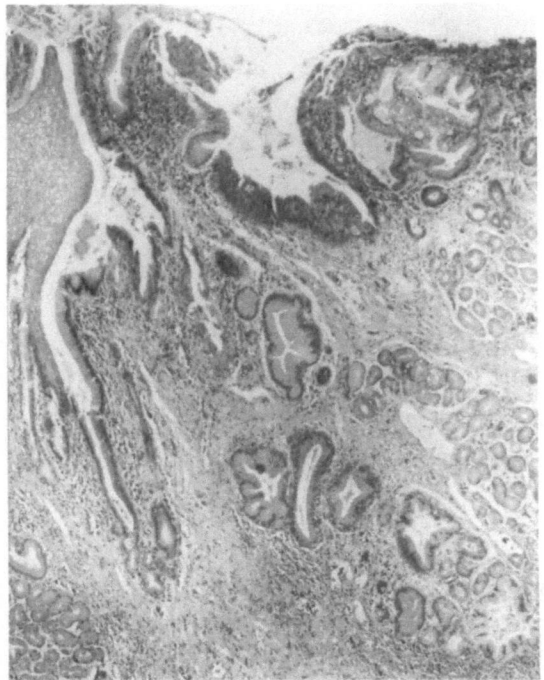

Figure 1-5. Gastroesophageal junction. Loosely packed cardiac glands, some cystic, are seen adjacent to esophageal squamous mucosa on the left. HPS, X40, reproduced at 80%.

Histology

Stomach

An up-to-date discussion of the normal histology of the stomach with special reference to features important to the pathologist can be found in the article by Owen.[10] The gastric mucosa is 0.5 to 1.5 mm in thickness, being thinnest in the cardiac region. Shallow grooves divide the mucosa into slightly bulging gastric areas 1 to 6 mm in diameter. With the dissecting microscope or hand lens, numerous surface indentations corresponding to the openings of gastric pits can be seen.[19,20] The gastric mucosa can be divided into a superficial layer, which has the same composition throughout the stomach, and a deep layer, which is composed of different spe-

cialized glands. Based on these differences, the gastric mucosa is divided into cardiac, body or fundic, and antral or pyloric types.

The superficial layer is composed of a single row of mucinous epithelial cells that line the surface and dip down to form pits or foveolae of varying length: In the cardiac mucosa pits constitute about one-half of the mucosal thickness, in the body about one-quarter, and in the antral mucosa at least one-half or more. Surface mucinous cells are formed in the deep part of the pits, the gastric neck glands, and are renewed every 3 days.[21] Surface and pit lining cells as well as mucous neck cells stain with periodic acid-Schiff and Alcian blue above pH 2.5, but not with mucicarmine.[10]

The cardiac mucosa covers the area around the cardioesophageal junction for a distance varying from 5 to 30 mm (see Fig. 1-3)[3]. The deep layer is composed of simple tubular or compound tubuloracemose type, sometimes cystic, glands, lined by simple mucus-secreting cells with bubbly cytoplasm (Fig. 1-5). Rare acid- and pepsinogen-secreting cells may be present. Glands are packed more loosely and the lamina propria is more abundant than in antral mucosa, which otherwise resembles cardiac mucosa.

The body mucosa covers the largest area of the stomach (see Fig. 1-3). Deep glands are called *gastric*, *body*, or *fundic glands* and are simple, straight, tightly packed tubules, one to four of which open into the bottom of a pit (Fig. 1-6). There are an estimated 35 million gastric body glands. They contain four cell types: the mucous neck cell, the parietal or oxyntic cell, the chief or zymogen cell, and the endocrine cell. Mucous neck cells are sparse and present only at the junction of glands and pits.

Parietal cells are most numerous and are found mainly in the upper portion of the body glands. They are large (20–35 μm), round or pyramidal, and acidophilic, and have a central nucleus (Fig. 1-6). They secrete hydrochloric acid, blood group substances, and intrinsic factor.[20] The parietal cell was the

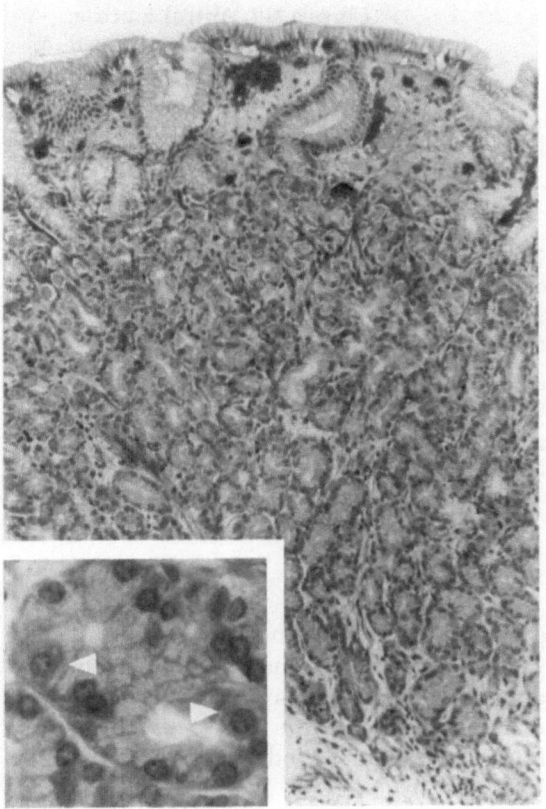

Figure 1-6. Body mucosa. Closely packed gastric glands occupy about three-quarters of the mucosal thickness. The pits are short and lined by mucinous epithelium. H&E, X100, reproduced at 90%. **Inset** Gastric glands. Parietal cells can be distinguished from chief cells by their central nucleus, pyramidal shape, and darker granular cytoplasm (*arrows*). H&E, X320, reproduced at 90%.

first vital hydrogen ion generator to be recognized, and the details of its cell biology are still under discussion.[22,23] The subcellular site of acid production is the secretory canaliculus, the volume density of which shows circadian variation that is highest at night and lowest during the day.[24]

Chief cells predominate in the lower half of the gastric body glands and in freshly fixed tissue show basophilic refractile granules that disintegrate almost immediately after death. The nucleus is basal (Fig. 1-6). Chief cells produce pepsinogen. Passing from the proximal to the distal body mucosa, parietal cells increase progressively while chief cells decrease progressively.[25]

Endocrine cells of the gastrointestinal tract have received increasing attention in the literature. With the help of new immunohistochemical techniques, new cells and cell products are continuously being discovered.[26,27,28] In the stomach, the antral mucosa contains most endocrine cells. In the body mucosa somatostatin-producing (D) cells, serotonin-secreting enterochromaffin (EC) cells, and enterochromaffin-like (ECL) cells have been identified.[28] Small numbers of X, P, and D cells contain an unknown product.[10]

The antral mucosa covers a roughly triangular area in the lower third of the stomach (see Fig. 1-5). There is marked individual variation, especially along the lesser curvature where pyloric glands may be found as high up as the cardia, particularly in women. Usually antral mucosa extends upward for about two-fifths of the length of the lesser curvature and for a much shorter distance along the larger curvature. The antral mucosa is thinner than the body mucosa and varies from 0.2 to 1.1 mm in thickness. Pyloric glands are simple or branched coiled tubules lined by mucinous cells indistinguishable from mucous neck cells (Fig. 1-7). Scattered parietal cells may be present near the boundary with the body mucosa as well as in the region of the sphincter.[20,22]

The antral mucosa has the highest concentration in the entire gastrointestinal tract of gastrin-producing (G) cells and D cells.[27,28,29] Of antral endocrine cells 50% are G cells, 30% are EC cells producing serotonin, and 15% are D cells.[10] The EC cells are argentaffin and stain with Fontana-Masson. The other cells, with the exception of some ECL cells, are argyrophil and stain with the Grimelius technique. Antropyloric gastrin cells have also shown immunoreactivity for enkephalin-like and adrenocorticotrophic

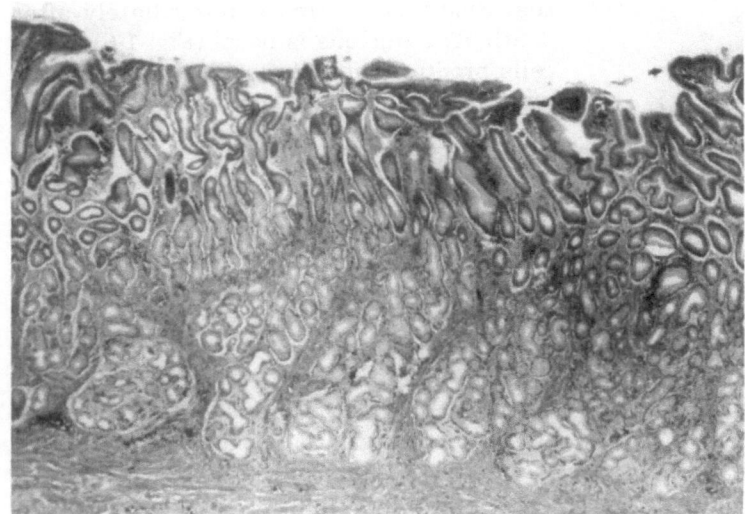

Figure 1-7. Antral mucosa. Coiled glands are arranged in lobules and occupy approximately one-half of the mucosal thickness. Pits are longer than in the body mucosa. H&E, X40, reproduced at 80%.

hormone-like substances and are the first gastrointestinal cells known to store different peptides. Bombesin cells have been identified in the stomach as well as in the duodenum. Each of these three polypeptides is also found in nerves and perhaps even in the central nervous system, and is thus part of the "gastrointestinal nervous system."[27]

Transitional mucosa is a term applied to the junction between the different types of gastric mucosa in which two types of glands may coexist.

The lamina propria is the connective tissue supporting the glands. It consists of reticulin, collagen, and elastic fibers, capillaries, arterioles, lymphatics, and nonmyelinated nerve fibers and, more so in the antral than in the body mucosa, also contains occasional fibroblasts, macrophages, eosinophils, plasma cells, mast cells, and lymphocytes. Lymphocytes of the lamina propria are primarily of B-cell type and produce immunoglobulin A, whereas rare lymphocytes within the epithelium are of T-cell type. Occasional lymphoid follicles are normally present in the deep mucosa of the antrum.[10] The lamina propria is most abundant in the superficial mucosa

between the pits. Strands of smooth muscle from the muscularis mucosae radiate upward between cardiac and antral glands, but in normal circumstances not between body glands. For a detailed description of the ultrastructure of the gastric mucosa, the reader is referred to the study by Day and Morson.[22]

The submucosa of the stomach contains blood vessels, lymphatics, venous plexuses, and the submucosal nerve plexus surrounded by fibrous tissue and a few fat cells. There are scattered mast cells, lymphocytes, and eosinophilic leukocytes.

The muscularis propria is composed of smooth muscle. Its organization is discussed in the chapter on anatomy. Close junctions between smooth muscle cells, called *nexuses*, are seen by electron microscopy and provide the morphologic basis for low-resistance electrical shunts.[11] The muscularis propria contains the myenteric plexus, which comprises three networks of nerve bundles and ganglion cells, all located in the same plane between the longitudinal and circular muscle coats. Cholinesterase and serotonin have been identified in the myenteric plexus.[11]

The serosa, the outermost layer of the stomach, is a thin layer of loose fibrous tissue covered by mesothelium.

Duodenum

Since this volume covers only localized duodenal pathology and not diffuse small intestinal diseases that may also involve the duodenum, detailed small intestinal histology is dispensed with and only the most important histologic features are discussed.

Due to the expansion of the resorptive surface by means of folds and villi, the duodenal mucosa covers an area of approximately 18 m².[9] Mucosal villi are most numerous in the duodenum and proximal jejunum, where they number 10 to 40 per mm². Duodenal mucosal villi are shorter (0.2 to 0.5 mm) than those in the more distal small intestine, more leaf-like (instead of finger-like), and more deeply creased.[30] They are lined by intestinal absorptive cells with a microvillous luminal border and irregularly scattered goblet cells. The surface epithelium invaginates to form tubular glands, the crypts of Lieberkühn (Fig. 1-8). Small intestinal epithelium is replaced entirely within 3 to 6 days[31] and regenerates itself in the lower half of the crypts of Lieberkühn, the only place where mitoses are seen in normal circumstances.[22]

Paneth cells occur in small numbers in the depth of the crypts. They show little or no cell turnover. They have large acidophilic granules and are rich in zinc.

The duodenal mucosa is rich in endocrine cells. A great variety of polypeptides has been identified: gastrin in G cells, most numerous in the bulb; secretin in S cells; cholecystokinin in I cells; gastrin-inhibiting peptide in K cells; somatostatin in D cells; substance P in EC_1 cells; motilin in EC_2 cells; neurotensin in N cells; and bombesin in P cells.[27] As indicated in the section on gastric endocrine cells, most of these polypeptides are also produced in the central and gastrointestinal nervous systems. Each endocrine cell has its specific ultrastructural granule

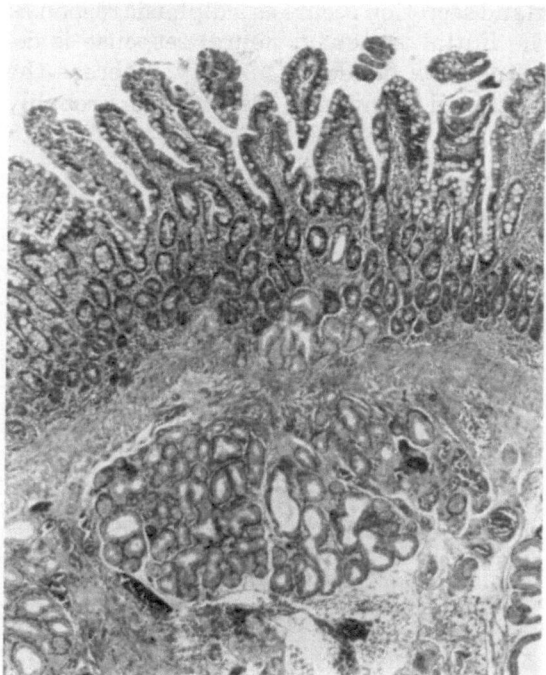

Figure 1-8. Duodenal mucosa. Villi, crypts of Lieberkühn and submucosal Brunner's glands are characteristic. H&E, X40, reproduced at 80%.

morphology, which, however, is not necessarily repeated by the tumors that may arise from these cells.

Brunner's glands are unevenly distributed in the duodenum. They are largest and most numerous in the proximal third, diminishing in size and finally disappearing in the distal portion. Their concentration tends to be highest in the core of the circular folds. They sometimes extend for a few centimeters into the pyloric region of the stomach. Although termed "submucosal," Brunner's glands are frequently also present in the mucosa (see Fig. 1-8). They are richly branched and coiled tubules arranged in lobules 0.5 to 1 mm in diameter. They produce alkaline mucus, which protects the duodenal mucosa from the corrosive effects of acidified gastric juice. Brunner's glands also contain G and EC cells in low to moderate numbers.[26] Brunner's gland secretion occurs as a diphasic response: the initial transient, neural response is dependent on duodenal motility, whereas the sustained hormonal response is probably mediated by secretin.[32]

References

1. Langman J: Medical Embryology. Human Development, Normal and Abnormal. Baltimore, Williams & Wilkins Co, 5th ed., 1985.

2. Hamilton WJ, Boyd JD, Mossman HW: Human Embryology: Prenatal Development of Form and Function, 4th ed. Cambridge, W Heffer & Sons Ltd, 1972.

3. Large-Hansen N: The Development and the Embryonic Anatomy of the Human Gastrointestinal Tract. A New Basis for the Study of Anomalies of the Gastro-intestinal Tract. Eindhoven, Centrex Publishing Co, 1960.

4. Heisler JC: A Textbook of Embryology. Philadelphia, WB Saunders Co, 1899.

5. Tandler J: Zur Entwicklungsgeschichte des menschlichen Duodenums im frühen Embryonalstadium. Morphol Jb 1900;29:187.

6. Willis RA: The Borderland of Embryology and Pathology, 2nd ed. London, Butterworths, 1962.

7. Fukamachi H, Takayama S: Epithelial-mesenchymal interaction in differentiation of duodenal epithelium of fetal rats in organ culture. Experientia 1980;36:335–336.

8. Goldsmith HS, Akiyama H: A comparative study of Japanese and American gastric dimensions. Ann Surg 1979;190:690–693.

9. Piersol GA: Human Anatomy, 8th ed. Philadelphia, JB Lippincott, 1923.

10. Owen DA: Normal histology of the stomach. Am J Surg Pathol 1986;101:48–61.

11. Christensen J: The controls of gastrointestinal movements: Some old and new views. N Engl J Med 1971;285:85–97.

12. Heading RC: Gastric motility. Front Gastrointest Res 1980;6:35–66.

13. Di Dio LJA, Christoforidis AJ, Chandani PC: Posterior gastric artery and its significance as seen in angiograms. Am J Surg 1980;139:333–337.

14. Pissus A, Dyon JF, Sarrazin R, et al: Le drainage lymphatique et l'estomac. J Chir (Paris) 1979;116:583–590.

15. Thailai Z, Junsheng T, Zuxun Z, et al: Vagus nerve anatomy at the lower esophagus and stomach. A study of 100 cadavers. Chin Med J 1980;93:629–636.

16. Skandalakis JE, Gray SW, Soria RE, et al: Distribution of the vagus nerve to the stomach. Am Surg 1980;46:130–139.

17. Compeanu ERR: The suspensory muscle of the duodenum. Rev Roum Morphol Embryol Physiol 1981;27:123–126.

18. Bloom W, Fawcett DW: A Textbook of Histology. Philadelphia, WB Saunders Co, 1986.

19. Szkudlaret R: Pancreaticoduodenal veins in man. Folia Morphol (Warsaw) 1980;39:15–28.

20. Goldstein AMB, Brothers MR, Davis EA Jr: The architecture of the superficial layer of the gastric mucosa. J Anat 1969;104:539–551.

21. Bloom W, Fawcett DW: A Textbook of Histology. Philadelphia, WB Saunders Co, 1975.

22. Day DW, Morson BC: Structure and infrastructure. Front Gastrointest Res 1980;6:1–19.

23. Sachs G, Berglindh T, Rabon E, et al: Aspects of parietal cell biology: Cells and vesicles. Ann NY Acad Sci 1980;341:312–334.

24. Jacobs DM, Sturtevant RP: Circadian morphometric variation in gastric parietal cell populations of the rat. Cell Tissue Res 1980;211:175–177.

25. Hogben CAM, Kent TH, Woodward PA, et al: Quantitative histology of the gastric mucosa: Man, dog, cat, guinea pig, and frog. Gastroenterology 1974;67:1143–1154.

26. Sjölund K, Sanden G, Hakanson R, et al: Endocrine cells in human intestine: An immunocytochemical study. Gastroenterology 1983; 85:1120–1129.

27. Larsson L-I: Pathology of gastrointestinal endocrine cells. Scand J Gastroenterol 1979; 53(suppl 14):1–8.

28. Lechago J: The endocrine cells of the digestive tract. Am J Surg Pathol 1987;11(suppl 1): 63–70.

29. Reichlin S: Somatostatin. N Engl J Med 1983;309:1495–1499.

30. Siew S, Goldstein ML: Scanning electron microscopy of mucosal biopsies of the human upper gastrointestinal tract. Scanning Electron Microsc 1981;4:173–181.

31. Heitz PU, Oberholzer M: Histologie, Ultrastruktur and Histochemie der Duodenalschleimhaut. Schweiz Rundsch Med 1981;70: 1375–1379.

32. Lang IM, Tansy MF: Neural and hormonal control of Brunner's gland secretion. Life Sci 1982;30:409–417.

CHAPTER 2

Physiology

The stomach functions as a reservoir for fluids and food, as a mill to reduce the size of ingested solids, as an initiator of the process of digestion of proteins, and as a mechanism to deliver slurried products in amounts and time adapted to efficient processing by the small intestine. These activities are complex; thus, the reader interested in further information should refer to general reviews of the subject, especially those by Davenport,[1] Heading,[2] Cohen and colleagues,[3] and Brooks,[4] from which we have drawn most of the material that follows.

Basic Gastric Motility

Gastric motility is governed by the inherent basic electrical rhythm of the gastric musculature. This consists of slow waves of polarization and depolarization, which are relatively constant at rest at a rate of about three per minute in humans. The fundus is electrically silent. These "pacemaker" waves begin at a point high on the greater curvature and sweep circumferentially and distally, increasing in velocity as they approach the antrum. The pacemaker waves only result in contraction when coupled with action potentials, termed *spikes*, which are the initiators of contraction. Spikes occur when the slow wave reaches an amplitude and duration above the local excitory threshold of the muscle. Therefore, only a certain variable percentage of slow waves are coupled with spikes and thus contractions. Since the phase lag of the smooth muscle is shorter distally and the antral musculature thicker, the end result is a series of contraction bands that deepen and widen and increase in velocity as they approach the antrum and pylorus, which contract almost, although not quite, simultaneously.

The activity of the pacemaker is an inherent property of muscle but is influenced somewhat by the vagus. Vagotomy results in disorganization of the pacemaker system and thus marked delay in gastric emptying of solids. After some months the basic pattern is reestablished. Propagation of the contraction bands is neurally dependent through the myenteric plexi.

The vagal nerves contain both efferent and afferent fibers. The efferent fibers, except for some postganglionic sympathetic fibers carried in the vagus, synapse with the myenteric plexi. This causes the ganglionic fibers to release either acetylcholine, which stimulates contraction, or an unknown inhibitory mediator, possibly dopamine or vasoactive intestinal peptide. Certain peptides recently isolated from the brain and gut influence gastric motility by functioning as neuromodulators of vagal reflexes in the brain stem and as hormones in the gut. These peptides include substance P, neurotensin, and cholecystokinin octapeptide. Their physiologic role remains poorly understood, but substance P is known to act directly on gastrointestinal smooth muscle and to exert an excitatory effect on neurons of the central nervous system (CNS) as well as on the myenteric plexus. Local gastric responses to substance P have been shown to affect neuronal activity in the tractus solitarius of the brain stem, where afferent vagal fibers terminate.[5]

Efferent sympathetic fibers either carried with the vagus or, in larger numbers, from the coeliac axis or splanchnic nerves are mainly inhibitory in effect. They suppress contractility and slow the basic electrical rhythm of the gastric musculature. Their importance physiologically is not great, since truncal sympathectomy does not greatly alter gastric motility.

The Fasting Stomach

During fasting there are intermittent bursts of myoelectric activity. The lower esophageal sphincter contracts, and waves of contraction occur at a rate of three per minute for 5 to 10 minutes. These waves increase in strength and velocity distally, and at this time any residual contents of the stomach, including large undigested objects, tend to be emptied into the duodenum. These are known as *housekeeper waves*. The peristaltic waves continue on to the ileocecal valve, at which time a new surge of activity begins in the stomach. Such contractions may or may not be accompanied by the sensation of hunger pains. The chief stimulant appears to be the hormone motilin.[1]

Response To Feeding

As food or fluid enters the stomach, or indeed with swallowing or with dilatation of the esophagus, the fundus and body relax, a reflex known as *receptive relaxation*. Both vagovagal and vagosympathetic reflex arcs are involved. Afferent impulses from mechanoreceptors in the gastric musculature and from receptors in the mouth,

pharynx, and esophagus result in excitation of inhibitory efferent vagal impulses to the stomach. The oblique muscle layer of the fundus and body is thought to be important in this regard.[2,3] The result is that intragastric pressure does not markedly increase until the volume exceeds about 1600 ml in the adult. Vagotomy interferes with receptive relaxation. Thus, after vagotomy gastric pressure rises at lower volumes and the reservoir function of the stomach is impaired.

Gastric Emptying

Tonic contractions of the proximal stomach are important for the transfer of liquids from the stomach to the duodenum. Peristaltic contractions of the distal stomach reduce the size of solid food particles and transfer solids to the duodenum.[6] The terminal antrum and pylorus contract nearly simultaneously; during most contractions some contents are extruded in spurts into the duodenal bulb, which holds 5 to 10 ml of fluid. Solids larger than about 2 to 3 mm are retained, compressed, and pushed proximally. The antrum thus acts as a "mill," grinding down solids to a size that permits their egress as well as mixing and churning the gastric contents. Little if any mixing occurs in the fundus and body. The contractions of the duodenal bulb are timed for the most part with pyloric–antral contractions against a closed pylorus. Whether the pylorus acts as a true sphincter or has its own contractile properties is somewhat controversial. It is rich in nerves containing enkephalin. Nalozone, an opioid receptor blocking agent, blocks the contractions of the pylorus to vagal stimulation. The pylorus also appears to respond differently than does the antrum to gastrin, secretin, and electrical stimulation.[4] Although only small slips of longitudinal muscle extend between the pylorus and duodenal musculator, these are sufficient to coordinate the timing of duodenal contractions so that the duodenal musculature does not contract against a relaxed pylorus. Normally there is little or no regurgitation. Such regurgitation is, however, frequent in patients with gastric ulcers.

The emptying rate of fluids from the stomach increases at an exponential rate with volume and is thus proportional to the amount of fluid left in the stomach at any one time. Gastric secretion adds an appreciable fraction to the gastric volume. Solids empty more slowly, at a linear rate, and, as stated previously, only pass when reduced to a certain small size except for those expelled during the interdigestive phase.

Proximal gastric motility is mainly under neural control. Acetylcholine, released by excitatory vagal neurons, stimulates the smooth muscle cells of the proximal stomach to contract. Cholecystokinin, secretin, and somatostatin inhibit proximal gastric contractions when administered exogenously. Distal gastric motility is also controlled by neural influences carried over the vagus, but is modified extensively by endogenous gastrointestinal hormones. Cholecystokinin and motilin stimulate peristaltic contractions, whereas secretin, gastric inhibitory polypeptide, and somatostatin inhibit these contractions.[6] Hypoglycemia induced by insulin increases antral activity, an effect blocked by vagotomy.[1]

Regulators of Gastric Emptying Time

The only known physiologic accelerator of gastric emptying is gastric distention. At least five factors are known to delay emptying of liquids: 1) Hyper- or hypoosmolarity, 2) duodenal acidity, 3) presence of fats, 4) tryptophan (alone among the amino acids), and 5) caloric density.[4] These factors act through receptors variously located in the duodenum and small intestine. Fat in the upper small intestine delays gastric emptying by producing prolonged pyloric closure.[7] Fat is without inhibitory effect in patients with pancreatic insufficiency, suggesting that lipid breakdown products are involved.[3] After truncal vagotomy, the delaying effects of hyperosmolarity and of fat are greatly

reduced.[4] In some patients rapid emptying may follow truncal vagotomy and pyloroplasty due to impaired receptive relaxation and an inadequate pyloric–sphincteric mechanism, contributing to the so-called *dumping syndrome*. Impaired gastric emptying occurs in many clinical situations; its mechanism is assumed to be a reflex inhibition of gastric peristalsis. Acoustic and cold stress increase gastric emptying, an effect apparently mediated at the level of the CNS by corticotropin-releasing factors.[8]

The myth that eating or drinking lipid-containing substances, such as patés and milk, protects against the immediate effects of alcohol remains just that, because although gastric emptying is delayed, some ethanol is directly absorbed through the gastric mucosa.

Retching and Vomiting

Vomiting is usually proceeded by retching. After a widespread autonomic discharge producing sweating, pallor, and a rapid heartbeat, a wave of reverse peristalsis occurs in the small intestine that causes its contents to reflux into the stomach. In prolonged vomiting even fecal material may be so refluxed. Deep inspiration and closing of the glottis results in a decrease in intrathoracic pressure. Contraction of the abdominal musculature increases the intrathoracic pressure. Contraction of the abdominal musculature increases the intraabdominal and, therefore, the gastric pressure so that a pressure differential of up to 200 mg Hg may occur. Strong antral contractions tend to divide the stomach; a portion of the stomach is forced through the hiatus, and the contents of the stomach are discharged into the esophagus. If, at this point, the abdomen relaxes and the thorax moves inward, the contents of the esophagus reenter the stomach. If there is a sudden increase in intrathoracic pressure in the presence of continued abdominal muscle contraction, the material is ejected through the cricopharyngeous sphincter and vomiting occurs.[1] The high pressure differential at one stage of this cycle explains the occasional occurrence of mucosal tears and bleeding at the gastroesophageal margin (Mallory-Weiss syndrome).

Regulation of Food Intake

Regulation of food intake has been thoroughly reviewed by Paintal.[9] It is clear that the CNS plays an important role since essential feeding patterns remain the same, even after vagotomy and gastrectomy. Various lesions of the CNS produce profound disturbances in the regulation of food and water intake. It has long been known that obesity and hyperphagia follow the experimental production of bilateral lesions of the ventromedial region of the hypothalamus in the rat. Electrical stimulation of these areas results in reduction of food intake. Lateral to this undefined "satiety center" are areas where destruction leads to failure to eat and stimulation to hyperphagia—the so-called *hunger centers.* Glucostatic, lipostatic, and thermostatic receptors have been postulated as serving a regulatory role in these "centers." Peripheral mechanisms are also important. Reduction of appetite is a feature common to many gastrointestinal disturbances thought to be produced by unidentified toxic chemicals carried via the blood to the brain and by sensory vagal and sympathetic impulses.

It is known that at least two types of receptors are present in the stomach that may be the peripheral triggers to the regulation of food and water intake. These are receptors responding to distention and mucosal chemoreceptors. The stretch receptors are present chiefly in the antropyloric region and are within the muscularis. The chemoreceptors appear to be mucosal. The evidence is strongest that the stretch receptors are involved in the sensation of immediate satiety. In dogs, distention of the stomach by a balloon or inert substances leads to reduced food intake. Various receptors have also been described in the small and large intestine that respond to tension or to the passage of fluids and may be associated with the sensation of anorexia.

It is hypothesized that the satiety neurons, acting either directly or through the inhibition of the "hunger" neurons, when stimulated by the peripheral receptors, particularly the gastric stretch receptors, act to produce the sensation of immediate satiety. It is also hypothesized that the glucostatic and other central receptors influence this system to regulate short-term satiation. Other areas of the brain are also involved since, for instance, prefrontal lobotomy reduces the anorexic effects of amphetamines. Cholecystokinin inhibits gastric emptying by binding to cholecystokinin receptors on the circular muscle fibers of the pylorus. Subsequent gastric distention may explain the satiety-provoking effect of this hormone.[10] Bombesin, a peptide present in high concentrations in the stomach, has also been shown to have a satiating effect.[11]

Gastric Secretion

The stomach secretes a wide variety of substances in carrying out its role as an initiator of digestion. These secretions include the hormone gastrin, the paracrine peptide somatostatin, mucins, pepsinogens, intrinsic factor, and various electrolytes, importantly hydrochloric acid. Secretion depends on a complex interplay of neural controls, hormonal controls, the direct effect of food, the state of distention of the stomach, and the stage of digestion, which results in the turning on or off of the secretory impulses. Several of these components will be discussed and their interrelationships reviewed as briefly as possible consistent with understanding. For further details, the reader should consult the review articles by Davenport,[1] Brooks,[4] Bonfils and colleagues,[12] Reichlin,[13] Piper,[14] and Johnson.[15]

Gastric Endocrine Components in Secretion

The dispersed endocrine system (APUD system) is important in the control of gastric secretion. These cells secrete biologically active polypeptides that produce their effect by either a hormonal or a paracrine mechanism. They are demonstrable by argentaffin or argyrophil staining or more specifically with immunoperoxidase techniques. A number of differing APUD cells are known to be present in the stomach. The most numerous and carefully studied are those producing gastrin (G cells) and somatostatin (D cells). In addition, similar peptides such as vasoactive intestinal peptide and others, the physiologic role of which remains undefined but is probably important, exist within the vagus. Peptides of intestinal origin will be discussed later.

Gastrin

G cells are present in large numbers in the antrum as well as in the duodenum, and in small numbers in the body of the stomach. Gastrins are polypeptides whose activity is determined by the terminal four amino acids, which are identical even though the length of the peptide chain varies. Antral G cells predominantly secrete a 17-amino-acid gastrin (G-17, or little gastrin), whereas those in the duodenum predominantly secrete a 34-amino-acid peptide (G-34, or big gastrin). Big gastrin is less active, but has a longer half-life (42 minutes) than little gastrin (7 minutes).[1] Other forms also occur. Cholecystokinin, an intestinal polypeptide, shares the terminal amino acid sequence with gastrin and is competitive for gastrin receptor sites. Gastrin 1) stimulates the secretion of hydrochloric acid; 2) stimulates the acidic receptors, which in turn stimulate pepsinogen via cholinergic reflexes; 3) stimulates the contraction of the gastric circular muscle; and 4) exerts a trophic effect on oxyntic cells, the exocrine pancreas, and intestinal mucosa.

The major stimulus for gastrin release is a neutral solution of certain L amino acids liberated by proteolysis from imbibed protein.[1] Microvilli of the G cell are exposed to luminal contents and act as a receptor to such stimuli. Impulses from the vagus may stimulate, possibly through a bombesin-like mediator,[16] or inhibit, through acetylcholine, the release of gastrin. Vagally released gastrin acts mainly as a permissive factor potentiating the direct vagal effect on the oxyntic cell.[12] Epinephrine may also release gastrin. There is also evidence of an adrenergic role in the control of gastrin, with β stimuli releasing gastrin and α-adrenergic stimuli inhibiting gastrin release. The major inhibitor of gastrin release is the presence of acid at a pH below 2.5.[4] In the presence of hypochlorhydria or achlorhydria, gastrin release is not inhibited and hypergastrinemia occurs. This is particularly true in such conditions as the atrophic gastritis of primary pernicious anemia, in which the antrum is relatively spared. Gastrin release also can be inhibited by somatostatin. With vagal stimulation, circulating gastrin levels rise and somatostatin levels fall.

Somatostatin

Somatostatin has been experimentally shown to inhibit gastrin release via a paracrine effect, that is, local release of the peptide at a site near or adjacent to the G cell. Acid secretion in response to histamine and pentagastrin is accompanied by a dose-dependent increase in somatostatin secretion. Acid secretion in response to neural stimuli is the result of direct action on acetylcholine on the parietal cell and its ability to eliminate the paracrine effect of somatostatin.[16] Somatostatin-producing cells (D cells) are present in the fundus as well as in large numbers in the antrum. They also contain microvilli, which may sense hydrogen ions and certain nutrients that play a role in the activation of its secretion.[13]

Mucin (Glycoprotein) Secretion

Glycoproteins are a heterogeneous group of chemicals sharing carbohydrate and amino acid compounds in variable proportion. The term *mucopolysaccharide* is used for those with a more prominent carbohydrate component linked covalently with serine. In the stomach the glycoproteins include the mucins, blood group antigens, intrinsic factor, and gastrone, a substance found in gastric juice that is known to depress acid secretion, although its role in normal human physiology is not clear.[14]

Mucin is secreted in a soluble form from mucous gland neck cells in the fundus and body as well as from the cardiac and pyloric glands, and in a gel form from the superficial epithelial cells throughout the stomach. Duodenal mucosa is also a source of mucin. The gel form of mucin forms a surface coating, the thickness of which is determined by the rate of secretion and the rate of dissolution by pepsin. Pepsin depolymerizes the mucin.

The production of mucins is under reflex control; both splanchnic and vagal impulses may stimulate its production, as well as mechanical injury. Histamine is variously stated to have no effect[1] and to stimulate mucin production.[14]

All investigators agree that mucin serves a lubricating function, and some believe that it also serves a protective function in that it may delay back-diffusion of H^+ into the mucosa. Since bicarbonate ion is secreted by surface cells, an unstirred layer of mucin will neutralize a proportion of H^+ and raise the pH at the cell surface level. Brooks[4] believes mucin may serve a protective role, at least during the fasting state.

Intrinsic Factor

Intrinsic factor is a glycoprotein secreted in humans by the oxyntic (parietal) cell. It combines with imbibed vitamin B_{12} to form a complex that permits its absorption in the ileum and thus the entry of vitamin B_{12}.

Secretion of intrinsic factor is linked to histamine and to cyclic AMP.[4]

Blood Group Antigens

Most individuals secrete ABH(O) glycoproteins into the gastric lumen. In some it is replaced by Lewis-a (LE^a) antigen. A few individuals lack ABH antigens (nonsecretors). Peptic ulcers are more frequent in blood group O nonsecretors. The explanation for this finding is not clear.[14]

Immunoglobulins

Immunoglobulins A, G, and M have been found in gastric juice. Their role is not defined.[14]

Pepsinogen Secretion

Pepsinogens are zymogens separated electrophoretically into two groups. Group I contains rapidly migrating proteins and group II slowly migrating proteins. These various pepsinogens differ when activated to pepsin in their pH optima and substrate specificity. The first group is secreted in the proximal stomach by chief cells and in low concentration by mucous neck cells. The second group is secreted most abundantly in pyloric mucosa and in Brunner's glands of the duodenum.[1] In the presence of acid pepsinogens are converted to pepsin, which acts as a proteolytic enzyme most active at pH 1 to 3.[1]

Pepsinogen is secreted continuously in small amounts under basal conditions; its secretion is stimulated most strongly through vagal stimulation, and thus by feeding. The effect is mediated by acetylcholine. Secretin, histamine, and the presence of acid in the lumen also stimulate pepsinogen release. The acid may act by stimulating the intramural complexes through diffusion of H^+ into the mucosa. It is also stimulated by gastrin through its effect on acid production and possibly independently. In general, pepsinogen secretion parallels that of acid except for the effect of secretin, which stimulates secretion of pepsinogen but inhibits that of acid.

Other Enzymes

A potent gelatinase, probably of chief cell origin, has been identified. A gastric lipase effective in hydrolizing short- and medium-chain fatty acids, such as those in milk, is also present, as is urease.[1]

Acid Secretion

Hydrochloric acid functions to activate pepsinogens to pepsin, to sterilize chyme, and to permit the normal absorption of nonheme dietary iron and the ferric form of iron.[4] It is secreted in an all-or-none fashion from the oxyntic cell (parietal cell), and the maximal acid output is thus dependent on the number of oxyntic cells present.

The mechanism of secretion of H^+ at the cellular level is complex; the reader is referred to Davenport[1] and Brooks[4] for details. It is an active process requiring energy derived from H^+, K^+-ATPase and the presence of oxygen. Its transfer to the lumen generates OH^- in the cell; OH^- combines with CO^2 in the presence of carbonic anhydrase to form HCO_3^-, which is in large part secreted into the blood. The H^+ is coupled with Cl^-, which is also actively secreted. Some K^+ also escapes from the oxyntic cell into the gastric juice. Thus, H^+ and Cl^- are both secreted into the lumen and removed from the plasma with enough water to keep the juice nearly isotonic (it is often slightly hypotonic, however, since HCO_3^- in the presence of H^+ in the gastric lumen forms CO_2, which escapes from the fluid).

Oxyntic cell secretion is activated by a triad of chemicals that potentiate each other's effect, that is, gastrin, histamine, and acetylcholine, for each of which receptors exist. In the case of histamine these are H_2 receptors which account for the effect of the H_2 blocking agent, cimetidine, in lowering acid secretion.

The composition of gastric juice varies with the rate of excretion. As the concentration of H^+ rises, the concentration of Na^+ falls. Theories differ as to whether the concentration of H^+, as it issues from the oxyntic cell, is a constant, and the discovered composition is a function of reaction and admixture with nonacidic compounds such as bicarbonate, or varies, having a higher Na^+ and a lower H^+ concentration at low levels of secretion. The secretory product is modified by diffusion of H^+ into the mucosa and of Na^+ into the lumen. Davenport[1] believes a combination of these hypotheses may be required to explain the facts.

Stimuli to Acid Secretion

As mentioned previously, gastrin, acetylcholine, and histamine are the final mediators of H^+ secretion. They potentiate each other's effect on the oxyntic cell. The source of gastrin is the G cell of the antrum and duodenal mucosa. Acetylcholine is secreted at nerve endings and histamine is presumed to be produced by cells, which are present in large numbers in the oxyntic mucosal lamina propria. Histamine is rapidly metabolized but is constantly present in the interstitial fluid about the oxyntic cell. The release of these compounds is controlled by humoral, paracrine, and neuronal mechanisms.

Calcium, whether in the lumen or under conditions of elevated serum concentrations, is known to liberate gastrin and thus increase acid secretion. Ethanol increases gastrin release in some animals. Its effects in humans are debatable.[10] The factors that damage mucosa and the mucosal barrier also increase acid via release of histamine on contact of mast cells by H^+ diffusing into the injured mucosa.

Gastric secretion is usually divided into cephalic, gastric, and intestinal phases, although these run nearly concurrently.

The Cephalic Phase

The cephalic phase is initiated by the thought, smell, taste, chewing, and swallowing of food and is mediated via chemoreceptors and mechanoreceptors that affect the vagal nuclei, which in turn activate efferent fibers to stimulate secretion. The cephalic phase is thus blocked by vagotomy. The vagus has a double effect, that is, release of gastrin and a direct effect on oxyntic cells via acetylcholine release. Only a small proportion of gastrin is released during this phase, perhaps in part because the fasting stomach is strongly acidic and H^+ inhibits gastrin release. In humans the completeness of vagotomy may be tested by the lack of effect of insulin-produced hypoglycemia, which also triggers the vagal efferent impulses.

The Gastric Phase

As food and fluid enter the stomach the buffering effect of the contents raises the pH, removing the inhibitory effect of the lower pH on gastrin release. Food itself, particularly peptides and certain amino acids, is the strongest stimulus to gastric secretion because it buffers acid and directly causes release of gastrin. This stimulus is not vagally dependent. The effect is abolished by acidification of the gastric contents. Since secretion is also suppressed by atropine and by H_2 antagonists, it is probably not due to a direct effect on oxyntic cells. Finally, distention of the stomach acting through mechanoreceptors, in addition to its effect on motility, stimulates acid release through long vago-vagal reflexes. It also acts through local distention reflexes of several types— thus, distention of an isolated denervated antral pouch stimulates acid release.

The Intestinal Phase

A less important role in acid secretion is mediated through release in the small intestine of an unknown peptide called *enterooxyntin*. The stimulus for its release appears to be the presence of peptones and some amino acids.[4,15]

Inhibition of Acid Secretion

As the stomach empties, it releases an unanalyzed substance termed *bulbogastrone*. This substance differs from secretin, which also inhibits acid secretions, and its importance in humans is not clear. The effect appears to be dependent on a neural mechanism. Other inhibitory hormones, generally *enterogastrones*, are liberated during the intestinal phase of digestion. Among these is secretin, which is known to inhibit acid release. In humans it may be important as an inhibitor, chiefly in the fasting state.[4] The presence of fat in the human jejunum inhibits acid secretion without altering gastrin levels. The factor released may be neurotensin. Cholecystokinin may also be a candidate for inhibition of acid secretion,[4] since it competes with gastrin for gastrin receptors due to its similar terminal amino acid sequence, but is pharmacologically less active in terms of acid secretory effects. The colon is also known to contain an unidentified substance capable of decreasing gastric secretion. In the stomach, somatostatin in D cells inhibits acid secretion both by a direct paracrine effect on G cells and by a direct effect on oxyntic cells.[4] The E_2 prostaglandins block histamine-stimulated production of cAMP and may have a local role in modulating production of HCl.[4]

Blood Flow

Gastric mucosal blood flow is increased by the presence of a meal, by histamine, by H^+, and by gastrin. It plays a permissive role in gastric secretion; it is stimulated by vagal excitation and inhibited by splanchnic excitation.

The Gastric Mucosal Barrier

One of the major problems in gastric physiology and pathophysiology is the elucidation of why the gastric mucosa is normally protected from autodigestion by gastric secretion. The answer is still not completely understood. The mucosal surface of the stomach is designed for minimal surface exposure to the mucosal elements. It is known that the normal surface mucosa is relatively resistant to back-diffusion of H^+ and to luminal diffusion of Na^+. Secretion of HCO_3^- by surface cells plus slowing of diffusion by the mucous coat is thought to play a role, at least in the fasting state.[4] Effective blood flow has been considered important, but only the combination of ischemia with the presence of acid and of bile has been experimentally shown to break the barrier.[1] Various prostaglandins appear to have a strong "cytoprotective" effect, even to agents such as absolute alcohol and boiling water. The mechanism is unknown.[1]

The barrier is broken by many nonionized fat-soluble acids such as butyric acid. Salicyclic and acetylsalicyclic acids, also fat soluble in acid solution, breach this barrier effectively. Bile acids and lysolecithin in an acid environment are also deleterious because of their detergent properties, as is ethyl alcohol. Regurgitation of duodenal contents including bile acids and lysolecithin is probably significant in the production of gastric ulcers.

In the duodenum, though the mucosal surface exposed is much greater, neutralization of acid is normally very rapid. Patients with duodenal ulcers are known to generally have both higher rates of acid secretion and an increase in the total amount of acid secreted, which may be sufficient to overcome the normal duodenal neutralization long enough for cell damage to occur. Once breached, a vicious cycle is established. Acid diffuses through the damaged mucosa, and surface cells are further damaged. Activation of pepsin by acid aggravates the problem. Histamine released by the effect of acid on mast cells both stimulates further acid secretion and increases capillary permeability. This results in edema and loss of proteins into the lumen, which may be considerable even in the absence of overt bleeding. This area will be further discussed in the chapter on peptic ulceration.

References

1. Davenport HW: Physiology of the Digestive Tract, 5th ed. Chicago, Year Book Medical Publishers, 1982, part II, pp 52–69, part III, pp. 103–113.
2. Heading RC: Gastric motility and emptying, in Sircus W, Smith AN (eds): Scientific Foundations of Gastroenterology. Philadelphia, WB Saunders Co, 1980, pp 287–296.
3. Cohen S, Long WB, Snape WJ Jr: Gastrointestinal motility, in Crane RK (ed): International Review of Physiology, Gastrointestinal Physiology III. Baltimore, University Park Press, 1979, vol 19, pp 118–132.
4. Brooks F: Movements and muscular activity in the gastrointestinal system, in West JB (ed): Physiological Basis of Medical Practice, 11th ed. Baltimore, Williams & Wilkins Co, 1985, chap 43.
5. Barber WD, Burks TF: Brain-gut interactions: brain stem neuronal response to local gastric effects of substance P. Am J Physiol 1987; (G)253:369–377.
6. Burks TF, Galligan JJ, Porreca F, Barber WD: Regulation of gastric emptying. Fed Proc 1985;44:2897–2901.
7. Kumar D, Ritman EL, Malagelada J-R: Three-dimensional imaging of the stomach: Role of pylorus in the emptying of liquids. Am J Physiol 1987;(G)253:79–85.
8. Gire M, Fiovamonti J, Bueno L: Comparative influences of acoustic and cold stress on gastrointestinal transit in mice. Am J Physiol 1987;(G)253:124–128.
9. Paintal AS: Regulation of food intake, in Sircus W, Smith AN (eds): Scientific Foundations of Gastroenterology. Philadelphia, WB Saunders Co, 1980, pp 123–129.
10. McHugh PR, Moran TH: The stomach, cholecystokinin, and satiety. Fed Proc 1986; 45:1384–1390.
11. Gibbs J, Smith GP: Satiety: The roles of peptides from the stomach and the intestine. Fed Proc 1986;45:1391–1395.
12. Bonfils S, Mignon M, Roze C: Vagal control of gastric secretion, in Crane RK (ed): The Inter-

national Review of Physiology, Gastrointestinal Physiology III. Baltimore, University Park Press, 1979, vol 19, chap. 2.

13. Reichlin S: Somatostatins. N Engl J Med 1983;309:1497–1499.

14. Piper DW: Mucus: Chemistry and characteristics, in Sircus W, Smith AN (eds): Scientific Foundations of Gastroenterology. Philadelphia, WB Saunders Co, 1980, pp 333–343.

15. Johnson LR: Gastrointestinal Physiology, 2nd ed. St. Louis, CV Mosby, 1979, chap. 7.

16. Giroud AS, Soll AH, Cuttitta F, et al: Bombesin stimulation of gastrin release from canine gastrin cells in primary culture. Am J Physiol 1987;(G)252:413–420.

17. Schubert ML, Edwards NF, Arimura A, et al: Paracrine regulation of gastric acid secretion by fundic somatostatin. Am J Physiol 1987;(G)252:485–490.

CHAPTER 3

Anomalies

Heterotopias

Heterotopia (Greek: *heteros* = other and *topos* = place) or ectopia (Greek: *ektopos* = displaced) refer to the presence of normal tissue in an abnormal location. Most heterotopias are considered congenital developmental anomalies caused by entrapment of embryologic cells in neighboring tissues during morphogenetic movements. This congenitally displaced tissue may differentiate in the course of organogenesis or perhaps later in response to an abnormal environment or nonspecific stimulus. The latter hypothesis would explain why most heterotopias become symptomatic only in adult life.

Heterotopic tissues found in the stomach and duodenum include pancreas, gastric mucosa in the duodenum, and Brunner's glands in the stomach.

Heterotopic Pancreas (Syn: Ectopic Pancreas, Aberrant Pancreas)

The most common heterotopic tissue found in the stomach and duodenum is pancreatic tissue. The incidence of heterotopic pancreas found at autopsy has been reported between 0.55 and 13.7%.[1] The most common sites of occurrence are the stomach (25 to 30%) and the duodenum (28 to 36%).[2] Men are affected more often than women. Lesions are most often detected in the fourth or fifth decade of life. The pathogenesis of ectopic pancreas may be explained in several ways, all of which support an antenatal origin. During the migratory phase of pancreatic development, small buds of the pancreatic anlage may become attached to and later incorporated into the gut. Alternately, lateral buds of rudimentary pancreatic ducts penetrate the intestinal wall and are carried by the longitudinal growth of the intestine upward and downward. Finally, pancreatic tissue could arise from multipotential cells in the embryonic gut.

In the stomach, heterotopic pancreas is most often found in the pylorus and antrum and along the greater curvature.[1] An exceptional location is the gastroesophageal junction.[3] In the duodenum, lesions occur mainly in the area proximal to the papilla and less often in the bulb.[4] Pancreatic tissue is usually situated in the submucosa (75%) and appears grossly as a broad-based, smooth nodule. Rarely, lesions are multiple, polypoid, or pedunculated.[3] In 25% the ectopic tissue is either intramuscular or subserosal and may produce only nonspecific thickening of the wall.[1,3] Most lesions are small, 0.5 to 1.5 cm in diameter,[5] but some as large as 6 cm have been reported.[4] Lesions are usually discovered incidentally, often in the course of ulcer disease.[5] Symptoms depend on the location and size of the mass. Lesions near the pylorus may produce gastric outlet obstruction; duodenal lesions near the ampulla of Vater may cause biliary obstruction.[6] Ulcera-

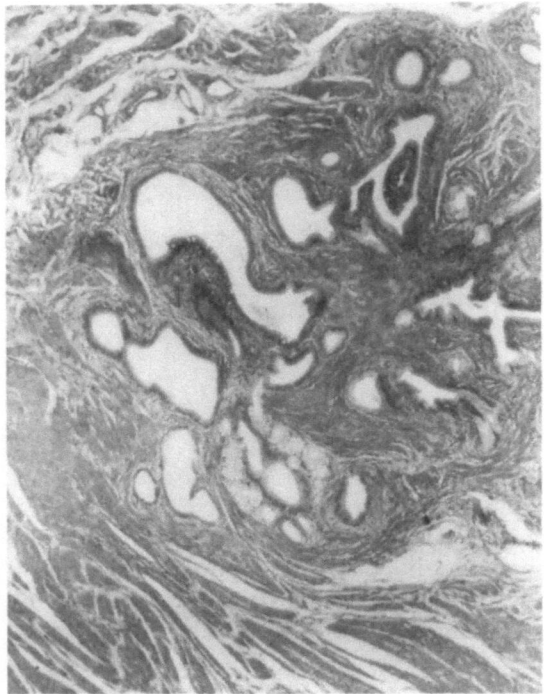

Figure 3-1. Heterotopic pancreas. Ducts and few Brunner-like glands are embedded deep into the muscularis propria. HPS, X50, reproduced at 80%.

tion and bleeding may occur. Rarely, there may be symptoms related to islet cell tumors developing in the heterotopic pancreas, such as hypoglycemia and the Zollinger-Ellison syndrome.[7,8]

The diagnosis may be made radiographically or by fiberoptic endoscopy, but is usually not definite until surgery. The classic radiographic appearance in a barium study is a broad-based or polyp-like fixed filling defect with a normal rugal pattern leading to it. Central umbilication appears as a point of retained barium.[1]

Histologic examination provides the definitive diagnosis. Endoscopic biopsies are usually insufficient to sample the intramural tissue, and surgical resection is usually necessary.

Most commonly there are ducts, acini, and Brunner-like glands (Fig. 3-1). Rarely, islets of Langerhans are seen.[4] A heterotopic

ampulla of Vater has been reported.[3] When accompanying smooth muscle proliferation becomes striking and the dominant feature, the lesions are also referred to as adenomyomas.[6,9] Degenerative changes within the heterotopic tissue include cyst formation, inflammation, ulceration, and hemorrhage.[10] Adenomas and carcinomas have been reported to originate in heterotopic pancreas.[7,8,11,12]

Pancreatic pseudocysts developing in the course of acute pancreatitis may rupture into the stomach or duodenum and present as intramural gastric or duodenal masses.[13,14] The second part of the duodenum, the nonperitonealized posterior surface of which is in direct contact with the head of the pancreas, is the most frequent site of involvement. These acquired pancreatic lesions must be distinguished from heterotopias.

Heterotopic Brunner's Glands

Brunner's type glands are often seen in heterotopic pancreas (Fig. 3-1).[3] Heterotopic lesions composed exclusively of Brunner's glands and smooth muscle occur in the pylorus and gastric antrum and are identical in appearance to Brunner's gland adenomas in the duodenum. Heterotopic duodenum, including mucosal villi, Brunner's glands, submucosa, muscularis, and serosa, has been reported in the cystic duct of the gallbladder.[15]

Heterotopic Gastric Mucosa
(Syn: Ectopic Gastric Mucosa)

Heterotopic gastric mucosa has been found in all segments of the digestive tract, including the esophagus, duodenum, small intestine, and rectum, but is most common in Meckel's diverticulum.[16,17,19-24] In the upper esophagus the incidence of gastric heterotopia was found to be 3.8% on endoscopy and biopsy.[16] Gastric heterotopia implies the presence of normal gastric mucosa, including mucinous surface epithelium, pits, neck glands, and body glands with parietal and chief cells. It is

Figure 3-2. Heterotopic gastric mucosa in duodenal villus. H&E, X63, reproduced at 80%.

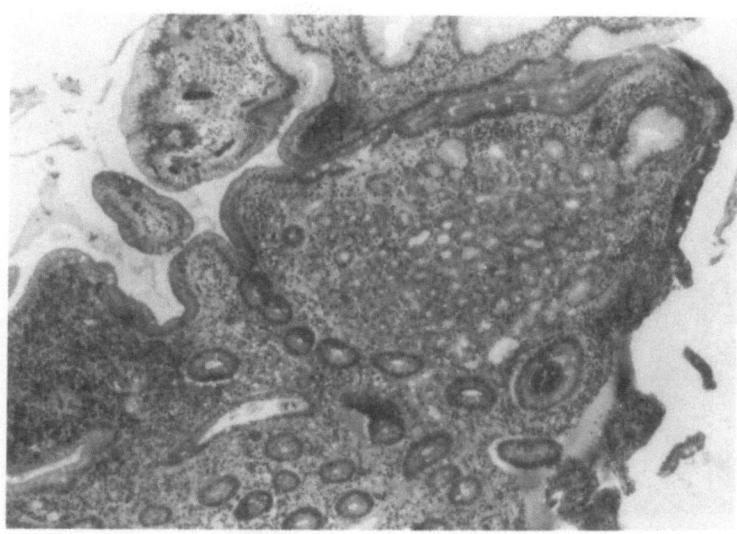

to be distinguished from gastric metaplasia associated with duodenitis, in which the resorptive surface epithelium is transformed into mucinous epithelium of the gastric surface and pits. Gastric heterotopia is also to be distinguished from pyloric metaplasia found in diverse inflammatory conditions of the small bowel, such as Crohn's disease or ischemic enteritis.[18]

Heterotopic gastric mucosa is common in the juxtapyloric portion of the duodenal bulb, where it was found in 30% of specimens obtained during gastrectomy, most of which were done for peptic ulcer disease.[19] Usually there is no grossly visible lesion and the diagnosis is made only microscopically. Recent endoscopic studies, however, have described rugose masses[20] and nodules and polyps[21,22] produced by heterotopic gastric mucosa in as many as 0.4 and 1% of upper gastrointestinal examinations, respectively. The most common location is the anterior wall of the first portion of the duodenum. Lesions are usually small, 1 to 6 mm in diameter, but may be extensive and involve most of the duodenal bulb. Tc-99m partechnetate abdominal scintigraphy and glucagon-induced duodenal hypotonia combined with a double-contrast technique have been used as diagnostic tools.[23] The endoscopic Congo red test was employed to demonstrate acid production.[24]

Histologically, heterotopic gastric mucosa is of body type, often associated with a stunted villous pattern on the surface (Fig. 3-2). Complications include ulceration and hemorrhage. Elsewhere in the small intestine, obstruction and intussusception may occur. Malignant transformation has not been described.

Diffuse Cystic Malformation of the Stomach

Diffuse cystic malformation of the stomach is rare; only 32 cases were found in the medical literature in 1975, 32 years after its first description in 1943.[25] The condition affects primarily men in the seventh decade of life and is not associated with cystic changes in other organs. Cysts are found mostly in the submucosa, but sometimes also in the muscularis mucosae, of the gastric body and antrum. They are thought to arise from heterotopic gastric or duodenal glands or pancreatic tissue and are lined by mucinous epithelium, sometimes interspersed with chief and parietal cells. Surrounding bundles

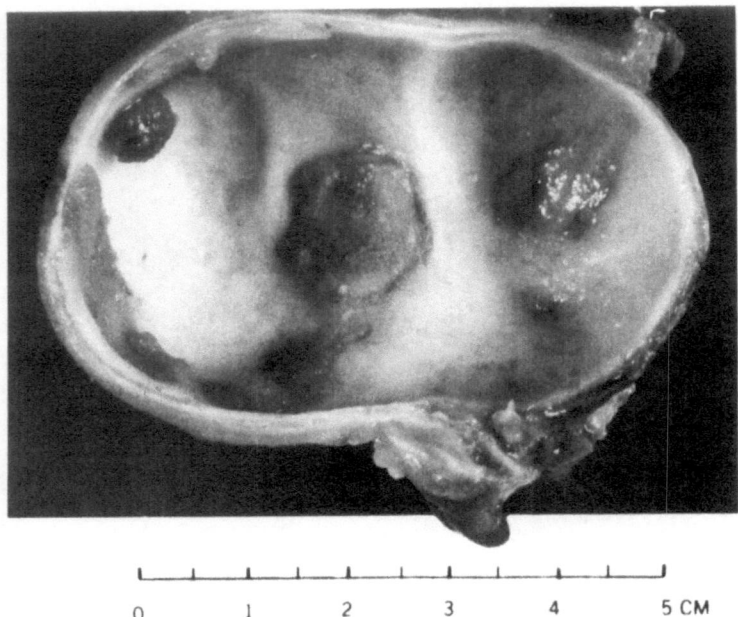

Figure 3-3. Gastric duplication cyst. The cyst lining is smooth except for areas of calcification on the left. Courtesy of Dr. R. Wieczorek, NYU Medical Center. From Wieczorek RL, Seidman I, Ranson JH, et al: Congenital duplication of the stomach. Am J Gastroenterol 1984;79:597–602. Reproduced by permission, American College of Gastroenterology.

of smooth muscle usually blend with the muscularis mucosae. Connection of the cysts with the gastric glands in the overlying mucosa may be seen. Cysts can be recognized grossly using a macrodissector or hand lens.[26] Gastric carcinoma was associated in several Japanese cases.[25]

Duplications

Intestinal duplications may be found anywhere from the base of the tongue to the anus, but are most common in the small intestine, particularly in the ileum. Gastric and duodenal duplications are rare and account for approximately 4 and 10% of all gastrointestinal duplications, respectively.[27,28] A total of 109 cases were found in the English literature in 1984.[29] Criteria for the diagnosis include the following: alimentary mucous membrane lining, a smooth muscle coat, and intimate attachment to the alimentary tract.[29] Duplications may be complete or incomplete, communicating or noncommunicating. Clinically, they may present as a double stomach or duodenum,[28,30] a diverticu-

lum, or an intramural cystic mass.[29,31,32] Most gastric and duodenal duplications are incomplete and noncommunicating, produce a cystic mass, and are detected in childhood or early adulthood. Rarely, symptoms appear as late as the seventh and ninth decade.[28] Vacchus and Blasius are credited with the first description of a double stomach in the cadaver of an 85-year-old man, and Wendel with the first surgical and histopathologic documentation.[33]

The most common location of gastric duplications is the greater curvature, and that of duodenal duplications the anterior wall of the first and second portions.[28,29] They measure from less than 3 cm to greater than 12 cm (Fig. 3-3).[29] Enteric cysts may be displaced proximally and present as gastrothoracic or mediastinal cysts,[32] or distally and posteriorly and produce retroperitoneal, mesenteric, pancreatic or bile duct cysts.[27] Infrequently, a tubular duodenal duplication extends through the diaphragm into the chest.[34] Other developmental anomalies occur in 35% of patients and are present primarily in the alimentary tract, including esophageal duplication, aberrant pancreas, malrotation of gut, and Meckel's diverticulum.[29] Vertebral anomalies are common, especially in the thoracic spine.[35] Rare coexisting abnormalities include pulmonary sequestration, accessory or abnormally shaped spleen, kidney or urinary tract abnormalities, Turner's syndrome, patent ductus arteriosus, and ventricular septal defect.[29,36] Abnormal communications with adjacent structures may result in pleural and pancreatic fistulas.[37] Communication of a duodenal duplication with the common bile duct secondary to erosion by a gallstone has been reported.[34]

The embryogenesis of enteric duplications may be explained in several ways. During the eighth to ninth week of embryonic development, epithelial cells fill the intestinal tube entirely and secretions accumulate in droplets or vacuoles, the coalescence of which later forms the lumen. Failure of vacuolar fusion could result in channels separate from the main lumen.[38] Another theory proposes infolding and fusion of longitudinal mucosal folds, followed by the muscularis, as a cause.[39] An alternate explanation is sequestration of embryonic tissue during embryonic movements.[40] Finally, abortive twinning at an early stage of cell division could result in enteric duplication.[41]

Gastric and duodenal duplications usually produce nonspecific symptoms, such as vomiting, pain, or hematemesis. A palpable abdominal mass is present in the majority of cases.[29] Duodenal duplications may be associated with pancreatic abnormalities and pancreatitis.[42,43] A filling defect, pyloric or duodenal stenosis, and rarely calcification are seen on radiologic examination.[27,44,45] Sonography discloses the cystic nature of the mass.[45]

Intramural cystic duplications are located in the submucosa or muscularis propria. The mucosa may differ histologically from the parent organ, and gastric and small intestinal epithelia may coexist. In gastric duplications, the gastric mucosa is often flattened and atrophic (Fig. 3-4). Components of the upper respiratory tract, including respiratory mucosa, cartilage, and seromucinous glands,

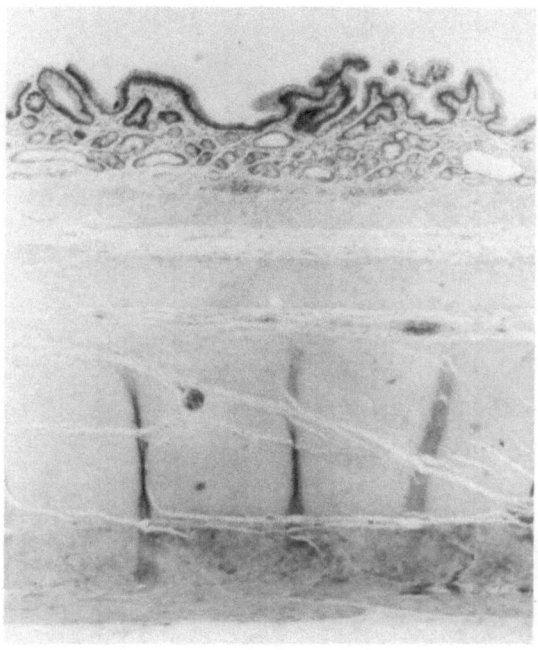

Figure 3-4. Gastric duplication cyst. The wall is composed of mucosa, submucosa, and muscularis propria. The mucosa is flattened and atrophic. H&E, X40, reproduced at 80%.

were present in an intramucosal cyst of the cardia.[41] Mucosa and submucosa usually show focal chronic inflammation. The muscularis propria is entirely present. Duodenal duplication cysts are lined by duodenal mucosa (Fig. 3-5) and in 13 to 15% also by gastric mucosa.[34] Ectopic pancreatic tissue and an adenomyoma have been found in a gastric duplication cyst.[31] Complications include inflammation, ulceration, bleeding, and rupture.[46] Carcinoma arising in a gastric duplication cyst has been described.[47]

Bile duct duplications are frequently associated with ectopic drainage of one duct into the gastric fundus.[48] The gallbladder and cystic duct may be absent.[49]

Diverticula

Diverticula of the upper gastrointestinal tract are much rarer than those of the lower gastrointestinal tract. Gastric diverticula

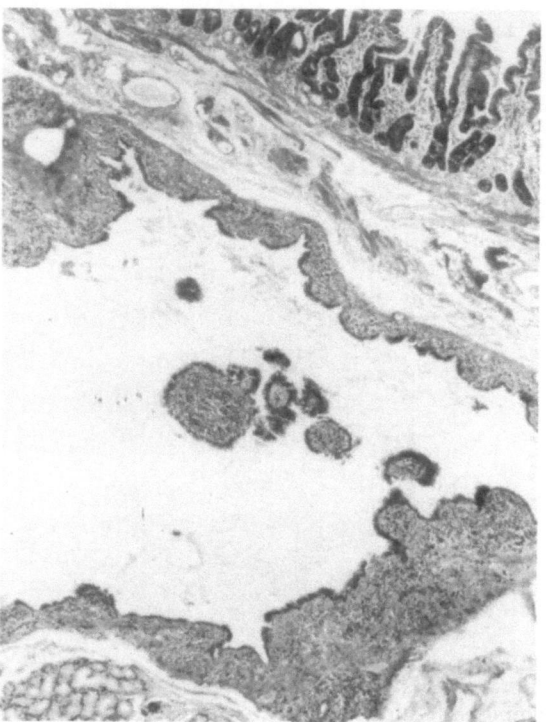

Figure 3-5. Duodenal duplication cyst. The cyst is lined by atrophic, chronically inflamed duodenal mucosa. A Brunner's gland is seen in the left lower corner. HPS, X40, reproduced at 80%.

are the rarest. Of 20 upper gastrointestinal diverticula, 6 were located in the esophagus, 2 in the stomach, and 12 in the duodenum.[50]

Gastric Diverticula

The first description of a gastric diverticulum was provided by Baillie in 1793.[51] The first review of gastric diverticula in 1951 cited 412 cases, 236 of which were diagnosed premortem and 176 postmortem.[52] The incidence at autopsy was found to be 0.02%, in upper gastrointestinal series 0.04%. More recent statistics, however, based on radiologic examinations in different projections report a much higher rate of 0.18%.[53]

The great majority of gastric diverticula are congenital, that is, they are true divertic-

ula with a wall composed of all layers of the normal stomach. The most common location is the posterior wall, close to the lesser curvature, just below the gastroesophageal junction.[53,54] They measure several centimeters, up to 7 cm in diameter.

Acquired diverticula are false diverticula (i.e., their wall is composed of mucosa and submucosa only and lacks a muscularis propria). False diverticula may be found at any location, but are most common in the distal one-third of the stomach, especially the prepyloric region.[55] They are caused by traction or pulsion secondary to inflammatory processes or tumors.

The diagnosis of gastric diverticulum is usually made incidentally at autopsy or in the course of radiologic examination for unrelated disease. Most gastric diverticula are asymptomatic, and complaints such as pain, epigastric fullness, or, rarely, bleeding are present in only 18%.[52] Posterior wall diverticula are easily missed by standard upper gastrointestinal series and require lateral oblique projections for visualization. Double-contrast barium meal allows for particularly good recognition of the luminal anatomy.[56] Intraoperative endoscopy has proved helpful for definite localization and for evagination to facilitate surgical resection.[57] Resection is necessary in only 10% of cases.[54] Complications of diverticula are rare and include bleeding, inflammation, and perforation. There are no reports of malignancies arising in gastric diverticula.

Duodenal Diverticula

The duodenum is second only to the colon as the most common site for diverticula in the gastrointestinal tract.[58] Duodenal diverticula were found in 1 to 5% of individuals undergoing barium meal study,[59] and juxtapapillary diverticula in as many as 3.2% of patients undergoing endoscopic retrograde cholangiopancreatography.[60] An incidence of 2.8% was found in an autopsy study in which diverticula were made to stand out by filling the small bowel in situ with water under moderate pressure.[61] More than 90% of diverticula are located along the concave border of the second or third portions and 60 to 80% occur in the second portion, especially near the ampulla. Juxtapapillary diverticula are associated with significant dysfunction of the choledochoduodenal sphincter. Muscular tone and contractile activity are decreased and rhythmic variations are fewer.[62] Sphincter dysfunction probably creates a predisposition to formation of biliary calculi and ascending bacterial infection of the bile ducts, both of which are common in patients with juxtapapillary diverticula.[63] Most duodenal diverticula are single, but 20% are multiple. Sizes are variable, ranging from very small to a capacity of up to 1000 ml.[64]

Most duodenal diverticula are acquired and represent extraluminal herniations of mucosa and submucosa through a weak point in the bowel wall.[65] Rarely, duodenal diverticula represent a developmental abnormality that is often associated with a duodenal diaphragm. Such intraluminal duodenal diverticula form slowly by the action of peristalsis on the diaphragm. Fewer than 50 cases have been reported.[66,67]

No definite symptom complex is associated with duodenal diverticula, and most cases are discovered incidentally. Pressure and inflammation may cause mild epigastric discomfort, which was found in 60% of patients.[50] Stagnation of intestinal contents in the diverticulum may lead to bezoar formation and small bowel obstruction.[68] Sphincter dysfunction, as already alluded to, creates a predisposition to cholelithiasis, cholangitis, and pancreatitis.[69] Hemorrhage is rare[66] and may be associated with ectopic gastric mucosa and peptic ulceration of the diverticulum.[70] Perforation is equally rare, and only 59 cases were found in the world literature in 1980.[71] Perforation into the aorta and formation of an aortoenteric fistula has been reported.[72] Finally, a bleeding polyp was discovered in a diverticulum.[73] Surgical intervention is required in only 2% of duodenal diverticula.[71]

Atresias, Stenoses, and Diaphragms

These congenital obstructive abnormalities of the gastrointestinal tract are most common in the anus, esophagus, and duodenum, in decreasing order of frequency.[74]

Several theories have been advanced to explain their pathogenesis. Tandler, in his classic study of duodenal development,[75] noted that during the second gestational month the duodenal lumen had no cavity but was filled with cells that later formed vacuoles, the coalescence of which reestablished patency. Failure to do so would result in atresia, stenosis, or diaphragm formation.

Prenatal vascular accidents may explain the majority of jejunoileal atresias, but seem to account for only a few duodenal atresias,[76] such as those associated with malrotation or intrauterine midgut strangulation by an omphalocele.[77] On the other hand, the common occurrence of atresia in the second part of the duodenum, which is the junctional zone between the vascular supply areas of the celiac axis and the superior mesenteric artery, suggests that ischemia may play a greater role than generally thought.[78] While the exact mechanism in individual cases remains obscure, there is general agreement that most cases of duodenal atresia represent early defects in embryologic development.[78-84] There is a high incidence of associated chromosomal defects. Maternal thalidomide intake during the 30th to 40th days of gestation, a time when duodenal differentiation is most active, has been shown to produce duodenal atresia.[78] Finally, a genetic origin is suggested by the familial nature of isolated duodenal atresia[85] and the hereditary nature of the syndrome of multiple intestinal atresias associated with pathognomonic intraluminal calcifications.[86]

Duodenal Atresia

Duodenal atresia is the most common type of fetal small bowel atresia. The incidence is reported variably between 1 in 6000 and 1 in 40,000 births.[79-81] Hydramnios was present in 53% of cases. Associated malformations were found in 48%. Down's syndrome was present in 33%.[80] Twenty-two percent had malrotation of the gut and 20% cardiovascular abnormalities. Combined esophageal and duodenal atresia has been reported.[82] There is an increased incidence of annular pancreas, biliary anomalies, and abnormal insertion of the ampulla of Vater in the medial wall of the duodenum. It is interesting that 37% of cases have anomalies of the vertebral column, which develops at approximately the same time as the duodenum.[78]

Duodenal atresia implies complete intrinsic luminal occlusion. Four types can be distinguished[79-80]:

1. The continuity of the gut is maintained.
2. Two blind ends are connected by a narrow solid string.
3. There is no continuity between the two blind ends.
4. There are multiple atresias of different types.

Duodenal atresia is fatal unless diagnosed and surgically treated promptly. Death occurs in the newborn secondary to vomiting, aspiration, and electrolyte imbalance. Distention of the stomach and esophagus with amniotic fluid may lead to spontaneous esophageal rupture.[87] The antenatal diagnosis can be made as early as in the 29th to 32nd week of gestation by means of ultrasonography.[88]

Duodenal stenosis accounts for about one-half of cases of neonatal duodenal obstruction[88] and is understood to be an incomplete form of atresia.

Mucosal Diaphragms

Mucosal diaphragms are membranous septa a few millimeters in thickness that may be congenital or acquired. Congenital diaphragms are considered incomplete forms of atresia.

Gastric Diaphragms

In the stomach, mucosal diaphragms occur most often at the pylorus and less frequently in the antrum.[89] In children, they are considered congenital; in adults, they are usually acquired secondary to peptic ulcer disease. It has been correctly pointed out, however, that peptic ulcers may also form as a complication of a congenital diaphragm, and that minor forms of congenital diaphragms may remain asymptomatic until complications ensue later in life. Fifty-six cases of antral diaphragms were collected from the English literature in 1981.[89] Clinically, these present with obstructive symptoms. Endoscopically, they are difficult to visualize unless the stomach is fully relaxed and distended. Most often there is a large mucosal fold with an aperture of constant size in the distal antrum. Apertures vary from 1 to 10 mm in diameter. Antral peristalsis stops abruptly at the diaphragm and proceeds normally beyond it. The surface is smooth and devoid of folds.

Pathologically, the resected stomach may show a serosal indentation at the level of the diaphragm. Histologically, the diaphragm is usually composed of antral type mucosa on both sides, with or without superimposed inflammation, and a central core of submucosal tissue. Rarely, ectopic pancreas is found within it.[89]

Duodenal Diaphragms

Duodenal diaphragms or congenital webs occur in about 1 of every 9000 to 40,000 births.[90,91] About 80% of reported cases involved the vicinity of the ampulla.[85] Postampullary lesions are twice as common as preampullary lesions. Rarely, the diaphragm is located elsewhere in the first or second portion. Obstructive symptoms usually appear in the newborn or pediatric population but may be detected only in adulthood, as late as the eighth decade.[90] Superimposed inflammation and scarring may lead to increasing narrowing of the lumen. In rare cases, chronic abdominal stasis leads to excessive antral stimulation, hyperacidity, and ulcer formation.[92,93]

The diagnosis can be made 95% of the time by hypotonic duodenography and 75% of the time with upper gastrointestinal series.[94] Endoscopically, duodenal diaphragms in adults have been described as circumferential cuffing of the duodenal mucosa with a narrow nipple-shaped lumen, the so-called *cervix sign.*

Pathologically, duodenal diaphragms are divided into complete and incomplete forms. A complete diaphragm occludes the entire lumen, but may tear and then have one or several apertures. An incomplete diaphragm involves only part of the circumference. Apertures vary from 1 mm to 3 cm.[91]

Histologically, diaphragms are composed of a central core or submucosal connective tissue and a covering of duodenal mucosa on both sides. Inflammation and scarring may be present in adults. Endoscopic resection of a diaphragm has been reported.[94]

Microgastria

Microgastria is a rare congenital anomaly, usually associated with other anomalies such as midgut malrotations, cardiac abnormalities, and asplenism.[95,96] An incompetent cardia and megaesophagus are secondarily acquired and revert to normal after successful surgical therapy.[97] Microgastria was first reported in 1894.[98] Symptoms usually appear in infancy and include failure to thrive, frequent vomiting, and recurrent aspiration pneumonia. A barium swallow demonstrates a small tubular stomach. A full-thickness biopsy of the stomach in one case showed no histologic abnormality, suggesting that microgastria represents hypoplasia of the entire stomach.[97]

Megaduodenum

Megaduodenum, a rare condition with a variety of causes, may be congenital or acquired.

Congenital enlargement of the duodenum may result from absence of ganglion cells, primary degeneration of the muscle layer, aplasia of the muscle layer, or have no recognizable cause.[99] Familial clustering of congenital megaduodenum has been noted. Megaduodenum may be associated with megaesophagus, megacolon, or megacystis.[100]

Megaduodenum may be acquired in the course of Chagas' disease, scleroderma, porphyria, and lupus erythematosus. Secondary duodenal dilatation because of distal obstruction may be congenital in cases of intestinal atresia or develop later in life due to any factors that can cause obstruction.

Dextrogastria

Dextrogastria is usually associated with total situs inversus, which occurs in approximately 1 of every 6000 to 8000 births.[101] Isolated situs inversus of the stomach and duodenum only, with normally positioned thoracic and remaining abdominal viscera, is extremely rare.[102] It occurs in two forms: the stomach lies either completely behind the liver (type I) or right above the liver, associated with eventration of the right hemidiaphragm (type II). Dextrogastria associated with an undescended or left-sided cecum has also been reported.[103,104]

Intrathoracic Stomach

Intrathoracic stomach is an infrequent but not rare anomaly caused by a congenital paraesophageal gap or a congenitally enlarged esophageal hiatus.[105] The herniated stomach lies anterior to the esophagus and may be accompanied by a colonic transverse loop or the spleen.[106] Symptoms often appear only late in life and are due to complications such as anemia, ulcer, or obstruction. One of the authors (H.R.) has seen a case of intrathoracic stomach associated with herniation of the entire mobile small and large bowel into the chest. The patient died of respira-

Table 3-1. Classification of Gastric Volvulus

---

1. Type
   a. Organoaxial
   b. Mesenterioaxial
   c. Combination of *a* and *b*
2. Extent
   a. Total
   b. Partial
3. Direction
   a. Anterior
   b. Posterior
4. Etiology
   a. Secondary
   b. Idiopathic
5. Severity
   a. Acute
   b. Chronic

---

tory insufficiency. The diagnosis of intrathoracic stomach was not made until autopsy. Computed tomography has proved helpful in the diagnosis of some cases.[105]

Gastric Volvulus

Gastric volvulus is an abnormal rotation of the stomach and may be classified according to type, extent, direction, etiology, and severity (Table 3-1).[107] The most common type, the organoaxial volvulus, occurs around a line from the pylorus to the cardia and is found in approximately 60% of reported cases. The second most common type, the mesenterioaxial volvulus, occurs around a line that runs from the center of the greater curvature to the porta hepatis and is found in 30% of cases. Rarely, both types are combined. In most instances, the volvulus is total and the entire stomach is involved. Partial volvulus commonly involves the greater curvature. Anterior rotation is present when the transverse colon comes to lie in front of the stomach in an organoaxial volvulus. Anterior rotation is much more common than posterior rotation.

Most cases of gastric volvulus occur in the presence of other intraabdominal anomalies, such as eventration of the left hemidiaphragm, adhesions, a lax esophageal hiatus, Bochdalek's hernia, or paraesophageal hiatus hernia, and are termed *secondary*.[108-110] In such cases, the rotated stomach may come to lie in the thoracic cavity. A gastric volvulus is primary in approximately one-third of cases and presumably is caused by considerable laxity of gastric ligaments. Although women apparently show greater mobility of retroperitoneal organs at laparotomy, the male/female ratio is approximately equal (46%/54%). Adults in the fifth and sixth decades of life are affected most often. Volvulus in the newborn is rare and usually associated with abnormalities of the diaphragm. Only 13 cases were found in the English literature in 1980.[109]

Cases of acute volvulus appear more often in the literature, probably due to a bias in reporting. Symptoms appear after a large meal and include epigastric abdominal distention, fruitless attempts at vomiting, and occasionally transient myocardial ischemia.[111] Attempts to pass a nasogastric tube are unsuccessful. Immediate surgery is required. Reported death rates for mesenterioaxial and organoaxial volvulus are 56 and 42%, respectively.[107] Death is caused by obstruction, strangulation, and ischemic necrosis of the stomach. Chronic volvulus may be complicated by pneumatosis cystoides intestinalis and pneumo-peritoneum.[110]

Gastroschisis

Gastroschisis is a congenital anomaly acquired during intrauterine life probably secondary to vascular injury to the abdominal wall during early embryogenesis.[112] Portions of the stomach, the small intestine, and the colon herniate through a defect in the abdominal wall lateral to the umbilical cord. In contrast to cases of omphalocele, in which the herniated intestine is protected from amniotic fluid by intact peritoneal and amniotic membranes, the abdominal wall defect is gastroschisis is complete and exposure to amniotic fluid occurs, resulting in thickening and edema of the gastric and intestinal walls and exudation of fibrin on their surfaces. Associated intestinal anomalies are common and usually include atresias of one or more portions of the small and large bowel and, less commonly, anomalies of the liver and biliary tract. Reduplication of the gallbladder has been reported.[113]

Right Paraduodenal Hernia

The right paraduodenal hernia belongs to the group of internal hernias that develop in the 10th week of intrauterine life in the course of the rapid, active rotational events around the axis of the superior mesenteric artery.[114] All or a portion of the small bowel or a single loop may become entrapped in the right paraduodenal area with the superior mesenteric artery forming the anterior portion of the hernia ring and the returning ascending colon and cecum the anterior wall of the sac. Fifty cases were found in the literature in 1979.[115] Symptoms are often chronic, consisting of vague abdominal pain and intermittent obstructive episodes, and medical attention is often sought only in adult life.

Congenital Duodenal Adhesions

Duodenal bands or adhesions result either from persistence of peritoneal bands and folds that appear during normal rotation or from peritonitis and localized enteritis during intrauterine life.[116] Adhesions can involve any part of the duodenum, including the ligament of Treitz. Symptoms appear in the early postnatal period, if obstruction is complete or nearly complete, or only in childhood or adulthood if obstruction is incomplete. Duodenal bands may occur isolated or in associa-

tion with intestinal malrotation, and rarely with a congenital duodenal diaphragm.[117] A barium meal shows dilatation of the duodenum proximal to the obstruction and sometimes dilatation of the stomach as well. Lysis of adhesions gives excellent results.

Anomalies of Duodenal Rotation (Syn: Intestinal Malrotation)

The distal portion of the duodenum, beginning at the middle third, is the most proximal part of the midgut and thus participates in the complex rotational movements of the midgut around the rotational axis formed by the superior mesenteric artery. Since the proximal (i.e., duodenojejunal or prearterial segment) and the distal (i.e., cecocolic or postarterial segment) do not rotate simultaneously but sequentially,[118] various combinations of rotational abnormalities may exist. In 1923, Dott[119] divided the rotational process into three stages. In the fifth week of gestation, the duodenojejunal segment rotates 90° counterclockwise, presumably secondary to pressure by the developing liver, and temporarily settles inferior and to the right of the superior mesenteric artery. In the eighth week the loop performs another counterclockwise 90° rotation and comes to lie slightly to the left of the superior mesenteric artery. In the 10th week the rotational process is completed by a final 90° rotation that occurs simultaneous with the return of the duodenojejunal loop from its temporary herniation into the umbilical cord, while the cecocolic loop is still located within the cord. Rotational abnormalities involving the duodenum include, in decreasing order of frequency: 1) Complete failure of rotation of the proximal and distal intestinal loops, 2) complete failure of rotation of the proximal loop with normal rotation of the distal loop, 3) complete failure of rotation of the proximal loop and partial rotation of the distal loop, and 4) partial failure of rotation of the proximal loop and normal rotation of the distal loop. Complete failure of rotation (i.e., nonrotation) is often associated with gastroschisis,[119] partial failure (i.e., incomplete rotation) with intestinal bands.[120] In cases with severe anomalies, symptoms of duodenal obstruction (i.e., bile-stained vomitus or gastric aspirate, often accompanied by midgut volvulus) appear early in infancy. In milder forms nonspecific symptoms of repeated intermittent obstruction may appear only in adulthood and remain unrecognized for long periods.[121] Diagnostic evaluation of rotational abnormalities should include radiologic examination of both the upper and lower gastrointestinal tract.[122]

Isolated Incomplete Duodenal Rotation

This form of partial duodenal nonrotation was first well delineated by Lewis in 1966[121] and has recently resurfaced in the literature as a cause of intermittent partial duodenal obstruction in childhood or adulthood.[122-124] The duodenojejunal junction is located on the right side of the abdomen instead of its normal position beneath and to the left of the superior mesenteric artery.[124] The duodenum is kinked upon itself and fixed by numerous adhesions incurring some degree of obstruction. Rotation of the colon is normal, although its fixation may be deficient. Intrinsic duodenal obstruction is found in 10%. Treatment consists of mobilization of the duodenum, lysis of adhesions, and ruling out an intrinsic duodenal obstruction.[124]

Defects of the Gastric Musculature

In 1943, Herbut[125] described congenital absence of the muscularis propria of the stomach at the site of perforation. A deficiency in the gastric musculature has been implicated in one-third of cases of gastric rupture in infants.[126] Histologically, gradual thinning of the muscle as the point of rupture was approached was observed. Since experimental rupture of normal stomachs was shown to produce the same changes, the concept of congenital absence of the gastric musculature is still controversial.[127] Most cases occurred in premature infants. For further discussion, see "Gastric Rupture," Chapter 12.

Hypertrophic Pyloric Stenosis

Hypertrophic pyloric stenosis exists in two forms: the more common, probably congenital, infantile form and the less common, probably acquired, adult form.[128] Both are characterized by localized muscular hypertrophy without associated inflammation or fibrosis. The pyloric channel is two to four times its normal length and its thickness exceeds 1 cm (normal, 4 to 8 mm).[129] Hypertrophy and hyperplasia affect primarily the circular muscle layer and, to a much lesser extent, the longitudinal layer. Mild mucosal and submucosal edema are usually present.

The infantile form occurs in approximately 1 of 400 to 500 individuals, shows a definite male predominance (male/female ratio, 4 or 5:1), and is often found in several members of the same family.[129,130] It is probably related to a congenital inability of the sphincter to relax. Muscle hypertrophy actually develops later in the postnatal period. Degenerated ganglion cells have been found in the myenteric plexus.[130] The infantile form manifests itself clinically between 4 and 6 weeks after birth, with vomiting and failure to thrive.

The adult form is less common. In some cases it is related to a preexisting infantile form. In the majority of cases it is associated with peptic ulcers, especially benign gastric ulcers, and appears to be acquired.[130,131]

Aganglionosis

Aganglionosis, or Hirschsprung's disease, is usually limited to the rectosigmoid; if more extensive, it involves the remaining colon and parts of the ileum.[132] Few cases of total aganglionosis of the entire intestine, including the duodenum, have been reported since the first description of this condition in 1951.[133,134] Involvement of the distal stomach is exceptional. Of 12 cases 6 occurred in siblings, suggesting autosomal recessive inheritance. The condition is not compatible with life, and infants die of intestinal obstruction shortly after birth. Aganglionosis may result in a megaduodenum.[99]

Vascular Malformations

Accessory Left Gastric Artery
(Syn: Accessory Left Hepatic Artery)

An accessory left gastric artery arising from the left hepatic artery is relatively common in the Japanese.[135] At Osaka University Hospital, 14.2% of hepatic angiograms demonstrated an accessory left gastric artery, producing a gastric wall stain that may mimic a hepatic tumor in the capillary phase. Blood may flow from the liver to the stomach or in the opposite direction. In the latter situation, the artery is called accessory left hepatic artery.

Submucosal Arterial Malformation
(Syn: Caliber-Persistent Artery,
Submucosal Aneurysm, Sclerotic
Submucosal Gastric Artery,
Abnormal Intramural Artery)

Submucosal arterial malformation,[136] also termed "caliber-persistent" artery,[137,138] submucosal aneurysm,[139] "sclerotic submucosal gastric artery,"[140] or abnormal intramural gastric artery,[141] is an uncommon yet potentially lethal vascular anomaly. A total of 47 cases were found in the literature in 1983.[136] The condition affects predominantly men, all ages, and is considered congenital. Normally, as arteries perforate the outer layers of the gastric wall, a simultaneous reduction of their caliber takes place with successive bifurcations.[137] Caliber-persistent arteries occur when this normal arterial branching

pattern is absent. Lesions may be single or multiple and are most commonly located in the proximal portion of the stomach. Typically, a mucosal erosion capped by thrombotic material overlying a ruptured submucosal vessel is seen. Histologically, unusually large, tortuous, muscular arteries with three well-defined layers are seen (Fig. 3-6). Atherosclerotic changes may be superimposed and cause a predisposition to rupture, but are not considered the cause of the malformation as such.[141] Loss or absence of the circular and inner muscular layers of the gastric wall adjacent to the abnormal submucosal artery was found in one case.[137] Hemorrhage following rupture of the abnormal vessel was fatal in 38 of 43 cases.[139]

Aneurysms

Aneurysms of the gastroduodenal arteries are rare compared with those of the splenic or hepatic arteries.[142,143] Most are atherosclerotic. Other etiologic factors include trauma, surgery, penetrating duodenal ulcer, carcinoma of the head of the pancreas,[143] alcoholic pancreatitis,[144] retroperitoneal tumor, and developmental medial defects.[142] The left gastric, gastroduodenal, pancreaticoduodenal, and gastroepiploic arteries have been affected.[143,145,146] Reported diameters range from 0.5 to 5 cm. Gastric arterial aneurysms may rupture into the stomach,[143] peritoneal cavity,[147] or bile duct.[145] Pancreatitis accounts for more than half of all gastroduodenal aneurysms, but only about 29% of pancreaticoduodenal aneurysms.[144] Almost all of these cases are accompanied by acute or chronic gastrointestinal bleeding. Selective mesenteric arteriography proved of greatest diagnostic specificity. Computerized axial tomography may be helpful. Mortality of 46% was reported.[147]

Gastric Varices

With the advent of flexible endoscopy and arteriography, gastric varices have been

Figure 3-6. Submucosal arterial malformation of the stomach. Ruptured, unusually large submucosal artery with superimposed intimal fibrosis. EVG, X40, reproduced at 75%.

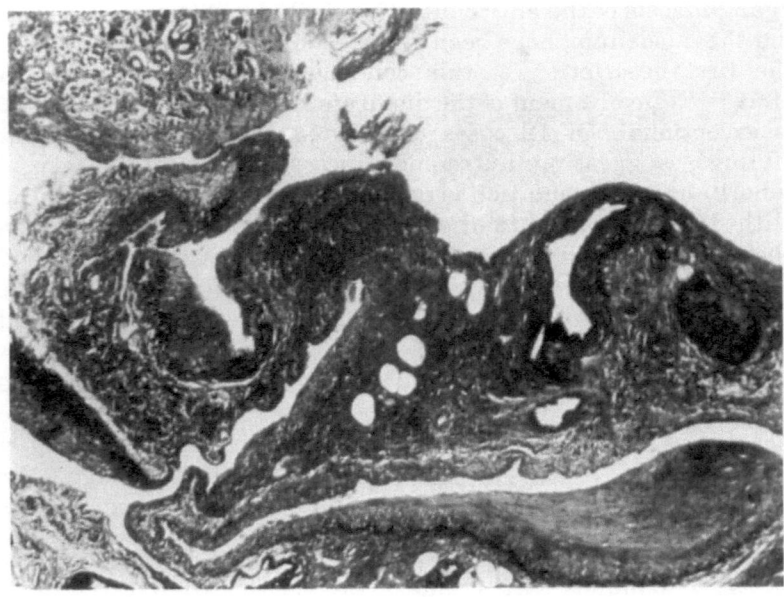

identified as a cause of gastrointestinal bleeding with increasing frequency.[148-154] Gastric varices, usually isolated (i.e., not accompanied by esophageal varices), develop secondary to splenic vein thrombosis[148-152] or as a complication of a wandering spleen.[153-154] Splenic vein thrombosis is usually associated with pancreatic disease, such as chronic pancreatitis, pancreatic pseudocyst, pancreatic abscess, pancreatic carcinoma, islet cell tumor, or retroperitoneal disease. Less commonly, splenic vein thrombosis is precipitated by myeloproliferative disorders or umbilical vein catheterization. Rarely, it develops spontaneously in the absence of other pathology. Regardless of its pathogenesis, splenic vein thrombosis produces a localized or left-sided form of portal hypertension, with splenic venous blood draining through the short gastric veins either into the right gastroepiploic vein or across the fundus of the stomach to the left gastric vein (coronary vein). Clinically, the diagnosis is suspected in any patient with gastrointestinal hemorrhage, pancreatic disease, and splenomegaly without other signs of portal hypertension. Gas-

tric varices secondary to a wandering spleen may be associated with gastric torsion.[154] In such cases the space beneath the left diaphragm contains the colon, which in turn pulls up the greater curvature of the stomach. Gastric varices develop due to obstruction of the venous drainage of the proximal stomach by a twisted splenic pedicle and gastric torsion. Radiologically, varices appear in the cardia or fundus as broad, serpentine, redundant folds or clusters of polypoid defects simulating thickened rugal folds. Double-contrast barium studies are suggestive in 74% of cases.[150] Angiography demonstrates occlusion of the splenic vein and the presence of collaterals. Endoscopy identifies gastric varices in only 40% of cases.[149] They are frequently misinterpreted as a gastric fundic mass or hypertrophic folds. Pathologically, gastric varices are either localized and polypoid or multiple and produce rounded submucosal projections. Due to the greater thickness of the gastric mucosa compared with the esophageal mucosa, a bluish tint or tortuous vessels are usually not seen. Treatment and cure is splenectomy.

Duodenal Varices

Duodenal varices, usually associated with portal hypertension, were found in almost 50% of patients undergoing splenoporto- grams.[155] Esophageal and gastric varices are often associated. Duodenal varices occur relatively more frequently in individuals with extrahepatic portal obstruction than in those with intrahepatic obstruction. Hepatic artery-portal vein fistula and congenital superior mesenteric vein obstruction may be associated. In most cases, bleeding does not occur because of the frequent deep intramural location of the collateral vessels. Submucosal bleeding varices, however, were identified in the duodenal bulb in one case by endoscopy[156] and below the papilla of Vater in another case at laparotomy.[157] Clinically, duodenal variceal bleeding is usually misdi- agnosed as a bleeding ulcer. Percutaneous transhepatic portography has been sug- gested as the diagnostic procedure of choice, and sclerotherapy via a flexible endoscope has been successful.[158]

Arteriovenous Malformations (Syn: Angiodysplasia, Telangiectasia, Telangiopathy)

Arteriovenous malformations of the gas- trointestinal tract have been classified into three types[159]: Type 1, also called angio- dysplasia, is probably acquired, affects elderly patients, is found primarily in the cecum, ascending colon, and ileum, and is commonly associated with some type of cardi- ovascular or pulmonary disease,[160] most nota- bly aortic stenosis.[161] Type 2 lesions are probably congenital, tend to affect a younger age group, are usually large and grossly visi- ble at laparotomy, and are most commonly found in the jejunum. Type 3 lesions are a manifestations of the Osler-Weber-Rendu syndrome, occur in association with respira- tory and cutaneous lesions, and are found throughout the gastrointestinal tract.

Although type 1 lesions are most common in the cecum, lesions in the stomach and duodenum have been reported with increas- ing frequency.[160-167] Hypoxygenation of the mucosa due to atherosclerotic peripheral vas- cular disease has been proposed as the most likely pathogenetic mechanism. Cholesterol emboli may be found in submucosal arter- ies.[162] The occurrence of lesions without a background of cardiovascular disease such as chronic hemodialysis[163] or with von Willebrand's disease,[165] however, throws doubt on the sole significance of this mechan- ism. Body, fundus, and antrum of the stomach and bulb, descending, and distal portions of the duodenum have been affected.[160,164] Lesions may be single or multi- ple. Bleeding is venous rather than arterial and mild and recurrent. In cases with aortic stenosis, valve replacement may stop[161] or initiate [166] bleeding. The diagnosis is best made by selective angiography.[167] Although endoscopic recognition is possible,[160,164] lesions are frequently missed on direct vision by the endoscopist, surgeon, and pathologist alike. Specimen angiography may be required to visualize their localization and extent.[168] In typical cases, lesions are red, flat or slightly raised, and measure 3 to 10 mm in diameter. Gastritis and traumatic hemor- rhage are common misinterpretations.[169] Sometimes the mucosa appears thickened and may become polypoid secondary to trac- tion during antral emptying, and the lesion is mistaken for a polyp. Histologically, there are distended, thin- and thick-walled vascu- lar spaces in the mucosa and/or submucosa (Fig. 3-7). Deeper layers are not involved. The simplest treatment consists of electrocoagu- lation via the endoscope, a procedure that may be repeated if initially unsuccessful.[160] Surgical resection should be restricted to cases that cannot be adequately visualized.

Type 2 arteriovenous malformations are rarer than the type 1 lesions, and only few cases with gastric and duodenal involvement have been reported.[169-171] Lesions are usually solitary and present with massive bleeding. The second portion of the duodenum seems to be involved preferentially. Large abnormal blood vessels may be seen at surgery in and

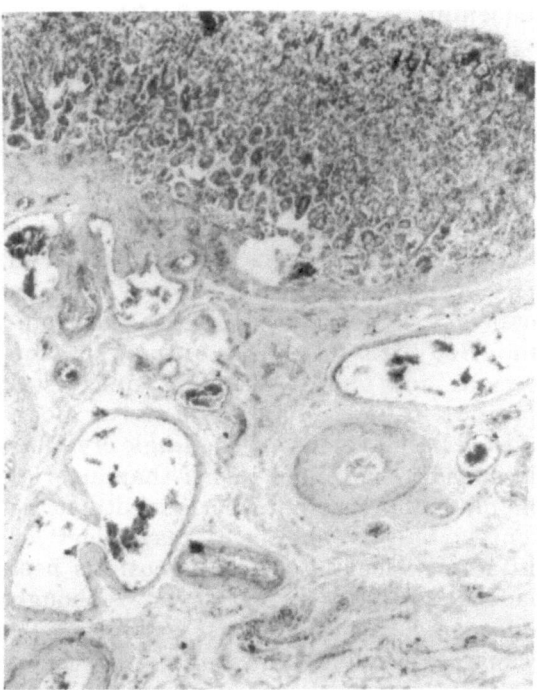

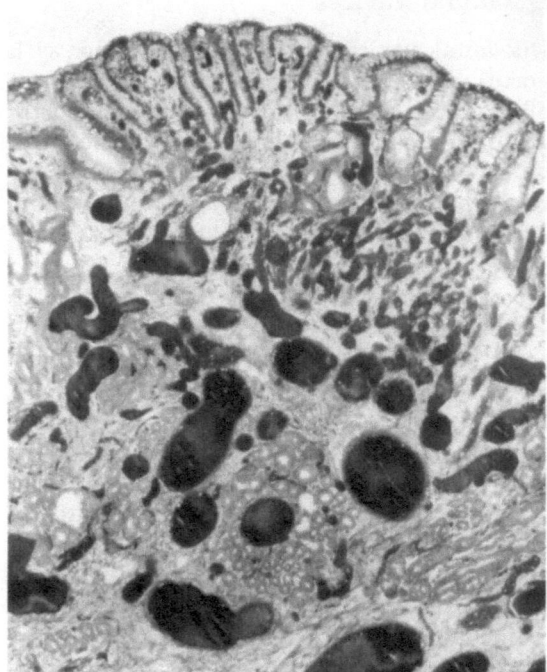

Figure 3-7. Angiodysplasia. Increased numbers of abnormally enlarged, thin- and thick-walled vascular spaces are present in the submucosa. HPS, X40, reproduced at 80%.

Figure 3-8. Telangiectasia. Thin-walled vascular channels are present in mucosa and submucosa. HPS, X40, reproduced at 80%.

around the duodenum, often extending into the head of the pancreas and the retroperitoneum. A pulsating mass may be palpable. Histologically, an increased number of small to medium-sized arteries and veins with a few arteries of larger caliber are seen in all layers of the duodenal wall. The mucosa may be ulcerated. Full-thickness excision of the duodenal wall or a modified Whipple procedure has been used to effect a cure.

Type 3 vascular malformations are more commonly known as telangiectasias. First described in the late 19th century and later elaborated by Osler,[172] hereditary telangiectasia is now known to be of autosomal dominant inheritance and to involve skin, alimentary tract, lungs, brain, retina, and liver.[173] Gastrointestinal bleeding is the presenting manifestation in 25% of cases, second only to epistaxis. Gastrointestinal

bleeding occurs at some time in 44% of patients. Its onset in the fifth decade of life is significantly later than that of epistaxis and is probably due to the additive effect of degenerative vascular changes. The earlier onset of epistaxis is explainable by the greater accessibility of nasal mucosal lesions to trauma. In a series of 68 symptomatic patients, gastrointestinal bleeding could be localized to the upper gastrointestinal tract in 40%, to the lower gastrointestinal tract in 10%, and was of uncertain origin in 50%.[173] Upper gastrointestinal endoscopy disclosed typical lesions most of them not actively bleeding, in the stomach of 70%. Coexisting duodenal ulcer disease was present in 9%, but no duodenal telangiectasias were seen. Gastrointestinal bleeding is particularly severe in cases with superimposed von Willebrand's disease.[174] Endoscopically, lesions can be seen best when they are not

Figure 3-9. Gastric antral vascular ectasia. In the mucosa capillaries are increased, glands are distorted, and the lamina propria is fibrotic. The muscularis mucosae is irregular. Submucosal arteries and veins are prominent. HPS, X40, reproduced at 85%.

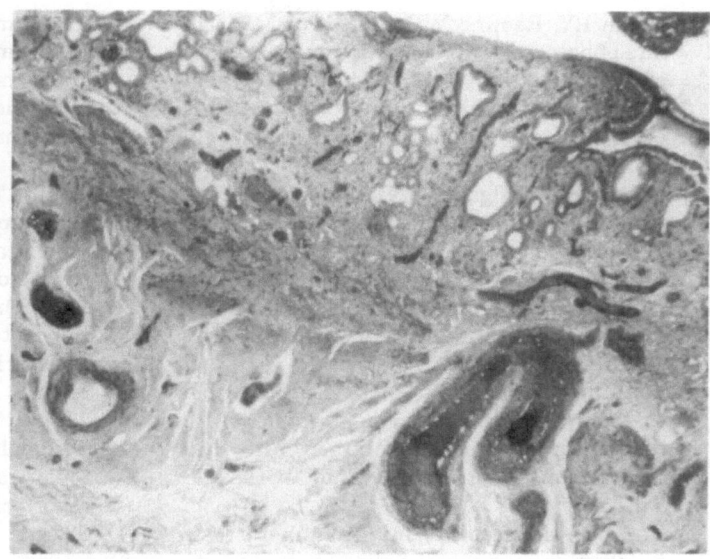

bleeding. They present as multiple isolated, discrete, reddened patches approximately 5 mm in diamter, with small vascular channels producing the appearance of spider angiomas, mostly along the greater curvature, in the cardia and in the body of the stomach.[174,175] Lesions are nonpulsatile, blanch with pressure, and bleed in an arterial fashion when traumatized. Biopsy should be avoided. Histologically, there are thin-walled distended vascular channels in the mucosa and submucosa (Fig. 3-8). Temporary therapeutic successes were achieved with electrocoagulation, laser photocoagulation, and radiotherapy.[175,176]

Gastric Antral Vascular Ectasia

This rare form of vascular malformation affects only the antrum and presents with bleeding and/or severe and persistent iron deficiency anemia.[177-179] Since its initial description in 1984, 15 such cases have appeared in the English literature as of late 1987.[179] The condition affects primarily elderly women and is most likely related to trauma, possibly intermittent prolapse of antral mucosa through the pylorus, as

demonstrated in some cases. Endoscopically, there are nearly parallel red stripes on the crests of mucosal folds converging toward the pylorus; as these stripes resemble the striped surface of a watermelon, the condition is also referred to as "watermelon stomach."[177]

Histologic hallmarks recognizable on endoscopic biopsy are increase and dilatation of mucosal capillaries, some containing fibrin thrombi, and fibromuscular hyperplasia of the lamina propria, that is, proliferation of smooth muscle cells and fibroblasts in the mucosa, accompanied at times by hyalinization (Fig. 3-9). The glandular architecture is usually distorted and a mild chronic inflammatory infiltrate is noted. Submucosal arteries and veins are prominent. Achlorhydria and gastric atrophy may be associated. Therapy varies: some patients need antrectomies, whereas others respond to sclerotherapy, thermocauterization, or steroids.[178,179]

References

1. Rose C, Kessaram RA, Lind JF: Ectopic gastric pancreas: A review and report of 4 cases. Diagn Imaging 1980;49:214–218.

2. Dolan RV, Remine WH, Dockerty MB: The fate of heterotopic pancreatic tissue: A study of 212 cases. Arch Surg 1974;109:762–765.

3. DeBord JR, Majarakis JD, Nyhus LM: An unusual case of heterotopic pancreas of the stomach. Am J Surg 1981;141:269–273.

4. Thoeni RF, Gedgandas K: Ectopic pancreas: usual and unusual features. Gastrointest Radiol 1980;5:37–42.

5. Stahlschmidt M, Schmitt-Köppler A, Mangold G: Versprengte Pankreaskeime im oberen Gastrointestinaltrakt. Zentrabl Chir 1979;104:588–591.

6. Kazuko B, Belber JB, Carson JW: Adenomyoma (pancreatic heterotopia) of the duodenum producing common bile duct obstruction. Gastrointest Endosc 1982;28: 182–184.

7. Bollinger J: Hypoglycemia from metastasizing insular carcinoma of aberrant pancreatic tissue in liver. Arch Pathol 1941;32:277.

8. Barrocas A, Fontenelle LJ, Williams MJ: Gastric heterotopic pancreas. A case report and review of the literature. Am Surg 1973;5:361–365.

9. Zarling EJ: Gastric adenomyoma with coincidental pancreatic rest: A case report. Gastrointest Endosc 1981;27:175–177.

10. Green PHR, Barratt PJ, Percy IP, et al: Acute pancreatitis occurring in gastric aberrant pancreatic tissue. Am J Dig Dis 1977;22: 734–740.

11. Tonimara A, Yamamoto H, Shibata H, et al: Carcinoma in heterotopic gastric pancreas. Acta Pathol Jpn 1979;29:251–257.

12. Goldfarb WE, Bennett D, Monefo W: Carcinoma in heterotopic gastric pancreas. Ann Surg 1973;158:56.

13. Radke HM, Bell JW: Gastric intramural pseudocyst in chronic pancreatitis. Am J Surg 1966;111:384–386.

14. Bellon EM, George CR, Schreiber H, et al: Pancreatic pseudocysts of the duodenum. AJR 1979;133:827–830.

15. Galloway PG: Heterotopic duodenum in the cystic duct. Arch Pathol Lab Med 1984; 1089:666–667.

16. Jabbari M, Goresky CA, Lough J, et al: The inlet patch: Heterotopic gastric mucosa in the upper esophagus. Gastroenterology 1985; 89:352–356.

17. Picard EJ, Picard JJ, Jorissen J, et al: Heterotopic gastric mucosa in the epiglottis and rectum. Am J Dig Dis 1978;23:217–221.

18. Yokoyama I, Kozuka S, Ito K, et al: Gastric gland metaplasia in the small and large intestine. Gut 1977;18:214–218.

19. Hoedemaeker PJ: Heterotopic gastric mucosa in the duodenum. Digestion 1970; 3:165–173.

20. Vizcarrondo FJ, Want TY, Brady PG: Heterotopic gastric mucosa: Presentation as a rugose duodenal mass. Gastrointest Endosc 1983;29:107–110.

21. Kondrotas LW, Camara DS, Meenghan MA, et al: Heterotopic gastric mucosa: A case report. Am J Gastroenterol 1985;80:253–256.

22. Spiller RC, Shousha S, Barrison IG: Heterotopic gastric tissue in the duodenum. A report of 8 cases. Dig Dis Sci 1982;27:880–883.

23. Lesselis AM, Martin DF: Heterotopic gastric mucosa in the duodenum. J Clin Pathol 1982;35:591–595.

24. Hamilton JW, Thune RG, Morrissey JF: Symptomatic ectopic gastric epithelium of the cervical esophagus: Demonstration of acid production with Congo red. Dig Dis Sci 1986;31:337–342.

25. Iwanaga T, Koyama H, Takahashi Y, et al: Diffuse submucosal cysts and carcinoma of the stomach. Cancer 1975;36:606–614.

26. Tschertkoff V, Wagner BM: Diffuse cystic malformation of the stomach. NY State J Med 1966;66:2049–2052.

27. Avni F, Kalifa G, Sauvegrain J: Les duplications gastriques et duodenales chez l'enfant. Ann Radiol 1980;23:195–202.

28. Fassbender CW, Gersmann A, Hausamen TU: Je ein Fall von vollständiger Duplikatur des Magens und des Duodenums. Fortschr Roentgenstr 1981;134:304–308.

29. Wieczorek RL, Seidman I, Ranson JH, et al: Congenital duplication of the stomach. Case report and review of the English literature. Am J Gastroenterol 1984;79:597–602.

30. Agha FP, Gabriele OF, Abdulla FH: Complete gastric duplication. AJR 1981;137: 406–407.

31. Floros D, Dosios T, Gourtsoyiannis N, et al: Gastric duplication associated with adenomyoma. J Surg Oncol 1982;19:98–100.

32. Case Records of the Massachusetts General Hospital No. 1, 1984. N Engl J Med 1984; 310:36–41.

33. Wendel W: Beschreibung eines operativ entfernten kongenitalen Nebenmagens. Arch Klin Chir 1911;95:895–899.

34. Knight J, Garvin PJ: Duodenal duplication in the adult. Mo Med 1981;78:644–646.

35. Torma MJ: Of double stomachs. Arch Surg 1974;109:555.

36. Thornhill BA, Cho KC, Morehouse HT: Gastric duplication associated with pulmonary sequestration: CT manifestations. AJR 1982;138:1168–1171.

37. Fitzgibbons RJ, Nugent FW, Ellis FH, et al: Unusual thoracoabdominal duplication associated with pancreaticopleural fistula. Gastroenterology 1980;79:344–347.

38. Keith A: Human Embryology and Morphology, ed 5. Baltimore, William Wood & Co, 1933.

39. Bremer JL: Diverticula and duplications of the intestinal tract. Arch Pathol 1944;38:132–140.

40. Dardik H, Klibanoff E: Retroperitoneal enterogenous cyst: report of a case and mechanisms of embryogenesis. Ann Surg 1965;162:1084–1086.

41. Shireman PK: Intramural cyst of the stomach. Hum Pathol 1987;18:857–858.

42. Jones PA, Knight MJ, Rayter Z, et al: Juxta-ampullary, bile filled duodenal duplication cyst: Another surgically correctable cause of acute pancreatitis. J R Soc Med 1982;75:662–664.

43. Hyman PE, Brennan MF, Head G, et al: Hyperamylasemia, duodenal duplication and pleural effusions in heriditary spherocytosis. Dig Dis Sci 1981;26:81–83.

44. Alford BA, Armstrong P, Franken EA, et al: Calcification associated with duodenal duplications in children. Radiology 1980;134:647–648.

45. Omojola MF, Hood IC, Stevenson GW: Calcified gastric duplication. Gastrointest Radiol 1980;5:235–238.

46. Kleinhaus S, Boley SJ, Winslow P: Occult bleeding from a perforated gastric duplication in an infant. Arch Surg 1981;110:122–123.

47. Mayo HW Jr: Carcinoma arising in reduplication of the stomach (gastrogenous cyst): A case report. Ann Surg 1955;141:550–555.

48. Sieber WK, Wiener ES, Chang J: Double choledochus with ectopic drainage into the stomach–a rare congenital anomaly of the biliary ductal system. J Pediatr Surg 1980;15:817–818.

49. Everett C, McCumber HE: Anomalous distribution of the extrahepatic biliary ducts. Ann Aurg 1942;115:472–474.

50. Sechas M, Karatzas G, Rigas A, et al: Diverticula of the upper gastrointestinal system. World J Surg 1981;5:731–732.

51. Baillie M: The Morbid Anatomy of Some of the Most Important Parts of the Human Body. London, J Johnson, 1793.

52. Palmer ED: Collective review: Gastric diverticula. Int Abstr Surg 1951;92:417–418.

53. Sommer AW, Goodrich WA Jr: Gastric diverticula. JAMA 1953;153:1424–1428.

54. Heijboer MP, Nieuwenhuizen LN: Gastric diverticula. Neth J Surg 1980;31:16–19.

55. Willard JH: Diverticula of the stomach, in Bacchus HL (ed): Gastroenterology. Philadelphia, WB Saunders Co, 1965, p. 893.

56. Wiljasalo M, Tallroth K, Korhola O, et al: A comparison of double contrast barium meal and endoscopy. Diagn Imaging 1980;49:1–15.

57. Anaise D, Brand DL, Smith NL, et al: Pitfalls in the diagnosis and treatment of a symptomatic diverticulum. Gastrointest Endosc 1984;30:28–30.

58. Juler GL, List JW, Stemmer EA, et al: Perforated duodenal diverticula. Arch Surg 1969;99:572–578.

59. Localio A, Stahl MW: Diverticular disease of the alimentary tract. Part II. The esophagus, stomach, duodenum, and small intestine. Curr Probl Surg, January 1968, pp 3–47.

60. Safrany L: ERCP in the diagnosis of juxtapapillary diverticulum causing pancreatobiliary diseases. Abstract, 3rd International Congress of Gastrointestinal Endoscopy, Mexico, 1974, p. 37.

61. Noer T: Non-Meckelian diverticula of the small bowel. Acta Chir Scand 1960;120:175–179.

62. Lotveit T, Oshes M, Aune S, et al: Studies of the choledocho-duodenal sphincter in patients with and without juxtapapillary duodenal diverticula. Scand J Gastroenterol 1980;15:875–880.

63. Oshes M, Lotveit T, Larsen S, et al: Duodenal diverticula and their relationship to age, sex and biliary calculi. Scand J Gastroenterol 1981;16:103–107.

64. Wolfe RD, Pearl MJ: Acute perforation of duodenal diverticulum with roentgenographic

demonstration of localized retroperitoneal emphysema. Radiology 1972;104:310–312.

65. Ryan ME, Hamilton JW, Morrissey JF: Gastrointestinal hemorrhage from a duodenal diverticulum. Gastrointest Endosc 1984; 30:84–87.

66. Griffin M, Carey WD, Hermann R, et al: Recurrent acute pancreatitis and intussusception complicating an intraluminal duodenal diverticulum. Gastrotinest Endosc 1981;81:345–348.

67. Fleming CR, Newcomber AD, Stephens DH, et al: Intralumenal duodenal diverticulum. Mayo Clin Proc 1975;50:244–248.

68. Shocket E, Simon SA: Small bowel obstruction due to enterolith (bezoar) formed in a duodenal diverticulum: A case report and review of the literature. Am J Gastroenterol 1982;77:621–624.

69. Thomas E, Reddy KR: Cholangitis and pancreatitis due to a juxtapapillary duodenal diverticulum. Am J Gastroenterol 1982;77: 303–304.

70. Gittel RB, Mudge TJ: The surgical significance of duodenal diverticula. N Engl J Med 1952;246:317–321.

71. Cox C: Perforated duodenal diverticulitis. South Med J 1980;73:830.

72. Rowlands BC, King PA: Duodenal diverticulum perforating into abdominal aorta causing fatal hemorrhage. Br J Surg 1954;41: 415–417.

73. Bradham GB, Martin JB: Massive bleeding from a polyp in a duodenal diverticulum. Ann Surg 1962;156:81–83.

74. Boyden EA, Cope JG, Bill AH: Anatomy and embryology of congenital intrinsic obstruction of the duodenum. Am J Surg 1967; 114:190–202.

75. Tandler J: Zur Entwicklingsgeschichte des menschlichen Duodenums im frühen Embryonalstadium. Morphol J 1900;29:187.

76. Gourevitch A: Duodenal atresia in the newborn. Ann R Coll Surg Engl 1971;48:141–158.

77. Shigemoto H, Horiya Y, Isomoto T, et al: Duodenal atresia secondary to intrauterine midgut strangulation by an omphalocele. J Pediatr Surg 1982;4:420–421.

78. Atwell JD, Klidjian AM: Vertebral anomalies and duodenal atresia. J Pediatr Surg 1982; 17:237–240.

79. Helbig D, Sallandt J: Duodenalstenose und

Duodenalatresia beim Neugeborenen. Muench Med Wochenschr 1980;122:704–708.

80. Fonkalsrud EW: Congenital atresia and stenosis of the duodenum. A review compiled from the members of the surgical section of the American Academy of Pediatrics. Pediatrics 1969;43:78–83.

81. Irving IM, Rickham PP: Duodenal atresia, stenosis and annular pancreas, in Rickham PP, et al (eds): Neonatal Surgery. London, Butterworth, 1978, pp 335–370.

82. Hayden CK Jr, Schwarts MZ, Davis M, et al: Combined esophageal and duodenal atresia: Sonographic findings. Am J Radiol 1983; 140:225–226.

83. Labko PI, Petrova RM, Chaika EN: Functional anatomy and physiology of atresia in human and mammal embryogenesis. Anat Anz 1979;145:338–352.

84. Louw JH, Barnard CN: Congenital intestinal atresia. Lancet 1955;2:1065–1067.

85. Mishalany HG, Der Kaloustian VM, Ghandour M: Familial congenital doudenal atresia. Pediatrics 1970;46:629–631.

86. Pombo F, Arnal-Monreal F, Soler-Fernandez R, et al: Multiple gastrointestinal atresias with intraluminal calcification. Br J Radiol 1982;55:307–309.

87. Nakamura H, Kanazawa Y, Hayano M, et al: Spontaneous oesophageal rupture with duodenal atresia in a new born infant. Arch Dis Child 1981;56:71–72.

88. Nelson LH, Clark CE, Fishburne JI, et al: Value of serial sonography in the in utero detection of duodenal atresia. Obstet Gynecol 1982;59:657–660.

89. Haddad V, Macopn WL, Islami MH: Mucosal diaphragms of the gastric antrum in adults. Surg Gynecol Obstet 1981;152:227–233.

90. Cooperman AM, Adachi M, Rankin GB, et al: Congenital duodenal diaphragm in adults: A delayed course of intestinal obstruction. Ann Surg 1975;182:739–742.

91. Economides NG, Fortner TM, Dunavant WD: Duodenal diaphragm associated with superior mesenteric artery syndrome. Am J Surg 1981;141:274–276.

92. Deitch EA, Harnar TJ: Congenital duodenal diaphragm in the adult: Report of two cases with associated prepyloric and duodenal ulceration. Am Surg 1981;47:363–365.

93. Airan B, Yadlav K, Yadlav RVS: Congenital incomplete duodenal diaphragm with pre-

diaphragmatic duodenal ulcer. Am J Gastroenterol 1979;72:426–427.

94. Turnbull A, Kussin S, Bain M: Radiographic and endoscopic features of a congenital diaphragm in an adult. A case report and review of the literature. Gastrointest Endosc 1980;26:46–48.

95. Kessler H, Smulewicz JJ: Microgastria associated with agenesis of the spleen. Radiology 1973;107:393–396.

96. Shackelford GD, McAlister WH, Brodeur AE, et al: Congenital microgastria. Am J Roentgenol 1973;118:72–76.

97. Neifeld JP, Berman WF, Lawrence W Jr, et al: Management of congenital microgastria with a jejunal reservoir pouch. J Pediatr Surg 1980;15:882–885.

98. Dide M: Sur un estomac d'adulte a type foetal. Bull Soc Anat Paris 1894;69:669–670.

99. Waldschmidt J, Charissis G, Berlien P, et al: Das Megaduodenum im Neugeborenenalter. Z Kinderchir 1980;30:197–209.

100. Law DH, Ten-Eyck EA: Familial megaduodenum and megacystis. Am J Med 1962;33:911–922.

101. Teplick J, Wallner LH, Teplick SK: Isolated dextrogastria. Am J Roentgenol 1979;132:124–126.

102. Hewlett PM: Isolated dextrogastria. Br J Radiol 1982;55:678–681.

103. Kinney LC: Congenital non-rotation of the stomach. Am J Roentgenol 1921;8:383–385.

104. Harris LI, Stivelman BP: Non-rotation of the stomach simulating spontaneous pneumothorax. JAMA 1927;89:1836–1837.

105. Schnyder PA, Candarjis G, Saegesser F: Intrathoracic stomach: CT evaluation of two cases. Diagn Imaging 1979;48:154–160.

106. Gerson DE, Lewicki AM: Intrathoracic stomach: When does it obstruct? Radiology 1976;119:257–264.

107. Wastell C, Ellis H: Volvulus of the stomach. A review with a report of 8 cases. Br J Surg 1971;58:557–562.

108. Patel NM: Chronic gastric volvulus: Report of a case and review of the literature. Am J Gastroenterol 1985;80:170–173.

109. Idowu J, Aitken DR, Georgeson KE: Gastric volvulus in the newborn. Arch Surg 1980;115:1046–1049.

110. Elidan J, Gimmon Z, Schwarz A: Pneumoperitoneum induced by pneumatosis cystoides intestinalis associated with volvulus

of the stomach. Am J Gastroenterol 1980;74:189–195.

111. Eagle KA: Transient myocardial ischemia resulting from gastric volvulus (letter). N Engl J Med 1985;312:121.

112. Case Records of the Massachusetts General Hospital No. 12, 1984. N Engl J Med 1984;310:774–781.

113. Ciardini A, Bini G: Gastroschisis and reduplicated gallbladder. Ital Chir Pediatr 1976;18:86.

114. Roberts WH, Dalgleish AE: Internal hernias of embryological origin. Anat Rec 1966;155:279–285.

115. Turley K: Right paraduodenal hernia. Arch Surg 1979;114:1072–1074.

116. Sekabuna JG: Congenital duodenal adhesions. East Afr Med J 1979;56:84–85.

117. Louw JH: Intestinal malrotation and duodenal ileus. J R Coll Surg Edinb 1960;51:101–126.

118. Snyder WH Jr, Chaffin L: Intermediate stage in return of intestines from umbilical cord. Anat Rec 1952;113:451–457.

119. Dott NM: Anomalies of intestinal rotations, their embryology, and surgical aspects with report of 5 cases. Br J Surg 1923;11:251–286.

120. Rees JR, Redo SF: Anomalies of intestinal rotation and fixation. Am J Surg 1968;116:834–841.

121. Lewis JE: Partial duodenal obstruction with incomplete duodenal rotation. J Pediatr Surg 1966;1:47–53.

122. Balthazar E: Intestinal malrotation in adults. Am J Roentgenol 1976;126:358–367.

123. Gage TP, Wind G: Intestinal malrotation demonstrated by small-bowel tube. J Clin Gastroenterol 1982;4:177–179.

124. Firor HV, Harris VJ: Rotational abnormalities of the gut: Re-emphasis of a neglected facet, isolated incomplete rotation of the duodenum. Am J Roentgenol 1974;120:315–321.

125. Herbut PA: Congenital defect in musculature of stomach with rupture in a newborn infant. Arch Pathol 1943;36:91–98.

126. Amadeo JH, Ashmore HW, Aponte GE: Neonatal gastric perforation caused by congenital defects of the gastric musculature. Surgery 1960;47:1010–1017.

127. Shaw A, Blanc WA, Santulli TV, et al: Spontaneous rupture of the stomach in the new-

born: a clinical and experimental study. Surgery 1965;58:651–671.

128. Balthazar EJ: Hypertrophic pyloric stenosis in adults: Radiographic features. Am J Gastroenterol 1983;78:449–453.

129. Bilodeau RG: Inheritance of hypertrophic pyloric stenosis. Am J Roentgenol 1971;113: 241–244.

130. Raia W, Curt P, Cardioso A: The pathogenesis of hypertrophic stenosis of pylorus in newborn and in the adult. Surg Gynecol Obstet 1956;102:705–712.

131. Larson IJ, Carlson HC, Dockerty MB: Roentgenologic diagnosis of pyloric hypertrophy in adults. Am J Roentgenol 1967;101:453–458.

132. Asch MJ, Weitzman JJ, Harp DM, et al: Total colonic aganglionosis. Arch Surg 1972;105: 74.

133. Saperstein L, Pollack J, Beck R: Total intestinal aganglionosis. Mt Sinai J Med 1980; 47:72–73.

134. Bodian M, Carter CO, Ward BCH: Hirschsprung's disease. Lancet 1951;1:302–309.

135. Nakamura H, Uchida H, Kuroda C, et al: Accessory left gastric artery arising from left hepatic artery: Angiographic study. Am J Roentgenol 1980;134:529–532.

136. Okada M, Iida M, Fuchigami T, et al: Submucosal arterial malformation of the stomach diagnosed endoscopically. Gastrointest Endosc 1983;29:30–31.

137. Molnar P, Miko T: Multiple arterial caliber persistence resulting in hematomas and fatal rupture of the gastric wall. Am J Surg Pathol 1982;6:83–86.

138. Dimjan L, Biliczki F, Lorand P, et al: Endoscopic diagnosis of "calibre-persistence," a rare cause of massive gastric hemorrhage. Endoscopy 1975;7:169–173.

139. Mohammad A, O'Neal RM: Fatal hemorrhage from a ruptured aneurysm. J Med Assoc G 1978;67:646–647.

140. Palmer ED, Boyce HW: Sclerotic submucosal gastric artery: A course of hemorrhage. Am Surg 1964;30:83–87.

141. Kung TM, Wong J: Arterial malformation of stomach: A cause of massive bleeding. Pathology 1982;14:81–84.

142. Ho K-L: Aneurysm of pancreaticoduodenal artery: Report of a case and review of the literature. Int Surg 1979;64:35–38.

143. Isaacson R, Delancy H: Intragastric rupture of a left gastric artery aneurysm. J Med Assoc G 1978;67:646–647.

144. Eckhauser PE, Stanley JC, Zelenock GB, et al: Gastroduodenal and pancreaticoduodenal artery aneurysms: A complication of pancreatitis causing spontaneous gastrointestinal hemorrhage. Surgery 1980;88:335–344.

145. Warmath M, Usselman JA: Hemobilia developing from an aneurysm of the left gastric artery. Gastrointest Radiol 1980;5:21–23.

146. Donaldson GA, Hamlin E: Massive hematemesis resulting from rupture of a gastric artery aneurysm. N Engl J Med 1950;243: 369–473.

147. Thomford NR, Yurko JE, Smith EJ: Aneurysm of gastric arteries as a cause of intraperitoneal hemorrhage. Ann Surg 1968;168: 294–297.

148. Keith RG, Mustard RA, Saibil EA: Gastric variceal bleeding due to occlusion of splenic vein in pancreatic disease. Can J Surg 1982;25:301–304.

149. Bachman BA, Brady PG: Localized gastric varices: Mimicry leading to endoscopic misinterpretation. Gastrointest Endosc 1983;30: 244–246.

150. Goldberg S, Katz S, Maidich J, et al: Isolated gastric varices due to spontaneous splenic vein thrombosis. Am J Gastroenterol 1984; 79:304–307.

151. Vos LJ, Potocky V, Broker FH: Splenic vein thrombosis with esophageal varices: A late complication of umbilical vein catheterization. Ann Surg 1974;180:152–156.

152. Marshall JP, Smith PD, Hoyumpa AM: Gastric varices. Problem in diagnosis. Am J Dig Dis 1977;22:947–955.

153. Sorgen RA, Robbins DI: Bleeding gastric varices secondary to wandering spleen. Gastrointest Radiol 1980;5:25–27.

154. Daneshgar S, Era P, Feldman S, et al: Bleeding gastric varices and gastric torsion secondary to a wandering spleen. Gastroenterology 1980;79:141–143.

155. Stephan G, Miething R: Röntgendiagnost varicöser Duodenalveränderungen bei portaler Hypertension. Radiologe 1968;8:90–95.

156. Rappazzo JA, Kozarek RA, Altman M: Duodenal varices: Endoscopic diagnosis of an unusual source of upper gastrointestinal hemorrhage. Gastrointest Endosc 1981;27: 227–228.

157. Aagaard J, Burcharth F: Bleeding duodenal varices demonstrated by transhepatic portography. Acta Chir Scand 1980;146:77–78.

158. Sauerbruch T, Weinzierl M, Mietrich HP, et al: Sclerotherapy of a bleeding duodenal varix. Endoscopy 1982;14:187–189.

159. Moore JD, Thompson NW, Appelman HD, et al: Arteriovenous malformations of the gastrointestinal tract. Arch Surg 1976;111: 381–389.

160. Gunnlaugsson O: Angiodysplasia of the stomach and duodenum. Gastrointest Endosc 1985;31:251–252.

161. Weaver GA, Allpern HD, Davis JS, et al: Gastrointestinal angiodysplasia associated with aortic valve disease: Part of a spectrum of angiodysplasia of the gut. Gastroenterology 1979;77:1–11.

162. Banks S, Aftalion B, Anfang C, et al: Gastric angiodysplasia due to cholesterol embolization in aortic stenosis (abstract). Gastrointest Endosc 1982;28:125.

163. Cunningham JT: Gastric telangiectasias in chronic hemodialysis patients: A report of 6 cases. Gastroenterology 1981;81:1131–1133.

164. Farup PG, Rosseland AR, Stray N, et al: Localized telangiopathy of the stomach and duodenum diagnosed and treated endoscopically. Endoscopy 1981;13:1–6.

165. Duray PH, Marcal JM, Livolsi VA, et al: Gastrointestinal angiodysplasia: A possible component of von Willebrand's disease. Hum Pathol 1984;15:539–544.

166. Keisler DS, Shay SS, Butler M: Bleeding from gastric angiodysplasia post aortic valve replacement. Gastrointest Endosc 1982;28: 118–119.

167. Roberts LK, Gold RE, Routt WE: Gastric angiodysplasia. Diagn Radiol 1981;139:355–359.

168. Baum S: Small bowel angiography, in Marshak RG, Lindner AE (eds): Radiology of the Small Intestine. Philadelphia, WB Saunders Co, 1976, p. 608.

169. Lewis JW, Mason EE, Jochimsen PR: Vascular malformations of the stomach and duodenum. Surg Gynecol Obstet 1981;153:225–228.

170. Criado FJ, Shureih SF, Howard WHB, et al: Arterio venous malformations of the duodenum: a report of 3 cases. Md State Med J 1972;21:63–65.

171. Case Records of the Massachusetts General Hospital No. 30, 1981. N Engl J Med 1981; 305:211–216.

172. Osler W: A family form of recurring epistaxis, associated with multiple telangiectases of the skin and mucous membranes. Johns Hopkins Hosp Bull 1904;12:333–337.

173. Reilly PJ, Nostrant TT: Clinical manifestations of hereditary hemorrhagic telangiectasia. Am J Gastroenterol 1984;79:363–367.

174. Schwartz JT, Patton GA, Graham DY, et al: Gastric radiotherapy as treatment of hereditary hemorrhagic telangiectasia. Am J Gastroenterol 1982;77:53–54.

175. Ona FV, Ahluwalia M: Endoscopic appearance of gastric angiodysplasia in hereditary hemorrhagic telangiectasia. Am J Gastroenterol 1980;73:148–149.

176. Weaver GA, Wilk HE, Olson JE: Successful endoscopic electrocoagulation of gastric lesions of hereditary hemorrhagic telangiectasia responsible for repeated hemorrhage. Gastrointest Endosc 1981;27:181–183.

177. Jabbari M, Cherry R, Lough JO, et al: Gastric antral vascular ectasia: The watermelon stomach. Gastroenterology 1984;87:1165–1170.

178. Kruger R, Ryan ME, Dickson KB, et al: Diffuse vascular ectasia of the gastric antrum. Am J Gastroenterol 1987;82:421–423.

179. Suit PF, Petras RE, Bauer TW, et al: Gastric antral vascular ectasia. Am J Surg Pathol 1987;11:750–757.

CHAPTER 4

Gastritis

Gastritis is generally classified according to etiology, clinical course, and microscopic appearance. We, therefore, distinguish between chronic idiopathic gastritis, acute hemorrhagic gastritis, infectious gastritis, granulomatous gastritis, and eosinophilic gastritis. Subgroups exist for each major type.

Chronic Idiopathic Gastritis

Chronic idiopathic gastritis is a common phenomenon, particularly in the older patient. It is important as a forerunner and/or associated lesion of pernicious anemia, gastric carcinoma, and iron deficiency anemia as well as other diseases.[1] The advent of the flexible endoscope has made it possible to obtain multiple biopsies of gastric mucosa with relative ease. This is helping to illuminate many problems concerned with the distribution, incidence, and progression of chronic idiopathic gastritis and is shedding light on its relationships to the disease entities mentioned. However, many problems as to the cause and effects of chronic gastritis remain to be completely elucidated. Both the collection of data for correlative studies and the obtaining of maximum information on an individual patient make definite demands on both the endoscopist and the pathologist.

General Comments on Biopsy Technique and Interpretation

Multiple biopsies are required for maximum information. A single biopsy may be quite misleading both as to the presence and the severity of chronic gastritis since the disease is often patchy and of variable severity from place to place.[2] The sites for biopsy should include the greater and lesser curvature of the antrum plus the fundic lesser and greater curvature at various levels. Mucosal biopsies should ideally be full thickness, including the muscularis mucosae. Special handling by the endoscopist is mandatory. The site of each biopsy should be carefully identified. The biopsy should be treated similarly to those of the small bowel. A dissecting microscope should be used, and the biopsy oriented mucosal side up, on a suitable substrate such as filter paper or a plastic mesh. Biopsies must be promptly fixed. In the laboratory, the orientation must be maintained during embedding in order that full-thickness vertical sections of the mucosa are obtained for the study. A reticulin stain is useful to detect minor atrophic changes and early fibrosis.[3] Metaplastic change may be more accurately detected and classified by the use of periodic acid-Schiff (PAS)-Alcian blue or high iron diamine stains. A Grimelius stain or immunologic staining technique may be desirable to evaluate increases or reductions of special-

Figure 4-1. Chronic superficial gastritis. Note increased infiltrate of plasma cells in superficial antral mucosa with relative sparing of deeper glands. Lymphoid reaction centers are prominent. H&E, X50, reproduced at 75%.

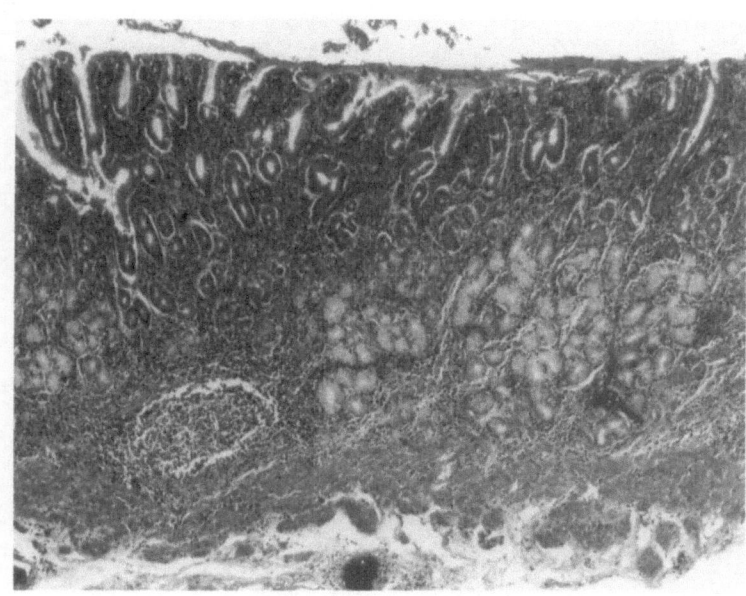

ized cells such as gastrin-producing cells. The pathologist should note the type and distribution of the chronic inflammatory infiltrate and the presence or absence of glandular atrophy, metaplasia, and dysplasia if present. The type of mucosa (i.e., antral or fundic) and the degree of "activity" as marked by the presence or severity of accompanying polymorphonuclear infiltrate should be part of the description.[3] In the past, pathologists have often been content to sign out such biopsies as "gastritis" or even "gastric mucosa—no tumor seen." This practice is archaic and not helpful.

Types of Chronic Gastritis

It has become customary to consider two types of chronic gastritis—chronic superficial gastritis and chronic atrophic gastritis. The latter is further classified by degree of atrophy (i.e., mild, moderate, or severe). The severe form is often referred to as gastric atrophy. These are not to be regarded as separate entities because there is evidence that chronic superficial gastritis may evolve into the chronic atrophic gastritis.[4] A similar evolution from mild to severe chronic atrophy may also occur. On the other hand, the type of gastritis may remain constant for long periods of time. Biopsies obtained at separate time intervals may show varying degrees of severity. In addition, a Type A and Type B gastritis and sometimes a Type AB chronic atrophic gastritis are recognized, based largely on the presence or absence of certain gastric autoantibodies to be discussed later in this chapter. It should be emphasized that these clinical types cannot be distinguished histologically and, for that matter, a considerable overlap occurs.[5] A marked increase in chronic inflammatory infiltrate is common to all except the most severe atrophic gastritis (gastric atrophy), in which the chronic inflammatory change may be sparse or indeed absent.

The term "hypertrophic gastritis" has been used in the past to indicate conditions where the mucosa is of increased thickness, such as in Menétrièr's disease, Zollinger-Ellison syndrome, and the Cronkhite-Canada syndrome. Actual gastritis is not a uniform feature of these disorders and the term "hyperplastic gastrophy" is preferable. These disorders are discussed elsewhere.

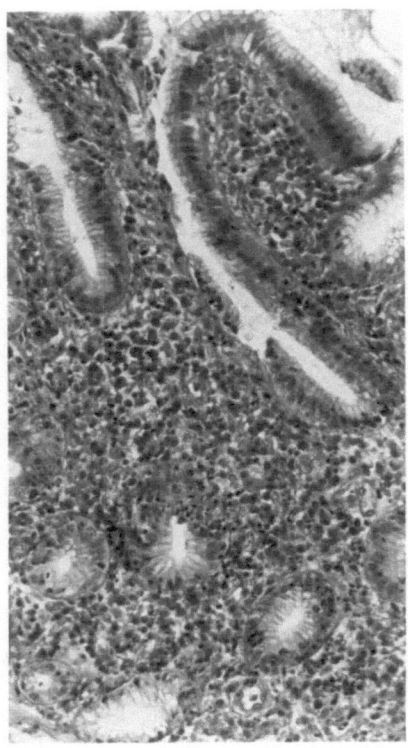

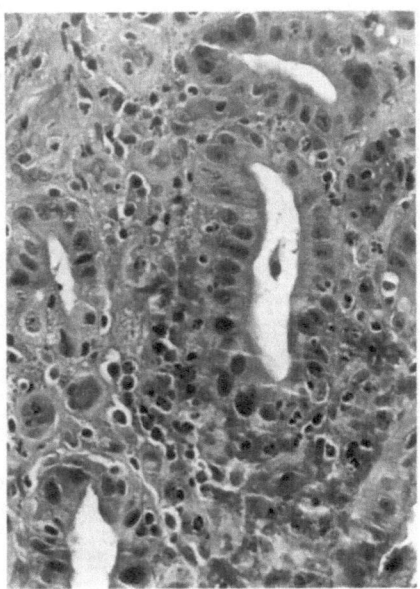

Figure 4-3. Regenerative epithelium in gastritis. Note well oriented but poorly differentiated glandular epithelium. The nuclei are somewhat vesicular and the nucleoli large. The patient had a gastric ulcer and no evidence of carcinoma. H&E, X250, reproduced at 75%.

Figure 4-2. Chronic gastritis (active). Note increase of both plasma cells and polymorphonuclear leukocytes in superficial mucosa. H&E, X160, reproduced at 75%.

Chronic Superficial Gastritis

The inflammatory reaction in chronic superficial gastritis, by definition, is restricted to the upper mucosal region (i.e., the area between the pits). The glands are intact. The more superficial mucosa shows a marked increase in chronic inflammatory cells in the lamina propria (Fig. 4-1). In addition, polymorphonuclear leukocytes may be present, both invading the mucous neck cells and the lumina, occasionally to the degree of forming small crypt abscesses (Fig. 4-2). Such acute inflammatory change should not lead to a diagnosis of acute gastritis when accompanied by a chronic inflammatory component, but rather taken as evidence of the continuing activity of the chronic gastritis. The epithelium shows progressive loss of mucin

secretion. The epithelial cells show various degenerative changes up to and including individual cell necrosis and sloughing. Large, plump, vesicular nuclei are usually present, indicating regenerative activity.[6] Nuclear hyperchromatism and pyknosis may be marked (Fig. 4-3), at times leading to confusion with in-situ carcinoma. Nuclear abnormalities roughly parallel the degree of inflammation in chronic gastritis, whereas in carcinoma there is usually a discrepancy. This discrepancy may be helpful.[5] In severe superficial gastritis, small shallow areas of ulceration may occur secondary to sloughing of epithelium. Stratification of nuclei may occur, and increased mitotic activity may be noted. Edema of the lamina propria between the pits may be seen in a patchy or diffuse distribution. However, the mid-portion (i.e., foveolar area) often gives the appearance of increased cellularity secondary to an inflammatory infiltrate in this area (Fig. 4-4).[7]

Figure 4-4. Chronic gastritis (active). Note both increased cellularity of the lamina propria with superficial edema and an increase of reaction centers. No metaplasia is seen in this area. H&E, X40, reproduced at 70%.

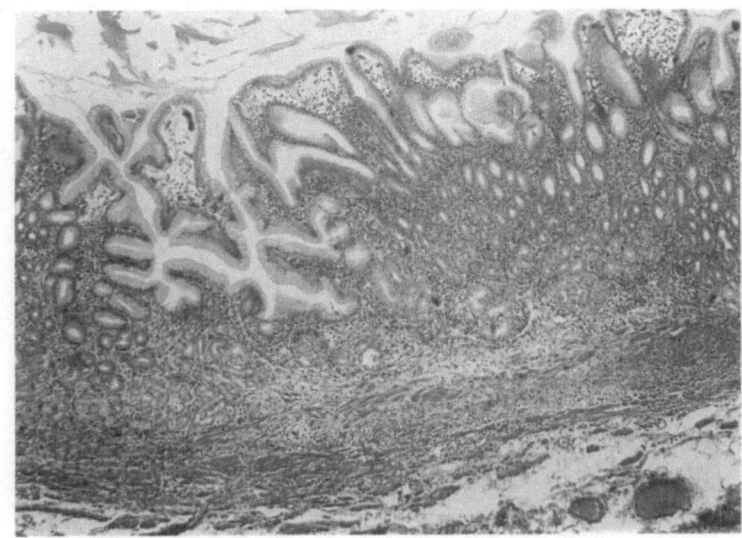

Chronic Atrophic Gastritis

In chronic atrophic gastritis, a chronic inflammatory process involves all layers of the mucosa. Acute changes, as in superficial gastritis, may also be present. Lymphoid follicles tend to be present in increased numbers and to have prominent germinal centers. When such changes are marked, some use the term "follicular gastritis." The muscularis mucosae becomes hypertrophied and often split. Strands of smooth muscle from the muscularis mucosae may extend into the lamina propria. The normal glands show increasing degrees of atrophy. In milder forms, this may be detectable only by condensation of reticulin about the glands along with a patchy increase of reticulin in the lamina propria, the latter being indicative of early fibrosis. The specialized cells of the glandular components tend to decrease or even nearly disappear (Fig. 4-5). Loss or marked reduction of parietal and chief cells has long been recognized in

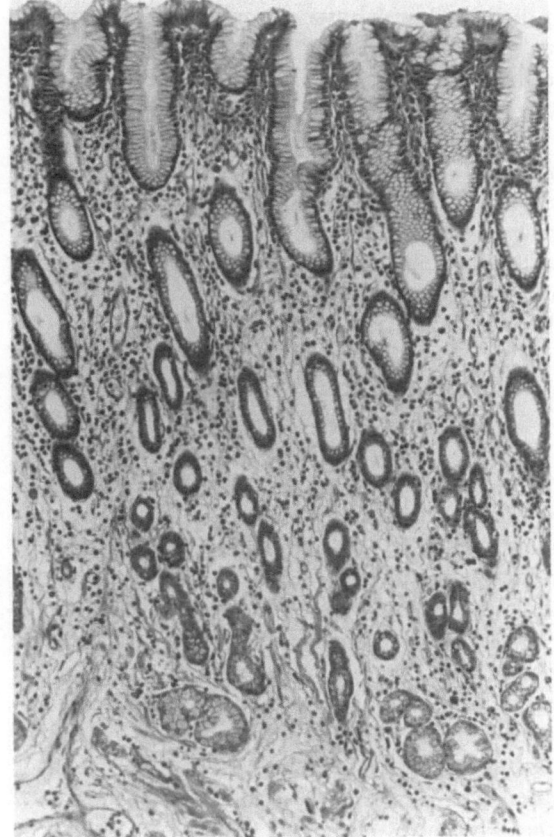

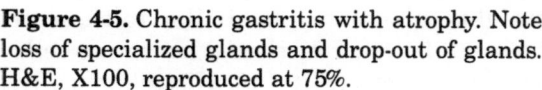

Figure 4-5. Chronic gastritis with atrophy. Note loss of specialized glands and drop-out of glands. H&E, X100, reproduced at 75%.

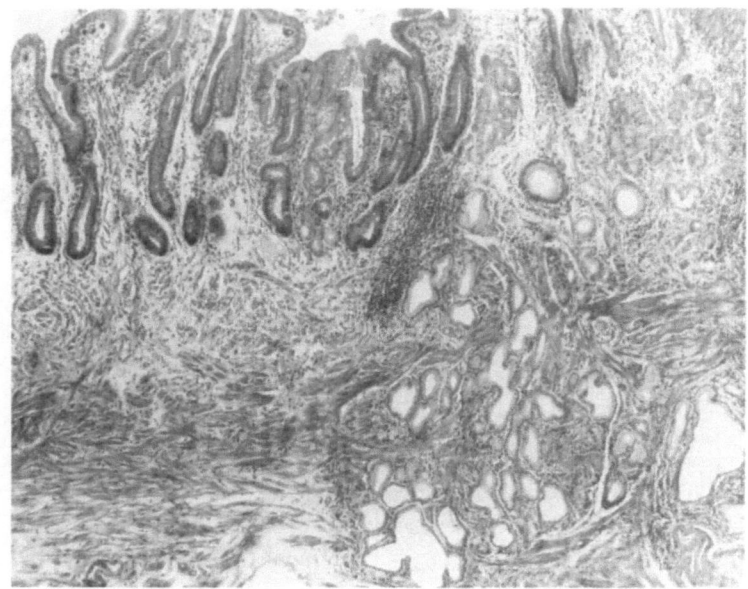

Figure 4-6. Chronic gastritis with intestinal metaplasia. Most of the surface epithelium is replaced by intestinal metaplasia (dark glands). Parietal cells are poorly preserved. Note extension of glands beneath abnormal muscularis mucosae in a section of fundic mucosa in patient with gastric carcinoma. H&E, X50, reproduced at 70%.

the fundic mucosa of chronic gastritis. Sloan and co-workers[8] have recently shown a similar patchy-to-marked reduction of gastrin cells in antral gastritis paralleling the severity of the gastritis. In contrast, in pernicious anemia where there is severe atrophic gastritis of the fundus but with relative sparing of the antrum, marked hyperplasia of the gastrin cells may occur, which is reflected in hypergastrinemia.[9] The deeper glands may become cystic. When marked, the term chronic cystic gastritis" is used by some.

Metaplastic Changes

The mucous neck glands may extend down and proliferate, replacing the specialized glands and producing a picture identical to that of antral mucosa. This is a so-called pseudopyloric "metaplasia." This makes identification as to the source of the biopsy difficult or impossible.

True metaplasia, referred to as intestinal metaplasia, is very common in atrophic gastritis. Its frequency more-or-less parallels the severity of the gastritis.[5] Intestinal metaplasia implies areas of transformation of gastric mucosa into cells resembling those of the small intestine or colon (Figs. 4-6 and 4-7). Jass[10] classifies such metaplasia into complete and incomplete types. In the complete type (Type I), goblet cells secreting acidic mucins and absorbtive cells with well developed brush borders are both present (Fig. 4-8). In the incomplete type (Type II), both neutral and acidic mucin-secreting goblet cells are present, but well developed absorptive cells are absent. The acidic mucins may be of the sialic acid type (Type IIA) or sulfated type (i.e., sulfomucin, resembling colon) (Type IIB). Type IIB intestinal metaplasia, also referred to as Type III, is the rarest type of intestinal metaplasia and is found in only 12% of biopsy specimens with intestinal metaplasia.[11] However, 90% of patients with Type III intestinal metaplasia have gastric carcinoma, especially of the intestinal type. Its presence should, therefore, prompt a careful search for coexisting carcinoma and close surveillance in the future if no tumor can be identified.

Sipponen[12] also recognizes a small intestinal and colonic type of metaplasia. The most common, the small intestinal type, is marked by the regular appearance of regular, straight, tubular crypts similar to those of the small bowel. Paneth and endocrine cells are also present (Fig. 4-9). Histochemically, enzymes typical of small intestine, such as

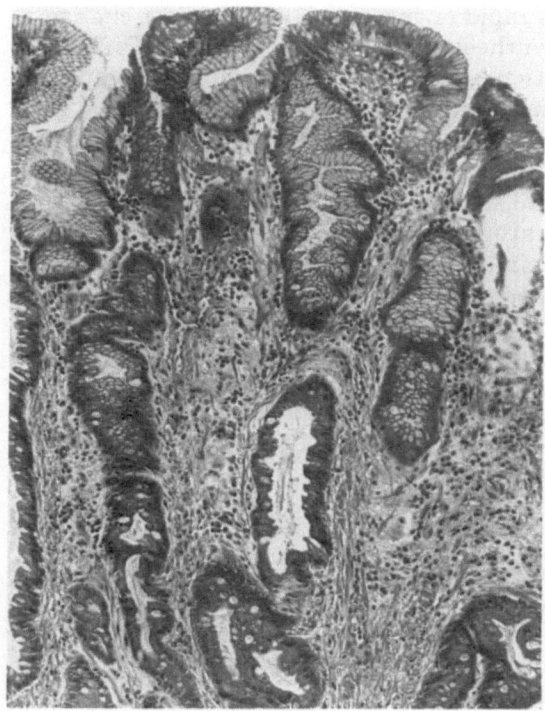

Figure 4-7. Chronic gastritis with intestinal metaplasia. Note contrast of residual normal mucous foveolar glands with dark metaplastic glands containing goblet cells. H&E, X100, reproduced at 70%.

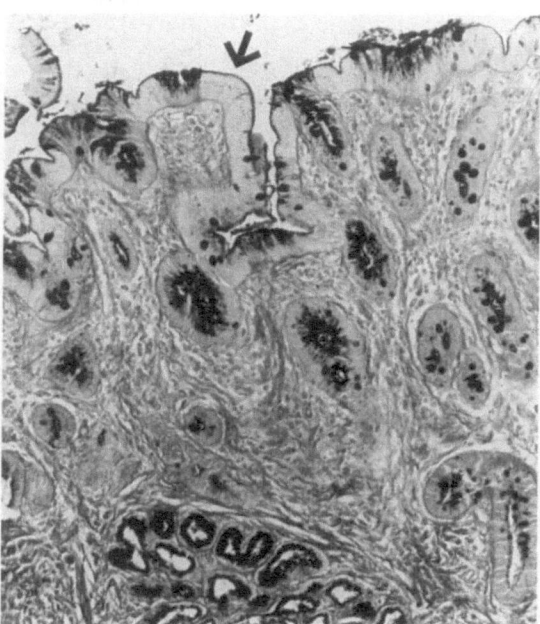

Figure 4-8. Intestinal metaplasia stained with a PAS-Alcian blue stain. The dark (blue) goblet cells seen are secreting acidic mucins. Interspersed are cells with well developed brush borders (*arrow*) representing absorptive cells. This is classified as complete metaplasia. Note persistence of glands with lighter-staining neutral mucin secretion (red). Most of these are immature cells with only some apical mucin secretion. X100, reproduced at 65%.

aminopeptides and alkaline phosphatase, can be demonstrated. The mucin is negative for sulfated mucopolysaccharides. Less commonly, a colonic type of metaplasia may be present. This has a more irregular glandular structure, which may show branching of the crypts. In some cases, the crypts may become cystic. Paneth and endocrine cells are reduced or absent, as are the small bowel type enzymes, and histochemically sulfated mucopolysaccharides may be demonstrated by the high iron diamine stain. He believes that the small intestinal type of metaplasia may progress to the colonic type, and this would appear to be the same lesion that Cuello and co-workers[6] refer to as "hyperplastic dysplasia." These authors, in addition, describe nuclear atypia ranging up to in-situ carcinoma in such metaplastic glands. They also de-

scribe an "adenomatous metaplasia." Certainly adenomatous change may be seen; however, we think this indicates a neoplasia and believe the term "adenomatous metaplasia" inappropriate.

It should be noted that intestinal metaplasia represents an absorptive surface and that various substances, including lipids, may be absorbed. This may explain the appearance of fat, which at times resembles that of xanthelasma being seen in collections of foamy histiocytes in the mucosa.

Gastric Atrophy

In the most severe form of chronic atrophic gastritis, the mucosa is thinner than normal. For the most part, the specialized glands are

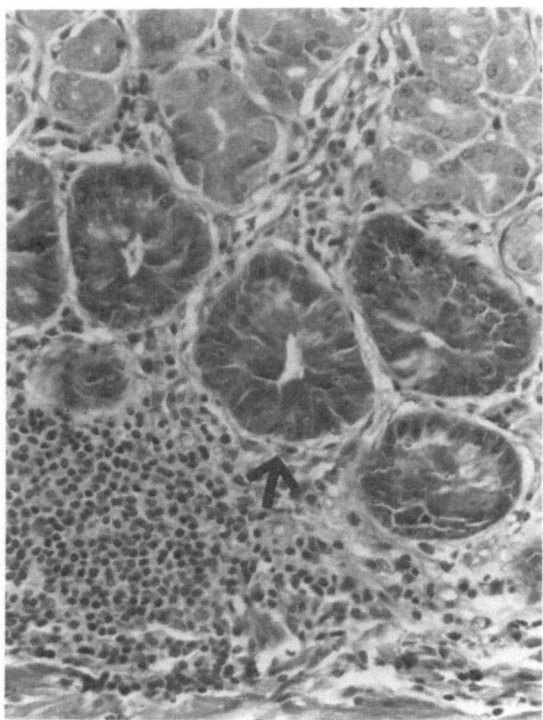

Figure 4-9. Chronic gastritis with Paneth cell metaplasia. Note dark metaplastic glands contrasting with paler fundic parietal/chief cells and multiple Paneth cells with supranuclear eosinophilic granules (*arrow*). H&E, X250, reproduced at 75%.

totally absent and replaced by intestinal metaplasia. Cystic changes may be seen. The lamina propria is prominent, and the inflammatory infiltrate is minimal. Lymphoid follicles are reduced, and occasionally fatty infiltrates can be seen.

Cell Kinetics

Cellular proliferation in the gastric mucosa, normally a very active process, is confined to the bottom of the mucous neck glands and neck area of the gastric glands. Cells so formed migrate upward as nonproliferative cells maturing as surface epithelium, and migrate downward maturing into the various cellular components of the specialized gastric glands. In chronic gastritis, cell proliferation

is rapid or increased. The earliest change is synthesis of DNA in surface cells. Differentiation is impaired, and the mucosa is replaced in the areas of intestinal metaplasia with cells of that type. Some of these remain immature and capable of DNA synthesis and mitosis. Thus, the cells fail to enter a mature nonproliferative state, a situation akin to that seen in colonic adenomas where there is again failure of repression of DNA synthesis and proliferative activity is no longer confined to the base of the crypts. In intestinal metaplasia, the maximum mitotic activity may be seen in the base of the crypts.

Cytology

In gastritis, cells obtained by lavage or brush techniques may show marked variation from normal and differentiation from malignancy may be difficult. Koss[13] notes that this is especially so in acute gastritis caused by aspirin where the differential diagnosis may only be made by finding rapid reversion to normal on repeat study within a few days. In general, in inflammatory conditions of the stomach, the cells tend to be shed in cohesive clusters and adjacent nuclei are more-or-less the same size with perhaps some increase in nuclear size to the periphery (Fig. 4-10A). In carcinoma, nuclear variation between adjacent cells is greater and cells tend to be shed singly or in small groups. In gastritis, Nieburgs and Glass[14] describe nuclei which are larger and more vesicular than normal. The nuclear borders tend to be regular and lack the irregularities and folding of the nuclear borders seen in malignant cells (Fig. 4-10B). Malignant cells tend to be more hyperchromatic, although this may not be true in certain well differentiated adenocarcinomas (Fig. 4-10C). However, it should be noted that in gastritis, single cells with more-or-less naked nuclei may be present in some numbers. Koss[13] states that in gastritis, only occasional nuclei are large, and emphasizes that the irregularities of increased size of nucleoli with some hyperchromatism and single cells make the differential diagnosis at times very

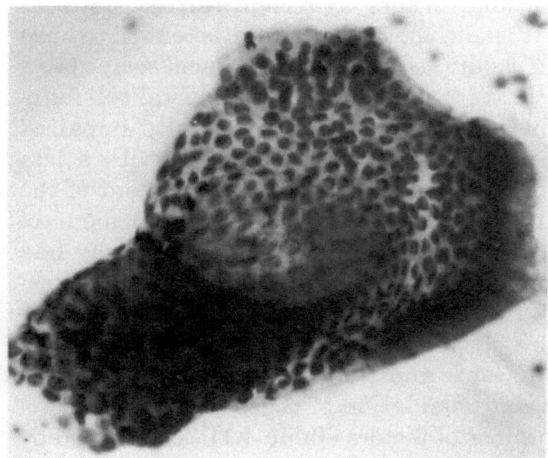

Figure 4-10.A. Cytology: Normal mucosal epithelium, gastric brush. Note cohesiveness of epithelium and regularity of nuclei. Papanicolaou, X250, reproduced at 75%.

hazardous. Intestinal metaplasia may be detected finding columnar cells larger than those of normal gastric cells and provided with an abundant somewhat opaque cytoplasm. The nuclei of such cells are round, even, and frequently larger and darker than those of the normal cell.[13] It should be recalled, however, that intestinal metaplasia is common in gastric carcinoma and identification of such cells does not rule out carcinoma. A conservative approach is certainly indicated since mistakes can be made even by those with considerable experience.

Endoscopy

The presence of erythema, per se, is a common and normal phenomenon in the stomach and should not be considered evidence of gastritis.[5] Endoscopic criteria generally accepted in the past have been 1) areas of pale gray, whitish blue mucosa; 2) a shiny translucent mucosa; and 3) the visibility of submucosal blood vessels. Of these, the last criterion is that most frequently quoted as being characteristic. More recent work[15] indicates that

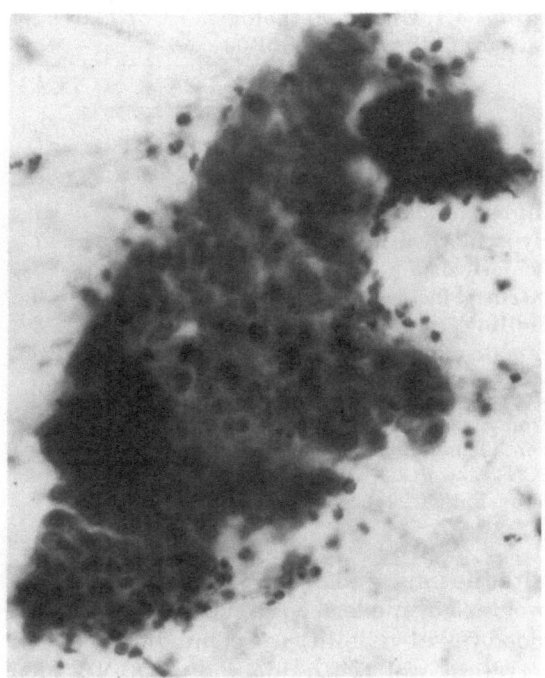

Figure 4-10.B. Cytology: Epithelial clusters in gastritis. The nuclei are larger and more vesicular with larger nucleoli than normal. Some size variation in the nuclei. Still fairly cohesive. Papanicolaou, X250, reproduced at 75%.

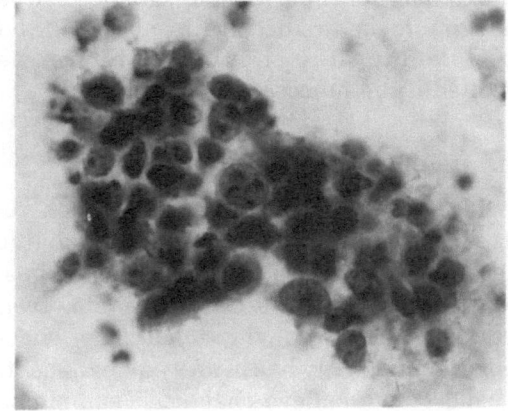

Figure 4-10.C. Cytology: Well differentiated adenocarcinoma. Note loss of cohesion and more variation of size and arrangement of nuclei as compared with (**B**). Papanicolaou, X250, reproduced at 75%.

Table 4.1. Clinico-Pathological Correlates of Parietal Cell Antibody Status

	PCA+	PCA−
No. of cases	30	40
Antral gastritis	4	37
Focal fundal gastritis	6	29
Diffuse fundal gastritis	24	11
Hypochlorhydria	4	17
Achlorhydria	26	23
Intrinsic factor antibody	9	0
Shilling test 5–10%	15	3
Female/male ratio	3/1	2/1
Mean age (yr)	50	55

From Strickland and Mackay.[18] Reproduced by permission, Plenum Publishing.
PCA+ and PCA− = a positive or a negative test for serum antiparietal cell autoantibodies.

with the improved illumination and visibility provided by modern equipment, focal areas of blood vessel visibility are common and do not correlate well with histology. Of 21 such cases of focal blood vessel visibility, 13 have had a normal histology on biopsy. However, Meshinpour and co-workers[15] believe that the finding of diffuse submucosal changes is significant. Current views are that although endoscopy is reasonably reliable in diagnosing extensive chronic atrophic gastritis, it is not reliable in predicting its absence, and multiple biopsies should, therefore, be obtained if the mucosa appears normal.[16]

Symptomatology

A wide variety of symptoms have been reported in patients with chronic gastritis. These include nausea and vomiting, epigastric pain, fullness, and flatulence. However, correlation between symptomatology, endoscopy, and histology has been weak or absent, and most now believe that such symptoms are not due to the chronic gastritis, per se, but are due to concomitant irritants such as bile reflux.[5,17]

Clinical Types of Gastritis

Correlative studies of histology of the gastric body (fundic) mucosa with function led earlier workers to recognize that patients with a diffuse fundal gastritis tended to have markedly reduced or absent acid secretion, a positive test for serum antiparietal cell autoantibodies (PCA), and eventually impaired vitamin B12 absorption. Those with a less advanced and multifocal involvement of the fundus had only moderate impairment of acid secretion, lacked PCA, and rarely had impaired vitamin B12 absorption. Strickland and Mackay[18] used the presence or absence of PCA to classify cases of gastritis into an A and B type, and noted the considerable correlation of these two types with a number of factors (Table 4-1). As outlined by Siurala,[19] Type A gastritis 1) mainly involves the fundus (body), 2) has low or absent acid secretion, 3) has high serum levels of gastrin, 4) has low pepsinogen I levels, and 5) often has evidence of circulating gastric autoantibodies (in particular PCA). In Type B gastritis, the gastritis 1) mainly involves the antrum with no or only patchy fundic involvement, 2) has normal or high acid secretion, 3) has a normal gastrin level, 4) has a normal or high pepsinogen level, and 5) lacks evidence of circulating gastric autoantibodies.

Despite the fact that these types seem to be of differing etiologies (as will be developed further on), there is considerable overlap (Table 4-1). The term "AB chronic gastritis" is used to include some of these variants. This is particularly true of acid secretion, which may be reduced in cases otherwise classified as Type B. It remains a useful concept.

The high gastrinemia in Type A (fundic) gastritis is not merely a matter of sparing of the antral G cell population. As mentioned previously, marked hyperplasia of G cells has been demonstrated in such gastritis, at least in pernicious anemia.[9] Also, hypochlorhydria in Type B gastritis (antral), despite sparing of the fundic mucosa, may be explained by the demonstrated loss of G cells.[8] It should be mentioned here that autoantibodies to gastrin have been demonstrated in 8 of 106 patients with otherwise antral Type B chronic gastritis.[20] Despite these exceptions, the evidence suggests that Type A chronic gastritis can be considered an autoimmune disease similar to chronic thyroiditis, and that Type B gastritis is likely the result of repeated mucosal insults such as reflux.[5,21]

Incidence and Progression of Chronic Idiopathic Gastritis

Most information on the incidence and progression of chronic gastritis has been obtained from the unparalleled studies by Siurala[19] who selected at random every fifth person for endoscopy from 1,000 of a total population of 1,300 inhabitants of a Finnish commune.[19] They reported chronic superficial gastritis in 25% and chronic atrophic gastritis in 28% of this biopsied population. In all, 53% of the group had some degree of gastritis, and there were four instances of severe gastric atrophy. There was no relation between symptomatology and severity. There are no comparable studies available for North American populations. It has been estimated from Siurala's reports[19] that the incidence in an adult Caucasian population of Type B gastritis is about 22% and that of Type A about 5 to 6%.

Repeat biopsy studies in this population at a 20-year interval showed that nearly half of those with superficial gastritis were found to have progressed to the atrophic form. Regression to normal was distinctly uncommon. In related studies, it has been shown that the incidence of chronic superficial gastritis does not increase with age although atrophy does, presumably through an initial stage of superficial gastritis.[22] The time required for such transformation has been estimated at about 17 years.[21] Intestinal metaplasia in Finland was found to increase from an incidence of 5% in the less than 30-year age group to 42% in those older than 65 years.[22] Similarly, a strong correlation between age and incidence of atrophic gastritis has been demonstrated in a Japanese population. In that country, with a high incidence of gastric carcinoma, less than 10% of individuals older than 60 years had a normal gastric mucosa.[2] There seems to be a marked difference in incidence of chronic gastritis by sex, although the severe atrophic form is more common in women.[22]

Loss of Gastric Secretions

Mild to complete loss of acid secretion correlates well with the extent and severity of chronic atrophic gastritis. Pepsin secretion may be normal in the presence of severe acid secretion failure, but also tends to decrease with severity and extent. Intrinsic factor is usually adequate, except in the gastric atrophy of pernicious anemia. It has been suggested that the sequence of secretion failure may relate to the more superficial site in the glands of most parietal cells as compared with chief cells. The relative sparing of intrinsic factor may relate to the fact that it is produced normally far in excess of need.[17]

Etiology

Both an autoimmune phenomenon and various irritants have been implicated in chronic gastritis. In Type B gastritis, in which a low incidence of autoantibodies is present, clearly other sources than autoimmune disease must be invoked. Alcohol, bile reflux, partial gastrectomy, and most recently *Campylobacter pylori* infection have been implicated. The latter is discussed later under the heading of "Infectious Gastritis."

The role of alcohol in chronic gastritis remains controversial. Obviously, alcohol may provoke acute gastritis and has been shown to markedly alter the gastric potential difference in man, as does aspirin and the presence of duodenal contents.[23] Some workers have concluded, however, that there is no relation of incidence between a control and alcoholic population if they are properly matched for age,[24] nor between a control group and patients with cirrhosis.[25] Others have found a correlation between incidence and severity of gastritis and the degree of alcoholism.[7,26] Glass and co-workers[7] found that while alcohol did not relate to fundal gastritis (Type A), the incidence of antral gastritis in alcoholics was twice that in a control group.

Bile Reflux

Experimentally, atrophic gastritis has been produced in dogs by chronic exposure to jejunal contents, pancreatic secretions, and bile.[27] A mixture of bile and pancreatic juice was most effective in producing gastritis. The most damaging agent appears to be lysolecithin, produced by the action of pancreatic phospholipase A on the lecithin in bile, a reaction activated by both trypsin and bile acids. Damage is most severe at a low pH, indicative of the role of acid.[5] The presence of duodenal gastric reflux correlates with antral gastritis, but again not with fundal gastritis, emphasizing the validity of separating chronic gastritis into types.[28] A high incidence of chronic gastritis following partial gastrectomy is well recognized.[29] This may, in large part, be explained by reflux, but it has also been suggested that it may be contributed to by a lack of gastrin-induced trophic factor. Considering the frequency of Type B atrophic gastritis, other factors are also likely involved, presumably other mucosal-damaging agents. A decrease in IgA-producing plasma cells and an increase in IgG- and IgE-producing plasma cells as well as in mast cells have been observed in the gastric mucosa of rats with bile reflux induced by gastroenteroanastomosis.[30] This allergic-type reaction may be responsible for the hyperplastic changes of the foveolar epithelium which accompany the atrophic changes of the deeper glands in experimental animals as well as patients after partial gastrectomy, especially Billroth II.[29] It has been suggested that this type of "reflux gastritis" can be recognized histopathologically by the combination of foveolar hyperplasia, vasodilatation, increased number of smooth muscle fibers in the lamina propria, and paucity of inflammatory cells.[31]

Etiology of Type A Gastritis

Parietal cell antibody has been found in atrophic gastritis in from 50 to 95% of patients with pernicious anemia (which is associated with the most severe form of Type A chronic gastritis) and in from 20 to 40% of cases of idiopathic chronic gastritis without pernicious anemia. Such autoantibodies are of the IgG class and, in most patients, react with the gastrin receptor on the surface of the parietal cell membrane. Such autoantibodies do not inhibit gastrin binding, per se, but interfere with gastrin-stimulated C^{14} aminopyrine accumulation. Both mechanisms of action result in a reduction of acid production by parietal cells.[32] The incidence of PCA in other forms of chronic gastritis, such as those associated with the usual gastric carcinoma, and in post gastrectomy states is low or absent.[7]

Autoantibodies to intrinsic factor have also been demonstrated. These are of two types: 1) a blocking antibody preventing binding of vitamin B12 to intrinsic factor, and 2) an antibody that binds either to intrinsic factor or to the intrinsic factor–vitamin B12 complex. The former is demonstrated in about two-thirds of patients with pernicious anemia; the latter is less common.

Other autoantibodies have also been demonstrated in atrophic gastritis, though uncommonly, such as to thyroglobulin, thyroid, pancreatic islet cells, and antinuclear antibodies.[20]

Lymphoblast transformation and leukocyte migration inhibition have been demonstrated in about one-third of patients with chronic gastritis when tested against crude homogenates of fundal and antral mucosa.[33]

It has been suggested that these antibodies may simply reflect a humoral response to injury of gastric cells. This is a possibility, but does not explain the low incidence of such antibodies in postgastrectomy fundic mucosa in which the histologic changes are identical to those of the Type A gastritis, in particular of those patients with pernicious anemia. Experimentally, PCA has been shown to bind to and destroy parietal cells. A decrease in complement level, fairly common in atrophic gastritis and pernicious anemia, suggests that immune complexes may form in vivo in parietal cells between PCA, PC antigen, and complement.[1] In rats, injection of PCA or intrinsic factor antibody (IFA) containing

IgG over a period of 6 weeks produced a reduction in acid secretion, pepsin secretion, and parietal cell mass and a thinning of the mucosa.[1] Chatterjee[21] also produced atrophic gastritis in the guinea pig by immunologic methods. In addition, there is evidence for a cellular hypersensitivity mechanism in chronic atrophic gastritis.[7]

It seems reasonable to conclude that classic atrophic gastritis in its Type A form is an autoimmune disease process akin to chronic thyroiditis or Sjögren's syndrome, mediated through both cellular and humoral factors.

Chronic Gastritis and Pernicious Anemia

Pernicious anemia is usually preceded by many years of gastritis and reduced or absent acid secretion. It is usually accompanied by severe chronic atrophic gastritis (gastric atrophy). However, severe chronic atrophic gastritis is not necessarily accompanied by nor progresses inexorably to pernicious anemia. Such atrophy is not caused by vitamin B12 deficiency since vitamin B12 therapy does not improve the gastritis and, very rarely, such deficiency may be accompanied by a normal stomach mucosa.[21] Nonetheless, as indicated, pernicious anemia seems to evolve as a rule from Type A atrophic gastritis. In Strickland and Mackay's study,[18] 16% of patients initially presenting with Type A atrophic gastritis developed pernicious anemia over a period of 2 to 24 years (mean of 8 years). This was not true of those with Type B gastritis. Intrinsic factor autoantibodies are a common but not invariable accompaniment of vitamin B12 malabsorption, nor does its presence necessarily indicate impaired vitamin B12 absorption.[18] Although intrinsic factor blocking agent Type 1 is seen in the majority of patients with pernicious anemia, it has also been reported in chronic thyroiditis and hypothyroidism without pernicious anemia.[1] As mentioned previously, hypergastrinemia due to hyperplasia of the antral G cells is common. In these instances, the gastritis does not involve the antrum. Pernicious anemia may arise following total gastrectomy or in patients with severe intestinal malabsorption. Congenital absence of intrinsic factor is also a rare cause. Also rare is the pernicious anemia-immune deficiency syndrome. In this condition, though most have a severe chronic atrophic gastritis, autoimmune antibodies are lacking. Most of these patients have severe diarrhea and giardiasis, and malabsorption of vitamin B12 is a feature.[34] This rare syndrome provides evidence that chronic gastritis may develop through the mechanism of cell-mediated hypersensitivity reactions since these were intact in these cases. Strickland and Mackay[18] considered the type of chronic gastritis so seen to be best thought of as an accelerated Type B gastritis since both antrum and body were involved in those that they studied.

It is agreed that the genetic factor is important in pernicious anemia, and the association of pernicious anemia with premature graying of hair, vitiligo, diabetes, and other endocrine problems is well known. Severe fundic atrophic gastritis, hypergastrinemia, and the presence of both gastric and thyroid autoantibodies are more common in relatives of pernicious anemia probands than in controls.[35] Whittingham and co-workers[35] believe that the gastric lesion of pernicious anemia is determined by both nonspecific damage from various environmental agents and an inherited defect in immune tolerance to the specific complex of antigens resulting in autoimmune reactions, and that both these factors must be present and interact for the transition of chronic gastritis to the gastric lesion of pernicious anemia.

Chronic Gastritis and Gastric Ulcer

Chronic gastritis is strongly associated with gastric ulcer, and the more proximal the ulcer, the more extensive the distribution of the gastritis and the impairment of acid secretion.[5,18] Also, the more proximal the ulcer, the greater the likelihood of an associated intestinal metaplasia.[36] Experimentally, the mucosa of atrophic gastritis is more susceptible to ulceration than is normal mucosa.[37] Healing of the gastric ulcer is not associated with an improvement of the gastritis. Gastric ulcers are usually found at the junction of antral and fundic-type mucosa. The hypothesis is that the sequence of events is reflux → gastritis → gastric ulcer, and that the ulcer does not precede the gastritis.[17] The associated gastritis is of the B type and is not autoantibody-associated.

Chronic Gastritis and Iron Deficiency Anemia

About 40% of patients with iron deficiency anemia without known cause have an associated chronic gastritis. Such gastritis does not improve with correction of the anemia. The incidence of chronic gastritis is lower in those with a known source of bleeding. Occult bleeding from superficial breaks in the gastric mucosa is a possible cause.[5] It has also been shown that gastric acid is important in absorption of non-heme iron, which in western diets supplies at least two-thirds of nutritional iron needs.[38] Thus, achlorhydria may contribute to the anemia. The associated gastritis may be either Type A or B.[18]

Chronic Gastritis and Gastric Polyps

Both hyperplastic and adenomatous polyps have a strong association with atrophic gastritis.[5] Marshak and Feldman[39] found that 91% of their series of gastric polyps had an associated achlorhydria. However, only 78 of their 138 cases of adenomatous polyps were associated with an atrophic gastritis. There is evidence that adenomatous polyps arise from a background of intestinal metaplasia (i.e., the so-called adenomatous dysplasis of Cuello and co-workers [6]). We have not been

impressed with marked chronic inflammation in the more common hyperplastic polyps, although it certainly may occur. We have not systematically studied their gastric mucosal environment. Considering the low incidence of gastric polyps compared with that of chronic gastritis it would appear to us, however, that the development of hyperplastic polyps at least must depend on some other factor or factors besides gastritis per se. A more direct regenerative response to injury may be such a factor. Thus, hyperplastic polyps at gastroenterostomy stomas, a site of maximum exposure to reflux, have been described as showing no evidence of atrophic gastritis or intestinal metaplasia elsewhere in the stomach.[40]

Chronic Atrophic Gastritis and Carcinoma

It has been accepted that patients with pernicious anemia are at an increased risk for gastric carcinoma. Such patients almost invariably have severe atrophic gastritis. Such risk was estimated by Lambert[17] as 21 times that of the general population, although much lower figures are also in the literature. Mosbech and Vitebaaek[41] reported a 10% incidence of gastric carcinoma in patients with pernicous anemia. Strickland and Mackay[18] believe that this figure is probably overstated. Although there is no doubt that a certain number of cases of gastric carcinoma are based on a background of pernicious anemia, this accounts for only a small portion of actual cases of gastric cancer. For instance, pernicious anemia is extremely rare in Japan and yet the incidence of gastric cancer in that country is extraordinarily high.

Setting aside the question of pernicious anemia, there seems to be no doubt that the incidence of gastric cancer in patients with atrophic gastritis is much higher than that in the general population. Siurala[19] reported a 10% incidence of gastric cancer in patients with atrophic gastritis who were followed up for 20 years compared with only a 0.6% incidence in those in whom the original biopsies were normal or showed only superficial gastritis. Follow-up studies from various countries have also established a higher incidence of atrophic gastritis in those with gastric cancer as compared with those without cancer.[17,18] It has been shown that the incidence of PCA antibodies is no higher in those with gastric cancer than in controls,[18] and it would seem that the association of chronic gastritis and gastric carcinoma is, for the most part, through Type B gastritis. In Strickland and Mackay's[18] Australian population, all of the patients with gastritis who developed gastric carcinoma had gastritis of this type. It should be recalled that Type B is far more frequent in all populations than Type A.

The evidence suggests that the linkage of chronic gastritis and carcinoma is via intestinal metaplasia.[5,10] All stages of dysplasia through to carcinoma in-situ have been demonstrated in intestinal metaplasia.[6] The evidence suggests that the colonic type of intestinal metaplasia is more strongly linked to gastric cancer than is the small intestinal type.[11]

Acute Hemorrhagic Gastritis

The terms "hemorrhagic gastritis," "erosive gastritis," and "stress ulceration" have been used somewhat interchangeably. As used here, hemorrhagic gastritis implies a diffuse mucosal lesion notable for erythema, petechiae, and larger mucosal hemorrhages. It nearly always is accompanied by focal erosions or acute ulcers. We have chosen to discuss erosions and acute ulcer in the chapter on peptic ulceration.

It has been estimated that acute hemorrhagic gastritis (AHG) is responsible for from 25 to 40% of massive bleeding episodes proximal to the ligament of Treitz.[42,43] Bleeding may range from occult to massive, and originates from the enumerable foci of mucosal damage.

Although the basic pathology is similar, AHG has usually been considered under two headings: 1) an acute self-limiting form secondary to ingestion of certain drugs, particularly salicylates and alcohol, plus various other injurious agents; and 2) those cases encountered as a compilation of trauma, uremic states, respiratory insufficiency, and sepsis, often with accompanying shock. This latter form is often very severe and bears an associated high mortality. Erosive gastritis with bleeding may also occur as a complication of intense physical activity, such as running.

Alcohol-Induced Hemorrhagic Gastritis

William Beaumont, the pioneer gastric physiologist of the early 19th century, noted mucosal erythema and superficial erosions plus cloudy viscid secretion in the gastric mucosa after alcoholic bouts by his famous patient Alexis St. Martin. Similar lesions have been produced experimentally in man by feeding alcohol at a rate of 1 gm/kg in known alcoholics. The mucosa in these experimental subjects was shown to be normal before alcohol administration and had returned to normal in several of the patients biopsied 3 days later. All developed moderate to severe eythema and friability of the antral mucosa. Two of the seven patients involved had patchy erosions and hemorrhages in the mucosa. Biopsy in four of the seven showed focal subepithelial hemorrhage into the superficial lamina propria associated with an infiltrate of eosinophils.[45] Gastric bleeding requiring transfusion has been described in alcoholics and appears to be associated in such instances with preexisting chronic gastritis ranging from chronic superficial gastritis to the severe atrophic form.[46] The effect of alcohol in the gastric mucosa seems to depend on a gastric alcohol concentration greater than 10% and not on the mere quantity of alcohol.[47] Alcohol is known to increase gastric permeability to hydrogen ion[48] and potentiates the effect of aspirin.[47] It has been reported that alcohol prolongs the bleeding time induced by aspirin, which may be a factor in such potentiation.[49]

Aspirin-Induced Gastric Erosions

Aspirin typically produces more focal lesions (i.e., erosions and acute ulcers) and is discussed in Chapter 5 (Peptic Ulceration). In some instances, ulceration may become extensive and bleed massively, particularly in the presence of other factors such as chronic gastritis, esophagitis, and peptic ulcer.[46]

Acute Hemorrhagic Gastritis Associated with Severe Illness (Stress)

Patients with various severe illness are at risk of massive gastric hemorrhage due to acute hemorrhagic gastritis. Trauma, sepsis, respiratory insufficiency, uremia, hypotensive episodes, and extensive burns are common background problems, alone or in combination.

Pathology
The gastric mucosa shows extreme congestion, edema, petechial hemorrhages, and small superficial ulcers (erosions) (Fig. 4-11). These are usually under 2 cm and rarely if ever penetrate the muscularis mucosae or perforate. The mucosa shows focal loss of epithelium with superficial deposits of fibrin and an acute inflammatory infiltrate, usually with sparing of the deepest glands. There is an accompanying intense engorgement of small mucosal vessels, with extravasation of blood into the lamina propria (Fig. 4-12). The erosions seen are most marked in the fundic area, but may spread to involve the entire stomach and, rarely, the duodenum as well. They are never restricted to the antrum alone.[50] Deep penetrating ulcers may occur under stress conditions such as Cushing's ulcer after head trauma, surgery, extensive burns, and activation of peptic ulcer after a renal transplant. Although these share some

of the background of acute hemorrhagic erosive gastritis, they differ in behavior by their tendency to be deep and penetrating and probably also in their pathogenesis. Silen and co-workers[50] point out that hypersecretion of acid and pepsin are common following neurosurgical injury, but unusual in stress ulceration, and that such cases often have high gastrin levels, again, not usually seen with acute hemorrhagic gastritis. Although, in a sense, they are part of the hemorrhagic stress syndrome, they will not be further considered here.

In a series of 42 patients with severe trauma, shock, or sepsis, endoscopy within 72 hours showed erosions in 100% of the cases, although not all had massive bleeding.[50] Massive bleeding under such conditions seems to occur as a later complication, usually 2 to 3 weeks after the stress injury.[51] Acute hemorrhagic gastritis occurs as a complication of trauma alone in from 1.5 to 5% of cases.[51] There is approximately a 5% incidence of such bleeding in patients in intensive care units and a 30 to 50% incidence in patients with a combination of sepsis with trauma or severe burns.[52] In patients with a combination of trauma, renal insufficiency, and sepsis, nearly all have bleeding episodes.[51]

Pathophysiology
It is agreed to by all that the presence of acid and probably pepsin is required for the appearance of AHG. Acute hemorrhagic gastritis can occur in the absence of luminal acid, but this is due not to a lack of secretion, but rather to resorbtion of secreted acid through an impaired mucosal barrier.[43] On the other hand, the amount of acid need not be excessive. Indeed, acid secretion correlates with blood flow and, as indicated, it may be decreased. Nonetheless, the presence of some acid secretion is necessary.[50] An increase in back diffusion of hydrogen ion may occur in the absence of obvious mucosal disruption and appears to be the initiating event. Neutralization of gastric acid prevents bleeding and erosions.[43]

Figure 4-11. Acute hemorrhagic gastritis—gross. This is a 28-year-old patient with esophageal varices and severe liver disease. Note hemorrhagic dark gastric mucosa sharply demarcated against white esophageal mucosa.

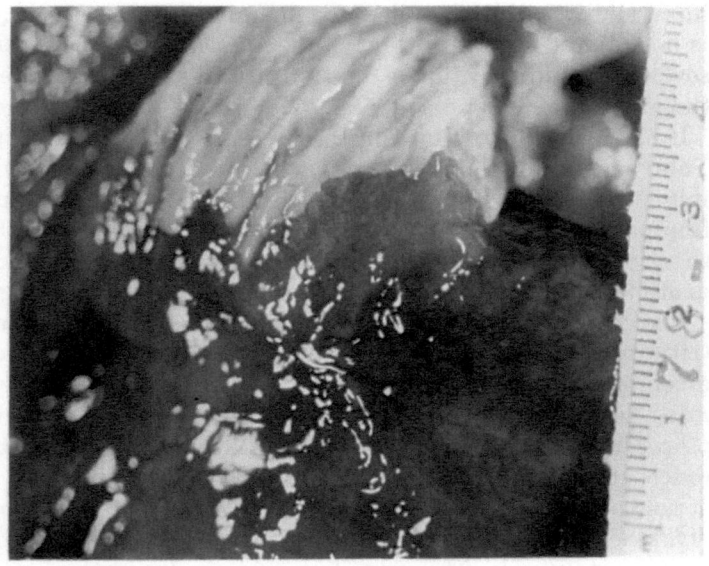

Mucosal ischemia is another common denominator of this condition, whether caused by generalized shock or by splanchnic shunting mechanisms. The maintenance of the mucosal acid barrier is strongly dependent on a normal mucosal blood flow. Both shock and sepsis cause redistribution of blood flow away from subepithelial capillaries. The resultant hypoxia may persist after recovery from shock. Hypoxia plus acid and bile lead to mucosal injury.[52] As in peptic ulceration, back diffusion of hydrogen ion causes histamine release, which increases capillary permeability and acid secretion.

The importance of bile reflux as a factor is strongly supported by experimental evidence. Hemorrhagic shock results in the appearance of stress ulcers in dogs and pigs, which is prevented by clamping of the pylorus, preventing bile reflux. Again, this factor is

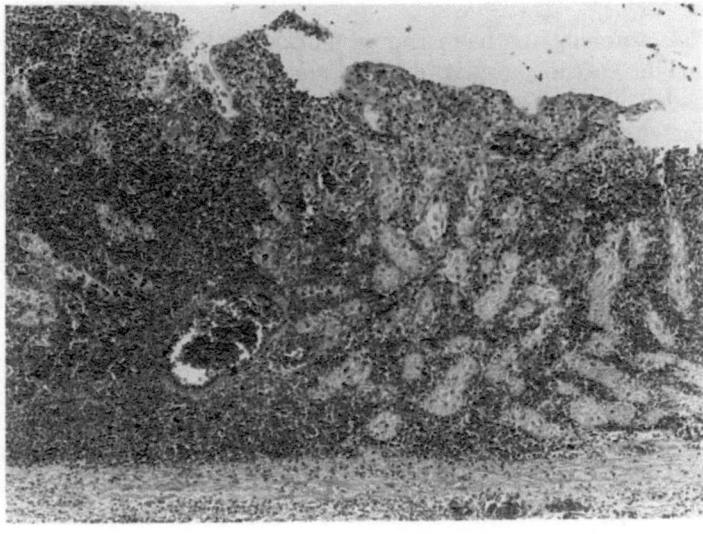

Figure 4-12. Hemorrhagic gastritis. Note superficial necrosis and mucosal hemorrhage. Multiple erosions were present. This is a section from a patient who died following an episode of cardiogenic shock. H&E, X100, reproduced at 66%.

interrelated with ischemia since the mucosa is not injured by bile without ischemia. The severity of injury by bile is also a function of the amount of acid present.[53]

It has been shown that shock reduces ATP. This reduction in the presence of acid leads to injury. Such reduction is more marked in the fundus than the antrum, which may explain the greater involvement of the fundic area in acute hemorrhagic gastritis.[50]

The development of acute hemorrhagic gastritis may thus be considered to be due to a complex interplay between mucosal ischemia, however caused, resulting in an impaired mucosal barrier, the accentuation of mucosal barrier permeability in the presence of acid and bile, all related in a vicious cycle of further damage. Histamine appears to play an important role. The role of steroids and prostaglandins, though no doubt involved, remains problematic.

The use of H_2 receptor-blocking agents (cimetidine) has proven effective in preventing the onset of stress ulcers in both animals and patients at risk. The use of this drug and other efforts to neutralize gastric acid is now considered effective prophylaxis in patients at risk of this serious disorder.[54]

Infectious Gastritis

General Remarks

The stomach has been thought of as both a barrier to the passage of bacteria and as a reservoir of bacteria and a source of infection elsewhere. These concepts are not mutually exclusive. The barrier function appears to be dependent on maintenance of normal acid secretion. Gastric juice, per se, is not bacteriocidal, though it is an effective bacteriocidal agent below the pH of four. The normal stomach is sterile or nearly so at acid levels of 20 to 30 mEq/liter.[55] There is both experimental and clinical evidence of the importance of gastric acid in protecting against such enteric pathogens as Salmonella, Shigella, and Vibrio cholera (i.e., increased threshold dose required for infection and a decrease in

the severity in such infections as may occur in those with a normally functioning stomach). There is also some evidence of a protective role of gastric acid against certain parasitic pathogens, especially Giardia. Patients with hypochlorhydria or achlorhydria are more subject to such enteric infections.[56,57] The subject is well reviewed by Gianella and co-workers.[57]

Normal gastric motility and emptying time also appear to serve a protective function. In the presence of pyloric obstruction, however caused, a wide variety of aerobic and anaerobic organisms have been cultured by gastric swab techniques. These include alpha-hemolytic streptococci, clostridia, and B proteus, even in the presence of normal acid secretion (perhaps secondary to the neutralization of acid by gastric contents). Postoperative sepsis in patients operated on for gastroduodenal disease has been shown to be usually due to endogenous gastric microflora and not to exogenous bacterial contamination.[58] The stomach has also been implicated as a reservoir for colonization of the esophagus and trachea in patients maintained on artificial ventilation,[59] and gastric microbial overgrowth is suspected of contributing to gastric and duodenal stress ulcers.[60]

Campylobacter pylori-Associated Gastritis

In 1983, Warren and Marshall[61] first isolated a previously unidentified curved Campylobacter-like bacterium from the stomach of humans with chronic gastritis in Australia. The organism was seen microscopically in surface and crypt mucus and could be cultured from gastric mucosal biopsies. Shortly thereafter, in order to prove that the bacterium was indeed the cause of gastritis and not merely an innocent bystander, Marshall ingested a culture of the organism, developed symptoms of acute gastritis 1 week later, had biopsy evidence of acute gastritis after 10 days, and spontaneous clearing of symptoms, infection, and gastritis after 2 weeks.[62] He postulated that acute colonization may either be followed by spontaneous clearing or result in permanent residence in the antrum and development of chronic gastritis. Acid production is reduced in the second week of infection, but returns to normal thereafter.[63] In retrospect, epidemic outbreaks of hypochloridia with concomitant gastritis have been attributed to *Campylobacter pylori*.

Since its initial description, the entity of *Campylobacter pylori*-associated gastritis has received steadily increasing attention in the medical literature.[64-70] Recent reviews are cited in reports by Marshall[71] and Blaser.[72] The organism is also referred to as *Campylobacter pyloridis*[73,74] or, because of its great phenotypic variability, as *Campylobacter*-like organism (CLO).[64,70] The most recently suggested name, *Campylobacter pylori* (*C. pylori*), is consistent with the terminology used for other *Campylobacter* species such as *C. jejuni*.[75] In spite of the wealth of information, the source and transmission of the organism are still unknown. *C. pylori* has been identified in large proportions of gastric biopsies of patients with dyspepsia from various parts of the world. The incidence was 69% in China,[64] 58% in Australia[61] and Denmark,[65] 54% in West Germany,[66] 47% in the United States,[67] 43% in Canada,[68] 40% in the United Kingdom,[69] and 38% in Finland.[70] It is noteworthy that Finland, a country with an unusually high incidence of chronic nonspecific gastritis, reports a relatively low incidence of *C. pylori* infection, suggesting that its etiologic significance for chronic gastritis at large still remains to be proven.

What is established by all of the above studies, however, is a statistically highly significant correlation with chronic gastritis— up to 95% of patients harboring the organism in the stomach have chronic gastritis and usually the gastritis is active.[72] Gastritis is not necessarily present at the same site where the bacteria are seen.[73] For example, *C. pylori* may be present on normal fundic mucosa when gastritis is present only in the antrum.[72,73] Correlation with peptic ulcer-

ation, especially duodenal ulceration, also exists, but may be due to concurrent antral gastritis. There is no correlation with gastric carcinoma.

The association with gastritis is specifically an association with antral gastritis (i.e., Type B gastritis as opposed to Type A gastritis). *C. pylori* is thought to first colonize antral mucosa and gradually extend along the lesser curvature into the body. In the antrum, it produces chronic active gastritis whether the mucosa was previously damaged or normal. In the body, preexisting chronic gastritis may be activated by *C. pylori*, but not induced de novo. Interestingly, patients with intestinal metaplasia have fewer organisms than do patients with the same degree of gastritis but without intestinal metaplasia. It has been suggested that gastric cells may carry receptors for *C. pylori*, while intestinal cells do not. In biopsies of duodenal ulcers, the organism is only present in areas of gastric metaplasia (i.e., where the surface epithelium is of gastric rather than small intestinal type).

The diagnosis of *C. pylori*-associated gastritis can be made by culture, the urease test, or biopsy. Mucosal biopsies rather than gastric juice are required for culture since the organism is located within the surface mucus and not in the gastric cavity. *C. pylori* is microaerophilic and slow growing and requires a selective culture medium.[72] The bacterium is a weakly gram-negative, 3.5 to 6 μm long, curved rod. Four sheathed flagellae, instead of a single unsheathed flagella characteristic of other *Campylobacter* species, allow for motility in a highly viscous environment. *C. pylori* produces large quantities of urease and catalase, which are essential for survival in the acidic environment of the stomach. Urease production is the basis of the so-called urease or CLO-test, in which a gastric biopsy is placed into a urea-containing solution with a pH indicator. *C. pylori* hydrolyzes urea and releases an alkaline product (ammonia), which raises the pH and produces a color change within less than 1 hour. The test is 100% specific and 91% sensitive.[73] In our

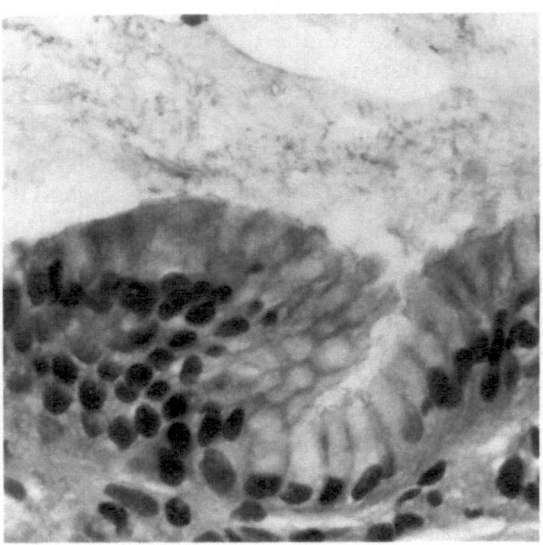

Figure 4-13. *Campylobacter pylori*-associated gastritis. Numerous curved rods are seen within the surface mucus as well as attached to the luminal side of epithelial cells. Giemsa, X500, reproduced at 75%.

experience, all cases that were biopsy-positive also had a positive urease test. However, some cases with only few bacteria on biopsy had a negative urease test.

The likelihood of finding *C. pylori* on a biopsy depends on the type of mucosa biopsied, the presence and severity of gastritis, and the age of the patient. Antral and cardiac mucosa are more likely to be positive than fundic type mucosa. Although normal mucosa may show the organism in the surface mucus (6%), inflamed mucosa has been reported positive in 58 to 95% of cases. There is a strong correlation between the number of bacteria and the severity of gastritis. Active chronic gastritis (i.e., with neutrophils) is more likely to be associated with *C. pylori* than is quiescent gastritis. The incidence of positivity increases with age, but children may be infected as well.[75]

Microscopically, curved rods can be seen singly and in clumps, within the surface mucus, as well as in the gastric foveolae. Single organisms are often seen along the luminal surface of foveolar epithelial cells, which are often mucin-depleted. In hematoxylin-eosin stained sections, organisms stain faintly blue. They are better seen in Giemsa (Fig. 4.13), Warthin-Starry silver, Gram, or acridine orange stains. Bacteria are not found in the deeper glandular portion of the gastric mucosa and usually do not invade. By electron microscopy, they may appear covered by microvilli and have been seen in neutrophils between epithelial cells.[72] Chronic active gastritis is characterized by polymorphonuclear leukocytes localized primarily to the gastric neck glands and a diffuse infiltrate of plasma cells and lymphocytes in the lamina propria. Atrophy of antral glands may or may not be present.

Acute infection may clear spontaneously. Chronic infection can be treated with bismuth salts or a variety of antibiotics.[72]

Phlegmonous Gastritis and Gastric Abscess

Diffuse infectious gastritis (phlegmonous) and gastric abscess are recognized as separate conditions although intergrades occur. Phlegmonous gastritis is now vanishingly rare, at least in the western world. Its first description is attributed to Cruveilhier.[76] Most of the over 400 cases reported to date were recorded prior to 1920. There is probably some confusion in the earlier literature between the infectious process (i.e., phlegmonous gastritis) and hemorrhagic gastritis. The disease has been associated with alcoholism, malnutrition, low socioeconomic status, and hypochlorhydria.[77] Most of the patients were between 30 and 60 years of age.[76] About 70% of the cases have been due to hemolytic streptococci, though pneumococci, staphylococci, *E. coli*, hemophilus influenza, and clostridia have also been reported.[76,78] The latter may produce gas in the gastric wall (acute emphysematous gastritis). The source of the bacteria is often hematogenous since cases have been pre-

ceded by erysipelas, furunculosis, scarlet
fever, and puerperal sepsis.[79,80] Other cases
occurred in patients with pneumonia, puru-
lent bronchitis, and pharyngitis, suggesting
swallowed infected sputum as the source of
bacteria.[77,78]

The course may be fulminating with shock
and death in a few hours, resembling a perforated viscus or, more often, there is an
acute illness of some days to a week with
fever, marked leukocytosis, abdominal pain,
and vomiting. More chronic forms may last
longer, localizing as an abscess. The presence of a normal amylase aids in differentiating the condition from acute pancreatitis.[76]

The process is usually sharply restricted to
the stomach which is atonic or rigid and
thickened with marked submucosal edema,
loss of rugae, hyperemia, and a fibrinous
serosal exudate. There is frequently thrombosis of veins in the greater curvature. Small
abscesses may be present. The major changes
are in the mucosa and submucosa.[79] The
mucosa shows necrosis of varying extent, and
the submucosa shows dense infiltration with
neutrophils (Fig. 4-14). Numerous bacteria
can be seen on Gram stain (Fig. 4-14 insert).
Bacteria may penetrate through the serosa
and induce peritonitis and ascites. Peritoneal
fluid was positive for the causative organism
in 75% of cases.[77] Mortality, even in the anti-
biotic era, remains high in the more acute
forms.[61] In one review, surgery reduced mortality to 18%.[77]

Gastric Abscess
Less severe and more localized forms of gastric infection also occur. These abscesses are
relatively small, usually being less than 5
cm. They primarily occur in the distal stomach. Roentgenographic studies may show a
filling defect.[81] Access of bacteria to the gastric wall may be direct (i.e., via injury by foreign bodies or corrosive material), hematogenous (as from endocarditis), or by adjacent septic foci usually cholecystitis or, more
rarely, pancreatitis.[82]

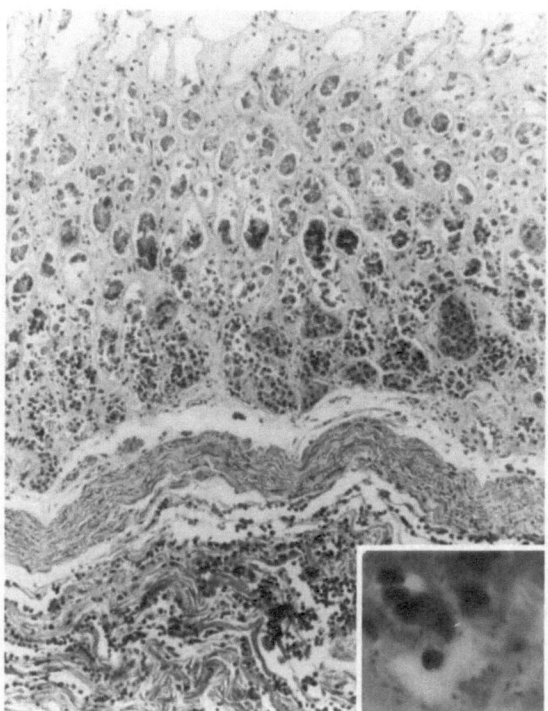

Figure 4-14. Phlegmonous gastritis. The mucosa
is largely necrotic and accompanied by a polymorphonuclear leukocyte infiltrate. The Gram stain
insert shows large numbers of gram-positive rods.
The patient was in renal failure and had had past
cellulitis of the leg. The terminal event was massive bleeding from the stomach, which was grossly
hemorrhagic. H&E, X100; Inset X630. H&E,
X100, reproduced at 66%; Inset X630, reproduced
at 66%.

Fungal Gastritis

Various fungi have been reported to infect
the stomach. By far, the most common is *Candida albicans. Candida* is an ubiquitous
organism which may be cultured from the
respiratory and gastrointestinal tract in a
large percentage of patients, usually without
associated clinical significance. The presence
of pseudomycelia, on the other hand, in
biopsy or cytologic material is considered
evidence of true "colonization" and requires
further attention. The gastrointestinal tract

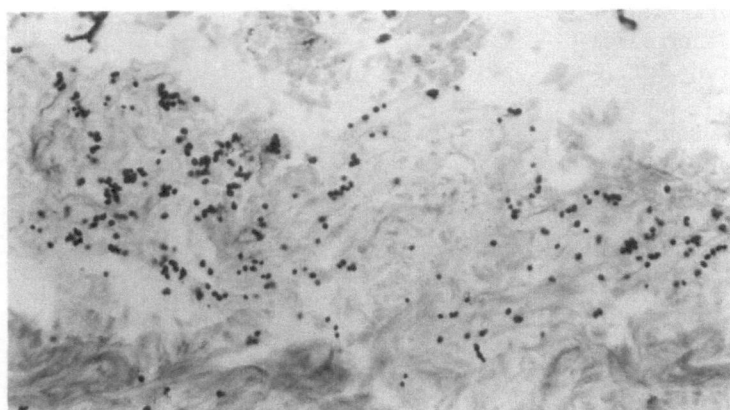

Figure 4-15. *Candida* coloniz-ing duodenal ulcer—yeast form. Gomori methenamine silver, X250, reproduced at 75%.

is thought to be the usual portal of entry of visceral candidiasis. The incidence of gas-trointestinal candidiasis in autopsy studies varies from 0.1 to 13%, the latter figure from a hospital treating a large proportion of patients with neoplastic disease.[83,84] Candidi-asis of the stomach, as in other visceral sites, is usually an opportunistic infection. It may be a complication in patients with neoplastic disease, especially myeloproliferative dis-eases, in patients with debilitating illness, or those with gram-negative sepsis with multi-ple exposures to antibotics, and with patients on steroid or intravenous therapy.[83,85]

More recently, it has been appreciated that *Candida* infection of the stomach may occur in the apparently immunocompetent host either as an isolated phenomenon[86] or as a surprisingly frequent colonizer of peptic ulcerations.[84] In peptic ulcer beds, such colonization may be superficial and perhaps of little or no significance (Fig. 4-15) or may extend deeply into the ulcer bed. Katzenstein and Maksem[84] reported a study of 72 peptic ulcers in which *Candida* was identified in 23 instances. In 13 of these cases, the organisms were numerous, and in 4 the pseudomycelia extended into the ulcer bed. They suggested that fungi may play a role in aggravating or perpetuating the ulcers in these circum-stances. Invasion of the wall of major arteries in peptic ulcer beds by *Candida* pseudomyce-

lia with arterial rupture and massive hemor-rhage indicates more directly that gastric candidiasis may be a significant factor in morbidity and mortality and not merely an innocent bystander (Fig. 4-16).[87] Secondary candidal invasion of gastric or duodenal ulcers is often associated with cimetidine therapy, probably because of the reduced acidity. Such ulcers may require antifungal therapy for healing to occur.[88]

Several forms of gastric candidiasis have been described. *Candida* infection of the stomach may be manifested by shallow ero-sions with a creamy exudative base (Figs. 4-17A and 4-17B) or in typical peptic ulcers, as already mentioned. It may also be mani-fested by small mucosal nodules with a ne-crotic tip (aphthoid ulcer). These may appear on roentgenographic studies as small bulls-eye defects. The nodules are due to microab-scesses in which pseudomycelia may invade and thrombose adjacent small vessels and these apparently coalesce to linear ulcera-tions, presumably secondary to the ischemia so caused.[89] Exophytic lesions up to several centimeters in size have also been reported.[90]

A peculiar form of candidiasis has been des-cribed in patients after undergoing gastric surgery—usually vagotomy and antrectomy with Billroth I anastomoses. In these pa-tients, the stomach has been dilated by large, semisolid, viscid masses of mucin and yeast,

Figure 4-16. Gastric candidiasis with pseudohyphae. Note invasion of artery tissue from site of previous gastrojejunostomy. Gomori methenamine silver, X250, reproduced at 70%.

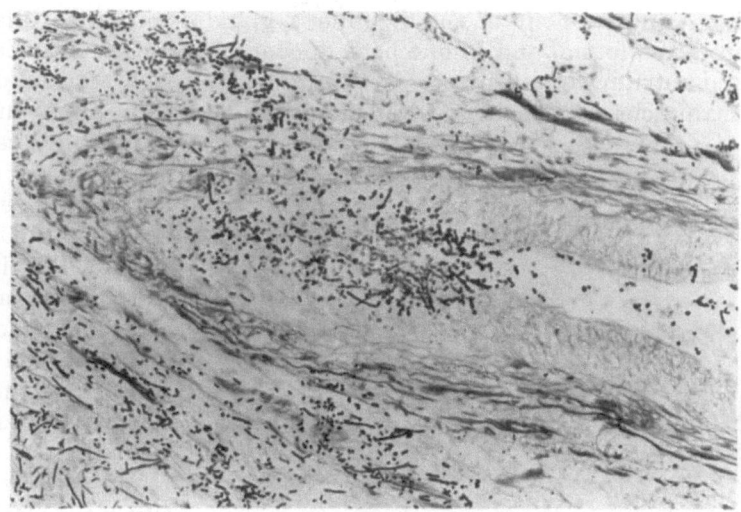

the so-called fungal bezoar. The typical barium appearance is that of a widely patent gastric outlet with an irregularly mottled, freely floating mass projecting into the fundal air bubble. *Candida albicans, Torulopsis glabrata,* or both have been cultured from such "bezoars."[91]

Histoplasmosis of the stomach has been very rarely reported, usually in patients with disseminated histoplasmosis. Involvement of small and large bowel is more common. It may produce a picture mimicking carcinoma, polyp, or hypertrophic gastropathy.[92] Actinomycosis in gastric ulcers has been rarely reported.

Zygomycotic gastric infections (formerly known as phycomycoses or mucormycoses) have also been reported rarely, especially from South Africa. These may or may not show the extensive blood vessel invasion by mycelia, which is usually seen in a more familiar pulmonary form of infection by these organisms. Cases with blood vessel invasion in the stomach have usually been fatal. Both tumor-like masses and perforated ulcers have been reported.[93,94]

Coccidoidomycosis, usually a pulmonary infection, rarely shows gastrointestinal dissemination.[95]

Viral Gastritis and Duodenitis

Viral gastritis is less common than fungal gastritis or viral esophagitis. Most of the cases reported have involved cytomegalovirus (CMV). The majority of patients with proven gastrointestinal CMV infections have been immunosuppressed due to steroids, chemotherapy, immunosuppressive therapy after renal transplantation, or infection with the human immunodeficiency virus (HIV).[96-99] Gastrointestinal CMV infection has also been reported in diabetics and in the CMV posttransfusion syndrome, which mimics infectious mononucleosis.[97] Most cases of gastric CMV infection in the past have been diagnosed in postmortem material. More recently, CMV is found with increasing frequency in gastrointestinal biopsies of patients with AIDS (Fig. 4-18). However, in AIDS, gastric CMV infection is much less common than is colonic CMV infection.[97]

Infection by CMV of the stomach and duodenum is probably not uncommon in other immunocompromised hosts and is frequently overlooked. Franzin and co-workers[99] performed endoscopic biopsies of the fundus, antrum, and duodenum in 12 patients after renal transplantation. In four instances, duodenal involvement of the Brunner's gland area was found, and in one both duodenum and antrum were involved. Cytomegalovirus intranuclear inclusions were identified in

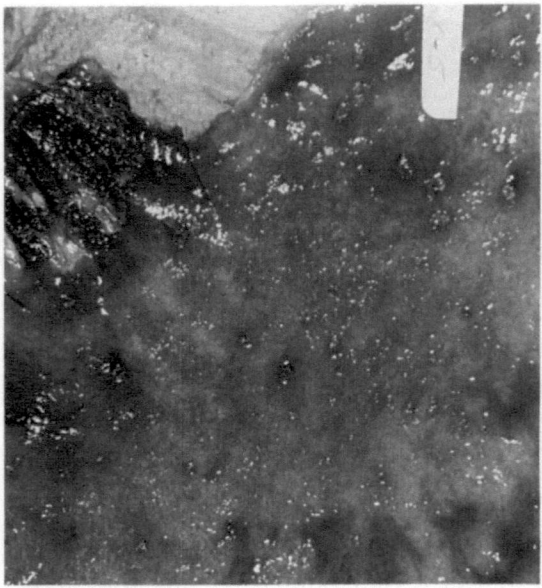

Figure 4-17.A. Gastric candidiasis—gross. Note multiple small grayish ulcers and "aphthoid nodules." The photograph is from a patient who had died with renal failure and FUO following chemotherapy for leukemia.

epithelial cells of Brunner's gland and in the antral crypt cells. On reexamination of multiple sections of the biopsies, three additional cases were encountered, usually consisting only of involvement of rare epithelial cells.[99] We have seen selective involvement of Brunner's gland epithelium by CMV in AIDS cases with CMV colitis (Fig. 4-19). More often, CMV inclusion bodies are found in fibroblasts, macrophages, smooth muscle cells, and endothelial cells, in intact mucosa, or in the bed of ulcers. In AIDS, epithelial cells show inclusion bodies much less frequently than mesenchymal cells. The role of CMV in the etiology of the gastric ulcers remains to be proven. Confirmation of identity of the CMV inclusion bodies by immunoperoxidase stains or in-situ DNA hybridization is possible, but is not necessary in typical cases. Cultures if taken, are usually positive, but rising titers of CMV antibodies are rarely demonstrable in patients with AIDS.[97]

Herpetic gastritis has been reported rarely as causing numerous ulcers or discrete plaques with ulcerated "volcanic tips," with cytologic confirmation of viral inclusions.[100] Several cases of herpes zoster have been reported.[101,102]

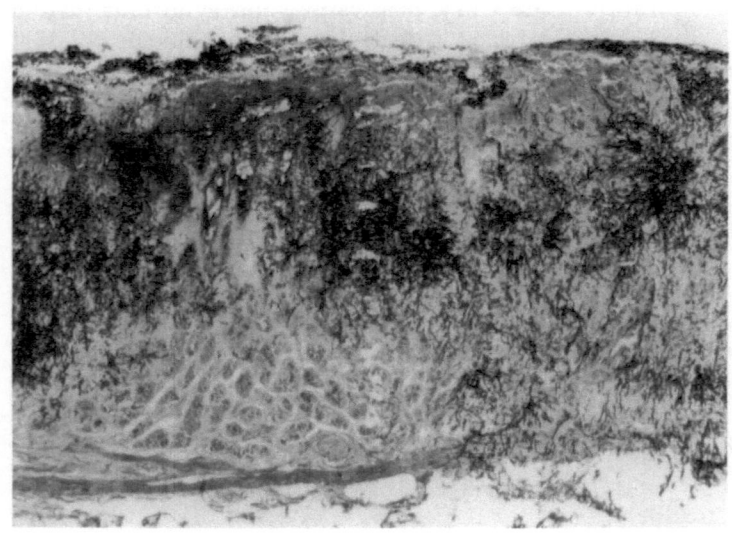

Figure 4-17.B. Gastric candidiasis—microscopic. Pseudohyphae infiltrate the partially necrotic mucosa. Gomori methenamine silver, X50, reproduced at 75%.

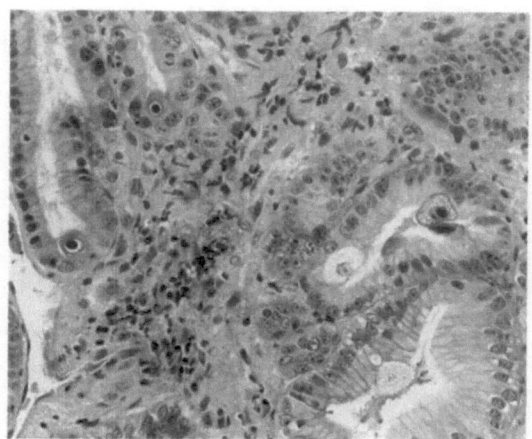

Figure 4-18. Cytomegalovirus infection of stomach. Note typical inclusions in epithelial cells. Gastric biopsy from patient with AIDS. H&E, X250, reproduced at 60%.

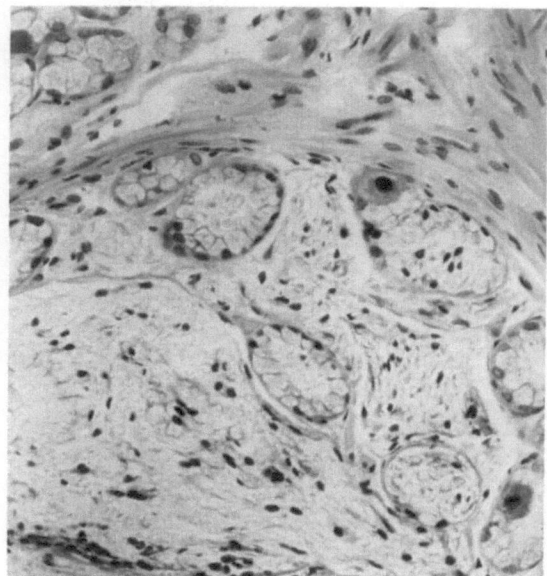

Figure 4-19. Cytomegalovirus infection of duodenum. Brunner's gland epithelium is involved. No inclusion bodies were seen in the surface epithelium. HPS, X250, reproduced at 70%.

Syphilitic Gastritis

The stomach is said to be the most common site of gastrointestinal involvement in syphilis.[103] It is still a rarely recognized condition. The diagnosis is, no doubt, missed on occasion, but should be considered, especially in relatively young men and women with abdominal pain, vomiting, weight loss, anorexia, and hypochlorhydria or achlorhydria.[104,105]

The earlier stages may be indistinguishable on gastroscopy from active superficial gastritis by showing extensive erosions, particularly in the antrum.[103] Later stages may show a linitis plastica-type picture on radiologic examination, the most typical appearance being a tapered antrum, although hourglass types of deformity and filling defects have also been reported.[106,107]

The histologic lesion is that of a heavy mucosal and submucosal infiltrate of plasma cells, sometimes vasocentric, with a proliferative endarteriolitis. Granulomas are distinctly not a feature, as emphasized by Haggitt.[108] A rare exception is a case with a gummatous granuloma, illustrated in the early literature.[109] When suspected, the spirochaetes can be demonstrated with the Dieterle stain or by specific immunofluorescent techniques.[105] Plaques with squamous metaplasia have also been described. We have seen one such possible case, although we were not able to demonstrate organisms (Fig. 4-20). A case of well differentiated gastric squamous cell carcinoma superimposed on such squamous metaplastic areas has been reported.[110]

Gastric Ascariasis

Ascaris lumbricoides, the most ubiquitous helminth infecting approximately 650 million people in the world, is a traditional inhabitant of the small intestine, but has occasionally been found in adjacent sites including the stomach. While worms are known to be expelled in vomitus and thus must have passed through the stomach, the term "gastric ascariasis" is confined to cases with a more permanent gastric lodgement

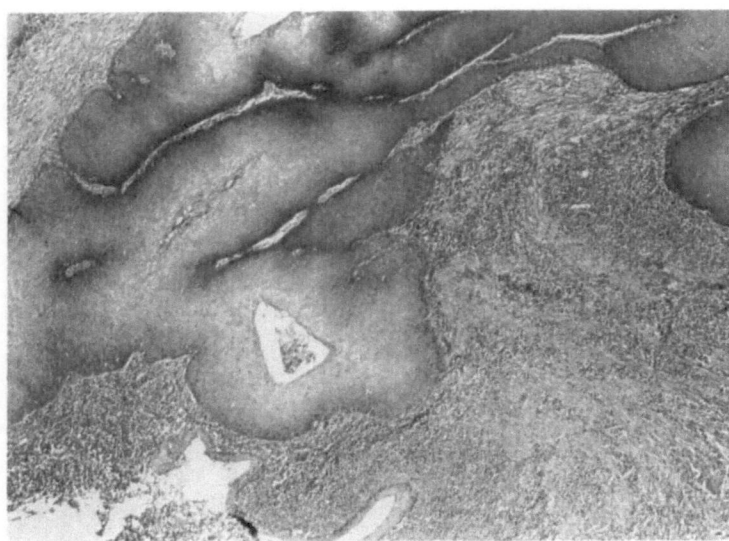

Figure 4-20. Extreme squamous metaplasia of stomach— probably luetic. This section is from the stomach of a middle-aged black male said to be luetic. Records not available. Courtesy of Dr. Jeffrey Myers. H&E, X40, reproduced at 66%.

that produces symptoms. Only four such cases were reported in 1986.[111] Gastric outlet obstruction by a mass of roundworms was characteristic. Treatment consists of endoscopic removal and antihelminthic medication. Histologic descriptions of the gastric mucosa are not available.

Certain other fungal, parasitic, and mycobacterial infections are discussed below.

Granulomatous Gastritis and Duodenitis

The term "granuloma" is, at times loosely used to the detriment of our understanding of the process involved (i.e., eosinophilic granuloma, once a popular term for what is now referred to as inflammatory fibroid polyp). We discuss here those conditions affecting the stomach or duodenum, which may show a granuloma defined as a compact (organized) collection of mature mononuclear phagocytes (macrophages or epitheloid cells) that may or may not be accompanied by necrosis or other inflammatory cells. Multinucleated histiocytes (giant cells) may or may not be a feature. A wide variety of causes for granuloma-

tous inflammation of the stomach and duodenum exist, many of them rare. Table 4-2 is modified from Haggitt's excellent chapter on gastrointestinal granulomas, eliminating only those reported from other parts of the gastrointestinal system.[108]

Care must be taken not to mistake tangential sections of the base of crypts, muciphages, focal nodular smooth muscle proliferation, epitheloid germinal centers, and clusters of ganglion cells. The latter may be surprisingly confusing in planes of section in which the large nucleoli are not obvious. It is our practice with any granulomatous process to perform the usual stains for fungi and acid-fast organisms. When these are negative, good practice includes examination with polarized light, which at times is helpful in detecting foreign material. Slightly racking down the condensor will also occasionally make obvious the presence of nonstaining foreign matter.

Tuberculous Gastritis and Duodenitis

Formerly, tuberculous involvement of the gastrointestinal tract was fairly common, but pasteurization of milk plus the advent of effective antituberculous drugs have now made this condition very rare, in the United States at least, though it is still a considerable problem in parts of Africa and Asia. Involvement of the upper gastrointestinal tract was always much less common than the more typical distal small and large intestinal sites.[112-114] In the stomach, three types have been described: 1) multiple small ulcers; 2) a hypertrophic type, mainly antral, with a heavy submucosal infiltrate leading to annular indurated thickening of the antrum; and 3) a form mimicking linitis plastica. Sinus tracts and fistulae may be present. It rarely may be a cause of pyloric obstruction.[114] Associated pulmonary tuberculosis, formerly usual, is now seen in less than half the cases. The disorder is usually confused with carcinoma or Crohn's disease.[112,113] The duodenum, when involved, is usually associated with disease in the stomach and is rarely involved alone.[115]

While caseating granulomas are the hallmark of tuberculosis, the lack of caseation (or even of granulomas) does not preclude tuberculosis. We have encountered a case of a patient who after renal transplantation developed abdominal pain, low grade fever, diarrhea, and vomiting. He had a past history of peptic ulcer. Vagotomy and antrectomy were performed, which included the proximal duodenal area. A deep ulcer was discovered with an accompanying massive infiltrate of macrophages, plasma cells, and polymorphonuclear leukocytes. This heavily involved the pyloric and duodenal area. No well defined granulomas were present, but innumerable acid-fast bacilli were demonstrated, which cultured as M. tuberculosis (Fig. 4-21) The ulcer was probably preexisting and peptic. He also had a tuberculosis peritonitis.

Similarly, infections with M. avium intracellulare (MAI) usually lack well defined granulomas. Infections with this organism of the intestine, including duodenum, are being reported especially in immune deficiency states, usually presenting with diarrhea and steatorrhea.[96,116,117] We recently encountered one such case, a 28-year-old

Table 4-2. Etiologic Classification of Granulomatous Diseases of the Stomach and Duodenum*

Infectious granulomas
  Bacteria
    Tuberculosis
    Syphilis[†]
  Fungi
    Histoplasmosis
    Paracoccidioidomycosis
    Phycomycosis
    Cryptococcosis
    Coccidioidomycosis
  Parasites
    Anisakiasis
    Fasciola hepatica infection
Foreign body granulomas
  Exogenous
    Food
    Barium
    Suture
    Cotton
    Talc
  Endogenous
    Mucin
    Altered muscle or collagen (?)
Miscellaneous granulomas
  Crohn's disease
  Isolated granulomatous gastritis
  Sarcoidosis
  Granulomatous vasculitis
  Chronic granulomatous disease of childhood
  Granulomatous reaction to carcinoma

*Modified from Haggitt.[108]
[†]Very rarely.

black male, who was a known homosexual with AIDS. He had the usual complex of infections, including cytomegalovirus, herpes, and *Pneumocystis carinii*. He developed severe diarrhea and at autopsy showed extensive involvement of the duodenum and small and large bowel with yellowish mucosal plaques and nodules. The histology, as in other reported cases, was that of a massive mucosal infiltrate of macrophages without granuloma formation (Fig. 4-22). Culture was positive for MAI. There was evidence of dissemination in many organs. The stomach was spared. Sparing of the stomach was also true of the case reported by Gillan and coworkers.[116] Their case, as ours, mimicked

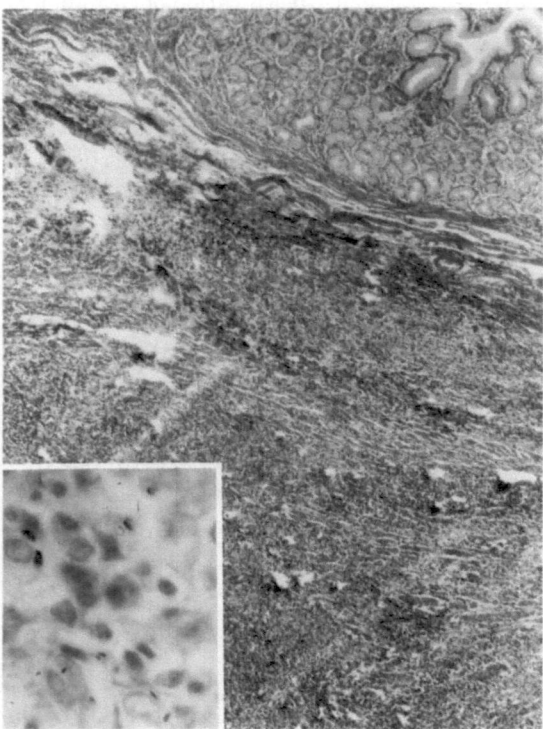

Figure 4-21. Tuberculosis of gastroduodenal area. Section is from the gastroduodenal junction of a renal transplant patient with a perforating ulcer. Note the ill-defined, heavy infiltrate of chronic and acute inflammatory cells without clear-cut granulomas. H&E, X50, reproduced at 70%. **Inset**: Acid-fast stain, showing acid-fast organisms cultured as *M. tuberculosis*. X630, reproduced at 70%.

Whipple's disease, at least superficially. Recently, we have seen a gastric biopsy with focal MAI-containing histiocytic infiltrates in a patient with widespread small and large intestinal and nodal mycobacteriosis (Fig. 4-23).

Fungal Granulomas

Candidiasis does not produce granulomas. South American blastomycosis (paracoccidioidomycosis) is rare in the stomach and, like mucormycosis, produces a suppurative inflammatory process with a granulomatous

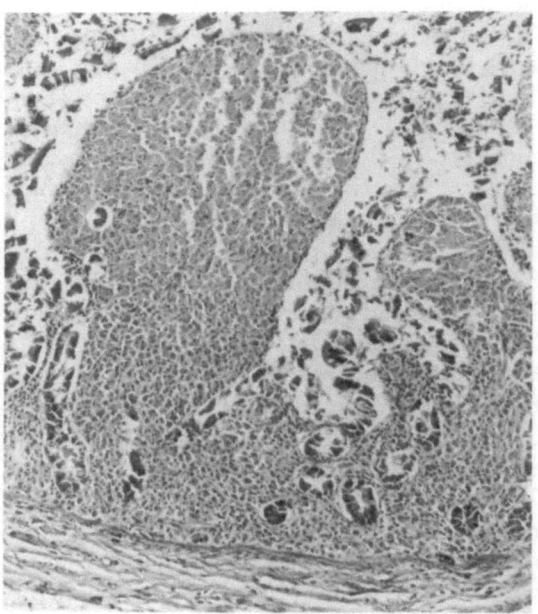

Figure 4-22.A. *Mycobacterium avium intracellulare* infection of duodenum and small intestine. The mucosa is largely replaced by masses of histiocytes in a pattern suggestive of Whipple's disease. No granulomas are seen. A PAS stain was positive. The section is from the jejunum. H&E, X630, reproduced at 80%.

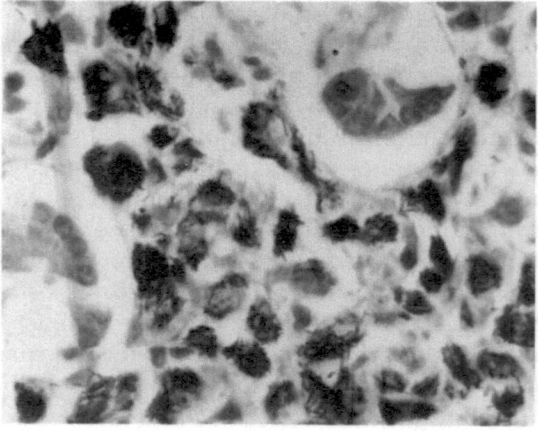

Figure 4-22.B. Acid-fast stain of same case (see Fig. 4-21). Note masses of acid-fast organisms cultured as *M. avium intracellulare*. The patient was a young man with AIDS. A major problem was chronic diarrhea. X100, reproduced at 75%.

reaction.[108] The other zygomycotic fungi are associated with granulomas and a more chronic inflammatory process. The granulomas of histoplasmosis, rare in the stomach, may be confused with those of sarcoidosis or Crohn's disease. The organisms can usually be demonstrated with appropriate stains. Coccidioidomycosis, although rarely affecting the gastrointestinal tract, is associated with granulometous inflammation.[95]

Parasitic Granulomatous Infections

Anisakiasis

This is the most commonly reported parasite associated with granulomas in the stomach and duodenum. It must be considered in any case characterized by a marked eosinophilic infiltrate and, indeed, is sometimes referred to as parasitic eosinophilic gastroenteritis.

Anisakiasis is an infection of the stomach or intestine caused by larval nematodes of the family Anisakidae. Three genera of nematodes within this family are known to infect man. Many saltwater fish act as the intermediate host. The infection occurs by eating salted, slightly pickled, or uncooked fish (such as Sushi in Japan), "green" herring in the Netherlands, and Ceviche in Latin America. The definitive hosts of the organism are marine mammals such as porpoises. The larvae do not mature in man, but burrow into the gastric or intestinal wall.

The disease first came to general attention in reports from Northern Europe as infestations of the upper small bowel.[118] Similar infestations were shortly recognized in Japan, where eating raw fish is popular. In Japan, over half of the reported cases have been in the stomach, possibly because of the frequency in that country of gastric hypochlorhydria or achlorhydria.[119,120] In North America, salmon are commonly infected and the disease has been identified here.[120]

The onset may be acute within 6 to 8 hours after ingestion of heavily infected fish. It is marked by colicky abdominal pain plus the finding of peripheral eosinophilia. Many patients, however, have some months of com-

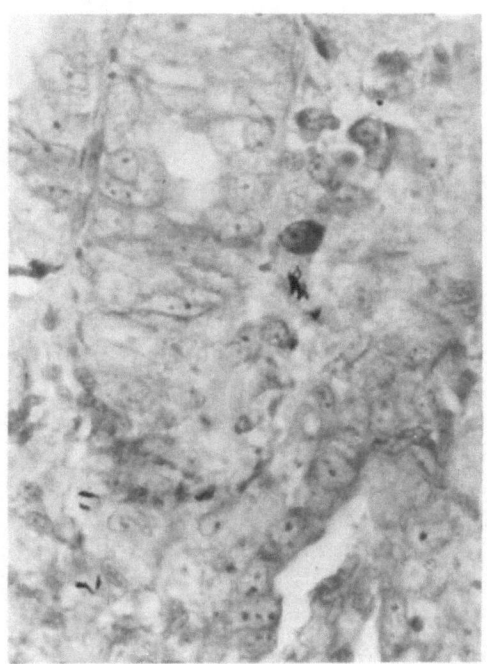

Figure 4-23. *Mycobacterium avium intracellulare* infection of stomach. The patient had AIDS and extensive MAI involvement of small and large intestine. Note rare clumps of bacilli in macrophages. Acid-fast stain, X630, reproduced at 75%.

plaints and a diagnosis of ulcer or tumor is suspected. Pyloric stenosis or gastric and duodenal ulcers may be present. At times, a tumor-like polyp may be seen. In the chronic stages, ulceration disappears and the symptomatology is more vague.[119,121]

In the early stages of the infection, the tissue reaction is similar to that of eosinophilic gastroenteritis (i.e., diffuse swelling or nodularity caused by tissue edema and heavy eosinophilic infiltrates). At this stage, viable nematodes may be detected by endoscopy or on air-contrast films. Later, the nematode dies, and foreign body granulomas to portions of the nematode may be seen. A phlegmon, abscess, or granulomatous picture may predominate.[119] The nematode larva is about 0.3 mm in diameter and from 15 to 50 mm in length. Lateral chords forming a Y-shaped figure are seen on cross-section (Fig. 4-24).[119]

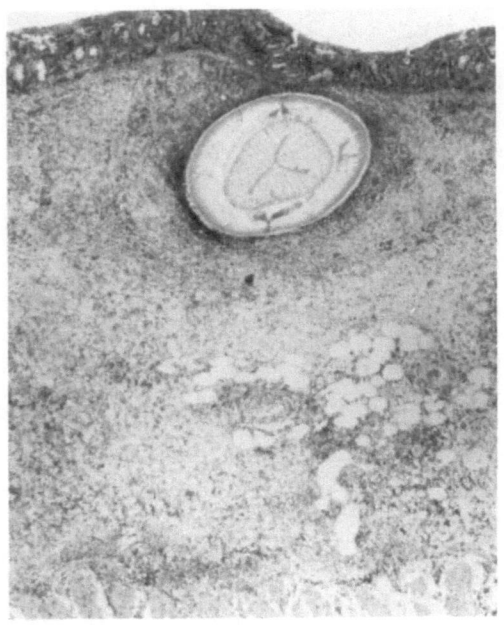

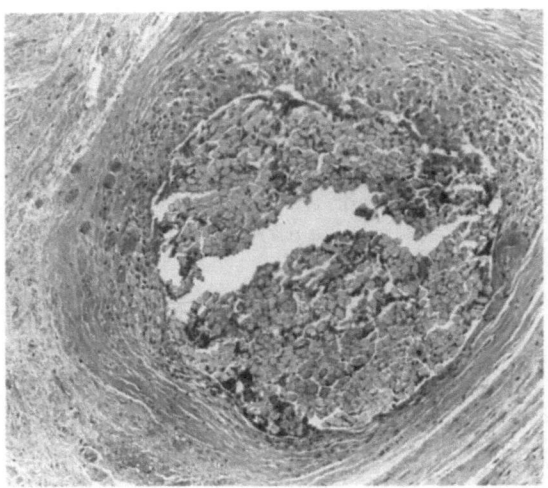

Figure 4-25. Suture granuloma (silk) of stomach. H&E, X50, reproduced at 60%.

Figure 4-24. Anisakiasis. The *Anisakis* larva is characterized by lateral chords (6 and 12 o'clock) and a thick-walled esophagus in the center. The submucosa is edematous and infiltrated with eosinophils. H&E, X40, reproduced at 75%.

Fasciola Hepatica Infestation

Although, as the name implies, the liver and gallbladder are the normal sites of involvement with this parasite, two cases have been reported in the stomach. Both cases had gastric ulcers and migratory tracks of the fluke in the stomach wall. The tracks were filled with necrotic debris and surrounded by eosinophils. The actual parasite is said to be rarely encountered in such tracks.[122]

Foreign Body Granulomas

Granulomatous inflammation has been reported from a variety of foreign material gaining entry into the gastric wall. This includes talc,[123] kaolin,[124] and food material, the latter being the most common. Granulomas secondary to food material are often associated with peptic ulceration, and may be seen in all layers of the stomach. They also may be found without any obvious entry site. Food particles acting as a stimulus to granuloma form amorphous eosinophilic masses surrounded by histiocytes and giant cells and often contain identifiable vegetable cellular debris as noted by the nonstaining thick cellular walls.[125] Such granulomas may be confused with sarcoidosis or Crohn's disease, but additional sections will usually demonstrate the foreign material.

Suture granulomas from prior operations on the stomach or on adjacent organs may present as masses composed of a dense fibrotic wall with a central abscess formation and a granulomatous response about the nonabsorptive suture material (Fig. 4-25).[126] A spectacular case of this nature was reported by Carsky and Haswell.[127] This was a 27 cm, 4,970 gm gastric mass due to an encapsulated laparotomy pad left in the abdomen 12 years previously. Barium granulomas more typically occur in the rectum, but have been seen in the stomach, one such case presenting as a 2 cm spherical submucosal nodule.[128]

"Endogenous" Foreign Body Granuloma

Moran and Sherman[129] reported a short series of cases of patients with peptic ulcer of the prepyloric area associated with peculiar granulomas containing central amorphous eosinophilic or basophilic material with surrounding macrophages, fibrosis, and eosinophils. These granulomas suggested allergic granulomatosis, but lacked peripheral eosinophilia. They reproduced the lesions experimentally by injection of gastric juice into the gastric wall of rabbits and considered that necrotic collagen or smooth muscle was acting as a foreign body. The patients did not have histories of allergies.

Allergic Granulomatosis

Abell and co-workers[130] describe a 53-year-old male patient who presented with anorexia and a 30% peripheral eosinophilia. The stomach showed obliteration of rugae and intramural nodules, especially in the region of the lesser curvature. Biopsy showed granulomas much like those reported by Moran and Sherman,[129] with central granular eosinophilic material surrounded by radially oriented proliferating histiocytes plus occasional giant cells. Masses of degenerating eosinophils were seen in what were considered to be the younger granulomata. The granulomas were stated not to be related to vessels. A dramatic response to steroids was reported.

Granulomatous Vasculitis

Gelb and co-workers[131] report a case of a 25-year-old female with abdominal pain, nausea and vomiting, and weight loss, who had an extensive erosive process of the stomach and duodenum related to a granulomatous vasculitis of the small muscular arteries in the submucosa and adjacent mesentery. There was no evidence of disease elsewhere (except liver) and no peripheral eosinophilia. A similar instance involving stomach and rectum can be found in the literature.[132] This case was also without evidence

of any widespread vasculitis. We have seen two examples of apparently isolated vasculitis involving the gastrointestinal tract—one in the gallbladder and one periappendiceal —though we have not seen cases in the stomach, such as these reported.

Granulomatous Gastritis Associated with Carcinoma

Rarely, granulomas have been seen in lymph nodes draining carcinomas and more rarely actually within a carcinoma. A case of superficial spreading adenocarcinoma of the stomach associated with such mucosal granulomas has been reported.[133] Haggitt[108] cautions that such should not be assumed to represent carcinoma secondary to Crohn's disease in the lack of other evidence.

Chronic Granulomatous Disease of Childhood

Chronic granulomatous disease of childhood is a rare, recessively inherited disorder of children. It is notable for repeated infections, lymphadenopathy, multiple abscesses, enlargement of liver and spleen, skin disorders, and chronic lung disease. It is due to the inability of phagocytes and polymorphonuclear leukocytes to kill certain ingested bacteria. Involvement of the small and large bowel is common, sometimes simulating Crohn's disease. Granulomas are a feature. A few cases involving the stomach have been reported in young boys, all with annular stenosis of the antrum and outlet obstruction. The submucosa and muscularis were chiefly affected with marked edema, granulomas, and collections of peculiar yellowish-brown pigmented histiocytes, probably containing lipofuscin. In one case, the gastric problem was the initial complaint.[134,135]

Gastric and Duodenal Crohn's Disease

Crohn's disease may occur in the stomach as well as in more typical sites. The histopathology of gastric Crohn's disease, as elsewhere, is not pathognomonic, but rather is based on a spectrum of changes. It is not surprising, therefore, that most reported cases have had supportive evidence of the disease elsewhere. The incidence of proven involvement of the upper gastrointestinal tract has ranged from 1.6 to 4%[136,137] of the total cases of Crohn's disease, but is probably much higher. Endoscopic study and biopsy of 43 patients with Crohn's disease elsewhere who had had normal upper gastrointestinal roentgenographic studies revealed 7 cases in which histologic evidence of involvement of the stomach existed (and 4 of the duodenum). The diagnosis was based on the finding of granulomas, microgranulomas, lymphangiectasia, or prominent submucosal chronic inflammation with lymphoid aggregates, though the mucosa often did not appear abnormal on endoscopy. The findings in these cases did not appear to correlate with clinical evidence of activity of the disease.[138]

Although in the vast majority of cases there has been evidence of more distal disease at the same time or previously, in a few cases, gastric or duodenal involvement has been the first indication of the disorder.[139,140] In one series,[140] the stomach was the only site of upper gastrointestinal involvement in 8 cases, the duodenum in 10, and both stomach and duodenum in 12 cases. In some, the involvement was secondary to contiguous diseased large or small bowel.

Aphthoid ulcers have been presumed to be the "earliest" lesion of Crohn's disease. There is some support for this in a case reported by Badley.[141] The patient, a 16-year-old girl, presented with epigastric pain and vomiting. Innumerable "aphthae" were seen on the apices of the gastric rugae by endoscopic examination. Six months later, typical Crohn's disease of the ileum developed, and 1 year later, antral biopsy revealed noncaseating granulomas.

The gross findings in the stomach have been that of thickening of the gastric wall, usually more marked distally, with thickened rugal folds and a granular mucosa.[136]

Pyloric obstruction may be a feature. Gastric ulcers may or may not be present, and gastrocolic fistulas occur. The histology is similar to Crohn's disease elsewhere, with deep ulcers, chronic inflammation, fibrosis, and granulomas in many cases.

In the duodenum, ulcers that may be distal have been reported. Deformity of the duodenum secondary to contiguous abscess and duodenal colic fistulas have been reported.[139] The duodenal mucosa may show cobble-stoning, thickened folds, and stenosis. On x-ray examination in those cases involving both the stomach and the duodenum, the antrum is narrowed and the pylorus patulous with apparent obliteration of the pyloric canal. According to Marshak and co-workers,[142] sinus tracts and fistulas rarely originate in the stomach and duodenum, but when found, are usually secondary to disease in the small or large bowel. Obstruction of the duodenal portion of the bile duct and pancreatitis secondary to bile reflux have also been observed in Crohn's disease of the duodenum.[143,144]

Biopsy diagnosis should rest on the finding of typical granulomas (Fig. 4-26) together with evidence of the disease in more usual sites. We believe that the granulomas of Crohn's disease, sarcoidosis, and isolated granulomatous gastritis cannot be reliably differentiated. All tend to be small, non-coalescing, and noncaseating and may contain crystalloids, Schaumann bodies, and asteroid bodies.

Clinically, the development of epigastric pain and/or symptoms of gastric obstruction in a patient with a past history of Crohn's disease should raise a strong suspicion of gastric Crohn's disease. Peptic ulcer, not infrequent in such patients, causes the most diagnostic difficulty.[137]

Sarcoidosis of Stomach and Duodenum

It is difficult to come to firm conclusions on the incidence and pathologic lesions of sarcoidosis as it affects of the stomach and duodenum. There are numerous cases so reported,

Figure 4-26. Granulomatous gastritis (Crohn's disease) of stomach. Note small discrete epithelioid granulomas. The patient is a 23-year-old male who had a clinical diagnosis of "gastric outlet obstruction." Later, typical Crohn's disease of colon was demonstrated, confirmed by biopsy. H&E, X100, reproduced at 70%.

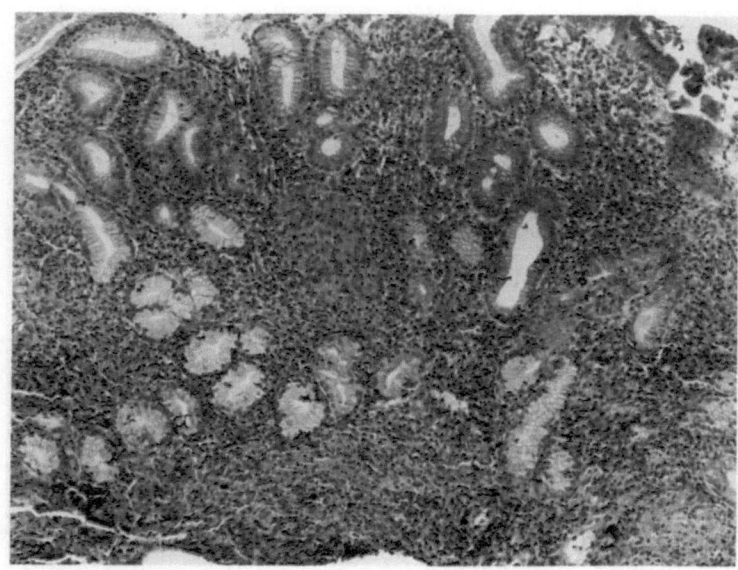

but reading the literature makes it clear that far fewer are acceptable and that there is confusion between gastric sarcoidosis, Crohn's disease, isolated granulomatous gastritis, and probably other entities. The problem is well addressed by Haggitt.[108] Although the stomach is considered a rare site for sarcoidosis, Palmer[145] found typical granulomas in endoscopic biopsies in 6 of 60 patients with known sarcoidosis. For the most part, these patients were without symptoms relating to the stomach. The term should be confined to those patients with gastric or duodenal granulomas of a characteristic appearance, with evidence of sarcoidosis elsewhere. The term "consistent with," though overused in other situations, is an appropriate one when pathologists are confronted with noncaseating, organism-negative gastric and duodenal granulomas. We have seen mucosal biopsies in acceptable cases, but have not had the opportunity of studying the whole organ (Fig. 4-27).

The mucosa is usually described as cobblestoned. Roentgenographic studies may show a cone-shaped antral deformity or a picture simulating linitis plastica.[146] Gastric peptic ulceration has been associated in about 25%

of the cases, sometimes accompanied by severe bleeding. Granulomas have been identified in the margins of such ulcers. Small multiple and persistent ulcers may be pre-

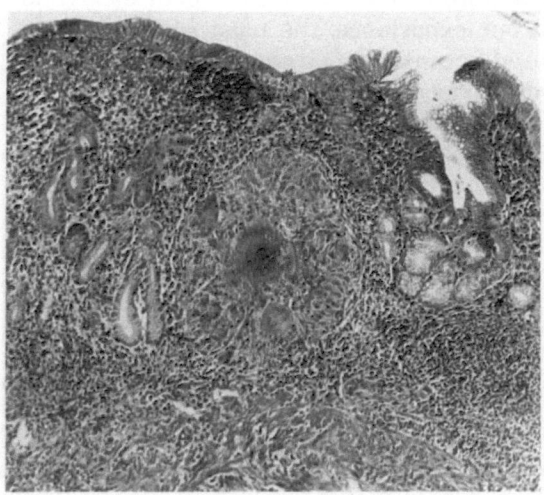

Figure 4-27. Granulomatous gastritis (consistent with sarcoidosis). The patient is a middle-aged female with cough and weight loss and "erosive gastritis" on endoscopy. Stains for organisms are negative. Clinical evidence of sarcoidosis. H&E, X100, reproduced at 60%.

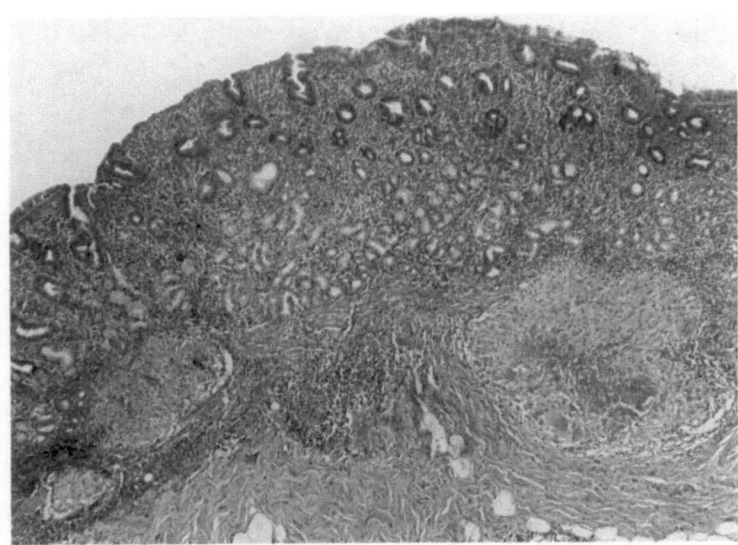

Figure 4-28. Granulomatous gastritis (isolated). The patient was a 66-year-old woman with a gastric ulcer and gastritis. A subtotal gastrectomy was performed. Multiple granulomas negative for organisms are seen. There was no evidence of sarcoidosis, tuberculosis, or Crohn's disease, and the patient is well 8 years later. Courtesy of Dr. David Hausman, Pennsylvania Hospital. H&E, X100, reproduced at 70%.

sent.[147] The term "gastric sarcoidosis" is strictly a diagnosis of exclusion, and the whole area is in need of critical review.

Isolated Granulomatous Gastritis

The third member of this trio of diseases and, in our experience, the most common is isolated granulomatous gastritis. The term was popularized by Fahimi and co-workers.[148] These workers critically compared the three diseases, all of which share a presentation of symptoms of pyloric obstruction, thickening and narrowing of the antrum, and noncaseating, organism-negative granulomas (Fig. 4-28). Since the etiologies of sarcoidosis,

Crohn's disease, and isolated granulomatous gastritis are equally in doubt, one must reserve judgment as to their real relationship or lack of relationship. Nonetheless, there are differences, which are summarized in Table 4-3.

As stated, the granulomas are similar to those of sarcoidosis and Crohn's disease. They are more common in the mucosa, but have been reported in all layers.[123] The lesions are most severe in the antrum and may mimic linitis plastica (as in sarcoidosis or Crohn's disease). The mucosa may show roughening, multiple small ulcers, or no obvious change.[149] In most cases, a partial gastrectomy has been performed. One peculiar case

Table 4-3. Comparison of Sarcoidosis, Crohn's Disease, and Isolated Granulomatous Gastritis (IGG)

	Gastric Sarcoid	Crohn's Disease	IGG
Age <20 yr	Occasional	Common	Not reported
Occurrence in Blacks	Common	Uncommon	Uncommon
Asymptomatic	Probably common	Probably common	0
Antral narrowing and thickening	Usual	Usual	Usual
Granulomas in lymph nodes*	82%	83%	34%
Involvement of lung, hilar nodes	90%	0	0
Involvement of intestine, colon	Rare	Usual	0

*From Fahimi et al.[148]

(atypical in involving only the gastroesophageal junction) is said to have subsided without therapy.[150] Whether this case is the same entity is problematic. The diagnosis is strictly that of exclusion. Tuberculosis, fungal infections, sarcoidosis, and Crohn's disease are the main diagnoses to be considered. It should be recalled that Crohn's disease may rarely present first as a gastric lesion. It is important, therefore, for an adequate negative follow-up of some years before that entity can be eliminated.

Eosinophilic Gastroenteritis

This uncommon and poorly understood condition is characterized by diffuse thickening of the stomach, segment of intestine (or commonly both), an infiltrate of eosinophils, and associated tissue edema. It was first reported by Kaijser[151] in 1937. A variety of terms has been used to designate it, which include "diffuse eosinophilic granuloma," "gastric Loeffler's syndrome," "pyloric hypertrophy with eosinophilic infiltration," and "infiltrative eosinophilic gastritis." The term "eosinophilic gastroenteritis" is now the term generally accepted. It should not be confused with the lesion that has been called localized eosinophilic granuloma, for which the current term is "inflammatory fibroid polyp." This is a completely different entity. The term also excludes certain eosinophilic infiltrates associated with nematode infestation, some cases of allergic vasculitis in which eosinophils may be prominent and the hypereosinophilic syndrome.

It is a rare condition. Johnstone and Morson[152] noted 120 cases in the literature as of 1978. It is twice as common in males than in females. It may occur at any age, but is most common in the third through fifth decades.

Clinical Presentation

The usual clinical picture is that of colicky abdominal pain, nausea and vomiting, and symptoms of obstruction (especially in those with involvement of the small intestine). The symptoms may be intermittent, and cases have been known to persist for 30 or more years.[152,153] Some may develop ascites notable for high eosinophilic content,[154] or, especially in children, diarrhea that may be accompanied by protein loosing enteropathy (see below).

In approximately 90% of the patients, there is an associated eosinophilia, usually with a moderately elevated total white cell count, with eosinophils ranging from 20 to 65% of the total count, often fluctuating markedly. The lower percentages are more typical. Such eosinophilia may wax and wane in the same patient. Absence of eosinophilia does not include the diagnosis. A family or personal history of allergy is common. In some cases there is intolerance to a particular food item.[155]

Site

The stomach may be the only organ involved, but in half of the patients, the duodenum and small intestine are also involved and, unusually, the disorder is restricted to the small intestine.[155] The colon is least often involved, but such involvement has been reported.[152,156,157] Rarely, the entire gastrointestinal tract may be involved.[157] Again, rarely other organs such as lung, liver, and bladder have been involved in the process, although widespread involvement of organs is usually considered part of the hypereosinophilic syndrome.[152] Everett and Mitros[153] reported one case and cited another with associated granulomas of the liver. These were also infiltrated with eosinophils. Interestingly, both cases had a history of disease for 30 years or more.

Roentgenographic Findings

The findings on roentgenographic studies are not specific. In the stomach, signs of pyloric obstruction and gastric retention are common, and nodular filling defects may be seen at times, which may be confused with

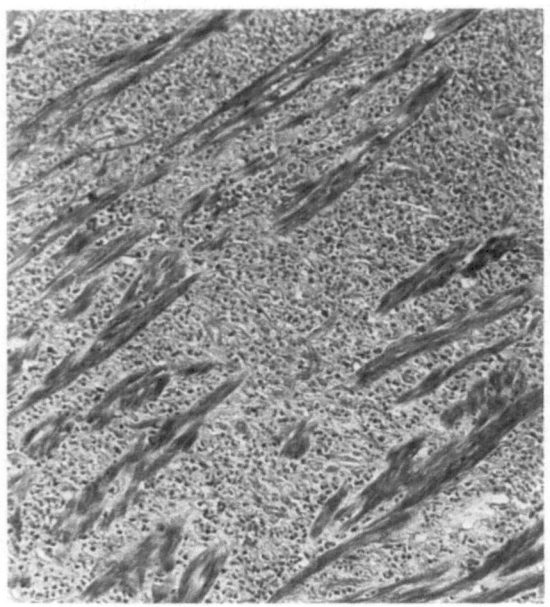

Figure 4-29. Eosinophilic duodenitis. Muscle bundles are widely separated by large numbers of eosinophils. HPS, X125, reproduced at 75%.

gastric carcinoma.[155] The small bowel may be dilated, suggesting obstruction or resembling regional enteritis. In children, a lacy irregular antral surface together with evidence of small bowel abnormalities is considered strongly suggestive.[158]

Pathology

The stomach is described as thickened with cobble-stone mucosa, sometimes with associated ulceration. The infiltrate chiefly involves the antrum and pylorus, although rarely the entire stomach may be involved. The eosinophilic infiltrate and edema are characteristically heaviest in the submucosa, muscle, and occasionally subserosa (Fig. 4-29). The mucosa is usually the least heavily involved. Despite this, it has been reported (in a pediatric age group) that gastric mucosal biopsy of the antral area is an effective diagnostic procedure. Such biopsies have shown a: 1) predominantly eosinophi-

lic infiltrate with some accompanying polymorphonuclear leukocytes, 2) necrosis and regeneration of the surface and glandular epithelium, and 3) in some cases, clumps of eosinophils (i.e., eosinophilic abscess).[159] It must be realized that some eosinophils are a normal finding in the gastric mucosa and, on the other hand, that the degree of eosinophilic infiltrate in a given case may vary widely.

The symptomatology varies with the level of maximum involvement (i.e., those with predominant mucosal involvement presenting with an iron deficiency anemia, hypoproteinemia, and symptoms of malabsorption; those with a predominant muscularis propria infiltration presenting with obstructive symptoms; and those with a subserosal infiltrate with an eosinophil-rich ascites). In children, growth retardation has been described.[158]

Pathogenesis

The pathogenesis remains obscure. From the initial case as evidenced by the title of Kaijser's[151] paper, the condition has been considered to be probably of an allergic nature. In some cases, the attacks are precipitated by certain foods. In young children, strong histories of an allergic diathesis are present (i.e., atopy, asthma, and food hypersensitivity). There is some question whether these pediatric cases are precisely the same disease process. Morson and Dawson[160] consider these pediatric cases presenting with anemia, edema, and protein-loosing enteropathy as a separate disorder, which they term "allergic gastroenteropathy." They point out that the eosinophilic infiltrate in such cases is only mucosal and may be scanty or absent.

In adults, an allergic diathesis has been noted in many, but in less than a majority, of patients. Again, subsets may be involved. Thus, 10 of the 11 cases with eosinophilic ascites had an allergic diathesis.[154]

An elevated IgE value (often increased in allergic states) has been reported in one of two patients.[161] The same authors found no food sensitivity or abnormal immunologic studies in an earlier group of seven patients.[162] Suen and Burton[163] suggest a relationship to allergic granulomatous angiitis of Churg and Strauss. While certain foods have been known to aggravate the condition, removal of the offending food does not result in cure.

Recently, a group of patients have been described who shared many features of eosinophilic gastroenteritis. These, however, were associated with connective tissue disease—chiefly scleroderma. The authors believe that these can be distinguished on biopsy by the presence of a band-like infiltrate of eosinophils and many mast cells between the bottom of the crypts of the small bowel and the muscularis mucosae. Where the muscularis was infiltrated, cytotoxic changes in the smooth muscle cells were identified. Hyperplasia and scarring of the muscularis mucosae were seen.[164] An increase in mast cells was not reported in the cases studied for such cells in other cases of eosinophilic gastritis.

It thus seems likely that with further study, eosinophilic gastroenteritis will no longer be considered a homogeneous disease entity, but rather one with subsets of varying etiology.

Although almost all cases have been responsive to steroids, surgery for gastric obstruction has been required in some. An occasional fatal outcome has been reported.[165]

In young patients with peripheral eosinophilia and gastrointestinal symptomatology, the diagnosis is usually clear. Eosinophilic infiltrates may be seen, however, with Crohn's disease, ulcerative colitis, adenocarcinoma, peptic ulceration, and, of course, parasitic infection. The diagnosis should be considered among the causes of pyloric obstruction, particularly those of a recurrent nature. A full-thickness surgical biopsy is usually required for diagnosis, since, as mentioned above, the most marked eosinophilic infiltrate, especially in cases presenting with obstruction, is intramural (Fig. 4-29).

Inflammatory Fibroid Polyp

Although many workers consider inflammatory fibroid polyp to be, as the name implies, a reaction of inflammation, we have chosen to consider it in the chapter on soft tissue neoplasms because of its tumor-like presentation.

Miscellaneous Types of Gastritis

Gastritis Cystica

Cystic glands within the mucosa are a common finding in a variety of pathologic conditions, including Ménétrier's disease, neoplastic as well as regenerative polyps, and in the mucosa adjacent to gastric cancer. The condition is sometimes referred to as gastritis cystica superficialis.[166] Gastritis cystica profunda describes the presence of cystic glands in the submucosa and is similarly associated with other pathologic conditions such as erosions and adenomas and particularly with polyps at gastroenterostomy sites (gastritis cystica polyposa).[151]

Chronic Erosive Gastritis

This relatively rare condition has been described in the European literature under a variety of names, including varioliform gastritis, complete erosions, chronic erosions, and gastric aphthous ulcers.[167,168] Abdominal pain is the most common presenting symptom. Endoscopically, there are one, several, or numerous—up to several hundred—erosions, each surrounded by a mound of elevated mucosa that is sharply separated from the surrounding mucosa. Most erosions are in the antrum, but in more than 50% of cases the body is involved as well. Microscopic findings are not specific and include sloughing of the superficial layer of the mucosa and a mixed infiltrate of plasma cells, lymphocytes, and usually also neutrophils, in the lamina propria. The diagnosis of chronic erosive gastritis is based on endoscopic findings and biopsy is not considered essential for the diagnosis.

The cause of the condition is unknown. Elevated serum levels of IgE and increased numbers of IgE plasma cells in the gastric lamina propria, described in some cases, suggest an allergic etiology.[168]

Chronic Ischemic Gastritis

While the role of acute ischemia in the pathogenesis of acute hemorrhagic gastritis is well established, the importance of chronic ischemia is less clear. A recent case report described diffuse erosive gastritis and duodenitis, unresponsive to conventional therapy, that healed after a revascularization procedure.[169]

References

1. .Glass GB: Immunology of atrophic gastritis. NY State Med J 1977;77:1697–1706.
2. Kimura K: Chronological transition of the fundic-pyloric border determined by stepwise biopsy of the lesser and greater curvatures of the stomach. Gastroenterology 1972;63:584–592.
3. Whitehead R, Truelove SC, Gear MWL: The histologic diagnosis of chronic gastritis in fiberoptic gastroscope biopsy specimens. J Clin Pathol 1972;25:1–11.
4. Siurala M, Isokoski AA, Varis K, et al: Prevalance of gastritis in a rural population. Bioptic study of subjects selected at random. Scand J Gastroenterol 1968;3:211–223.
5. Owen DA: The diagnosis and significance of gastritis. Pathol Annu 1979;14(part 1):247–271.
6. Cuello C, Lopez M, Correa P, et al: Histopathology of gastric dysplasias: Correlations with gastric chemistry. Am J Surg Pathol 1979;3:491–500.
7. Glass GB, Pitchomoni CS: Atrophic gastritis: Structural and ultrastructural alterations, exfoliative cytology and enzyme cytochemistry and histochemistry, proliferation kinetics, immunological derangements and other causes and clinical associations and sequelae. Hum Pathol 1975;6:219–250.
8. Sloan JM, Buchanan KD, McFarland RJ, et al: A histologic study of the effect of chronic gastritis on gastrin cell distribution in the human stomach. J Clin Pathol 1979;32:201–207.
9. Polak JM, Hoffbrand AV, Reed PI, et al: Qualitative and quantitative studies of antral and fundic G cells in pernicious anemia. Scand J Gastroenterol 1973;8:361–367.
10. Jass JB: The role of intestinal metaplasia in the histogenesis of gastric carcinoma. J Clin Pathol 1980;33:801–810.
11. Silva S, Filipe MI: Intestinal metaplasia and its variants in gastric mucosa of Portuguese subjects: A comparative analysis of biopsy and gastrectomy material. Hum Pathol 1987;17:988–995.
12. Sipponen P: Intestinal metaplasia and gastric carcinoma. Ann Clin Res 1981;13:139–143.
13. Koss KG: Diagnostic Cytology. 3rd Edition, Volume 2. Philadelphia, Toronto: JB Lippincott, 1979, pp. 835–837.
14. Nieburg HE, Glass GBJ: Gastric cell maturation disorders in atrophic gastritis, pernicious anemia, and carcinoma. Am J Dig Dis 1963;8:135–156.
15. Meshkinpour H, Orlando RA, Arguello JF, et al: Significance of endoscopically visible blood vessels as an index of atrophic gastritis. Am J Gastroenterol 1979;71:376–379.
16. Fung WP, Papadimitriou JM, Matz LE: Endoscopic histological and ultrastructural correlations in chronic gastritis. Am J Gastroenterol 1979;71:269–279.
17. Lambert R: Chronic gastritis: a critical study of the progressive atrophy of gastric mucosa. Digestion 1972;7:83–126.
18. Strickland RG, Mackay IR: A reappraisal of the nature and significance of chronic atrophic gastritis. Dig Dis 1973;18:426–440.
19. Siurala M: Gastritis, its fate and sequelae. Ann Clin Res 1981;113:111–113.
20. Vandelli C, Bottazzo GE, Doniach D, et al: Autoantibodies to gastrin producing cells in antral (type B) gastritis. N Engl J Med 1979;300:1406–1410.
21. Chatterjee D: Idiopathic chronic gastritis. Surg Gynecol Obstet 1979;143:986–1000.
22. Villako K, Siurala M: The behavior of gastritis and related conditions in different population series. Ann Clin Res 1981;13:114–118.
23. Gael MG, Phillips SF, Summerstkill DM: Profile of gastric potential difference in man—effects of aspirin, bile, and endogenous acid. Gastroenterology 1970;48:437–443.
24. Cheli R, Giacosa A, Marenco G, et al: Chronic

gastritis and alcohol. Z Gastroenterol 1981; 19:459–463.

25. Brown RC, Hardy GJ, Temperly JM, et al: Gastritis and cirrhosis–no association. J Clin Pathol 1981;34:744–748.

26. Segawa K, Nakazawa S, Tsukamoto Y, et al: Chronic alcohol abuse leads to gastric atrophy and decreased gastric secretory capacity: A histological and physiological study. Am J Gastroenterol 1988;83:373–380.

27. Lawson HH: The production of chronic gastritis under experimental conditions. Scand J Gastroenterol 1981;16(suppl 67):91–98.

28. Cheli R, Giacosa A, Molinari F: Chronic atrophic gastritis and duodenogastric reflux. Scand J Gastroenterol 1981;16(suppl 67): 125–127.

29. Bechi P, Amorosi A, Mazzanti R, et al: Gastric histology and fasting bile reflux after partial gastrectomy. Gastroenterology 1987; 93:335–343.

30. André F, André C, Saoui H, Cavagna S: Effects of experimental gastroduodenal reflux on density of mast cells and plasmacytes in the fundic mucosa of the rat. Digestion 1987;37:10–14.

31. Dixon MF, O'Connor HJ, Axon ATR, et al: Reflux gastritis: Distinct histopathological entity. J Clin Pathol 1986;39:524–530.

32. De Aizpurua HJ, Ungar B, Toh B-H: Autoantibody to the gastrin receptor in pernicious anemia. N Engl J Med 1985;313:479–483.

33. Uibo R, Salupere V: Immunobiology of chronic gastritis. Ann Clin Res 1981;13: 130–132.

34. Twomey JJ, Jordan PH, Jarrold T, et al: The syndrome of immunoglobulin deficiency and pernicious anemia: A study of 10 cases. Am J Med 1969;47:340–350.

35. Whittingham S, Ungar B, Mackay IR, et al: The genetic factor in pernicious anemia. Lancet 1969;1:951–956.

36. Stemmerman GN, Ishidate T, Samloff M, et al: Intestinal metaplasia of the stomach in Hawaii and Japan: A study of its relation to serum pepsinogen I, gastrin, and parietal cell antibodies. Am J Dig Dis 1978; 23:815–820.

37. Ritchie WP, Delaney JP: The susceptibility of experimental atrophic gastritis to ulceration. Gastroenterology 1971;60:554–559.

38. Skikne BS, Lynch SR, Cook JD: Role of gastric acid in food iron absorbtion. Gastroenterology 1981;81:1068–1071.

39. Marshak RH, Feldman F: Gastric polyps. Am J Dig Dis 1965;10:909–934.

40. Stemmerman GN, Hayashi T: Hyperplastic polyps of gastric mucosa adjacent to gastroenterostomy stomas. Am J Clin Pathol 1979; 71:341–345.

41. Mosbech J, Vitebaaek A: Mortality in and risk of gastric carcinoma among patients with pernicious anemia. Br Med J 1950;2: 390–394.

42. Ritchie WP: Introduction to symposium on stress ulcer and erosive gastritis. World J Surg 1981;5:135–137.

43. Ivey JJ: Acute hemorrhagic gastritis: modern concepts based on pathogenesis. Gut 1971; 12:750–754.

44. Cooper BT, Douglas SA, Firth LA, et al: Erosive gastritis and gastrointestinal bleeding in a female runner. Gastroenterology 1987; 92:2019–2023.

45. Gottfried EB, Korsten MA, Zieber CS: Alcohol-induced gastric and duodenal lesions in man. Am J Gastroenterol 1978;70:587–592.

46. Winawer SJ, Bejar J, McCray RS, et al: Hemorrhagic gastritis: importance of associated chronic gastritis. Ann Intern Med 1971;127: 129–131.

47. Fromm D: Drug-induced gastric mucosal injury. World J Surg 1981;5:199–208.

48. Skillman JJ, Gould SA, Chung RSK: The gastric mucosal barrier, clinical and experimental studies in critically ill and normal man and the rabbit. Ann Surg 1970;172: 564–584.

49. Deykin P, Janson P, McMahon L: Ethanol potentiation of aspirin induced prolongation of the bleeding time. N Engl J Med 1982; 306:852–854.

50. Silen W, Merhav A, Simson JNL: Pathophysiology of stress ulcer disease. World J Surg 1981;5:165–174.

51. Lucas CE: Stress ulceration, the clinical problem. World J Surg 1981;5:139–151.

52. Bowen JC: Comment on pathogenesis and pathophysiology of stress ulcer disease. World J Surg 1981;5:174.

53. Ritchie WP: Role of bile acid reflux in acute hemorrhagic gastritis. World J Surg 1981; 5:189–195.

54. Gurll NJ, Damianos AJ: Role of histamine receptors in pathogenesis and treatment of erosive gastritis. World J Surg 1981;5:181–186.

55. MacGregor AB, Ross PW: Bacterial content of gastric juice. Br J Surg 1972;59:443–445.

56. Buchin PJ, Andriole VT, Spiro HM: Salmonella infection and hypochlorhydria. J Clin Gastroenterol 1980;2:133–138.

57. Gianella RA, Broitman SA, Zamchek N: Influence of gastric acidity on bacterial and parasitic enteric infections: A perspective. Ann Intern Med 1973;78:271–276.

58. LoCicero J III, Nichols RL: Sepsis after gastroduodenal operations: Relationship to gastric acid, motility, and endogenous microflora. South Med J 1980;73:878–880.

59. Atherton ST, White DJ: Stomach as a source of bacteria colonizing respiratory tract during artificial ventilation. Lancet 1978;2: 968–969.

60. Brooks DA: Stomach as a reservoir for respiratory pathogens. Lancet 1978;2:1147–1148.

61. Warren JR, Marshall B: Unidentified curved bacilli on gastric epithelium in active chronic gastritis. Lancet 1983;2:1273–1275.

62. Marshall BJ, Armstrong JA, McGechie DB, et al: Attempt to fulfill Koch's postulates for pyloric Campylobacter. Med J Australia 1985;142:436–439.

63. Morris A, Nicholson G: Ingestion of Campylobacter pyloridis causes gastritis and raised fasting gastric pH. Am J Gastroenterol 1987;82:192–198.

64. Jiang SJ, Liu WZ, Zhang DZ, et al: Campylobacter-like organisms in chronic gastritis, peptic ulcer, and gastric carcinoma. Scand J Gastroenterol 1987;22:553–558.

65. Raskov H, Lanng C, Gaarslev K, et al: Screening for Campylobacter pyloridis in patients with upper dyspepsia and the relation to inflammation of the human gastric antrum. Scand J Gastroenterol 1987;22:568–572.

66. von Wulffen H, Heeseman J, Butzow GH, et al: Detection of Campylobacter pyloridis in patients with antrum gastritis and peptic ulcers by culture, complement fixation test, and immunoblot. J Clin Microbiol 1986;24: 716–720.

67. Buck GE, Gourley WK, Lee WK, et al: Relation of Campylobacter pyloridis to gastritis and peptic ulcer. J Infect Dis 1986;153: 664–669.

68. Taylor DE, Hargreaves JA, Ng L-K, et al: Isolation and characterization of Campylobacter pyloridis from gastric biopsies. Am J Clin Pathol 1987;87:49–54.

69. Pearson AD, Bamforth J, Booth L, et al: Polyacrylamide gel electrophoresis of spiral bacteria from the gastric antrum. Lancet 1984; 1:1349–1350.

70. Karttunen T, Niemelä S, Lehtola J, et al: Campylobacter-like organisms and gastritis: Histopathology, bile reflux, and gastric fluid composition. Scand J Gastroenterol 1987; 22:478–486.

71. Marshall BJ: Peptic ulcer: an infectious disease? Hosp Pract 1987; Aug 15, pp 69–78.

72. Blaser MJ: Gastric Campylobacter-like organisms, gastritis, and peptic ulcer disease. Gastroenterology 1987;93:371–383.

73. Hazell SL, Borody TJ, Gal A, Lee A: Campylobacter pyloridis gastritis I: Detection of urease as a marker of bacterial colonization and gastritis. Am J Gastroenterol 1987;82: 292–296.

74. Hazell SL, Hennessy WB, Borody TJ, et al: Campylobacter pyloridis gastritis II: Distribution of bacteria and associated inflammation in the gastroduodenal environment. Am J Gastroenterol 1987;802:297–301.

75. Drumm B, Sherman P, Cutz E, Karmali M: Association of Campylobacter pylori in the gastric mucosa with antral gastritis in children. N Engl J Med 1987;316:1557–1561.

76. Starr A, Wilson JM: Phlegmonous gastritis. Ann Surg 1957;145:88–93.

77. Miller AI, Smith B, Rogers AI: Phlegmonous gastritis. Gastroenterology 1975;68:231–238.

78. Tierney LM, Gooding G, Bottles K, et al: Phlegmonous gastritis and Hemophilus influenzae peritonitis in a patient with alcoholic liver disease. Dig Dis Sci 1987;32:97–101.

79. Gonzalez-Crussi F, Hackett RL: Phlegmonous gastritis. Arch Surg 1966;93:990–995.

80. Chen ST, Kawai S, Matsumoto H, et al: Acute diffuse phelgmonous gastritis. Jpn J Surg 1980;10:155–158.

81. Murphy JF, Graham DY, Frankel NB, et al: Intramural gastric abscess. Am J Surg 1976; 131:618–621.

82. Weiner CI, Kumpe DA, Diaconis JN: Idiopathic gastric abscess: a bizarre intramural lesion. Am J Gastroenterol 1975;64(6):452–459.

83. Eras P, Goldstein MJ, Sherlock P: Candida infection of the gastrointestinal tract. Medicine 1972;51:367–369.

84. Katzenstein AA, Maksem J: Candidal infection of gastric ulcers, incidence and clinical

significance. Am J Clin Pathol 1979;71:137–141.

85. Parker JC, McCloskey JJ, Knaver KA: Pathobiologic features of human candidiasis. Am J Clin Pathol 1976;65:991–1000.

86. Nelson RS, Bruni H, Goldstein HM: Primary gastric candidiasis in uncompromised subjects. Gastrointest Endosc 1975;22:92–94.

87. Peters M, Weiner J, Whelan G: Fungal infection associated with gastroduodenal ulcerations: Endoscopic and pathologic appearance. Gastroenterology 1980;78:350–354.

88. Thomas E, Reddy KR: Nonhealing duodenal ulceration due to candida. J Clin Gastroenterol 1983;5:55–58.

89. Cronan J, Burrell M, Trepeta R: Aphthoid ulceration in gastric candidiasis. Radiology 1980;134(1):607–611.

90. Piken E, Dwyer R, Zablenma, et al: Gastric candidiasis. JAMA 1978;240:2181–2182.

91. Konok G, Haddad H, Strom B: Post operative gastric mycosis. Surg Gynecol Obstet 1980;150:337–341.

92. Fisher JR, Sanowski RA: Disseminated histoplasmosis producing hypertrophic gastric folds. Am J Dig Dis 1978;23:282–285.

93. Lawson HH, Schmaman A: Gastric phycomycosis. Br J Surg 1974;61:743–746.

94. Dennis JE, Rhodes KH, Cooney DR, et al: Nosocomial rhizopus infection (zygomycosis) in children. J Pediatr 1980;96:824–828.

95. Weisman IM, Moreno AJ, Parker AL, et al: Gastrointestal dissemination of coccidioidomycosis. Am J Gastroenterol 1986;81:589–593.

96. Rotterdam H: Tissue diagnosis of selected AIDS-related opportunistic infections. Am J Surg Pathol 1987;11(suppl):3–15.

97. Hinnant KL, Rotterdam H, Bell ET, et al: Cytomegalovirus infection of the alimentary tract: a clinico-pathological correlation. Am J Gastroenterol 1986;81:944–950.

98. Campbell DA, Piercey JRA, Schnitka TK, et al: Cytomegalovirus associated gastric ulcer. Gastroenterology 1977;72:533–535.

99. Franzin G, Novelli P, Fratton A: Histologic evidence of cytomegalovirus in the duodenal and gastric mucosa of patients with renal allograft. Endoscopy 1980;12:117–120.

100. Sperling HV, Reed WG: Herpetic gastritis. Am J Dig Dis 1977;22:1033–1035.

101. Khilnani MJ, Keller RJ: Roentgen and pathological changes in the gastrointestinal tract in herpes zoster generalization: A unique case and brief review. Mt Sinai Med J 1971;38:303–310.

102. Wisloff F, Bull-Berg J, Myren J: Gastric involvement in herpes zoster. Endoscopy 1980;12(3):134–135.

103. Butz WC, Watts JC, Rosales-Quintana S, et al: Erosive gastritis as a manifestation of secondary syphilis. Am J Clin Pathol 1975;63(2):895–900.

104. Besses C, Sans-Sabraten J, Badia X, et al: Ulcero-infiltrative syphilitic gastropathy: Silver stain diagnosis from biopsy specimen. Am J Gastroenterol 1987;82:773–775.

105. Sacher D, Klein R, Swerdlaw F: Erosive syphilitic gastritis: Dark field and immunofluorescent diagnosis from biopsy specimen. Ann Intern Med 1974;80:512–515.

106. Coley RN, Childers JH: Acquired syphilis of the stomach. Gastroenterology 1960;39:201–207.

107. Morin ME, Tan, A: Diffuse enlargement of gastric folds as a manifestation of secondary syphilis. Am J Gastroenterol 1980;74:170–172.

108. Haggitt RC: Granulomatous diseases of the gastrointestinal tract. In: Ioachim HL (ed), Pathology of Granulomas. New York: Raven Press, 1983:257–305.

109. Eusterman BG: Gastric syphilis: observations based on ninety-three cases. JAMA 1931;96:173–179.

110. Vaughn WP, Straus FH, Paloyan D: Squamous carcinoma of the stomach after luetic linitis plastica. Gastroenterology 1977;72:945–948.

111. Chondhuri G, Sohass, Tandon RK: Gastric ascariasis. Am J Gastroenterol 1986;81:788–790.

112. Palmer ED: Tuberculosis of the stomach and the stomach in tuberculosis. Am Rev Tuberculosis 1950;61:116–130.

113. Keenan DJM: Tuberculous pyloric stenosis. Br J Surg 1981;68:44.

114. Suberi I, Attar B, Schmitt G, et al: Primary gastric tuberculosis: A case report and literature review. Am J Gastroenterol 1987;82:769–772.

115. Misra RC, Agarwal SK, Prakash P: Gastric tuberculosis. Endoscopy 1982;14:235–237.

116. Gillan JS, Urmacher C, West R: Disseminated mycobacterium intracellulare infection in acquired immunodeficiency syndrome,

mimicking Whipple's disease. Gastroenterology 1983;85:1187–1191.

117. Hawkins CC, Gold JWM, Whimbey E, et al *Mycobacterium-avium* complex infections in patients with the acquired immunodeficiency syndrome. Ann Intern Med 1986;105: 184–188.

118. Kuipers FC, Vanthiel PH: Eosinophilic phlegmon of the alimentary canal caused by a worm. Lancet 1960;2:1171–1173.

119. Yokogawa M, Yoshimura H: Clinicopathologic studies on larval anisakiasis in Japan. Am J Trop Dis Hyg 1967;16:723–728.

120. Pinkers GS, Coolidge C, et al: Intestinal anisakiasis: First case reported from North America. Am J Med 1975;59:114–120.

121. Dooley JR, Neafie RC: Anisakiasis. In: Binford CH, Conner DH (eds), Pathology of Tropical and Extraordinary Diseases. Atlas, Volume 2. Washington: AFIP, 1976:475–484.

122. Acosta-Ferveira W, Vercelli-Retta J, Falconi LM: Fasciola hepatica human infections. Virch Arch Pathol Anat Histol 1979;383: 319– 327.

123. Khan MH, Lam R, Tamoney HJ: Isolated granulomatous gastritis. Am J Gastroenterol 1979;71:90–94.

124. Wadina GS, Melamed A: Gastric granuloma (sarcoidosis ?). Am J Gastroenterol 1966;45: 11–39.

125. Morson BC, Dawson IMP: In: Gastrointestinal Pathology. 2nd Edition. Oxford, London, Edinborough, Melbourne: Blackwell Scientific Publications, 1979:112–115.

126. Harned RK, Anderson JK, Owen DR: Suture granulomas following splenectomy. Am J Gastroenterol 1979;72:302–305.

127. Carsky EW, Haswell DM: Huge laparotomy pad simulating a gastric wall tumor. Am J Radiol 1978;131:909–910.

128. Marek J, Jurek K: Comparative light, microscopical and x-ray microanalysis study of barium granuloma. Pathol Res Pract 1981; 71:293–302.

129. Moran TJ, Sherman FE: Production of granulomas of the stomach: Experimental production by intramural infection of foreign material including gastric juice. Am J Clin Pathol 1954;24:422–433.

130. Abell MR, Limond RV, Blamey WE: Allergic granulomatosis with massive gastric involvement. N Engl J Med 1970;282:665–668.

131. Gelb AM, Solan A, Gluck E: Granulomatous vasculitis of the upper gastrointestinal tract: A case report. Mt Sinai J Med 1978;45: 172–178.

132. Lemoine F, Benatre A, Metman EH: Gastrite granulomateuse revelatrice d'une vascularite granulomateuse digestive. Gastroenterol Biol 1983;7:546–548.

133. Scully RE, NcNeely BU: Case records of the Massachusetts General Hospital. N Engl J Med 1974;291:1127–1133.

134. Griscom NT, Kirkpatrick JA, Girdany BR: Gastric antral narrowing in chronic granulomatous disease of childhood. Pediatrics 1974;54:456–460.

135. Johnson FE, Humbert JR, Kuzela DC: Gastric outlet obstruction due to X-linked classic granulomatous disease. Surgery 1975;78: 217–233.

136. Haggitt RC, Meissner WA: Crohn's disease of the upper gastrointestinal tract. Am J Clin Pathol 1973;59:613–622.

137. Fielding JF, Toye DKM, Beton DC, et al: Crohn's disease of the stomach and duodenum. Gut 1970;11:1001–1006.

138. Korelitz BI, Waye JD, Kreuning J, et al: Crohn's disease in endoscopic biopsies of the gastric antrum and duodenum. Am J Gastroenterol 1981;76:103–109.

139. Kyle J: Gastroduodenal involvement in Crohn's disease. J Royal Coll Surg 1982;27: 327–333.

140. Rutgeerts P, Onette E, Vantrappen G: Crohn's disease of the stomach and duodenum: A clinical study with emphasis on the value of endoscopy and endoscopic biopsies. Endoscopy 1980;12:288–294.

141. Badley BWA: Gastric apthae: An initial manifestation of Crohn's disease. Lancet 1981;1: 785–786.

142. Marshak RH, Maklansky D, Kurzban JD: Crohn's disease of the stomach and duodenum. Am J Gastroenterol 1982;77:340–345.

143. Foutch PG, Ferguson DR: Duodenal Crohn's disease complicated by common bile duct obstruction: Report of a case and review of the literature. Am J Gastroenterol 1984;79: 520–524.

144. Altman H, Phillips G, Bank S: Pancreatitis associated with duodenal Crohn's disease. Am J Gastroenterol 1983;78:174–177.

145. Palmer ED: Note on silent sarcoidosis of the gastric mucosa. J Lab Clin Med 1958;52: 231–234.

146. Konda J, Ruth M, Sassaris M: Sarcoidosis of the stomach and rectum. Am J Gastroenterol 1980;73:516–518.

147. Ona FV: Gastric sarcoid: Unusual cause of upper gastrointestinal hemorrhage. Am J Gastroenterol 1981;75:286–288.

148. Fahimi OD, Deren JJ, Gottlieb LS: Isolated granulomatous gastritis: Its relationship to disseminated sarcoidosis and regional enteritis. Gastroenterology 1963;45:161–175.

149. Schinella RA, Ackert J: Isolated granulomatous disease of the stomach: Report of three cases presenting as incidental findings in gastrectomy specimens. Am J Gastroenterol 1979;72:30–35.

150. Weinstock JV: Idiopathic isolated granulomatous gastritis: Spontaneous resolution without surgical intervention. Dig Dis Sci 1980;25:233–235.

151. Kaijser R: Zur Kenntnis der allergischen Affektionen des Verdauungskanals vom Standpunkt des Chirurgen aus. Arch Klin Chir 1937;188:36–64.

152. Johnstone JM, Morson BC: Eosinophilic gastroenteritis. Histopathology 1978;2:335–348.

153. Everett GD, Mitros FA: Eosinophilic gastroenteritis with hepatic eosinophilic granulomas. Am J Gastroenterol 1980;74:519–521.

154. McNabb PC, Fleming CR, Higgins JA: Transmural eosinophilic gastroenteritis with ascites. Mayo Clin Proc 1979;54:119–122.

155. Blackshaw AJ, Levison DA: Eosinophilic infiltrates of the gastrointestinal tract. J Clin Pathol 1986;39:1–17.

156. Haberkern CM, Christie DR, Haas JE: Eosinophilic gastroenteritis presenting as ileocolitis. Gastroenterology 1978;74:896– 899.

157. Levinson JD, Ramanathan VR, Nozick JH: Eosinophilic gastroenteritis as ascites and colon involvement. Am J Gastroenterol 1977;68:603–607.

158. Teele RL, Katz AJ, Goldman H, et al: Radiographic features of eosinophilic gastroenteritis (allergic gastropathy) of childhood. Am J Radiol 1979;123(2):575–580.

159. Katz AJ, Goldman H, Grand RJ: Gastric mucosal biopsy in eosinophilic (allergic) gastroenteritis. Gastroenterology 1977;73:705–709.

160. Morson BC, Dawson IMP: In: Gastrointestinal Pathology. 2nd Edition. Oxford: Blackwell Scientific Publications, 1979:316.

161. Caldwell JH, Sharma HM, Hurtubise PE: Eosinophilic gastroenteritis in extreme allergy. Gastroenterology 1979;77:560–564.

162. Caldwell JH, Mekhjian HS, Hurtubise PE: Eosinophilic gastroenteritis with obstruction: Immunologic studies of seven patients. Gastroenterology 1977;74:825–829.

163. Suen KS, Burton JD: The spectrum of eosinophilic infiltration of the gastrointestinal tract and its relationship to other disorders of angiitis and granulomatosis. Hum Pathol 1979;10:31–43.

164. DeSchryver-Keeskemeti K, Clouse RE: A previously unrecognized subgroup of "eosinophilic gastroenteritis": Association with connective tissue diseases. Am J Surg Pathol 1984;8:171–180.

165. Konrad EA, Meister P: Fatal eosinophilic gastroenteritis in a two-year-old child. Virch Arch A Pathol Anat Histol 1979;382:347–353.

166. Franzin G, Novelli P: Gastritis cystica profunda. Histopathology 1981;5:535–547.

167. Elta GH, Iawaz KA, Doyal Y, et al: Chronic erosive gastritis–a recently recognized disorder. Dig Dis Sci 1983;28:7–12.

168. Gallagher CG, Lennon JR, Crowe JP: Chronic erosive gastritis: A clinical study. Am J Gastroenterol 1987;82:302–307.

169. Højgaard L, Krag E: Chronic ischemic gastritis reversed after revascularization operation. Gastroenterology 1987;92:226–228.

CHAPTER 5

Peptic Ulceration

History

Peptic ulcers, like the poor, seem to have always been with us. Gaius Pliny, in the 1st century (as translated in the 17th century) stated that "receits for the paine of stomake and loines—If there be an ulcer growne in the stomacke, drinke the milke of an asse or cow and it will heal it."[1] Galen recognized gastric ulcer from autopsy studies. The first complete description of the pathology and symptoms is attributed to Matthew Ballie in 1793.[2] Cruveilhier differentiated ulcer from gastric ulcer. In 1817, Trevers,[3] described very clearly the finding of sharply marginated small perforating ulcers at autopsy in fatal cases of perforated ulcer of the stomach and duodenum, and differentiated such ulcers from those of scrofula and dysentery. He also reported a case in which the peritoneum had sealed off a deep ulcer of the stomach in an elderly patient who died of another unstated cause.

Most attention in the 19th century was directed to gastric rather than duodenal ulceration, although Curling, in his classic paper of 1842, described typical duodenal ulcers occurring 7 to 17 days after extensive burns. In one such ulcer, he noted a large open vessel in the base. He stated that "the origin of the mischief must be referred to some sympathetic cause," i.e., compensatory oversecretion of Brunner's glands compensating for "suppression of exhalation from the skin."[4]

In the mid 19th century, two views on pathogenesis were current. Virchow favored factors of vascular insufficiency or occlusion leading to mucosal damage as being the initiating cause. In contrast, Rokitansky is quoted as viewing peptic ulceration as secondary to morbid conditions of innervation resulting in excessive acidification of the stomach.[5] However, it would seem that he was referring to gastromalasia in newborns or cachetic individuals and, at least in that book, did not offer opinions on the cause of the common chronic ulcer. Cushing[6] drew on Rokitansky's views when he published his famous series of cases of peptic ulceration associated with central nervous system disorders. These ulcers were variously situated in the esophagus, stomach, and duodenum. Although some of these were peptic ulcers, for the most part acute, others were erosions or what could probably be referred to now as hemorrhagic gastritis.

By the end of the 19th century, the consensus was that peptic ulcer was secondary to excessive acidity and gastric secretion—a view that we now realize is not valid for many ulcers. For further information, the reader is referred to Zucker and Clayman's interesting recent historical review.[2]

We would close this brief account with two quotations that in some respects are still apropos. In 1842, Curling[4] stated: "In no part of the alimentary canal are the diseases to which it is liable as obscure, both in their origin and diagnosis, as in the duodenum."

Second, Cushing,[6] writing in 1932, made the interesting observations: "Old hypotheses, long forgotten, are from time to time reviewed. The fact that in defense of each one a strong brief could be written indicates that in all probability, more than one causative element be concerned. It is indeed possible that several hypotheses, i.e., vascular, traumatic, bacterial, biochemical and so on are capable of being harmonized." The remainder of this chapter will attempt to summarize current information and views and certainly support his multifactorial view of the situation, although total consensus has yet to be accomplished.

Definition

Peptic ulceration may be broadly, though negatively, defined as circumscribed mucosal defects of the gastrointestinal tract not secondary to neoplasm, infection, or obvious infarction. In general, such ulcerations require the presence of an acid/pepsin mix as one factor in their pathogenesis. Well documented exceptions do occur, particularly with certain erosions and extremely rarely in chronic peptic ulcer.[7,8] However, in general, the adage "no acid no ulcer" remains valid. Ulcers so defined may occur at any site subject to exposure to an acid/pepsin mix (i.e., esophagus, stomach, and small intestine) either at sites normally exposed to acid, or via reflux or in mucosa adjacent to areas of gastric parietal cell ectopia—as in Meckel's diverticulum. This does not imply that the acid/pepsin mix in contact to such damaged mucosa is necessarily of abnormal amount or concentration, as will be developed below.

Peptic ulceration is divided into the categories of erosions, acute ulcers, and chronic ulcers. We will follow Morson and Dawson's definitions,[9] which have the virtue of simplicity.

Erosion: A circumscribed loss of mucosa not involving the full thickness of the mucosa.

Acute Ulcer: A circumscribed lesion involving the full thickness of the mucosa and which may or may not involve deeper layers but is not accompanied by an appreciable fibrotic reaction.

Chronic Peptic Ulcer: A circumscribed defect of variable depth of the wall of the viscus in which a fibrotic reactive process is readily apparent.

These categories should not be thought of simply as stages of chronic ulcer since there are sharp differences in site, clinical milieu, and pathogenesis between erosions and acute ulcers on the one hand and chronic peptic ulcer on the other. This is not to deny that any ulcer, chronic or not, must presumably begin as an erosion.

Erosions and Acute Peptic Ulcer

Erosions are sharply demarcated circular or ovoid lesions usually of only a few millimeters in diameter (Fig. 5-1). They vary somewhat in appearance, and endoscopists have classified them into a so-called complete type (type I)—a lesion with an elevated border and flat base—and an incomplete (type II)—a lesion that is flat—as well as a type III erosion, which is basically a hemorrhagic spot (Fig. 5-2). The complete type is considered to be a more chronic phase.[10] The ulcer bed may be composed of blood clot or consist of a grayish necrotic area of slough. In some, cystic dilatation of adjacent foveolae has been reported.[10] Erosions are said to appear within several days, as judged by endoscopy, and frequently disappear rapidly, leaving no residual scar. They may occur anywhere and commonly in acid-secreting areas of the mucosa. For a discussion of chronic erosive gastritis, see Chapter 4.

Acute ulcers, since they are of deeper penetrance (Fig. 5-3), should heal with some residua. Perhaps these explain the endoscopic finding of small scars in acid-secreting areas of the stomach that have been identified endoscopically with the use of installation of Congo Red—which turns blue at low

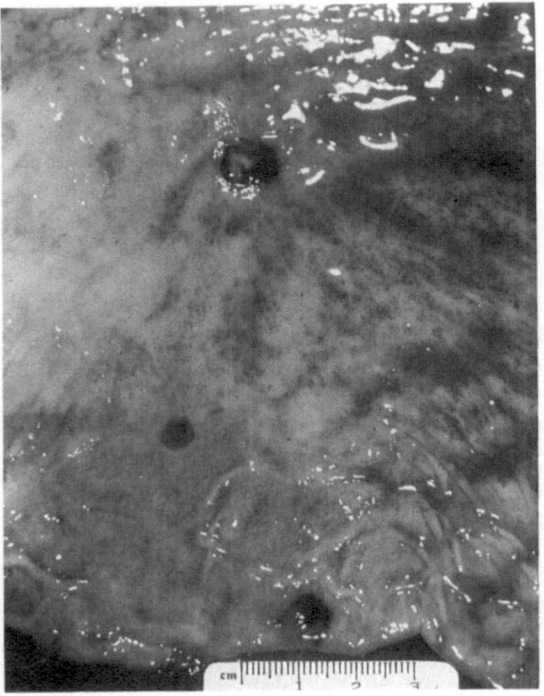

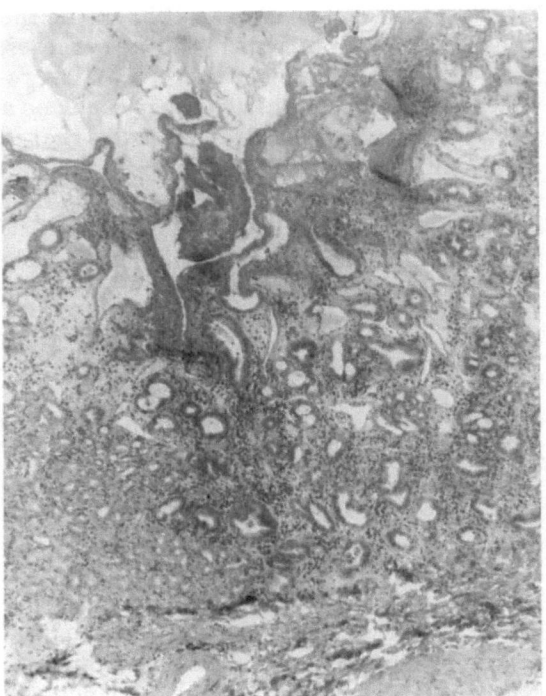

Figure 5-1. Acute ulcers and erosions from a patient who died of cardiogenic shock.

Figure 5-2. Erosion of fundic mucosa showing fibrin, drop-out of glands, and early regeneration in a patient with a past history of massive bleeding and multiple transfusions. H&E, X63, reproduced at 60%.

pH—a site not typical for chronic peptic ulcer.[11]

Erosions shade into hemorrhagic erosive gastritis on the one hand and into acute ulcer on the other. They were originally an observation made at autopsy and considered of debatable significance. Since then, the term has often been used almost interchangeably with "stress ulcer" and "hemorrhagic gastritis." However, erosions appear in differing settings:

1. as a component of the "stress syndrome,"
2. associated with chronic peptic ulceration and/or antral gastritis, and
3. secondary to aspirin or other agents known to impair the "mucosal barrier."

The first is closely linked with the so-called "stress syndrome" (i.e., in patients severely ill after massive trauma, extensive burns, cachetic states, major operative procedures,

sepsis, shock, or hemorrhage). In all of these conditions, as in hemorrhagic gastritis, multiple erosions or acute ulcers may form in the stomach or a single acute ulcer may occur in the duodenum, often with an associated acute gastritis or duodenitis. Ulcers in this background tend to be painless and asymptomatic until the onset of major hemorrhage or complications secondary to perforation, which may occur rapidly.

In the past, the incidence of stress ulceration has been understated. In those instances where routine gastroscopy has been performed in the presence of a major risk factor (such as those mentioned above), it has been high. Thus, in a study of adults with major burns, 86% developed erosions for the most part within the first several days following the burn.[12] Similarly, acute lesions were identified endoscopically in 75% of patients with major head injury.[13] Many of these cases were silent, and the erosions and ulcerations were often difficult to pick up on radiologic examinations. Such erosions can apparently appear and disappear rapidly, to some degree paralleling the patient's general well-being. Bleeding may be extensive from such erosions.

The pathogenesis remains obscure. It is definitely not related to abnormal increases in acid secretions, with the possible exception of those occurring after certain head injuries with presumed vagal stimulation. On the other hand, the presence of acid seems essential in most cases, and management efforts to lower acid secretion and neutralize or remove acids from the stomachs of patients at high risk have both been advocated and appear effective in preventing the occurrence of the ulcerations.[14] The common denominator in most cases is hypovolemia, either on the basis of shock or splanchnic shunting of blood. It is thought that the preferential site of such ulcers in the acid-secreting portions of the mucosa may relate to high demands for oxygen of the parietal cells, causing them to be more susceptible to ischemic damage. The loss of blood flow would also produce a relative acidosis of the mucosa and prevent rapid dilution of backed-diffusing hydrogen ions. Similarly, blood flow would also reduce the availability of bicarbonate ion HCO_3^- and ATP (see Fig. 5-4).

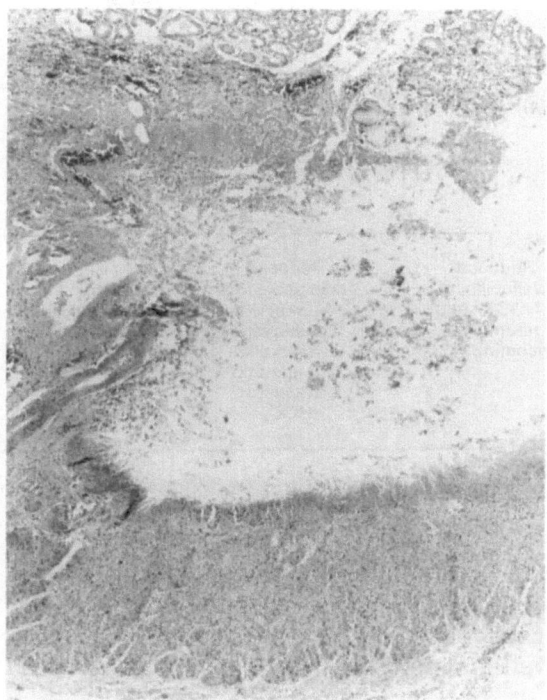

Figure 5-3. Acute ulcer of duodenum. Note necrosis extending into muscularis and necrosis of artery in ulcer bed. Patient was a 39-year-old male who died after brain surgery, in part from massive duodenal hemorrhage. H&E, X40, reproduced at 60%.

"Nonstress" Erosions and Acute Ulcers

Not all erosions occur in this setting. Karvonen and co-workers[10] reported on a very large series of patients undergoing elective gastroscopy. Presumably, all of these patients had some type of gastrointestinal problem, although this was not elucidated. A history of present or past peptic ulceration was reported in 30% of the cases. Among their very large series of patients, 10% were shown to have erosions, either small erosions scattered about the fundus or larger and fewer erosions in the prepyloric area, or both. Nine of their cases were said to be achlorhydric, whereas those erosions nearer the pylorus tended to be associated with acid secretion and peptic ulceration.

Morgan and associates[15] reported a group of patients with histories of dyspeptic symptoms, negative findings on barium meal examination, and multiple erosions in the antral lesser curvature. These seemed to relate to acute superficial gastritis. The erosions (acute ulcers?) did not respond well to conventional ulcer therapy and tended to persist. Obvious bleeding was lacking, and several patients required surgical therapy (highly selective vagotomy) for relief of symp-

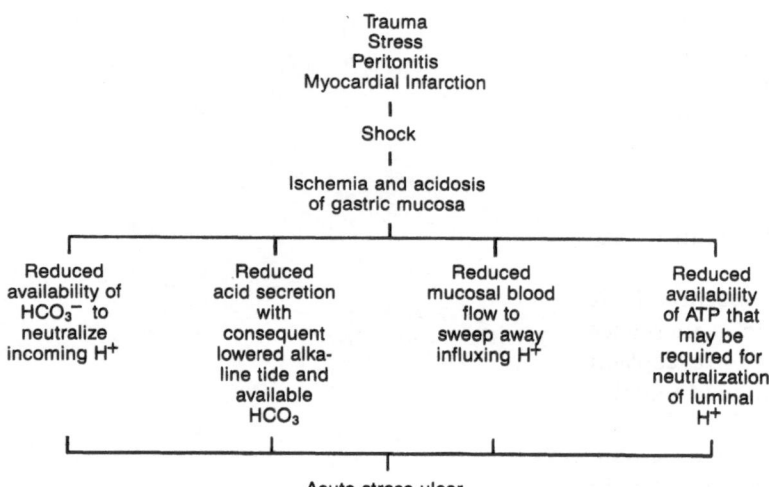

Trauma
Stress
Peritonitis
Myocardial Infarction
|
Shock
|
Ischemia and acidosis
of gastric mucosa

Reduced availability of HCO_3^- to neutralize incoming H^+

Reduced acid secretion with consequent lowered alkaline tide and available HCO_3

Reduced mucosal blood flow to sweep away influxing H^+

Reduced availability of ATP that may be required for neutralization of luminal H^+

Acute stress ulcer

Figure 5-4. Factors and mechanisms for the production of stress ulcers. From Silen,[14] with permission.

toms. Although all of these erosions appear similar, it is clear there must be varying mechanisms of pathogenesis that are still not well understood.

Aspirin-Related Erosions and Ulceration

Although the association of aspirin with chronic peptic ulcer is debatable, there is no doubt that aspirin in the presence of acid will rapidly produce erosions and subsequent blood loss. This has been shown both experimentally and clinically. Oral intake of aspirin nearly always produces some gastric bleeding, usually in the magnitude of a few milliliters per day. This has been noted by experimental studies[16-18] using chromate-labeled red cells. Such bleeding is not prevented by simultaneous ingestion of milk or food. It is greater in the presence of preexisting lesions such as chronic gastritis,[19] peptic ulcer,[20,21] or esophageal varices.[16] In some instances, massive hemorrhage has been precipitated by aspirin ingestion, usually only in those who have such associated lesions, particularly peptic ulcer.[21,22]

Disruption of the apical membrane of surface cells has been demonstrated by scanning electron microscopy (EM). Minute erosions were seen endoscopically in 60% of healthy volunteers 15 minutes after administration of 600 mg of aspirin.[18] Acute erosions have also been observed endoscopically near particles of aspirin in the stomach.[20] There is no correlation between the occurrence of hemorrhage and known aspirin intolerance.[20] The damage is rapidly reversible within 24 to 48 hours. Although the mechanism is not totally understood, the usually accepted view is that aspirin at a pH above 3.5 is largely ionized and water soluble. At a lower pH it is nonionized and lipid soluble. Under these circumstances, it dissolves the protein lipid membrane of gastric cells and diffuses into the cell. In the higher intracellular pH of the cell environment, it ionizes and produces cell damage leading to hydrogen ion ($H+$) leakage through the damaged mucosa. This, in turn, causes histamine release, which stimulates acid secretion and increases capillary permeability. Duggan,[23] in a critical review, pointed out that this mechanism does not explain experimental mucosal damage by intravenous salicylates in cats, in which no alteration of the mucosal potential difference occurs, nor does it explain the potentiating effects of alcohol. He supports the idea that nonsteroid antiinflammatory compounds (such as aspirin) concentrate in secretory and absorptive tissue (such as gastric and small intestinal mucosa), producing cellular damage that may be mediated by the effect of aspirin in reducing prostaglandin E, under which circumstances, increased acid secretion and vasoconstriction would be expected. This cytotoxic effect is prevented or reduced by histamin (H-2) blocking agents and prostaglandin E_2. One effect, at least in the case of aspirin, appears to be the breakdown of the macromolecules of glycoprotein (i.e., the mucosal barrier).[24,25] Experimentally, glucagon protects against salicylate damage, perhaps by inhibition of acid secretion.[18]

Alcohol and caffeine may potentiate damage by increasing the need of surface tissue for oxygen in the presence of vasoconstriction. Certain other drugs (such as indomethecin, tolmetin, and proprionic acid derivatives) also may damage gastric mucosa, although the effect is less severe than that of salicylates.

Chronic Peptic Ulcer

Incidence

Peptic ulceration is a major health problem, particularly in regard to morbidity and with a much lower, but significant, mortality. Incidence and prevalence of gastric and duodenal ulcers differ sharply, reflecting the fact that in many respects they represent different diseases. These differences vary interestingly in a historic manner. In the 19th century, duodenal ulcer, as stated above, was almost disregarded, and gastric ulcer was considered the predominant type of peptic ulceration, usually in women. The early records, of course, mainly reflect prevalence figures from autopsy populations. Ivy and coworkers (quoted by Spiro[26]) reported that prior to 1900, duodenal ulcer was noted only in 0.1 to 0.3% of autopsies, a figure that increased to about 1% at the turn of the century and, after 1913, ranged from 2.2 to 3.9%. Autopsy records during the 1930s[27] and 1950s[28] indicated a prevalence of from 3.7 to 4% of either gastric or duodenal ulcers. Other reports have ranged up to the extraordinary figure of 24% from The Netherlands. More current figures of incidence in the general population from the United States and the United Kingdom range in males from 1 to 3.5 per thousand per year for duodenal ulcers and about 0.5 per thousand per year for gastric ulcer, with the figures for females being about 25 to 40% those of males in the duodenum and 60 to 80% in the stomach.[29] Although the male/female ratio for duodenal ulcer has always been much higher than that for gastric ulcer, with figures as high as 6 to 1 reported from Hong Kong, the male/female ratio appears to be declining.[30] There have been a number of recent reports citing sharp declines in hospital admissions and ulcer mortality in the United Kingdom. Kurata[30] discussed this critically, pointing out that there are problems in knowing whether this is a true decrease in incidence due to fewer presumptive diagnoses of ulcer since endoscopy has been more widely used, or a decrease reported as a result of changes in hospitalization criteria and coding practices. He pointed out that hospitalization rates and mortality are by no means uniform. Sonnenberg and Fritsch indicated that in Germany during the period of 1955 to 1975, the rates of absenteeism for peptic ulceration had actually increased while the rate of hospitalization has remained the same. Figures from Hong Kong[32] from 1970 to 1980 show a 21% increase in admissions and a 14% decrease in mortality during that period. Thus, it would certainly be premature to state that duodenal ulcer, in particular, is a passing disease, although there is some evidence to suggest a decrease in some parts of the world. Mortality rate estimates given by Kurata and coworkers[33] for 1982 are 3 per 100,000. Again, in the United States admissions for duodenal ulcer have decreased by 41% and death due to peptic ulcer, in general, by about 30% in recent decades. This decline appears to have begun before the use of cimetidine. As already stated, above, there may be many factors involved in this, and Karata and co-

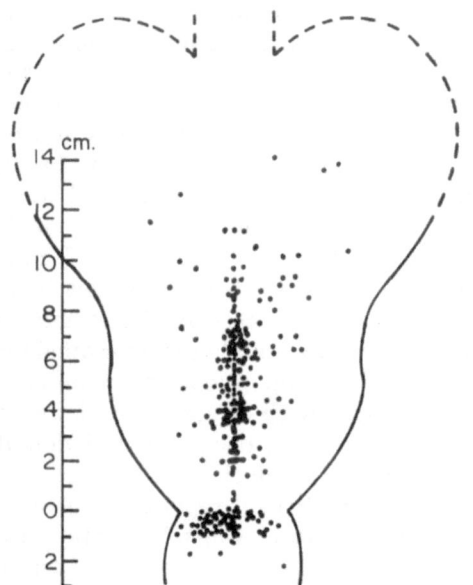

Figure 5-5. The location of duodenal and gastric ulcers. Location of 170 ulcers in stomach alone in 140 resected specimens, and of 93 ulcers in duodenum alone in 80 resected specimens (cases of associated gastric and duodenal ulcers are omitted). From Oi and Sakurai,[36] with permission.

workers[33] suggest that the situation needs critical review.

In a study covering the years 1922 to 1927, gastric ulcer was said to predominate by a four to one margin, especially in males. In contrast, in a very large necropsy study in Chicago and published in 1938,[37] duodenal ulcer was found to be more common than gastric. Gastric ulcer, in addition to showing a reduced male to female sex ratio, tends to occur in an older age group. It is estimated that about 1 in 10 American males will develop a peptic ulcer at some stage of their life.

Spiro[36] points out marked variations in race. For instance, in Sumatra, 11% of the Chinese are said to have peptic ulcer, in contrast to less than 1% in Javanese. In Africa, duodenal ulcer in blacks is rare in some areas, although there seems to be little or no racial difference in the United States.[34] The ratio of gastric to duodenal ulcer also

appears to vary sharply; for instance, in the Andes, gastric ulcer is said to be 20 times more common than duodenal ulcer.

Site

Stomach and duodenum are, of course, the major sites of peptic ulceration, in sum being 98 to 99% of the total.[35] Peptic ulcer occurs also, of course, in the esophagus secondary to reflux, in the ileal mucosa adjacent to Meckel's diverticulum secondary to ectopic acid-secreting mucosa, and in the jejunum in hypersecreting states such as the Zollinger-Ellison syndrome.

It has been realized for many years that chronic peptic ulceration of the stomach is concentrated along the lesser curvature and is rare at or near the greater curvature. In the duodenum, the vast majority are within 1 cm of the pyloric ring. This is well shown in the diagram of plotted ulcer locations in Figure 5-5. As Kirk[37] states, "Ulcers extend in a continuous band from high in the gastric lesser curvature to the angulus, where there is a concentration and then along the roof of the antrum through the pylorus to a second concentration in the upper half of the proximal duodenal bulb."

The factors influencing the site of ulceration are of interest and shed light on the pathogenesis, which will be discussed in more detail later. Oi and co-workers[36,38] were perhaps the first to emphasize that in the stomach, peptic ulcers are usually just distal to the border zone between the acid-secreting glands and the pyloric antral type of mucosa. It has been shown that this border zone is quite variable, with much individual variation as well as extension with age. Similarly, in the duodenum, the ulcer tends to be very close to the junction of duodenal and pyloric mucosa.

In the stomach, chronic ulcers generally are not only found in nonacid secreting mucosa, but also in mucosa showing evidence of chronic gastritis.[39]

The localization of ulcer in the antral-type mucosa may indicate a lesser resistance of

Table 5.1. Peptic Ulceration in Childhood and Infancy*

Age	Number	Primary	Secondary	Gastric	Duodenal
1 mo	23	6	17	19	4
1 mo–1 yr	6	0	6	0	6
1 yr–18 yr	32	25	7	10	22

*Modified from Tolia et al.[44] Reproduced by permission. JB Lippincott.

injury of this mucosa, but more likely relates to the accompanying chronic gastritis that is frequently associated with intestinal-type metaplasia. Since the latter has absorptive elements, it is presumably more permeable to acid than would be normal mucosa. Such a relation to chronic gastritis has been shown in studies from many parts of the world. Similarly, evidence from endoscopic studies indicates a high association of surrounding duodenitis as well as gastritis with duodenal ulcer, the duodenitis often showing evidence of gastric metaplasia.[40]

There can well be arguments as to whether the gastritis or duodenitis is cause or effect. The evidence suggests that chronic inflammation may persist or even advance despite ulcer healing, indicating that it is not at least directly caused by the ulceration.[39]

Since ulcers develop not in acid-secreting mucosa but in the antral-type mucosa, close to its border with acid-secreting mucosa, it follows that the more distal the ulcer, the greater the mass of acid-secreting mucosa that relates directly with parietal acid secretion. Thus, other factors must be involved since if there were simply the gastritis, per se, one would expect a more random pattern within the antral gastritis, which is not the case.

Of course, there are exceptions to the above. Benign gastric ulcers do occur in the greater curvature, though rarely.[41] It is not clear whether such cases are necessarily in fundic-type mucosa or whether they may reflect a very extensive gastritis and "antral metaplasia."

In the duodenum, the site is not determined by a jet stream effect from gastric contents hitting the duodenal wall.[42] The many factors involved in the site of ulceration are well reviewed by Kirk.[42]

Multiplicity

From 20 to 40% of gastric ulcers are reported as multiple, with the higher figure reported from a Japanese population.[38] Most commonly, only two such ulcers are present, although rarely more may occur. Duodenal ulcers are still more frequently solitary, although "kissing" anterior and posterior duodenal ulcers certainly occur. About 6% of patients will have simultaneous gastric and duodenal ulcers.[38]

Age

Peptic ulceration may occur at any age, though it is rare in those younger than 30 years of age. Autopsy studies suggest a peak incidence of duodenal ulcer at about age 30 and of gastric at about 50.[37] Peptic ulceration in infancy and childhood is rare but well recognized, and differs in some respects in its presentation and complications from that of the more usual type. In infancy, there is a higher incidence of single and perforating ulcers than in the adult.[43] Most ulcers during early infancy are secondary to other disease entities (such as sepsis) and belong with the more acute stress-type ulceration pattern. Nearly one-third of cases of children with so-called primary peptic ulceration (i.e., ulceration not associated with the "stress syndrome" such as sepsis and trauma) have a positive family history for peptic ulcerations (Table 5.1).[45]

Most reports of early onset peptic ulceration have emphasized the tendency for mas-

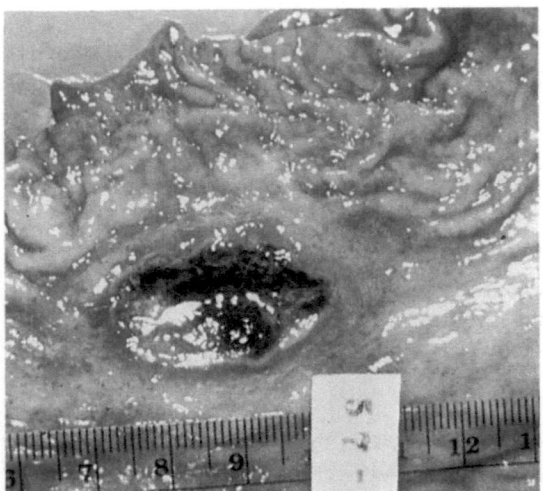

Figure 5-6. Typical peptic ulcer of stomach. Note sharp margins and flat base covered with grayish exudate.

sive hemorrhage and perforation. Thus, in Johnson and co-workers' report of cases occurring before 11 weeks of age,[46] 7 of the 16 cases had rapid onset of gastrointestinal (GI) bleeding and/or perforation. Recurrent vomiting may also be a presenting feature.

Gross Findings

Gastric ulcers are usually 2 cm or less in diameter (Fig. 5-6). However, the old dictum that any ulcer larger than 5 cm was, of necessity, malignant is not true. Gigantic ulcers of the stomach have been reported enlarging in a saddle-shaped manner across the antral lesser curvature or in a longitudinal fashion, the so-called "trench ulcer"[47] (Fig. 5-7). The edges of such ulcers are clear-cut and sharp and have a flat grayish base of necrotic debris, often described as "cookie cutter" ulcers. In an endoscopic study, Gear and associates[39] stated that ulcers of the body tend to be distinctly larger than those of the prepyloric area, averaging 1 to 3 or 4 cm, in contrast to 0.5 to 1 cm for those in the prepyloric region.

Histology

The histology has been well defined for many years and is summarized by Trier[48] as showing four distinct layers, the most superficial being a mesh of fibrin with admixed acute and chronic inflammatory cells. Beneath this is a zone of more or less amorphous granular

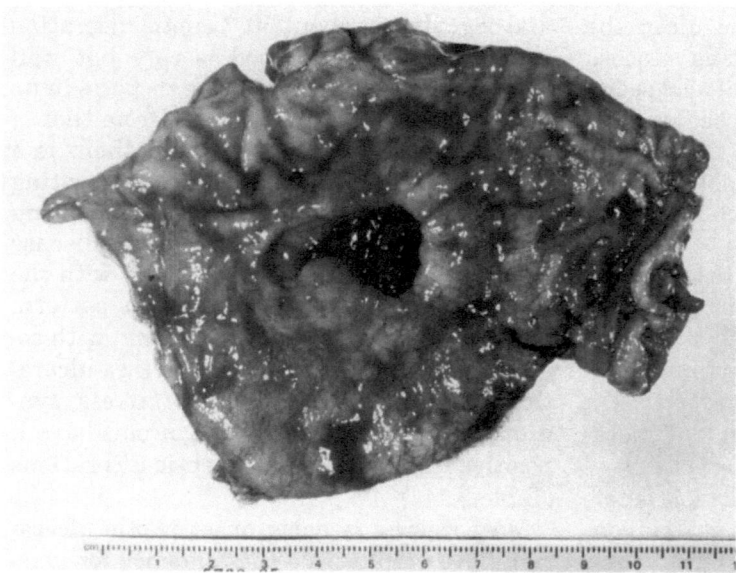

Figure 5-7. Chronic gastric ulcer, enlarging in a longitudinal fashion.

Figure 5-8. Typical bed of chronic ulcer. Note layers of necrotic debris and fibrin, granulation tissue, and fibrosis. H&E, X63, reproduced at 60%.

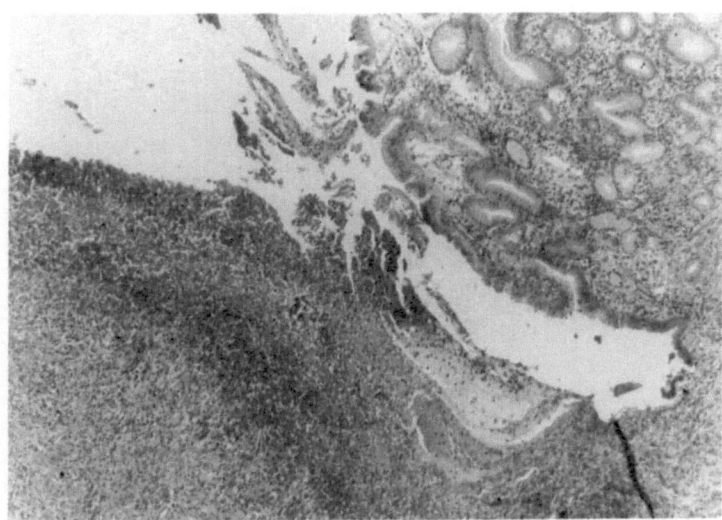

eosinophilic material representing necrotic debris. Deep to this layer is a layer of granulation tissue, which fades into a dense fibrotic layer (Fig. 5-8). The muscularis propria is usually sharply interrupted (Fig. 5-9) and replaced by fibrous tissue. The "cut" end of the muscularis propria is frequently pulled up and fused with the muscularis mucosae. The vessels are often prominent in the fibrotic base and may show thrombi in various stages of organization or occasionally, in rapidly advancing ulcers, acutely necrotic walls. The amount of fibrosis around the vessels is impressive, which possibly contributes to the degree of hemorrhage by preventing the normal retraction and contraction of a vessel when it is cut or, in this case, destroyed by acid (Fig. 5-10). The ulcers are of various depths, and it is not uncommon for the ulceration to extend well out into the surrounding adventitia of the stomach, even in patients without a history of perforation. In such

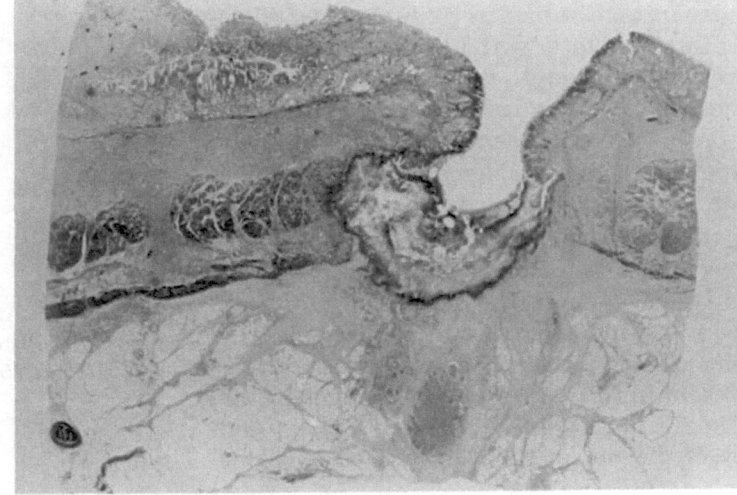

Figure 5-9. Whole-mount section of chronic gastric ulcer extending to adventitia. Note sharp separation (*dark line*) of necrotic debris and underlying granulation tissue and fibrosis. Note sharp "cut off of muscularis." Trichrome.

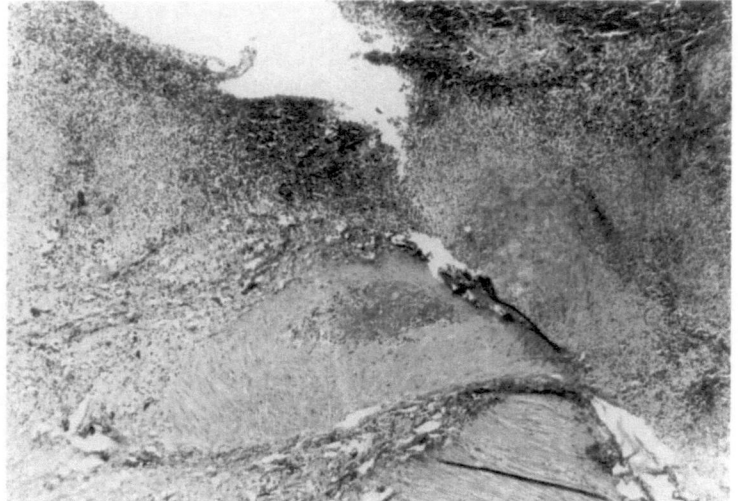

Figure 5-10. Erosion of artery in bed of chronic gastric ulcer. H&E, X50, reproduced at 60%.

cases, factors of repair and fibrosis at least balance those concerned with ulceration.

As has been mentioned before, the surrounding mucosa is rarely of the parietal type, but rather is composed of mucosa showing chronic gastritis and, very commonly, intestinal metaplasia. The gastritis is evidence by an increase of lymphocytes and plasma cells in the lamina propria, with a variable number of polymorphonuclear leukocytes which may, if marked, accumulate in the form of microabscesses.[49] As ulcers heal, the necrotic zone is replaced by granulation tissue and fibrosis, and the epithelium regenerates—at first as a simple layer of epithelium and later with all mucosal elements present, although to a usually reduced degree. The specialized glands may be poorly represented or absent. Parietal cells and chief cells are occasionally seen, although not usually associated with well defined parietal type glands. Intestinal metaplasia is common in such regenerated epithelium and tends to reflect the metaplasia of the surrounding mucosa.[49] As in any regenerated epithelium, a certain degree of atypism is present in the earlier phases of regeneration (Fig. 5-11). Attention to the vesicular quality of the nuclei and the lack of a marked

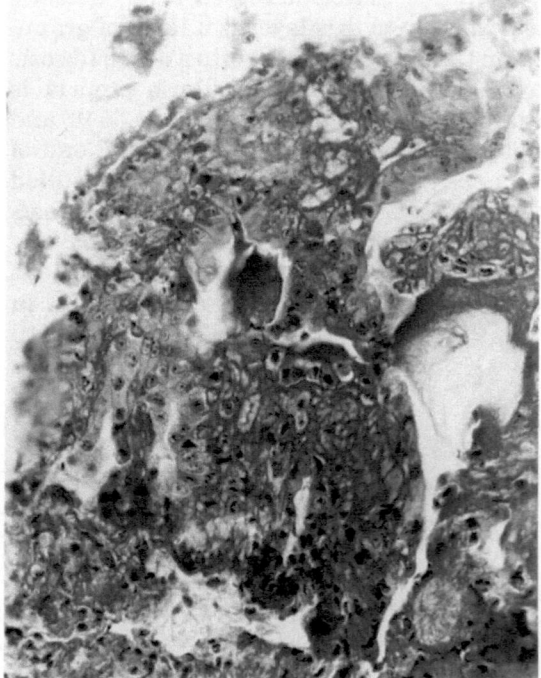

Figure 5-11. Atypical regenerating epithelium growing into fibrin. Section from biopsy of ulcer edge. H&E, X250, reproduced at 60%.

increase in the nuclear/cytoplasmic ratio should prevent mistaking such epithelium for carcinoma in biopsy material. At times, this can be a difficult problem. A conservative attitude is urged (see the section Relationship of Peptic Ulcer to Gastric Carcinoma). Evidence of old scars from past ulceration are not uncommon in gastrectomy specimens in which an unhealed ulcer is present. There is usually some distortion of the rugae forming a radiating pattern from such old ulcers (Fig. 5-12).

Duodenal Ulcers

Duodenal ulcers are grossly and histologically very similar to those of the stomach, although perhaps more often somewhat irregular. The site, as previously mentioned, is close to the pyloric ring as a rule and usually in the anterior or posterior aspect of the first portion of the duodenal bulb. Again, as in gastric ulcer, there is commonly a surrounding chronic duodenitis.[40] Most duodenal ulcers are very modest in size, averaging less than 1 cm. So-called giant duodenal ulcers are reported, however, ranging in size from 2 to 5 cm. These latter are more often located in the posterior wall or beyond the bulb.[50]

Complications of Peptic Ulceration

Complications may be listed as:

1. hemorrhage,
2. perforation,
3. obstruction, and
4. pancreatitis.

Hemorrhage of massive amount occurs in from 15 to 20% of patients. Bleeding from a gastric ulcer tends to be more frequent than from a duodenal ulcer, more massive when it occurs, and with a tendency to recur in over half the cases.[51] Perforation occurs in less than 10% of cases, usually from the anterior aspect of the antral lesser curvature (Fig. 5-13) or from the anterior aspect of the duodenal bulb (Fig. 5-14). In about 5% of cases, deep penetration, well beyond the serosa, occurs without actual perforation.[52] Penetration may present in bizarre forms and has been described as extending into the spleen,[53] pericardium, and heart,[54] and even into the subcutaneous tissue in a case of ulcer

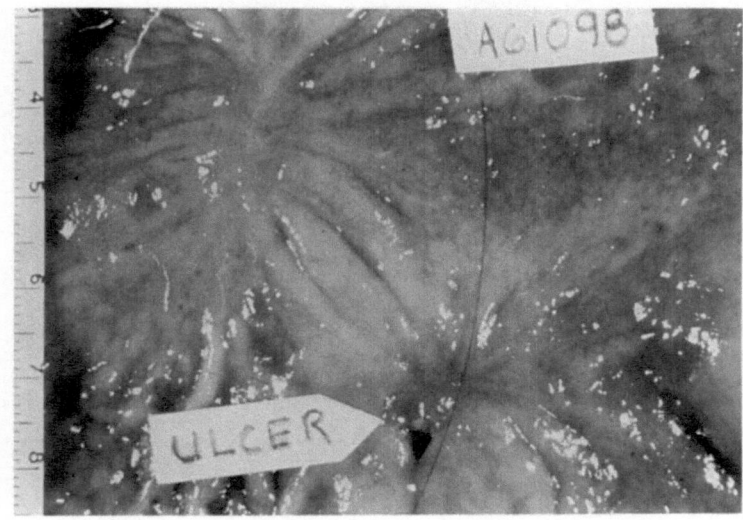

Figure 5-12. Active and healed gastric ulcer. Note radiating folds of mucosa centering on healed ulcer.

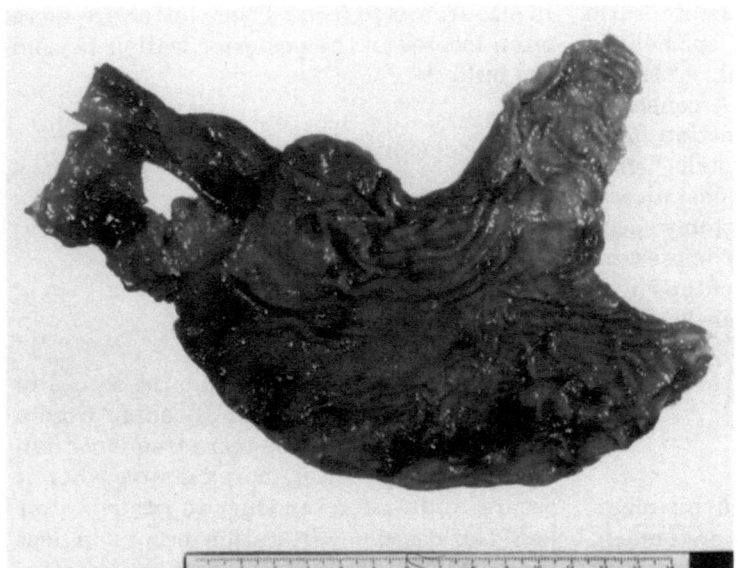

Figure 5-13. Perforated gastric ulcer of the antrum.

in an incarcerated hiatal hernia.[55] Penetration into the liver may yield liver tissue in an endoscopic biopsy (Fig. 5-15).

Acute pancreatitis is a more common finding and usually associated with the more acute variants of duodenal ulcer. It may, of course, frequently be a fatal complication.

Perforation is uncommon in those younger than 40 years of age, with an increasing incidence in those who are older than 40 years. Spillage is initially sterile. In a review of 150 perforated duodenal and 32 perforated gastric ulcers, Fong[56] reported only 22 cases of postoperative abscesses, 26 cases of wound

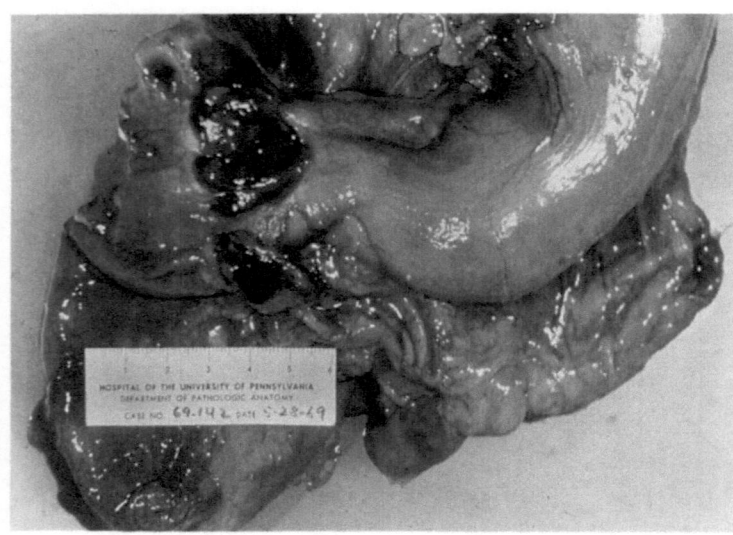

Figure 5-14. Large perforated duodenal ulcer with pancreatitis.

infection, and 18 cases of peritonitis, usually in those with delay in diagnosis or operation.

Obstruction is unusual. It is reported in less than 5% of cases and, as might be expected, is seen chiefly in prepyloric and high duodenal ulcers.

A "double pylorus" has been reported,[57] which may represent a rare complication of deeply penetrating pyloric and prepyloric ulcers. However, it is possible that some such cases may be congenital.[57]

Pathogenesis of Peptic Ulcer

Introduction

It is impossible to define any one factor as common to all peptic ulcers, whether gastric or duodenal, unless it be the presence of at least some acid/pepsin mix in contact with the ulcerated mucosa. As already mentioned, there are even a few rare exceptions to this. The situation is much more complex than previously thought, and most concur with Rotter[58] that peptic ulcer is a group of diseases having in common a hole in the gastrointestinal lining. Therefore, one cannot expect one explanation to cover all cases, just as very diverse factors may lead to anemia. Certainly gastric and duodenal ulcers must be considered separately, and gastric ulcers themselves do not represent a uniform set. As Carter[29] suggests, no single theory of pathogenesis can explain gastric or duodenal ulcer. In the final analysis, the cause of chronic ulceration must be found in the interplay between factors causing digestion of mucosa, factors resisting digestion (the mucosal barrier) and, as Wormsley[59] stresses, factors aiding or preventing the healing of mucosal breaks. We will attempt to review this situation, realizing these difficulties. For those wishing to delve further into this complex area, refer to the references, particularly the review references.[29,58,60]

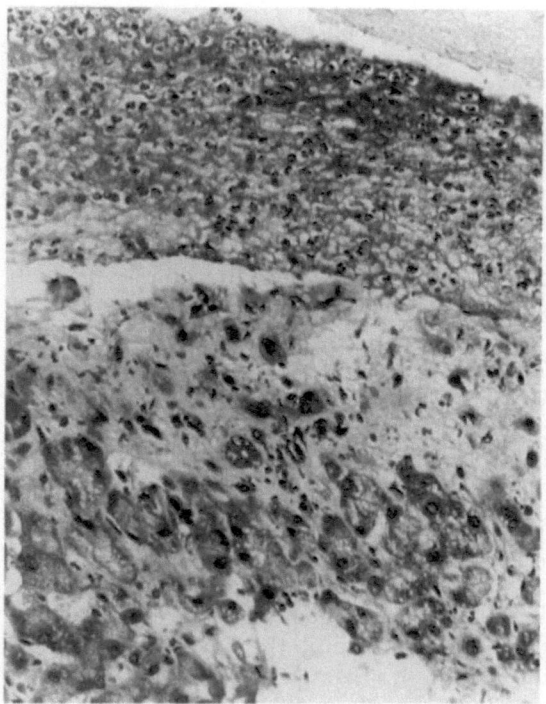

Figure 5-15. Liver tissue in an endoscopic biopsy from the base of a penetrating gastric ulcer. HPS, X250, reproduced at 60%.

Pathogenesis of Gastric Ulcers

In a much quoted article, Johnson[61] subdivided gastric ulcers into three types—type I being those ulcers occurring in the body of the stomach without evidence of ulceration or scarring in the prepyloric or duodenal area; type II being those ulcers in the body of the stomach associated with and perhaps secondary to an ulcer or scarring in the duodenum; and type III, prepyloric ulcers occurring to the right of the gastric angulus in the lesser curvature. In a review of 5000 cases of gastric ulcer, 57% were of type I, 22% of type II, and 20% of type III. Type I was characterized in general by low fasting and maximum acid output, while the other two types shared many features in common with duodenal ulcers (such as a higher than expected incidence of blood group 0 and a tendency toward hypersecretion). Thus, ulcerogenic factors in these latter two types have been thought to have more in common with those considered important in duodenal ulceration.

In the type I ulcer, at least, acid and pepsin secretion is either normal or reduced. Thus, one must look elsewhere to understand such gastric ulceration.

The Mucosal Barrier

We will first consider the factors involving the so-called mucosal barrier. This is a convenient concept, containing those facts and ideas that are envisioned as being protective against autodigestion. A transmucosal potential difference has been used as a rough measure of the integrity of the mucosal barrier. This has already been considered in part in Chapter 4. In sum, the factors considered important in the stomach have been: 1) the presentation of a minimal cell surface with tight cell junctions not normally absorptive; 2) the maintenance of adequate circulation to facilitate neutralization of hydrogen ions that may diffuse through the cell border and to permit surface secretion of bicarbonate and maintain metabolic energy requirements necessary for rapid cell replication of gastric mucosa; 3) the debated, but probable, role of the viscid mucus layer in the stomach in creating a pH gradient from lumen to cell surface; 4) the cytoprotective role of prostaglandins, in particular PGE_2; 5) the growth-promoting action of epidermal growth factor (EGF), and 6) the negative feedback mechanisms on secretion.

As stated in Chapter 4, interruption of the relatively impermeable surface cell layer by any means increases back-diffusion of H^+, causing the release of histamine, an increase in capillary permeability, edema, and cell damage. Another effect of histamine is that of further increasing acid/pepsin secretion through its action on the parietal cell. Thus, a vicious cycle is set up of increasing cell damage and ulceration. There are many sources for this. For instance, aspirin and certain other lipid-soluble drugs are known to damage the cell after absorption through the lipoprotein cell membrane of the surface cells. Obviously, protective mechanisms must come into play. Otherwise, the no doubt numerous evanescent focal surface injuries would always result in chronic or perforating ulcers.

Clearly, maintenance of an adequate circulation is important. Hypovolemia and splanchnic shunting have been implicated in the acute ulcers of shock, burn, and other major stress factors. Major vascular disease does not seem important in the usual gastric ulcer, though if experimental work from the duodenum[60] can be extrapolated from, relative ischemia of the most superficial mucosa may be a factor in the localization of gastric ulcers.

There is increased acceptance of the importance of an unstirred mucus gel layer as protective of gastric mucosa. The mucus glycoproteins are secreted as a polymer of four equal-sized subunits joined by disulfide bonds. This polymerized form presents as a thick tenacious mucoid gel. Its thickness and structure vary with acid and pepsinogen secretion since it is degraded by pepsin in the presence of acid (i.e., there is normally a balance between mucus secretion and degradation). Stimulants of mucin secretion are vagal stimulation, acetyl choline, as well as certain prostaglandins. Thus, mucin secretion, to some degree, parallels acid/pepsin secretion. Since carbonic acid (H_2CO_3) is secreted by surface cells and is at its highest concentration at or near the luminal surface, it has been suggested that the unstirred mucus layer probably does create a pH gradient, although it is permeable to acid ion.[62] Younan and co-workers[63] have shown that samples of mucin from patients with gastric ulcer contain about 65% of depolymerized glycoproteins as compared with 33% in a control group. Samples of gastric mucin from patients with duodenal ulcer fell between these values at about 50% degradation. Thus, patients with peptic ulcer may have a weak mucus gel structure.

Prostaglandins

Human gastroduodenal tissue produces prostaglandins, especially prostaglandin E_2 (PGE_2) and prostaglandin F_2 (PGF_2). These chemicals have powerful effects, although the mechanism of these effects is poorly understood. They have been shown to 1) inhibit basal and stimulate gastric acid secretion, 2) stimulate H_2CO_3, 3) stimulate mucin secretion, 4) possibly have a trophic effect on mucosal epithelium, and 5) are strongly cytoprotective even at levels below the threshold necessary for antisecretory effects. Experimentally, certain prostaglandins appear to protect the mucus gel layer in the rat against the effect of various damaging agents.[64] Prostaglandins therefore seem to mobilize all known defense mechanisms against ulceration.[65]

Epidermal Growth Factor

Epidermal growth factor (EGF) is a polypeptide similar in composition and biologic action to urogastrone, which was originally extracted from the urine of pregnant women and demonstrated to have a beneficial effect on the healing of chronic ulcers.[66] The major sources of EGF in the gastric and duodenal lumen are the submandibular salivary glands and Brunner's glands. EGF is resistant to degradation by gastric proteases and absorption from the intestine. Luminal EGF increases DNA and RNA synthesis in the gastric mucosa and stimulates mucosal cells to take up and incorporate glucosamine into glycoproteins, which, as mentioned above, are the main constituents of the protective mucus gel of the gastric and duodenal surface. The gastroprotective activity of EGF is limited to aspirin- and stress-induced ulcerations, in contrast to prostaglandins, which also protect against ethanol injury. The protective effect of EGF is independent of its antisecretory activity, which is expressed only after large doses.

Stasis

Dragstedt's views,[67] influential in their time, are summarized in his statement that "80% of gastric ulcers are caused by hypotonus of the vagus nerves, evidenced by decreased basal secretion and gastric stasis secondary to functional or structural pyloric damage. Prolonged contact of food with antral mucosa causes hypersecretion of gastric juice of humoral origin and prolonged contact with acid gastric contents produces ulcers in the stomach." He excluded the prepyloric ulcer from this concept. He backed up this idea with a considerable amount of experimental work. This concept (i.e., basically hypergastrinemia secondary to stasis) has been disproven because there is no evidence of antral stasis, hypergastrinemia secondary to antral distention, or acid hypersecretion in at least the type I gastric ulcer.[68]

The Role of Gastritis

The relative reduction in acid/pepsin secretion may reflect a loss of parietal cell mass, in turn secondary to the extensive atrophic or superficial gastritis that is nearly invariable in type I chronic gastric ulcer (nonaspirin-associated). The frequently accompanying intestinal metaplasia seen in chronic gastritis as well as the inflammatory infiltrate may well increase the back-diffusion of acid and thus permit ulceration, even in the absence of abnormal amounts of acid and pepsin. This does not explain the fact that ulcers, although occurring in areas of gastritis, are not randomly distributed within the areas of gastritis, but rather occur in a narrow band near the margin with the acid-secreting mucosa. So, again, other factors must be operative. It has been fairly well documented that the gastritis present is not secondary to the ulcer, since it usually persists and may become of even more severe grade despite healing of ulcers under medication.[63]

Bile Reflux

Gastritis follows procedures designed to cause reflux in animals and is a common sequel of gastric surgery in man, especially after gastrojejunal anastomoses.[62] Since bile is known to be disruptive to the mucosal barrier, it is tempting to consider it a factor in gastric ulcer, and many believe that it is, indeed, such a factor. Bile reflux is known to occur in patients with chronic gastric ulcer. However, bile reflux has been demonstrated in subjects without ulcer, and its practical role in the production of gastric ulcer is still not well defined.

Other Factors

The role of aspirin as a direct damaging agent in acute ulceration has already been mentioned and has been well demonstrated experimentally. Some studies indicate a significant association of aspirin abuse and chronic gastric ulcer, especially in prepyloric ulceration.[69] The role of alcohol, steroids, smoking, and diet has not been firmly established.

The recent discovery of *Campylobacter pylori* in gastric ulcer borders as well as in the adjacent antral mucosa has led to speculations of a causal role of bacterial infection in ulcerogenesis.[70] While some believe that the association is due to coexisting antral gastritis, others have hypothesized that *Campylobacter* may digest the mucus layer and thus deprive the gastric mucosa of its natural protection.[70] The incidence of *Campylobacter pylori* infection in patients with gastric ulcer has been reported to be between 58 and 70% and is significantly greater than that in patients with nonulcer dyspepsia.[70]

Summary

Although acid/pepsin is necessary for gastric ulceration, no consistent abnormality of secretion are noted unless it be for the tendency for reduced secretion. Abnormal pyloric function seems to occur in some patients and may, through increased bile reflux, play a role, but this is not well defined. Hypergastrinemia, though often present, is probably secondary to reduced acid secretion

rather than a primary factor. Aspirin may be a factor in many ulcers, but certainly not in all. The role of prostaglandins is becoming appreciated, but still is not clarified.

Pathogenesis of Duodenal Ulcer

Although some of what has been discussed under the heading of gastric ulceration applies to the duodenum, there are many differences—one of them certainly being the mucosa, which, quite the opposite of the gastric mucosa, is arranged for maximal surface and is absorptive in nature, so that there is essentially no block to diffusion of acid. Protection is indeed thought to be due to the rapid diffusion and neutralization of acid within the duodenal mucosa plus neutralization from biliary and pancreatic secretions in the lumen.

Compared with gastric ulceration, the study of duodenal ulceration has an advantage since there are experimental models available for study. The ulcerogenic substance cysteamine has been perhaps most widely used in studying pathogenetic factors. This drug very closely reproduces duodenal ulcer in many respects, including the anterior and posterior sites of involvement. In the rat, cysteamine has been observed to cause channeling of duodenum (i.e., the formation of a flat tube so that gastric secretions can only pass in the anterior and posterior planes). Szabo[60] has submitted experimental evidence that this site predilection has to do with the anatomic confinement of the duodenum. Mobilization of the duodenum by severing the surrounding ligaments produces irregular duodenal ulcers in addition to (or instead of) the usual anterior and posterior ulcers. The main observed difference between cysteamine and naturally recurring ulcers is the high frequency of adrenal cortical lesions associated with cysteamine-induced duodenal ulceration. Although there is some support for a link between adrenal lesions and duodenal ulceration in man, particularly in children, it is certainly not the case in most patients with duodenal ulcer. Injections of cysteamine have shown the initial changes to be release of stainable mucin within 1 or 2 hours, followed by electron microscopic changes revealing openings of the intercellular junctions and disarray of microvilli. This is followed by shortening of the villi and necrosis of the most superficial portion of the mucosa, with progression toward the crypts. At the chemical and hormonal level, cysteamine has been shown to acutely increase serum gastrin levels in rats (an effect further augmented by peptone or food administration) and to decrease plasma secretin levels (secretin being inhibitory to acid secretion). It also appears to deplete immunoreactive somatostatin in gastric and duodenal mucosa in the pancreas and hypothalamus. These interrelationships are well discussed in Szabo's review.[60] Cysteamine is also known to increase gastric secretion in a reproducible way and delay gastric emptying. The effect of cysteamine, however, must be more complex than the simple increase in acid secretion. In rats with a chronic gastric fistula experiments by Kirkegaard and co-workers[71] have shown that, although cysteamine both produced ulcers and markedly increased acid secretion, ulcers were not produced by a similar amount of acid secretion induced by pentagastrin without cysteamine.

On the average, patients with duodenal ulcers differ from those with type I gastric ulcers in that they show evidence of hypersecretion of acid and pepsin. However, this is not seen in all patients (only in perhaps half of the total patients with duodenal ulcer) and cannot be the only factor involved. Indeed, none of the changes described in duodenal ulceration apply uniformly across the board, again indicating heterogeneity in duodenal ulcer disease. Table 5-2 is modified from Holt and Isenberg's review[72] in which the various factors are listed. They emphasize that only 20 to 50% of all patients will show any given change of any one of the abnormalities listed.

Table 5.2. Physiologic Defects in Patients with Duodenal Ulcer*

1. Increased number of parietal cells (and thus secretory capacity).
2. Increased pepsinogen I.
3. Increased basal secretion of acid and pepsin.
4. Increased parietal cell sensitivity to gastrin.
5. Decreased acidic inhibition of gastrin.
6. Increased gastrin release (meal-stimulated).
7. Increased acid and pepsin in duodenum.
8. Increased rate of gastric emptying.

*Modified from Holt and Eisenberg.[72]

These factors are all on the "aggressive side." It is clear that mucosal defense factors must also be considered. The roles of prostaglandins, abnormal duodenal motility, *Campylobacter pylori* infection, and reduced duodenal bicarbonate secretion have been explored. It has been shown (as discussed under the heading of gastric ulcer) that PGE_2 is strongly cytoprotective, and that duodenal and gastric mucosa of patients with duodenal ulcer may be defective in its ability to synthesize prostanoids such as PGE_2.[73] Ahlquist and co-workers[74] suggest that while in the healthy, mucosal prostaglandin generation is induced after eating in relation to acid load, in patients with duodenal ulcer there may be a defect in this mechanism.

Recent studies have demonstrated abnormalities of duodenal motility having the net effect of delaying distal migration of acid in the duodenum and proximal migration of pancreatic and biliary bicarbonate, thus increasing the depth and duration of lowered pH in the upper duodenum. This may be a critical factor in duodenal ulcer genesis, and would explain duodenal ulcer even in those cases in which hypersecretion of acid and pepsin is not a factor.[60,75,76]

Campylobacter pylori infection may interfere with mucosal defense mechanisms, as previously mentioned. The organism is present in the stomach and duodenum in 77 to 93% of patients with duodenal ulcer (i.e., with greater frequency than in patients with gastric ulcer).[60,70] Impaired proximal duo-

Table 5.3. Ulcer Site in Twins with Ulcer*

Ulcer Site in Twin No. 1	Total No.	Ulcer Site in Twin No. 2		
		Duodenal	Prepyloric	Gastric
Duodenal	69	55	10	4
Prepyloric	6	4	2	0
Gastric	10	3	1	6

*From Jensen KG: Scand J Gastroenterol 1980;15(suppl 63):11–14. Reproduced by permission, Norwegian University Press.

denal mucosal bicarbonate secretion was demonstrated in all 12 subjects tested and represents another factor that decreases mucosal defenses.[77]

It seems clear that simple hyperacidity in itself is not the explanation for duodenal ulcer. The answers are tied into very complex interactions of the neuroendocrine status, of anatomic and vascular factors, and of mucosal defense mechanisms, some of which are still poorly understood.

Genetic Aspects of Peptic Ulcer

It has long been realized that near-relatives of patients with peptic ulcer have a higher than expected incidence of peptic ulceration (on the order of two to three times the expected incidence).[58,78] Furthermore, it has been shown that the association is site-specific (i.e., that propositi with gastric ulcer have close relatives at higher risk of gastric ulcer, and relatives of propositi with duodenal ulcer again at higher risk for duodenal ulcer).[79,80] While proving that a familial factor is present, such information does not distinguish between the relative roles of environmental and genetic factors. This has been clarified by studies of twins, various blood groups, and certain other parameters.

Blood Group and Secretor Status

This area has been well reviewed by Jensen.[78] In summary, in patients with blood group O, there is an increased risk of ulcer in the duodenum, the prepyloric area, and of com-

bined gastric-duodenal ulcer, but not of isolated ulcer of the body of the stomach.[58] The patients with blood group 0 have about a 35% increased change of developing a duodenal ulcer. Nonsecretors of blood group substances have about a 50% increased risk, over secretors. These differences have been confirmed in many geographic areas despite large variation in the ABO secretor/non-secretor status from one area to another. The mechanism responsible for this is not clear and obviously other factors must be involved since not all group 0 non-secretors develop ulcer, nor is duodenal ulcer confined to that group.

Twin Studies

Studies from Denmark of twins with confirmed peptic ulceration (chiefly duodenal), including zygosity diagnosis of the twins via serologic analysis, showed that of 38 monozygotic twins with ulcer, 20 of their twin partners also had ulcer. In a dizygotic group of 67 propositi with ulcer, 21 of their partners developed ulcer.[78]

In another study of twins, there was considerable concordance of ulcer site (Table 5-3).

There may also be a relation with HLA antigen B₅.[78] It should be added that certain inbred strains of mice (NZB strain) have an ultimate incidence of duodenal ulcer in close to 100% of the animals.[58] Jensen[78] concludes that approximately equal importance should be placed on inheritance and environment.

The mode of inheritance of ulcer, however, it not clear. The preceding results could be explained on a polygenic basis, that is, 1) the combined effect of multiple genes resulting in ulcer predisposition, or 2) the alternative view, exposed by Rotter and co-workers,[58,81] that peptic ulcer is a heterogeneous group of diseases, some at least genetically determined, which have as a common expression peptic ulceration. This view has gained considerable though not universal acceptance. A contrary view is, for instance, expressed by Wormsley,[59] in his nihilistic review, who comments on the pathophysiologic heterogeneity hypothesis as:

...in other words, whatever apparent disturbance of function one happens to find, that particular dysfunction is somehow implicated in the genesis of the ulcer disease, and if one does not find anything, then (presumably) lack of defensive factors—which are unmeasurable—must be responsible.

The hypothesis is based in part on the fact that certain clearly genetic syndromes have a high association with ulcer, though acting through diverse mechanisms. The best established of these is the Zollinger-Ellison syndrome, as part of the multiple endocrine adenopathy complex (MEA₁), the ulcer-tremor-nystagmus syndrome, and systemic mastocytosis.

The Zollinger-Ellison syndrome may be present in up to 0.1 percent of all patients with duodenal ulcer disease in the United States.[82] Considered to be commonly of sporadic occurrence, with only about 20% of the cases of Zollinger-Ellison Syndrome associated with MEA₁, carefully obtained family histories have shown that the actual association is probably much higher, somewhere around 60%.[83] The effect of the tumor-produced gastrin acts both directly to increase acid/pepsin secretion and through its trophic effect on fundic mucosa.

Systemic mastocytosis is also associated with ulcer. Six of eight monozygotic twins with this rare disorder had peptic ulceration. A number of familial cases have been reported. This presumably has its effect through local histamine excess.[58]

A family kindred of a syndrome associated with nystagmus, essential tremor, duodenal ulcer, and narcolepsy has also been reported, in which of 17 affected members, 8 had duodenal ulcer, all in those members with the neurologic symptoms.[84] Other associations that have been reported, but that are not as well established include familial amyloidosis Type IV, and the so-called stiff man syndrome.

Another line of investigation has been the use of subclinical markers associated with ulceration (i.e., a parameter used to detect an abnormal genotype in the absence of the full phenotype, such as abnormal parathyroid hormone levels in MEA₁). Studies have considered such markers as maximal acid secretion, gastric emptying time, gastrin response to a meal, and serum pepsinogen 1 levels. Of these, the latter has been the most clear-cut.

Elevated serum pepsinogen 1 levels have been found in about two-thirds of the cases of duodenal ulcer.[85] Serum pepsinogen 1 (PG-1) has been shown to be inherited as an autosomal-dominant trait. Since serum PG-1 is elaborated from the gastric fundic mucosa, it equates with parietal cell mass, which thus may have a genetic basis. In patients with duodenal ulcer but with normal serum PG-1 levels who have siblings or twins with ulcers, such siblings have also been shown to have a normal PG-1 level. Rotter and co-workers[86] have suggested that such patients may have a distinct but separate genetic basis for duodenal ulcer.

Rotter[81] has classified peptic ulcer in a detailed list (Table 5-4), which is best interpreted as indicating the diversity of presentations of peptic ulcer. Not all of the listed associations are accepted as more than chance.

Diseases Associated with Peptic Ulceration

Peptic ulcer is a common disease and may coexist with other common diseases. An association has been claimed and denied with cardiovascular disease, chronic pulmonary disease (in particular emphysema), cirrhosis, hyperparathyroidism, renal disease, diabetes, and rheumatoid arthritis, as well as with other less common disorders (such as the MEA₁ complex) which are discussed elsewhere.[87-89] There are many problems in interpreting such reports (i.e., whether the disease is directly contributory, whether influenced by therapy such as the use of steroids and aspirin in rheumatoid arthritis, and so forth). As Langman and Cooke[89] stated, "assess-

Table 5.4. Classification of Peptic Ulcers*

I. Peptic ulcer associated with rare genetic
   syndromes
   A. Relationship established
      1. Multiple endocrine adenomatosis,
         type I (gastrinoma)
      2. Systemic mastocytosis
      3. Tremor-nystagmus-ulcer syndrome
      4. Amyloidosis, type IV
   B. Relationship suggested
      1. Hyperparathyroidism
      2. Cystic fibrosis
      3. Alpha-1-antritrypsin deficiency
      4. Carcinoid syndrome
      5. Stiff skin syndrome
      6. Pachydermoperiostosis
      7. Multiple lentigines-ulcer syndrome
II. Esophageal ulcer
III. Gastric ulcer
   A. Accompanied by chronic gastritis
   B. Secondary to use of aspirin[†]
IV. Combined gastric and duodenal ulcer
V. Hyperpepsinogenemic I duodenal ulcer[‡]
   A. Without postprandial hypergastrinemia
   B. With postprandial hypergastrinemia
   C. Secondary to retained antrum
VI. Normopepsinogenemic I duodenal ulcer
   A. Without rapid gastric emptying
   B. With rapid gastric emptying
VII. Childhood or early-onset duodenal ulcer[§]
   A. Normal acid secretion
   B. Elevated acid secretion
VIII. Immunologic forms of duodenal ulcer[§]
   A. Antibody to secretory IgA
   B. Immunoglobulin-stimulated acid secre-
      tion
IX. Peptic ulcer associated with other chronic
    diseases[§]
   A. Peptic ulcer and chronic lung disease
   B. Duodenal ulcer and renal stones (with-
      out hyperparathyroidism)
   C. Duodenal ulcer and coronary artery
      disease
X. Meckel's diverticulum

From Rotter.[81] Reproduced by permission, Raven Press.
[†]Also occurs with other non-steroidal antiinflammatory
agents.
[‡]Also usually acid hypersecretors.
[§]Tentative subdivision.

ments of associated diseases are hindered by lack of controls, or by inadequate controls and bias—few bear examination." They concluded that the evidence is not strong for an association with cardiovascular disease and that although the prevalence of ulcer in patients with chronic respiratory problems is twice that of people without it, this may reflect that both are more common in men. They accept a probable real association with chronic renal failure, and a possible one in hyperparathyroidism, cardiovascular disease, cirrhosis, and chronic respiratory disease. In a study of physicians with and without a duodenal ulceration, chronic pulmonary disease was significantly more common in patients with duodenal ulcer, even after adjustment for cigarette smoking and age. There was not a statistically significant difference in association with coronary artery disease and rheumatoid arthritis with ulcer.[87] Of course, the Zollinger-Ellison syndrome is both associated and etiologic, and, so are by extension, certain other polyendocrine adenopathies (i.e., MEA₁).[90] Some relationship of the MEA_1 syndrome and peptic ulcer may exist, independent of gastrinoma. Forty-nine of 85 patients of a kindred with the MEA_1 syndrome, but without the Zollinger-Ellison syndrome, have been shown to have peptic ulcer disease.[91] In addition, certain rare genetic complexes (such as Neuhauser's syndrome, stiff skin syndrome, and others) seem established.[58] Diabetes mellitus actually may show a negative association, secondary to decreased acid production, except late in the course of the disease.[92] Chronic hyperparathyroidism has been reported to be associated with intractable duodenal ulcer. According to Spiro,[93] the prevalence appears higher than normal, especially in males, but needs better controlled studies.

Zollinger-Ellison Syndrome and Related Disorders

Zollinger-Ellison Syndrome

The Zollinger-Ellison syndrome, though rare, has created a great deal of interest, in part

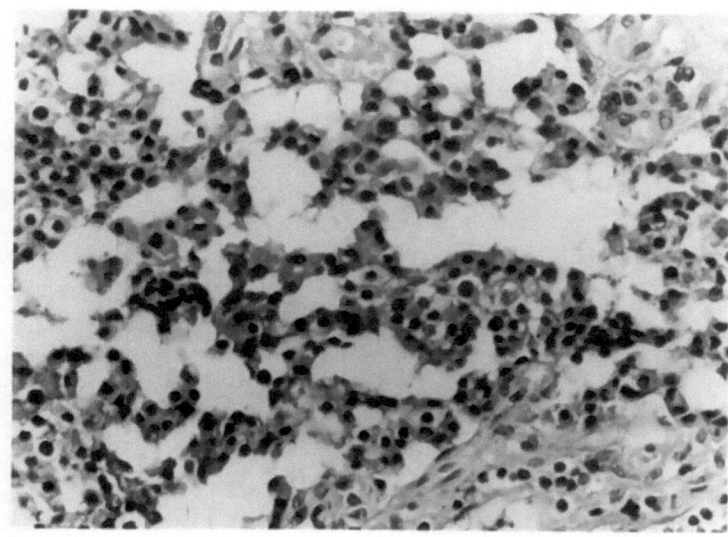

Figure 5-16. APUDoma of duodenum with positive staining with anti-gastrin antiserum. Immunoperoxidase technique. X400, reproduced at 60%.

because of its elegant pathophysiologic chain of events and in part because of certain genetic implications. It was first presented by Zollinger[94] at a meeting of the American Surgical Association in Philadelphia in 1955. As originally described, this syndrome included 1) a fulminating ulcer diathesis with excessive gastric secretions of 2 to 3 liters/day; 2) rapidly recurrent ulcerations, often multiple and at unusual sites despite medical therapy; and 3) the presence of non-beta cell tumors of the pancreas (or duodenum). Since then, the syndrome has been modified somewhat in that by no means do the patients necessarily present in a fulminating manner and that diarrhea is now recognized as frequent accompaniment of the syndrome. The peak years are in the third to fifth decades of life, with a strong male predominance by a ratio of at least 2:1. Gastrointestinal hemorrhage and complications secondary to bowel perforations are present in nearly 33% of the patients.[95] By 1960, it was realized that most of the non-beta cell tumors associated with the disorder were producers of gastrin (i.e., gastrinomas) (Fig. 5-16).

The incidence of Zollinger-Ellison syndrome is reported at about 1/500,000 per year or 0.1% in duodenal ulcer patients in the United States.[82] This syndrome occurs both as a sporadic finding and as part of the multiple endocrine adenopathy complex (MEA₁).

The familial MEA$_1$-associated cases tend to occur at an earlier age and are more likely to have associated benign tumors. Most patients will have an associated well defined tumor, with an "islet cell" pattern either of the pancreas or of the duodenum, but occasional cases have been reported with tumors showing a ductular pattern, with multiple microadenomata of the pancreas or with a nesidioblastosis.[96]

The associated gastrinomas may, as other Amine Precursor Uptake and Decarboxylation (APUD) cell tumors, be capable of forming other hormones as well. Somewhat more than half of the tumors reported have been malignant — 59% in Wilson's review.[95]

The ulcers in half the cases are multiple or are in unusual sites such as distal duodenum or jejunum — presumably secondary to the voluminous acidic secretions overwhelming the neutralization effects of the alkaline pancreatic and biliary secretions. Inactivation by the acid duodenal contents of pancreatic lipase and precipitation of bile acids give rise to malabsorption steatorrhea and account, at least in part, for the diarrhea.

The gastrin is, for the most part, secreted in the form of G34, although relatively inactive gastrin fragments may also be produced. The presence of excessive gastrin not only drives

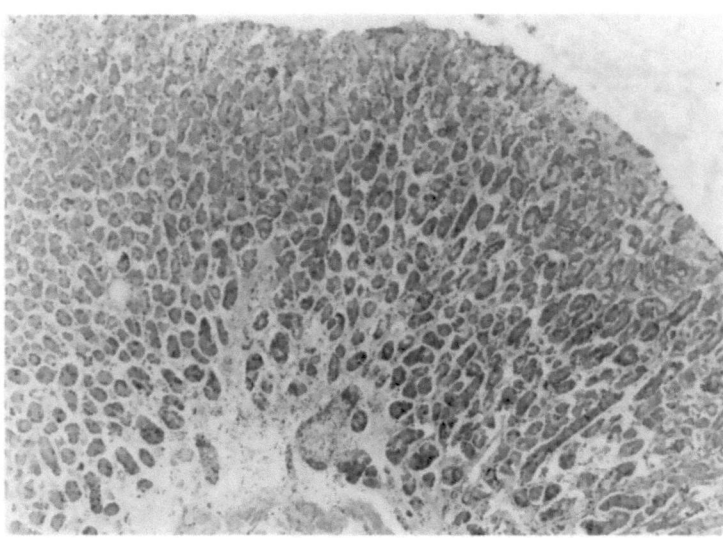

Figure 5-17. Marked parietal cell hyperplasia from gastrectomy. The patient was a 34-year-old male with recurrent ulcers of stomach and the gastrojejunostomy, an APUD tumor of the pancreas, papillary carcinoma of the thyroid, and para- thyroid hyperplasia. The APUD tumor was negative with anti-gastrin peroxidase stain, though the patient had a marked hypergastrinemia (Zollinger-Ellison syndrome with multiple endocrine adenopathy). H&E, X50, reproduced at 60%.

acid/pepsin secretion but also, through the trophic effect of gastrin, increases the total parietal cell mass so that patients with the disorder, in well developed forms at least, will also show a "giant rugal hypertrophy" pattern akin in size and mucosal thickness to that seen in Ménétrier's disease. On biopsy, these are easily distinguished because of the relatively marked increase in chief and parietal cell hyperplasia over that of the mucus neck glands in the Zollinger-Ellison syndrome (Fig. 5-17). In addition to ulceration, blunting of villi, inflammation, and edema of the mucosa have been described in the upper small bowel, presumably secondary to duodenal acidification.[97]

The size of the tumors is extremely variable, ranging from a few millimeters up to perhaps 3 or 4 cm. About 10% of the tumors will be found outside the pancreas, either in the duodenum (the most common site) or in the pylorus or peripancreatic area. At least 20% of the patients will have the MEA_1 syndrome and will show a tendency toward multiple tumors as opposed to the sporadic cases.

Average survival is stated to be about 90 months without liver metastases and 72 months with such metastases.[98] Wilson[95] recorded a 29% survival rate in patients with tumors producing multiple hormones as opposed to 55% in those with tumors producing only gastrin. Part of this mortality rate is derived from older reports prior to the advent of cimetidine, when total gastrectomy was considered imperative.

Zollinger-Ellison Variants
An interesting case of the Zollinger-Ellison syndrome has been reported in which the source of the gastrin was an ovarian cystadenocarcinoma.[99] Other cases presenting with a similar syndrome of hypergastrinemia and hypersecretion have been reported in which the source of the gastrin was retained antrum after unsuccessful or incomplete gastric surgery. Still another group[100] has shown exaggerated gastrin response to meals without response to secretin stimulation and lack of tumor but with hyperplasia of the antral G cells. Similar cases with presumed hyper-

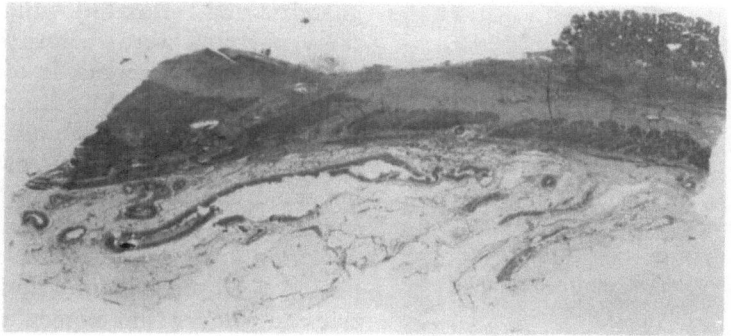

Figure 5-18. Adenocarcinoma arising at the margin of a chronic peptic ulcer. Whole-mount section of ulcer with scar tissue at the base, exudate on the surface, and carcinoma arising at the margin (see Fig. 5-17).

function but without demonstrable hyperplasia of the G cells are also reported in the literature.[101] Still other associations have been observed in patients with short bowel syndrome and in patients with renal failure.[102]

Relationship of Peptic Ulcer to Gastric Carcinoma

There are three areas to be considered here: 1) the proportion of gastric carcinomas that appear to arise directly from a preexisting peptic ulcer; 2) whether or not individuals who have had partial gastrectomy for peptic ulceration of stomach or duodenum are at a higher risk for carcinoma; and 3) the purely diagnostic problem of differentiating carcinoma from regenerative epithelium in biopsy material.

The earlier literature suggested that gastric peptic ulcer was a rather important source of gastric cancer, the figures suggesting that from 5 to 10% of gastric cancers had such origin. It is clear that much of this was earlier confusion between ulcerated gastric cancers and peptic ulcers with carcinoma arising from them. With more accurate radiologic and endoscopic techniques, the confusion between peptic ulcer and gastric carcinoma has been reduced so that diagnostic error is probably now only in the neigh-

borhood of about 1.5%.[103] Rarely, one may encounter a case that, grossly at least and by radiologic studies, is indistinguishable from peptic ulcer (i.e., having sharp margins and a flat base). Does gastric carcinoma ever arise from peptic ulcer? The answer must be yes, but rarely. To be convincing, such a case should have 1) a history of peptic ulceration and good histologic evidence of chronic peptic ulcer (i.e., a flat-based ulcer with the usual zones of necrosis, granulation tissue, and fibrosis, and with fusion of the muscularis mucosa to the muscularis propria); 2) a small carcinoma clearly continuous with the edge of such an ulcer (which would exclude large carcinomas that happened to border on such an ulcer); and 3) an absence of carcinoma in the base of the ulcer in question. Such cases are certainly reported[101,102] but the percentage thought to so arise has decreased sharply over the years. In 1967, Willis[104] reported figures from the literature of about 6%, although in his own personal experience, he considered it highly unusual.[104] Morson and Dawson[105] stated that unequivocal evidence of previous peptic ulcer at the site of a proven carcinoma is probably less than 1%, and caution that one should recall that chronic ulcer and gastric cancer may coexist without necessarily being causally related. It has certainly been unusual in our experience. Nonetheless, we have seen a rare convincing case (Figs. 5-18 and 5-19). Such carcinomas seem to

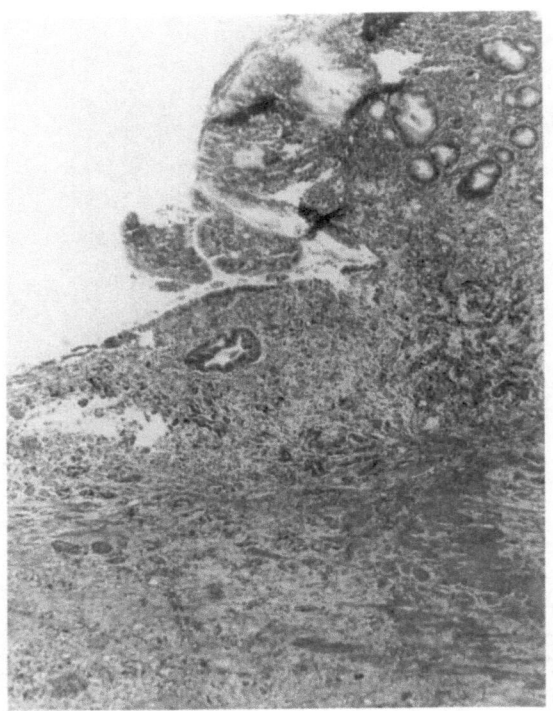

Figure 5-19. Edge of ulcer with dark-staining carcinoma cells infiltrating between regenerating foveolae. HPS, X50, reproduced at 60%.

have a predilection to be of the superficial spreading type.[106,107]

Another question for consideration is whether the presence of peptic ulcer, whether gastric or duodenal, or perhaps the presence of a history of partial gastrectomy for such an ulcer increases the incidence of a later carcinoma in the stomach. There is certainly evidence on both sides of this question.[108-111] In the series reported by Helsingen and Hillestad,[108] of 200 patients followed up for an average of 20 years, 11 cases of carcinoma were found as opposed to 5 expected. The series of Stalsberg and Taksdals,[109] an autopsy study with age- and sex-matched controls, indicated there was about a six times greater incidence of gastric cancer in those followed up for 25 years after operation. The risk was about the same for stomach and duodenal ulcer. More of these cases had had a Billroth II than a Billroth I operation, and Stalsberg and Taksdals' findings suggested that the

gastritis and reflux following gastroenterostomy perhaps were factors in the development of later carcinoma. In contrast, another study[110] of some 200 patients followed up with 98% success for almost 20 years found only one case of carcinoma as opposed to two expected. Similarly, a Mayo Clinic study of a series of 338 patients, of whom 63% were followed up until death (with a mean follow-up period of 17 years), found no increase in gastric cancer over that expected.[111] It is hard to draw conclusions from this except that the risk of increased cancer, if present at all, occurs only after a very long postoperative period, certainly in excess of 15 years and probably of 20 years.

Finally, considerable atypism may be discovered at the margins of peptic ulcers, at least of the stomach. This certainly is not a unique problem and occurs in any chronic ulcerated area in any part of the body. However, the problem is particularly acute when one is dealing with small endoscopic biopsies. Regenerative epithelium tends to show a smaller nucleo-cytoplasmic ratio than does carcinoma. The nuclei tend to be more vesicular than in carcinoma and, of course, the cells seen are not found as isolated cells within the lamina (Fig. 5-11). Even so, all surgical pathologists who see a fair amount of gastric material encounter cases in which doubt may exist on biopsy material, and we urge a conservative attitude and a request for further biopsies in such instances. Cytology also may be quite helpful.

Another problem arises in patients after undergoing chemotherapy. Weidner and co-workers[112] reported that biopsy of five of nine peptic ulcers, which developed as complications following hepatic arterial chemotherapy infusion, showed marked atypia with swollen hyperchromatic smudged nuclei and were differentiated with difficulty from carcinoma, though again these cases showed a lower nucleo-cytoplasmic ratio than is usual in carcinoma. This situation is like that seen in biopsy material from other sites after chemotherapy. Such a history should alert the pathologist to take a conservative stance in diagnosis.

References

1. Pliny G: The Historie of the World (Commonly called the Natural Historie). Volume 2. Holland, P. (trans). London: Adam Islip, 1601:329.
2. Zucker GM, Clayman CB. Bertram W: Sippy and ulcer disease therapy. JAMA 1983;250: 2198–2202.
3. Trevers B. (and Cramptom J): Rupture of the stomach and escape of contents. Med Chir Trans London 1817;8:228–245.
4. Curling TB: On acute ulceration of the duodenum in cases of burn. Med Chir Trans London 1842;25:260–281.
5. Rokitansky C: In: Handbuch der Pathologischen Anatomie (1841–46)–Section on ulcerative processes of stomach (quoted by Cushing).
6. Cushing H: Peptic ulcers and the interbrain. Surg Gynecol Obstet 1932;55:1–34.
7. Korn ER, Foroozan P: Pyloric channel ulcer with betazole-fast achlorhydria. Gastroenterology 1974;67:1248–1249.
8. Duberstein DL, Efrusy ME: Benign gastric ulceration with pentagastrin-fast achlorhydria. Gastroenterology 1977;72:1369–1370.
9. Morson BC, Dawson IMP: Gastrointestinal Pathology, 2nd Ed., Oxford: Blackwell Scientific Publications, 1979:123–124.
10. Karvonen AL, Sipponen P, et al: Gastric mucosal erosions–an endoscopic, histologic and functional study. Scand J Gastroenterol 1983;18:1051–1056.
11. Tatsuta M, Okuda S: Gastric ulcers in the fundic gland area. Gastroenterology 1976; 71:16–18.
12. Czaja AJ, McAlhany JC, et al: Acute gastrointestinal disease after thermal injury. N Engl J Med 1974;291:925–929.
13. Kamada T, Fusamoto H, et al: Acute gastroduodenal lesions in head injury. Am J Gastroenterol 1977;68:249–253.
14. Silen W: The prevention and management of stress ulcers. Hosp Pract 1980;March:93–103.
15. Morgan AG, McAdam WAF, et al: Multiple recurring gastric erosions (apthous ulcers). Gut 1976;17:633–639.
16. Grossman M, Matsumoto KK, Lichter RJ: Fecal blood loss produced by oral and intravenous administrations of various salicylates. Gastroenterology 1961;40:383–388.
17. Pierson RN, Holt PR, Watson RM, et al: Aspirin and gastrointestinal bleeding. Am J Med 1961;31:259–265.
18. Tarnawski A, Krause WJ, Ivey KJ: Effect of glucagon on aspirin induced gastric mucosal damage in man. Gastroenterology 1978;74: 240–245.
19. Winawer SJ, Benar J, McCray RS, et al: Hemorrhagic gastritis: Importance of associated chronic gastritis. Ann Intern Med 1971;127: 129–131.
20. Weiss A, Pitman ER, Graham EC: Aspirin and gastric bleeding: gastroscopic observations and review of the literature. Am J Med 1961;31:266–278.
21. Alvarez AS, Summerskill WHJ: Gastrointestinal hemorrhage and salicylates. Lancet 1958;2:920–925.
22. Roth JLA, Valdes-Dapens, A., et al.: Topical action of salicylates in gastrointestinal erosion and hemorrhage. Gastroenterology 1963;44:146–158.
23. Duggan JM: The pathogenesis of the aspirin related gastric lesion. J Roy Coll Phys Lond 1981;15(2):117–118.
24. Sarosiek J, Slomiany BL, et al: Effect of acetyl salicylic acid on the constituents of the gastric mucosal barrier. Scand J Gastroenterol 1984;19:150–153.
25. Asuumi Y, O'Hara S, et al: Topical aspirin plus HCL gastric lesions in the rat: Cytoprotective affect of prostaglandin, cimetidine and probanthine. Gut 1980;21:533–536.
26. Spiro HM: Duodenal Ulcer, Chapter 14. In: Clinical Gastroenterology. London: Collier-MacMillan Ltd., 1983:304–354.
27. Portis SA, Jaffe RH: A study of peptic ulcer based on necropsy records. JAMA 1938;110: 6–13.
28. Ellison EH, Abrams JS, et al: A post mortem analysis of 812 gastro-duodenal ulcers found in 20,000 consecutive autopsies with emphasis on associated endocrine disease. Am J Surg 1959;97:17–30.
29. Carter DC: Aetiology of peptic ulcer. In: Sircus W, Smith AN (eds). Scientific Foundations of Gastroenterology. Philadelphia: W.B. Saunders Co., 1980:344–357.
30. Kurata JH: What in the world is happening to ulcers? Gastroenterology 1983;84:1623–1625.
31. Sonnenberg A, Fritsch A: Changing mortality of peptic ulcer disease in Germany. Gastroenterology 1983;84:1553–1557.
32. Koo J, Ngan YK: Trends in hospital admis-

sions, perforation, and mortality of peptic ulcer in Hong Kong from 1970–1980. Gastroenterology 1983;84:1588–1562.

33. Kurata JH, Honda GD, et al: Hospitalization and mortality rates for peptic ulcers: A comparison of a large health maintenance organization and United States data. Gastroenterology 1982;83:1008–1016.

34. Kurata JH, Hasle BM: Racial differences in peptic ulcer disease, fact or myth? Gastroenterology 1982;83:166–172.

35. Robbins SL, Cotran RS: In: The Pathologic Basis of Disease. 2nd Ed. Philadelphia: W.B. Saunders Co., 1979: p. 928.

36. Oi M, Sakurai Y: The location of duodenal ulcer. Gastroenterology 1959;36:60–64.

37. Kirk RM: Factors determining the site of classic gastroduodenal ulcers – a review. Hepatogastroenterol 1982;29:75–85.

38. Oi M, Oshida K, et al: The location of gastric ulcer. Gastroenterology 1959;36:60–64.

39. Gear MWL, Truelove SC, et al: Gastric ulcers and gastritis. Gut 1971;12:639–645.

40. Greenlaw R, Sheahan DG, et al: Gastroduodenitis: a broader concept of peptic ulcer disease. Dig Dis Sci 1980;25:660–672.

41. Findley JW: Ulcers of the greater curvature of the stomach. Gastroenterology 1961;40:183–187.

42. Kirk RM: Does the jet of acid emergence through the pylorus determine the site of duodenal ulcer? Br J Med 1975;3:629–630.

43. Bell MJ, Keating JP, et al: Perforated stress ulcers in infants. J Pediatr Surg 1981;16:998–1001.

44. Tolia V, DuBois RS: Peptic ulcer in children and adolescents. Clin Pediatrics 1983;22:665–669.

45. Nord KS, Rossi TM, et al: Peptic ulceration in children. Am J Gastroenterol 1981;75:153–157.

46. Johnson D, Heureux L, et al: Peptic ulcer disease in early infancy: Clinical presentations and roentgenographic features. Acta Paed Scand 1980;69:753–760.

47. Morson B, Dawson IMP: In: Gastrointestinal Pathology, 2nd Ed. Oxford; Blackwell Scientific Publications, 1979:125.

48. Trier JS: Morphology of the gastric mucosa in patients with ulcer disease. Am J Dig Dis 1976;21:138–140.

49. Oohara T, Tohma H, et al: Intestinal metaplasia of the regenerative epithelia in 549 gastric ulcers. Hum Pathol 1983;14:1066–1071.

50. Jaszewski R, Crane SD, et al: Giant duodenal ulcers. Dig Dis Sci 1983;28:486–488.

51. Spiro HM: In: Clinical Gastroenterology. London: 1983: Collier-MacMillan Lmt., Chapter 15, pp. 355–368.

52. Thompson WM, Kelvin FM, et al: Radiologic investigation of peptic ulcer disease. Radiol Clin North Am 1982;20(4):704–720.

53. Joffe H, Antonioli DA: Penetration into spleen by benign peptic ulcers. Clin Radiol 1981;32:177–181.

54. West AB, Nolan N, O'Briain DS: Benign peptic ulcers penetrating pericardium and heart: Clinicopathological features and factors favoring survival. Gastroenterology 1988;94:1478–1487.

55. Johnson CA, Dufresne CR, et al: Intraabdominal perforation of gastric ulcer: A complication of incarcerated epigastric hernia. Am Surg 1980;46:418–421.

56. Fong W: Septic complication of perforated peptic ulcer. Can J Surg 1983;26:370–372.

57. Kothandaraman KR, Kutty KP: Double pylorus – in evolution. J Clin Gastroenterol 1983;5:335–338.

58. Rotter JE: The genetics of peptic ulcer: More than one gene, more than one disease. In: Steinberg AG, Childs B (eds). Progress in Medical Genetics, Volume 4 (new series). Philadelphia: W.B. Saunders and Co., 1980.

59. Wormsley KG: Duodenal ulcer: Does pathophysiology equal etiology? Gut 1983;24:775–780.

60. Szabo S: Pathogenesis of duodenal ulcer disease. Lab Invest 1984;51:121–147.

61. Johnson HD: Gastric ulcer classification. Blood group characteristics, secretion patterns and pathogenesis. Ann Surg 1965;162:996–1004.

62. Kauffman GL Jr: Gastric mucus and bicarbonate secretion in relation to mucosal protection. J Clin Gastroenterol 1981;3(Suppl 2):45–50.

63. Younan F, Pearson J, et al: Changes in the structure of the mucus gel on the mucosal surface of the stomach in association with peptic ulcer disease. Gastroenterology 1982;82:827–831.

64. McQueen S, Hutton D, et al: Gastric and duodenal surface mucus gel thickness in rats: effects of prostaglandins and damaging agents. Am J Physiol 1983;245:G388–393.

65. Johansson C, Bergstrom S: Prostaglandins and protection of the gastroduodenal mucosa.

Scand J Gastroenterol 1982;HR77 (Suppl): 21–46.

66. Konturek SJ: Role of epidermal growth factor in gastroprotection and ulcer healing. Scand J Gastroenterol 1988;23:129–133.

67. Dragstedt LR: Peptic Ulcer – an abnormality of secretion. Am J Surg 1969;117:143–156.

68. Olbe L: The pathophysiology of gastric ulcer. Scand J Gastroenterol 1979;55(suppl):49–51.

69. Cameron AJ: Aspirin and gastric ulcer. Mayo Clin Proc 1975;50:565–570.

70. Marshall BJ: Peptic ulcer: An infectious disease. Hosp Pract 1987;Aug 5:69–78.

71. Kirkegaard P, Paulsen SS, et al: Cysteamine induced duodenal ulcer and acid secretion in the rat. Scand J Gastroenterol 1980;16:621.

72. Holt KM, Isenberg JI: Peptic ulcer disease: Physiology and pathophysiology. Hosp Pract 1985;Jan 15:89–106.

73. Sharon P, Cohen F, et al: Prostanoid synthesis by cultured gastric and duodenal mucosa: Possible role in the pathogenesis of duodenal ulcer. Scand J Gastroenterol 1983;18:1045–1049.

74. Ahlquist DA, Dozois RR, et al: Duodenal prostaglandins synthesis and acid level in health and duodenal ulcer disease. Gastroenterology 1983;85:522–528.

75. Szabo S, Pihan G, et al: Role of local secretory and motility changes in the pathogenesis of experimental duodenal ulcer. Scand J Gastroenterol 1984;92:106–111.

76. Pihan G, Dupuy D, et al: Duodenal hypermotility impairs acid neutralization in experimental duodenal ulcerations. Gastroenterology 1984;86:1210.

77. Isenberg JI, Selling JA, Hogan DL, Koss MA: Impaired proximal duodenal mucosal bicarbonate secretion in patients with duodenal ulcer. N Engl J Med 1987;316:374–379.

78. Jensen KG: Genetics of peptic ulcer – a brief survey. Scand J Gastroenterol 1980;15(Suppl 63):11–14.

79. Doll R, Kellock TD: The separate inheritance of gastric and duodenal ulcer. Ann Eugenics 1951;16:231–240.

80. Monson RR: Familial factors in peptic ulcer, the occurrence of ulcer in relatives. Am J Epidemiol 1970;91:453–466.

81. Rotter JI: The genetics of gastritis and peptic ulcer. J Clin Gastroenterol 1981;3(Suppl 2):35–43.

82. Wolfe MM, Jensen RT: Zollinger-Ellison syndrome: Current Concepts in diagnosis and management. N Engl J Med 1987;317:1200–1209.

83. Lamers CB, Stadil F, et al: Prevalence of endocrine abnormalities in patients with the Zollinger-Ellison syndrome in their families. Am J Med 1978;64:607–612.

84. Neuhauser G, Daly RF, et al: Essential tremor, nystagmus, and duodenal ulceration. Clin Genet 1976;9:81–91.

85. Samloff IM, Liebman WM, et al: Serum group I pepsinogens by radioimmunoassay in control subjects and patients with peptic ulcer. Gastroenterology 1975;69:83–90.

86. Rotter JI, Sones JQ, et al: Duodenal ulcer disease associated with elevated serum pepsinogen I, an inherited autosomal dominant disorder. N Engl J Med 1979;300:63–66.

87. Wood WN: Chronic peptic ulcer in 94 diabetics. Am J Dig Dis 1947;14:1–11.

88. Glick DL, Kern F Jr: Peptic ulcer and chronic obstructive bronchopulmonary disease. Gastroenterology 1964;47:153–160.

89. Langman MJS, Cooke AR: Gastric and duodenal ulcer and their associated diseases. Lancet 1976;1:680.

90. Monson RR: Duodenal ulcer as a second disease. Gastroenterology 1970;59:712–716.

91. Frame B: The polyendocrine syndromes. Henry Ford Hosp Med Bull 1966;14:17–76.

92. Forqacs S, Vertes L, et al: Peptic ulcer and diabetes mellitus. Hepatogastroenterology 1980;27:500–504.

93. Spiro HM: Hyperparathyroidism, parathyroid "adenomas" and peptic ulcer. Gastroenterology 1960;39:544–552.

94. Zollinger RM: The Zollinger-Ellison syndrome. World J Surg 1981;5:173–175.

95. Wilson SD: Ulcerogenic tumors of the pancreas: The Zollinger-Ellison syndrome. In: Carey LC (ed). The Pancreas. St. Louis: C.V. Mosby Co., 1973:295–318.

96. McCarthy DM: The Zollinger-Ellison syndrome. Annu Rev Med 1982;33:197–215.

97. Jensen RT: The Zollinger-Ellison syndrome: Current concepts and management. Ann Intern Med 1983;98:59–75.

98. Friesen SR: Treatment of the Zollinger-Ellison Syndrome – 25 year assessment. Am J Surg 1982;143:331–338.

99. Bollen ECM, Lamers CBH, et al: Zollinger-Ellison syndrome due to gastrin producing ovarian cystadenocarcinoma. Br J Surg 1981;68:776–777.

100. Friesen SR, Tomito T: Pseudo Zollinger-

Ellison syndrome: hypergastronemia, hyperchlorhydria without tumor. Ann Surg 1981; 194:481–493.

101. Taylor LL, Calaim J, et al: Familial studies of hypergastrinemic, hyperpepsinogenic duodenal ulcer. Ann Intern Med 1981;95:421–425.

102. Walsh JH, Nair PK, et al: Pathologic acid secretion not due to gastrinoma. Scand J Gastroenterol 1983;18:45–58.

103. Spiro HM. In: General Considerations, Chapter 8. Clinical Gastroenterology. London: Collier-Macmillan Co., 1983:186–206.

104. Willis RA: In: Pathology of Tumors, 4th Ed. London: Appleton-Century-Crofts, 1967:392.

105. Morson BC, Dawson IMP: Gastrointestinal Pathology, 2nd Ed. Oxford: Blackwell Scientific Publishers, 1979:130.

106. Friesen G, Dockerty MB, et al: Superficial carcinomas of the stomach. Surgery 1962;51:300–312.

107. Bralow SP, Collins M: The relationship of peptic ulcer to superficial spreading carcinomas of the stomach. Gastroenterology 1957;32:1152–1161.

108. Helsingen M, Hillestad L: Cancer development in the gastric stump after partial gastrectomy for ulcer. Ann Surg 1956;143:173–179.

109. Stalsberg H, Taksdals S: Stomach cancer following gastric surgery for benign conditions. Lancet 1971;2:1175–1177.

110. Hankilvoto A: Long-term follow-up study of patients operated on for benign peptic ulcer. Ann Chir Gynaecol 1976;65:361–368.

111. Schafer LW, Larson DE, et al: The risk of gastric cancer after surgical treatment for benign ulcer disease. N Engl J Med 1983;309:1210–1213.

112. Weidner N, Smith JG, et al: Peptic ulceration with marked epithelial atypia following hepatic arterial infusion chemotherapy. Am J Surg Pathol 1983;7:261–268.

CHAPTER 6

Hyperplasias and Benign Epithelial Tumors

Hyperplastic Gastropathy (Syn: Hypertrophic Gastropathy, Hypertrophic Gastritis, Giant Mucosal Hypertrophy)

This term includes a group of uncommon to very rare disorders having in common the accentuation of the rugal folds, in part by an increased thickness of the gastric mucosa and in part, as Appelman[1] points out, by exaggeration of the submucosal folds. It includes at least four clinical and histologic entities to which a bewildering prolixity of terms have been applied. The best defined of these is the Zollinger-Ellison syndrome, which is discussed in Chapter 5 on peptic ulceration. Appelman has critically reviewed many of the problems of nomenclature and lack of clear criteria which seem to serve chiefly to illustrate, and perhaps even contribute to, the lack of understanding of the disorders discussed. The mucosa in these diseases is hyperplastic and not hypertrophic,[2] although the term "hypertrophic gastropathy" and many variants, including the term "hypertrophy," are ingrained in the literature.

For at least a partial classification, in Table 6-1 we present a classification modified from that of Appelman.[1]

The gross or endoscopic finding of giant gastric folds is not synonymous with hyper-

plastic gastropathy. The majority of such patients, on biopsy, will be found to have other diseases including chronic nonspecific gastritis, gastric polyposis, carcinoma, lymphoid hyperplasia, lymphoma, and a variety of other less specific conditions.[2] Only a large particle or "snare" biopsy provides enough tissue to allow for a distinction between these possibilities.

Table 6-1. Classification of Giant Gastric Folds

1. Normal variant – exaggeration of submucosal ridges
2. Parietal and chief cell hyperplasia
   A. With hypergastrinemia (Zollinger-Ellison syndrome)*
   B. Without hypergastrinemia ("hypertrophic" hypersecretory gastropathy)
3. Mucous cell hyperplasia with atrophy of parietal and chief cells
   A. With protein-losing gastropathy, chiefly adult (Ménétrier's disease)
   B. Without protein-losing gastropathy, chiefly adult (probable Ménétrier's disease)
   C. With local and/or peripheral eosinophilia, children (transient hypertrophic gastropathy of childhood)*
4. Mixed mucous cell and parietal/chief cell hyperplasia with protein-losing gastropathy ("hypertrophic" hypersecretory and protein-losing gastropathy)†

*Terms in parenthesis indicate clinical terms in use.
†See Discussion.

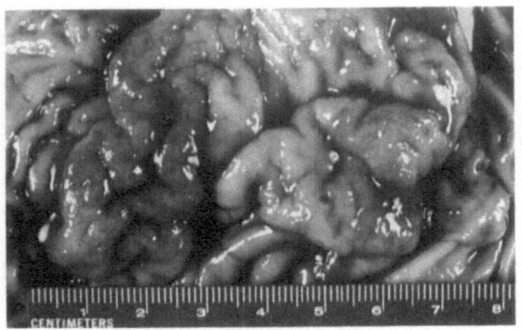

Figure 6-1. Ménétrier's disease. Gastric rugae of the body of the stomach are markedly enlarged as compared with the normal antral folds.

Zollinger-Ellison Syndrome

Hypertrophy of mucosal folds is due to hyperplasia of parietal and chief cells, resulting in hyperacidity and peptic ulceration. This glandular type of hyperplastic gastropathy occurs usually secondary to a gastrin-producing tumor,[3,4] but is also seen in association with other endocrine tumors,[5] in the absence of any detectable endocrine tumor,[6] and secondary to antral G-cell hyperplasia.[7,8] Inflammation is usually absent. One case with a mixed lymphoplasmacytic and neutrophilic infiltrate showed spontaneous recovery.[9] For additional discussion of this syndrome, see Chapter 5.

"Hypertrophic" Hypersecretory Gastropathy

This rare condition is distinguished from the Zollinger-Ellison syndrome by the lack of hypergastrinemia. Appelman[1] suggests that it be considered a form fruste of that entity.

Hypertrophic Hypersecretory Gastropathy with Protein-Losing Gastropathy (Mixed Type of Hyperplastic Gastropathy)

The only four reported cases of this entity are summarized by Appelman,[1] and it remains ill-defined. Hypertrophy of folds is due to hyperplasia of mucous cells as well as parietal and chief cells. Depending on the degree of hyperplasia and the relative proportion of cell types, there may be no symptoms, hypersecretion and protein loss, or hypersecretion without protein loss.[10]

Ménétrier's Disease

The terms "hypertrophic" gastropathy or "idiopathic hypertrophic" gastropathy have been used for those cases with mucous gland hyperplasia and atrophy (at least spotty) of parietal and chief cells, both with and without protein loss. The term "Ménétrier's disease" is usually restricted to cases with protein loss. However, it is impractical to separate out as entities those with and without overt protein loss since protein loss may be absent or remit despite retention of the mucosal changes, and protein loss may occur despite the absence of hypoproteinemia when the liver is able to compensate for such loss.[11]

When Ménétrier[12] described the condition of "polyadenomes gastrique" in 1888, he did not stress the protein loss, but rather was concerned with the possible precancerous nature of the disease. It should also be recalled that protein loss and gastric mucosal thickening are not pathognomonic for Ménétrier's disease, but are also present in the Cronkhite-Canada syndrome.[1] Ménétrier's disease is the most common type of hyperplastic gastropathy and accounts for 66% of such cases.[13]

Clinical

The disease is three times more frequent in men than women and is usually encountered in patients who are middle-aged or older,[13] although it is reported at all ages including in children.[14] The clinical symptomatology in order of decreasing frequency is abdominal pain, weight loss, edema, occult bleeding, vomiting, and overt bleeding.[11] Diarrhea may also occur, as may a macular papular skin rash. Hypersensitivity to foods and eosinophilia have been described.[15] Protein loss and hypoalbuminemia are present in about 80% of cases, and hypochlorhydria in about 75%.[15]

Figure 6-2. Ménétrier's disease. The mucosa of the hypertrophic folds is about five times thicker than the adjacent normal mucosa. H&E, X4.

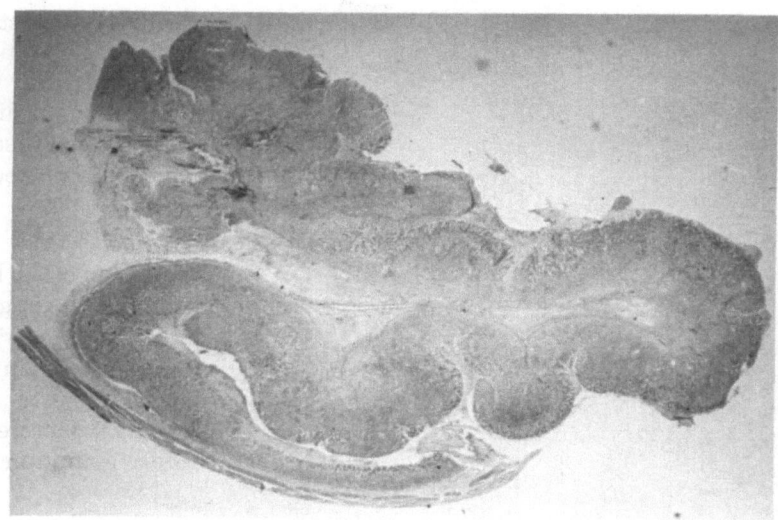

Pathology

The gastric rugae are conspicuously enlarged in the body and fundic area, with relative sparing of the antrum (Fig. 6-1). By endoscopy, they appear cerebriform, with heights varying from 4 mm to 4 cm,[13] being greatest along the greater curvature.[17] The mucosa may be nodular. Material aspirated from the stomach is viscid and of low acidity. Acid secretion is usually, though not always, reduced. The presence of large folds, especially of the greater curvature, disappearing at the antrum suggests the diagnosis radiographically, though the accumulated thick mucin covering the mucosa may complicate the radiographic picture, which at times may be mistaken for tumor, particularly lymphoma.[2,11,18]

Microscopically, the changes are restricted to the mucosa and muscularis mucosae (Fig. 6-2). The latter may be distorted and fragmented. The mucin-secreting cells are hyperplastic and tend to extend down the glands, replacing parietal and chief cells which may be strikingly reduced or, indeed, focally absent (Fig. 6-3). The mucous neck glands and foveolar pits are elongated and tortuous, producing a corkscrew effect. Cystic dilatation of the glands, especially near or at the base of the mucosa, is a feature of variable prominence. Such glands may extend through the muscularis mucosae into the submucosa, and strands of smooth muscle cells may extend up into the lamina propria. The changes, as described, may vary from area to area, with sparing of parietal and chief cells in places. This may explain those reported cases in which there is no obvious reduction of acid on presentation. Occasionally, areas suggestive of hyperplastic polyps may be seen, producing a certain nodularity.[1] Intestinal metaplasia has been described, and regression from the hyperplastic picture to that of an atrophic gastritis reported.[19] Such changes appear to correlate with clinical remission.[20] Variable infiltration of the lamina propria by lymphocytes, plasma cells, and polymorphonuclear leukocytes including eosinophils[15] may be seen. Granulomas have been described in cases with spontaneous resolution. Lymphangiectasia was seen in the mucosa and submucosa in two of three cases by Miura and co-workers.[21]

Pathogenesis

The pathogenesis of this condition is unknown. An animal model in cattle has been reported, which reproduces many features of the disease and is caused by infestation of nematodes of the genus *Osterogia*.[22] This is clearly not the case in man. Homogenates

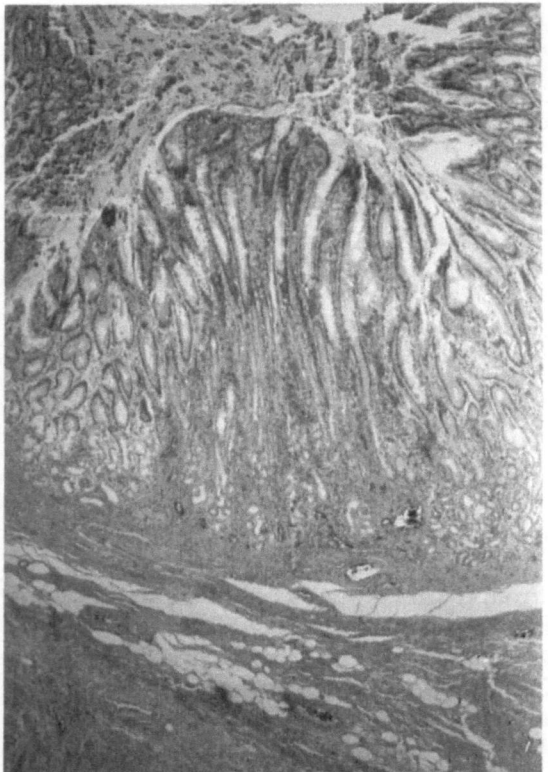

Figure 6-3. Ménétrier's disease. Mucosal thickening is due to foveolar hyperplasia. HPS, X40.

of course, suggests that a hereditary factor is involved. The report, however, does not make it clear whether these were really examples of Ménétrier's disease.[26] The association of anorexia nervosa and Ménétrier's disease has been reported.[27]

Prognosis
Remission of the hypoproteinemia may occur, although the rugal hypertrophy may persist for long periods.[18] Ten cases of remission in adults have been reported as of 1981,[28] and a few cases have improved after cimetadine therapy.[29] Gastrectomy is often required to relieve symptoms.

Relation to Carcinoma
Ménétrier commented on the possible relation of the disorder to carcinoma, and such concern may be justified since some 30 cases of association with carcinoma can be found in the literature.[30] However, the degree of risk is problematic since it is not clear how many of these patients had carcinoma initially and there are few long-term follow-up studies of those patients who did not have gastrectomies. The incidence of malignancy is estimated to be 5%.[13]

and extracts of mucosa have been reported to possess fibrinolytic activity from an endothelial-derived plasminogen activator, possibly causing protein loss by increasing mucosal permeability.[23] However, this may simply be secondary to increased vascularity.[24] Widening of the tight junctions of surface cells has been described at the ultrastructural level, and a decrease induced by anticholinergic drugs is associated with a reduction in protein leakage.[25]

Prostaglandin E_2 has been found in high concentrations in the gastric lumen. Its etiologic importance is suggested by the known inhibition of gastric acid secretion and increase in mucosal permeability.[13] Hyperplastic gastropathy has been described in two brothers, both suffering from pachydermoperiostosis, a hereditary condition which

Transient "Hypertrophic" Gastropathy of Childhood

There are reports in the literature of Ménétrier's disease of childhood.[14] It would appear that these cases do share many features of Ménétrier's disease of adults, such as giant rugae, mucous cell hyperplasia, and protein-losing gastroenteropathy. However, the reported cases, which are few, have shown eosinophils in the lamina propria and most have also had peripheral eosinophilia. Most of these patients had an abrupt onset, diarrhea, and anasarca. All but one apparently recovered on a variety of regimens. The course thus differs sharply from the adult form of Ménétrier's disease, and it is best considered separately. The cause is unknown. Its possible relationship to allergic gastroenteropathy as described by Morson and Dawson[31] is unclear.

Endocrine Cell Hyperplasia

The stomach is rich in endocrine cells. At the time of writing, the secretory product is known in only three of the seven types of cells recognized ultrastructurally (see Chapter 1).[32] Hyperplasia involves mostly the gastrin-producing G cell and rarely the enterochromaffin-like cells and somatostatin-producing D cells. The increasing use of immunohistochemistry, however, will surely result in the recognition of other types of endocrine cell hyperplasia in the future.

Gastrin (G)-Cell Hyperplasia

G-cell hyperplasia occurs in a primary and secondary form. Secondary G-cell hyperplasia can be induced by vagotomy and hypercalcemia[33], and be associated with pernicious anemia, atrophic gastritis, retained antrum, acromegaly, hyperparathyroidism, uremia, and antacid treatment.[7,8,9,32,34,35] In hypercalcemia, antropyloric G-cell counts were 48.2 cells per 0.25 mm² of mucosa as compared with 5.8 cells in normocalcemic control patients.[34]

Primary G-cell hyperplasia is defined as hypergastrinemia in the absence of gastrinoma or any of the above conditions.[7] Clinically, there are persistent peptic ulcers and hyperchlorhydria. The condition occurs predominantly in young males with a strong family history of ulcer disease and is resistant to medical therapy. Characteristic laboratory findings include a modestly increased basal gastrin value, an exaggerated gastrin response to feeding, a minimal response to secretin, and a variable response to calcium infusion. In contrast, patients with gastrinoma have a high basal gastrin value, no exaggerated gastrin response to feeding, but a marked response to secretin and calcium. Patients with common duodenal ulcer also lack an exaggerated gastrin response

to a test meal. G-cell counts in primary hyperplasia have shown more than twice as many antral G-cells than in a variety of normal and abnormal controls, the latter including patients with common peptic ulcer.[7] G-cell hyperplasia was fairly uniform except for low counts over lymphoid follicles. The recognition of G-cell hyperplasia requires immunoperoxidase or immunofluorescence techniques, which can be performed on gastrectomy specimens or endoscopic biopsies. G cells are concentrated in the lower portion of the middle-third of the antral mucosa. Electron microscopically, abnormally lucent endocrine granules were seen, suggesting peptide depletion.[7] Postulated pathogenetic mechanisms of primary G-cell hyperplasia include excess of an as yet unidentified trophic factor, excessive neurogenic stimulation, and inappropriate physiologic response. Considering the diagnosis of primary antral G-cell hyperplasia is of practical importance to a patient suspected of having a gastrinoma, since antrectomy is the treatment of choice in the former and total gastrectomy accompanied by surgical exploration in search for the gastrinoma in the latter.[36]

Hypergastrinemia, regardless of its cause, is associated with the appearance of immunoreactivity for the alpha-subunit of human chorionic gonadotropin (α-HCG) in endocrine cells of fundic type mucosa. Such cells may proliferate and account for 8 to 45% of argyrophil cells. Normal mucosa in normogastrinemic patients shows no α-HCG immunoreactivity.[37]

Enterochromaffin-Like (ECL) Cell Hyperplasia

ECL cells normally occur in the acid-producing gastric mucosa. Their hormonal product is still unknown. ECL cell hyperplasia has been observed after long-term hypergastrinemia and in patients with a portocaval shunt. The trophic effect of gastrin may explain ECL cell hyperplasia in hypergastrinemia, but no mechanism is known to explain the association with portocaval shunt.[38]

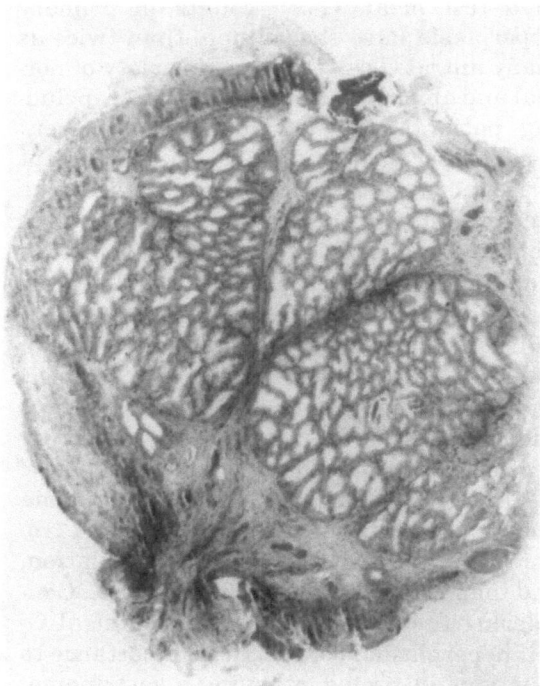

Figure 6-4. Brunner's gland hyperplasia, nodular type. Enlarged lobules are present in the submucosa. The mucosa is eroded. H&E, X40, reproduced at 85%.

Somatostatin-Immunoreactive D-Cell Hyperplasia

D cells are present in the normal oxyntic and pyloric mucosa and in the duodenum. A marked increase, 39-fold and 25-fold respectively in either location, was demonstrated in an unusual case of a woman with dwarfism, obesity, goiter, and dryness of the mouth. Antral G cells were increased only 2-fold.[39]

Brunner's Gland Hyperplasia

Hyperplasia of Brunner's glands was first described by Feyrter[40] in 1934. He distinguished three types: 1) diffuse nodular hyperplasia affecting all Brunner's glands and producing coarse mucosal folds; 2) circumscribed nodular hyperplasia affecting only

isolated Brunner's glands in the suprapapillary portion of the duodenum, while intervening glands may be atrophic; and 3) adenomatous hyperplasia characterized by single nodules of Brunner's glands varying in size form a "pea to a hazelnut." These frequently contain cystic dilatations.

Brunner's glands secrete an alkaline mucus that serves as the physiologic buffer of gastric acid and protects the duodenal mucosa from gastric acid digestion. Brunner's glands also produce urogastrone and epidermal growth factor (see Chapter 5), both inhibitors of gastric acid secretion.[41] Glandular activity is regulated by a combination of luminal, hormonal, and neural factors. Secretion is stimulated by gastric acid, mechanical distention, the vagus nerve, secretin, histamine, vasoactive intestinal polypeptide (VIP), gastric inhibitory polypeptide (GIP), glucagon, and cholecystokinin (CCK) and inhibited by somatostatin and the sympathetic nerve. Hyperplasia is an adaptive phenomenon frequently associated with hyperacidity. It has been suggested that a diagnosis of Brunner's gland hyperplasia can be made when gastric hyperacidity is found in the presence of roentgenologically demonstrable multiple duodenal nodules in a patient with a vague history of abdominal distress.[42]

Of 206 cases of nodular hyperplasia, all occurred in male patients with increased gastric acid secretion after pentagastrin stimulation.[43] Nodules are restricted to the first part of the duodenum and have a reddened surface. Other frequently associated endoscopic findings include chronic gastric erosions, a cobblestone pattern of the gastric body mucosa, and duodenal ulcer. Association with the Zollinger-Ellison syndrome and regression after cimetidine treatment have also been reported.[44] Other commonly associated conditions include chronic pancreatitis[41] and chronic renal failure.[45] In chronic pancreatitis, increased Brunner's gland secretion compensates for the loss of pancreatic alkaline juice and hyperplasia is always diffuse. In chronic renal failure, urea is secreted into the gastrointestinal lumen and serum concentrations of gastrin and group I pepsinogen are raised. Uremic patients with Brunner's gland hyperplasia have a higher gastric juice pH than do those without. Hyperplasia is of the circumscribed nodular type (Fig. 6-4). Hyperplastic Brunner's glands may reach a diameter of up to 15 mm and may be umbilicated as a result of erosion.[42] Histologically, the submucosal and mucosal portions of the gland are enlarged, but are cytologically normal (Fig. 6-5). In the lamina propria, Brunner's glands may extend up to the surface epithelium.

Gastric Polyps

Definition

The word "polyp" is derived from the Greek *"polypus,"* meaning many-footed, and is often loosely applied to any lesion that produces an elevation of the mucosa, including those that arise in the submucosa. Polyps discussed in this chapter are exclusively mucosal and of benign epithelial or mixed epithelial-mesenchymal origin.

Incidence and Clinical Presentation

The incidence of epithelial gastric polyps is low–0.4% at autopsy and approximately 5% among patients undergoing gastroscopy.[46,47] The endoscopic detection rate, however, is increasing year by year, and was 1.4% in 1967 and 8.7% in 1979.[47] Polyps are solitary in 50 to 87% of cases.[48,49] In 9%, there are two or three polyps, and in 4% there is generalized polyposis.[45] Gastric polyps are found in all age groups, with a peak incidence in the fifth to seventh decades, except for cases of polyposis that present at a younger age.[50] Polyps occur with equal frequency among men and women. In almost half of all cases, there are no symptoms.[49] If symptoms are present, they tend to be vague and nonspecific. Pedunculated polyps may prolapse through the pylorus and cause obstruction.[51] Bleeding may occur, but is usually mild and leads to hematemesis in only 10% of patients. Eighty-

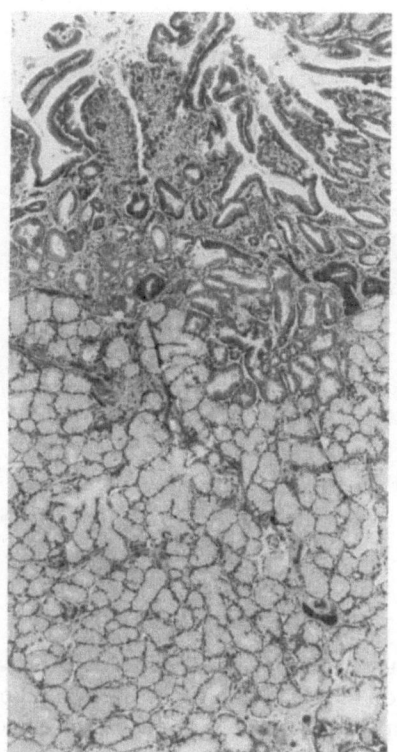

Figure 6-5. Brunner's gland hyperplasia. Cytologically normal glands are closely packed in the submucosa and mucosa. HPS, X60, reproduced at 70%.

five percent of patients with benign gastric polyps have achlorhydria. Conversely, polyps are common in patients with atrophic gastritis and pernicious anemia (5%).[49]

Diagnosis

The diagnosis of gastric polyps can be made radiologically with upper gastrointestinal tract double-contrast barium techniques in 70 to 90% of cases.[52] Fiberoptic endoscopy, however, is the diagnostic procedure of choice, since tissue diagnosis and definite therapy can be accomplished simultaneously. Whenever feasible, polyps should be removed in toto, since biopsies rarely are representative of the whole lesion, as reflected in a 70% dis-

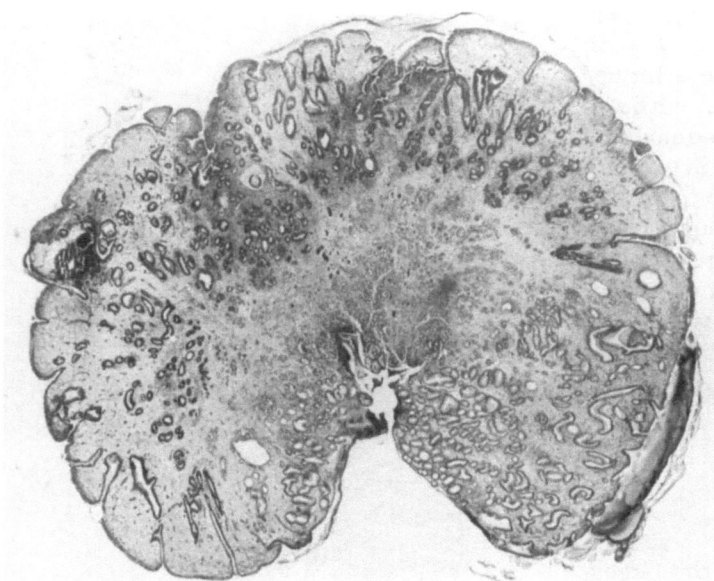

Figure 6-6. Gastric stomal polypoid hyperplasia—a form of hyperplastic polyp occurring at anastomotic sites. Foveolae are elongated and irregular; the stroma is edematous. HPS, X20, reproduced at 70%.

crepancy rate between histologic diagnoses based on biopsies and those based on polypectomy specimens.[53] The appearance on routine endoscopy usually does not allow for distinction of different types of polyps. Magnifying fiberoptic endoscopy, using magnification of up to X30, as employed in Japan, enables the endoscopist to correlate deformities of areolae and gastric pits with the histologic type of polyp.[54]

Classification and Pathology

Classification of gastric polyps is based on their histologic features. Since their first description as "fibroadenomas" by Borrmann[55] in 1926, a variety of nomenclatures has been used.[48,50,56-59] All classification systems agree on the importance of separating hyperplastic from neoplastic lesions because of their different precancerous potentials. Disagreement persists as to the existence of the hybrid form, called hyperplastic-adenomatous polyp,[58] which is not included in all classification systems. Difficulties also exist in classifying lesions that do not readily fall into any of the most commonly used categories.[56-59] The recently proposed classification scheme of Snover[50] takes these issues

into account, appears most practical and complete, and is used in the following discussion.

Gastric Hyperplastic Polyp (Syn: Regenerative Polyp,[56] Hyperplasiogenous Polyp,[59] Hyperplastic-Adenomatous Polyp[58])

Hyperplastic polyps represent the most common type of benign gastric epithelial polyp and comprise between 70 and 90% of all gastric polyps.[50,58] They may be solitary or multiple and occur in all parts of the stomach, most frequently, however, in the antrum. Unusual locations include the gastroesophageal junction[60] and anastomotic sites. Polyps at anastomotic sites occur between 1 and 18 years after Billroth II gastrectomy, are often multiple and confluent, cause obstruction, and have become known as gastritis polyposa[61] or gastric stomal polypoid hyperplasia[62] (Fig. 6-6).

Usually, hyperplastic polyps are less than 2 cm in diameter and sessile, although sizes of up to 4 cm diameter have been reported.[63] A change from a sessile semispherical to pedunculated type was noted with increasing size and follow-up time.[47] Men and women are affected with equal frequency at a median age of 69 years.[47] The youngest reported patient with a solitary hyperplastic polyp was a 12-year-old girl.[63] Chronic atrophic gastritis is associated in 72% of cases.[50]

Histologically, a hyperplastic polyp is composed of elongated tortuous, sometimes cystically distended faveolae and an edematous lamina propria with distended angiomatous vessels (Fig. 6-7). There may be an infiltrate of lymphocytes, plasma cells, eosinophils, and occasionally polymorphonuclear leukocytes. Bundles of smooth muscle radiate upwards from a splayed muscularis mucosae. The deep portions of the polyp contain cytologically normal antral glands, regardless of whether the polyp arose in the cardia, fundus, corpus, or antrum. Occasionally, typical fundic glands with parietal and chief cells can be seen. Thus, hyperplastic polyps may be divided into a pure antral-type and a mixed fundic/antral-type.[50] Erosion of the surface and subsequent regeneration may produce reactive atypia of the surface lining, characterized by cytoplasmic acidophilia, a large central nucleus, and a cuboidal cell shape not to be confused with precancerous atypia. Rarely, erosions of hyperplastic polyps may be associated with atypia of mesenchymal cells that exhibit marked nuclear pleomorphism and atypical mitotic figures. Such cells blend with typical granulation tissue and appear to be related to repeated trauma, especially in polyps near the cardia.[64] It may be difficult to distinguish pseudostratification of regenerating foveolar epithelium from adenomatous epithelium, but if found adjacent to typical acidophilic regenerating cells, should be interpreted as reactive. Intestinal metaplasia is found in approximately 10 to 27% of hyperplastic polyps[50,65] and reflects coexisting chronic atrophic gastritis. After polypectomy, there is a high incidence of recurrence (32.5%) at different locations in the stomach. Endoscopic follow-up for 5 to 12 years after a biopsy diagnosis of hyperplastic polyp showed enlargement of the biopsied polyp in 25% of cases, a decrease in size in 5%, and spontaneous disappearance in 3%.[47]

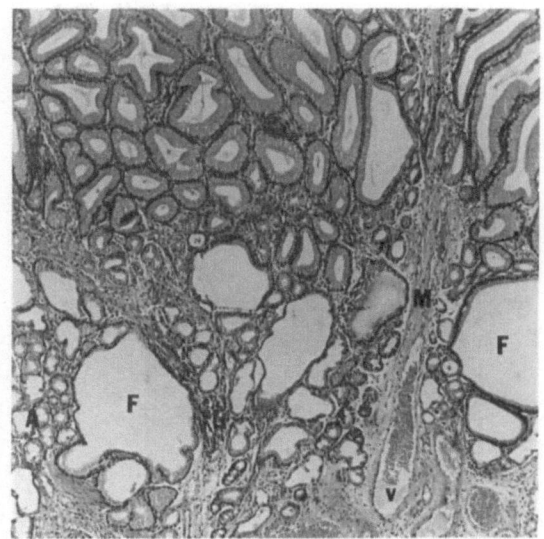

Figure 6-7. Hyperplastic polyp of the stomach. Characteristic microscopic features include elongated and cystic foveolae (F), preserved antral glands (A), angiomatous vessels (V), and smooth muscle fibers radiating upwards (M). HPS, X40, reproduced at 65%.

For the pathologist, it is important to recognize hyperplastic gastric polyps as distinctly different from adenomatous polyps because of the much weaker association with carcinoma of the former as compared with the latter. Carcinoma may be present elsewhere in the stomach and was found in 7%,[56] 12%,[50] and 28%[57] of three large series of hyperplastic polyps. Carcinoma is rarely found within a hyperplastic polyp.[50,65] In some such cases, it remains unclear whether carcinoma truly arose in the polyp or invaded it secondarily. Since most patients with hyperplastic polyps also have chronic atrophic gastritis, which by itself leads to carcinoma in 8% of cases,[66] there is most likely no causal relationship between hyperplastic polyps, per se, and carcinoma. The majority of associated carcinomas were of the diffuse type.[50] Long-term follow-up study of patients with gastric polyps, most of which were hyperplastic, showed only a 1.7% incidence of carcinoma developing within 1 to 7 years after polypectomy.[67]

Gastric Adenomatous-Hyperplastic Polyp

This polyp represents a hybrid of two different growth patterns. The base is identical to

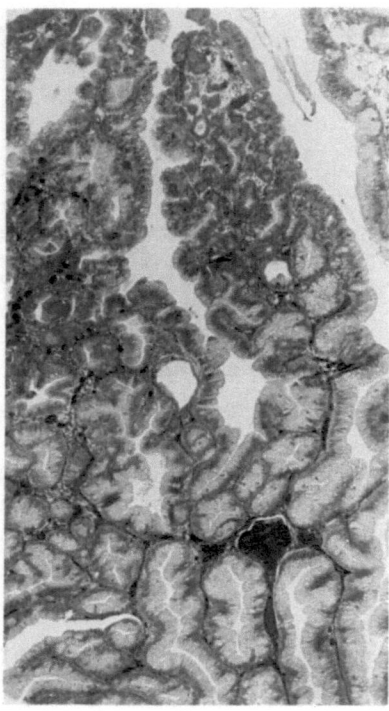

Figure 6-8. Adenomatous-hyperplastic polyp of the stomach. The base is composed of pale hyperplastic foveolae, the tip of dark-staining adenomatous glands. HPS, X40, reproduced at 70%.

a hyperplastic polyp, while the superficial portion is composed of adenomatous epithelium (Fig. 6-8). In contrast to the purely adenomatous polyp, the adenomatous-hyperplastic polyp is more often multiple. Four percent of all gastric polyps and 50% of all neoplastic polyps are of this type.[50]

Gastric Adenomatous Polyp
(Syn: Adenoma, Tubular Adenoma)

This term is frequently used to include all benign neoplastic gastric polyps (i.e., the adenomatous-hyperplastic polyp, the villous or villoglandular polyp, and the adenomatous polyp).[57] The term should be restricted to those polyps that are composed of tubular glands lined by adenomatous epithelium. In histology and behavior, the gastric adenomatous polyp resembles its colonic counterpart. The incidence varies with the definition of the term and has been reported between 8%[50] and 25%.[48,56,57] Patients with adenomatous polyps range in age from 22 to 84 years, and have a median age of 69 years. There is a slight male predominance (1.5:1, M:F), paralleling the higher incidence of gastric carcinoma in men. Adenomatous polyps are usually solitary and, if multiple, often part of a polyposis syndrome (see below). Most are located in the antrum. The average size is considerably larger than that of hyperplastic

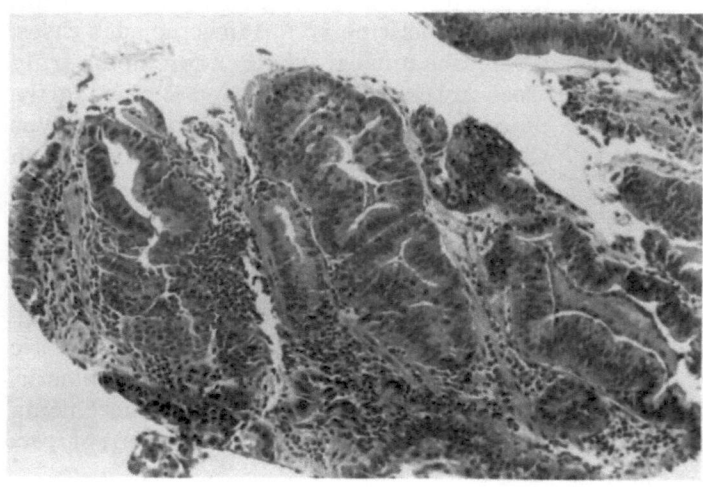

Figure 6-9. Adenomatous polyp of the stomach. Tubular glands are lined by pseudostratified dark-staining columnar cells. H&E, X100, reproduced at 85%.

polyps. Fifty percent have a diameter greater than 4 cm,[58] although reported average sizes tend to be smaller with the increased use and greater diagnostic yield of biphasic contrast examinations.[68]

Histologically, the entire polyp is composed of one type of epithelium that has no counterpart in the normal gastric mucosa. Pseudostratified columnar epithelial cells with dark-staining cytoplasm are arranged in closely packed glands (Fig. 6-9). Nuclei are elongated and hyperchromatic and show mitoses at all levels. Mucin is generally absent, except in areas of intestinal metaplasia. Varying numbers of argyrophil cells and lysozyme-containing cells may be present.[69] All degrees of dysplasia may be seen and correlate with increased nuclear DNA and aneuploidy in severe dysplasia.[70] Carcinoma in situ was found in 25%.[50] Independent synchronous invasive adenocarcinoma elsewhere in the stomach has been reported in 25 to 59% of cases.[50,56,57] Carcinoma was mostly of the diffuse type (Fig. 6-10).

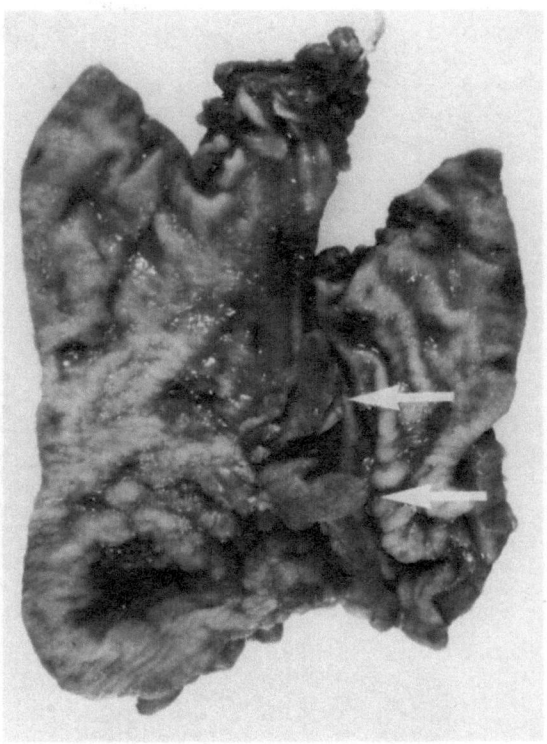

Figure 6-10. Adenomatous polyps (*arrows*) adjacent to an ulcerated gastric carcinoma.

Gastric Villous Adenoma (Syn: Papillary Adenoma)

Villous adenomas are rare, and only about 100 cases were found in the English medical literature in 1980.[71] In a more recent review of gastric polyps, the relative incidence was 0.6%.[50] Villous adenomas may be sessile, broad-based, or pedunculated. They may reach large sizes—the largest reported polyp was 21 cm in diameter[71]—and, perhaps because of their size, are more often associated with significant clinical symptoms than are other gastric polyps. Over half of all patients have weakness and weight loss. A palpable mass is present in one-third.[72] Almost all patients have achlorhydria; half are anemic. On upper gastrointestinal radiography, villous adenomas produce a characteristic fine or coarse lacy soap-bubble pattern.[71] Histologically, they are composed of papillary projections separated by deep fissures and lined by single layered or pseudostratified adenomatous epithelium (Fig. 6-11). Some villous adenomas show areas of glandular differentiation as seen in adenomatous polyps, and have been designated as villo-glandular polyps.[50] They are as rare as pure villous adenomas. Although their malignant potential increases with size,[73] not all large villous adenomas harbor a carcinoma.[71] Malignancy arising in a villous adenoma has been reported in 25 to 75% of cases.[58,73]

Gastric Fundic Gland Polyp (Syn: Fundic Gland Hyperplasia, Oxyntic Gland Polyp, Gastric Glandular Cysts, Cystic Glandular Fundic Polyps, Gastric Hamartomatous Polyp, "Drüsenkörperzysten")

Fundic gland polyposis was first described by Japanese and European authors[74,75] as a benign entity to be distinguished from other polyposis syndromes. It is now recognized with increasing frequency also in the United

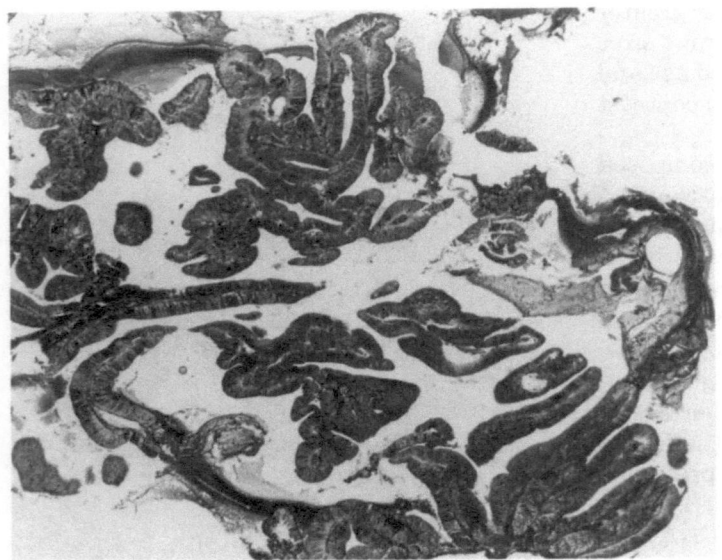

Figure 6-11. Villous adenoma. HPS, X80, reproduced at 70%.

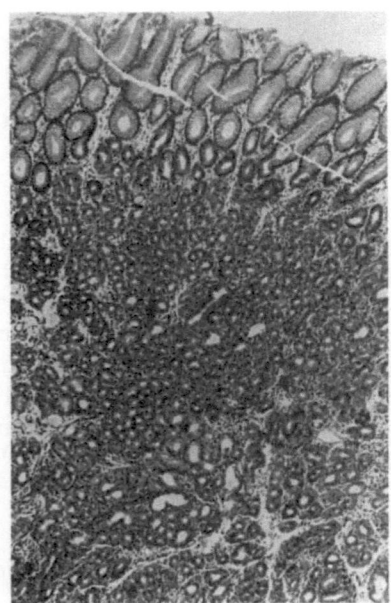

Figure 6-12. Fundic gland polyp. Fundic glands are increased in number and focally reach the surface. Cystic foveolae and cystic fundic glands are characteristic. H&E, X40, reproduced at 70%.

States.[50,76-78] Although most common in patients with either familial adenomatosis coli[79,80] or Gardner's syndrome,[76,80] the majority of cases of fundic gland polyposis show no such association.[50,79] In Japan, 39% of patients with familial adenomatosis coli had fundic gland polyps as compared with 0.085% of nonadenomatosis coli individuals.[79] Sporadic cases are three times more common in women than in men and affect patients approximately 50 years of age. Adenomatosis-associated cases show no such female predominance and tend to occur at an earlier age (25 years). The youngest affected patient was 8 years old.[78]

Fundic gland polyps are not uncommon and constitute 13% of all gastric polyps.[50] They are almost always multiple and restricted to the body and fundus of the stomach. They are small sessile lesions of 1 to 10 mm diameter and are composed of parietal and chief cells (Fig. 6-12). Many of these polyps, especially when present in large numbers, contain cysts lined by mucinous cells as well as by a few parietal and chief cells, imparting a hamartomatous appearance (Fig. 6-13). In contrast to true hamartomatous polyps, however, fundic gland polyps contain no smooth muscle.

Figure 6-13. Fundic gland polyp. Cystic glands are lined by both mucinous foveolar epithelium and parietal and chief cells. H&E, X400, reproduced at 70%.

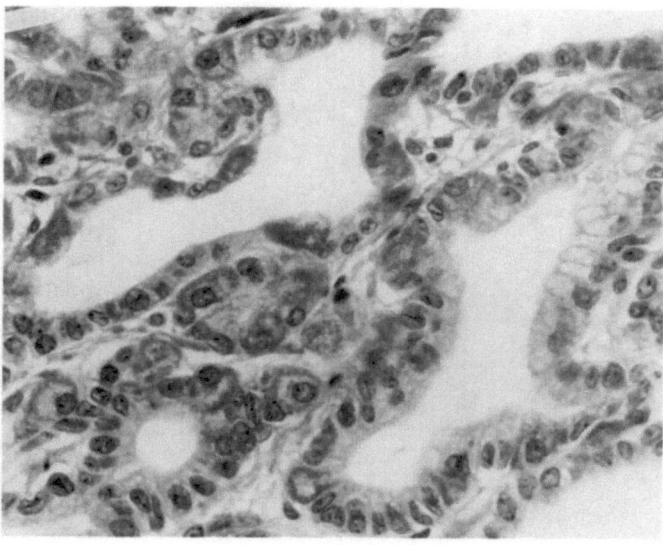

If solitary or present in small numbers, they may not contain cysts and can be composed of completely normal fundic glands that may be indistinguishable from normal mucosa in an endoscopic biopsy. Frequently, however, fundic glands occupy the full thickness of the mucosa, extending to the surface epithelium between the foveolae, where they are normally not present. Atrophic gastritis may be associated, and intestinal metaplasia may secondarily involve the polyp itself.[50] Adenocarcinoma, found elsewhere in the stomach in one case, was thought to be related to atrophic gastritis. Acid secretion by fundic gland polyps can be demonstrated by the endoscopic Congo red test[74] or by enlargement of the polyp, demonstrable by x-ray, after pentagastrin stimulation.[75]

Fundic gland polyposis has no known precancerous significance, and is understood as a hyperplastic rather than a neoplastic process. Spontaneous disappearance within 9 to 34 months has been observed in some cases.[81]

Rare Gastric Polyps

Foveolar hyperplasia has been described as distinct from hyperplastic polyp and differs from the latter by the absence of a smooth muscle core. It is characterized by elongation of foveolae and normal underlying glands (Fig. 6-14). Such lesions are found in all parts of the stomach, are usually multiple, and account for 5% of all gastric polyps.[51] A probably related lesion is the so-called *foveolar adenoma*. A single case has been described.[50] An 8 cm solitary lesion in the body of the stomach was composed of tightly packed glands lined by normal foveolar epithelium.

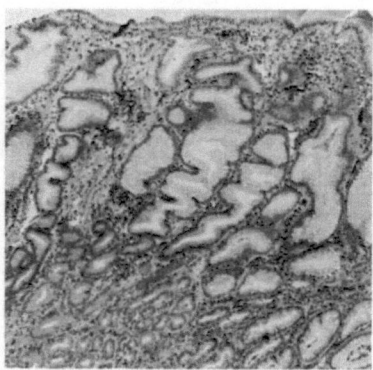

Figure 6-14. Foveolar hyperplasia. Foveolae are elongated and tortuous. In contrast to hyperplastic polyps, there are no cysts and no radiating smooth muscle bundles or angiomatous blood vessels. HPS, X40, reproduced at 70%.

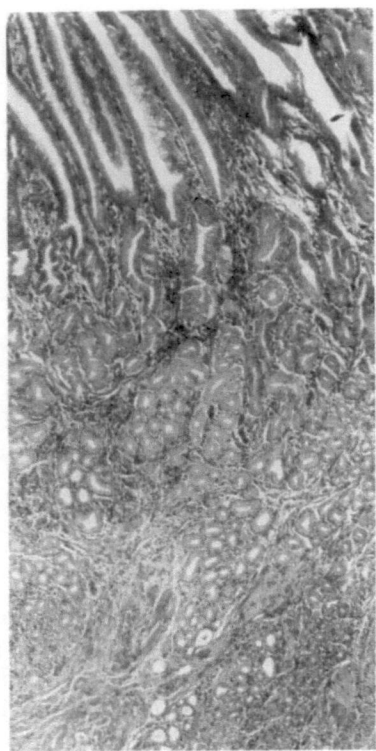

Figure 6-15. Antral gland hyperplasia. HPS, X40, reproduced at 70%.

Antral gland hyperplasia, also called heterotopic adenomatous polyp or Brunner's gland adenoma,[50] shows clusters of antral glands surrounded by bundles of smooth muscle (Fig. 6-15). These polyps range in size from 1.2 to 2 cm, are found exclusively in the antrum, and account for 2% of gastric polyps.

Hamartomatous polyps are rare, and only 1 was found in a series of 182 gastric polyps.[50] Most hamartomatous polyps occur as part of a polyposis syndrome, usually the Peutz-Jeghers syndrome, and less commonly Gardner's and Cronkhite-Canada syndromes.[58,82] The Peutz-Jeghers syndrome involves the stomach in 24% of cases.[58] Isolated gastric hamartomatous polyps have been described in the antrum,[82] and may reach sizes of up to 7 cm diameter. Histologically, they are composed of lobules of mucinous glands arranged around a center of radiating smooth muscle bundles.

Pseudopolyps are lesions that appear as polyps to the endoscopist but histologically present with normal gastric fundic-type mucosa.[83] Such pseudopolyps are found in chronic atrophic gastritis of the fundus and corpus, also called "type A gastritis," as opposed to "type B gastritis" that primarily involves the antrum. Atrophy affects the fundic mucosa unevenly, and endoscopically residual unaffected mucosa resembles a polyp in contrast to the surrounding flattened mucosa. Such pseudopolyps are usually multiple and are then referred to as "pseudopolyposis." They disappear spontaneously as atrophy spreads.

Polyposis Syndromes

Juvenile polyposis primarily affects the colon, but at times involves the entire gastrointestinal tract[84] or presents as isolated gastric juvenile polyposis.[85] Polyps may be present in early infancy[86] or, more commonly, are discovered in childhood or early adulthood. A family history of juvenile polyps is present in half of the cases, suggesting an autosomal-dominant mode of inheritance.[87] A genetic relationship with adenomatous polyposis has been postulated on the basis of the coexistence of both syndromes in the same family and within the same patient.[88] Gastric polyps may cause blood and protein loss, necessitating total gastrectomy.[85] Whereas intestinal juvenile polyps are most commonly solitary and not part of a polyposis syndrome, it is uncertain whether gastric juvenile polyps ever occur as a sporadic event. All reported cases were associated with polyposis syndromes.[50]

The stomach may show only few minute polyps[84] or be covered by numerous smooth-surfaced nonlobulated polyps (Fig. 6-16).[85] The duodenum may be involved.[84] Histologically, juvenile polyps are characterized by abundant loose stroma infiltrated by a variable number of lymphocytes, plasma cells, neutrophils, and eosinophils and by dilated,

Figure 6-16. Juvenile polyposis of the stomach. From Snover.[47] Reproduced by permission, Appleton-Century-Crofts.

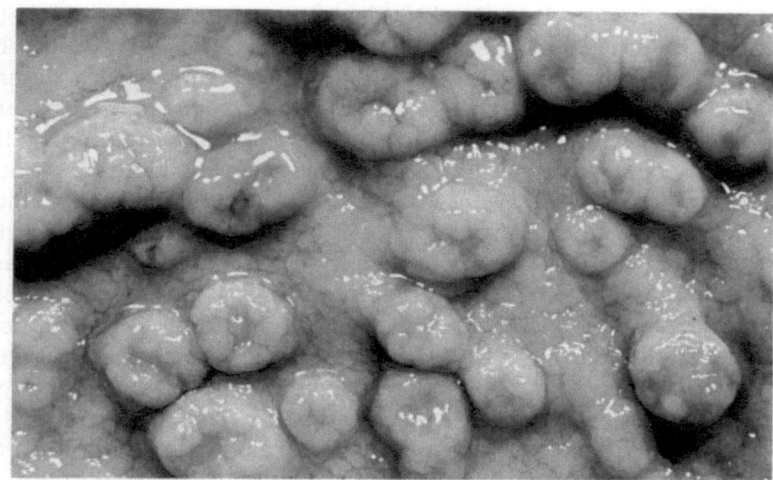

often cystic, mucinous glands. The latter feature explains the term "retention polyp," often used as a synonym for juvenile polyp. Juvenile polyps may coexist with adenomatous and hyperplastic polyps. Rarely, mixed polyps with both adenomatous and juvenile features have been described.[87] Marked hyperplasia of argentaffin and argyrophil cells was found in the latter case. Familial juvenile polyposis carries an increased risk of gastrointestinal carcinoma in the affected patient as well as in family members.

Familial polyposis coli with gastric and duodenal involvement has been described repeatedly in the past two decades, but only since the use of endoscopic surveillance has the high frequency of such an occurrence been appreciated.[89-90] In seven of nine patients, duodenal and gastric adenomas were detected during a 2- to 6-year period of yearly endoscopy and biopsy. These adenomatous polyps were single or multiple and varied in size from 2 to 8 mm. In the stomach, adenomatous polyps were found primarily in the antrum. In the duodenum, the third portion was preferentially involved. Polyps in the gastric body and fundus also occur, but are not adenomatous being either hyperplastic, lymphoid, or fundic gland hyperplasia.[92] Fundic gland polyps, as described above, are found in almost half of all patients with

colonic polyposis. Fundic gland polyps associated with familial polyposis coli differ from sporadic cases in their content of O-acylated sialic acid, a component of mucin present only in the intestine and not in the normal gastric foveolar cell.[92] The presence of O-acylated sialic acid in a fundic gland polyp should prompt an examination of the colon and rectum.

Familial gastric polyposis without colonic involvement is rare. Carcinoma of the stomach coexisted in both reported cases.[93]

Gardner's syndrome is a dominantly inherited polyposis syndrome that was originally described in 1953 by Gardner and Richards[94] as the triad of multiple polyposis coli, osteomas, and soft tissue tumors. Since then, the spectrum of lesions associated with the syndrome has markedly expanded and now includes small intestinal and gastric polyps, periampullary carcinoma of the duodenum, carcinomas of thyroid and adrenal glands, tumors of the central nervous system, skin and mucous membrane pigmentation, trichoepitheliomas, and abnormal dentition.[76,95-97] The great variety of organs and tissues involved lends support to the concept of a generalized defect in growth regulation based on chromosomal abnormalities.[95]

Gastric and duodenal polyps were found in more than half of the 11 affected members of the originally described Gardner's syndrome kindred.[96] Gastric polyps are mostly of the fundic gland-type, but numerous adenomas may also occur.[97] Duodenal polyps are more frequent than gastric polyps and have always been adenomas. One patient had 256 duodenal adenomas.[97]

Cronkhite-Canada syndrome, first described in 1955,[98] is characterized by gastrointestinal polyposis, hyperpigmentation, alopecia, and nail dystrophy. The condition is nonfamilial and rare—55 cases were found in a literature review of 1982.[99] The etiology is unknown. Almost half of all reported cases occurred in Japanese.[100] Symptoms such as abdominal pain, diarrhea, and protein-losing enteropathy develop late (i.e., at a mean age of 59 years).[51] Radiographically, there are enlarged gastric rugae, polyps, and "whiskering" produced by trapping of barium between enlarged areae gastricae.[101]

Polyps are found most often in the stomach and colon, but in some cases also in the small intestine.[94] Gastric lesions, reported in 90% of patients,[101] are basically retention polyps composed of elongated and cystically distended foveolae lined by cytologically normal mucinous epithelium (Fig. 6-17). The stroma is edematous and often infiltrated with plasma cells, neutrophils, and eosinophils. Rugae are hypertrophic, similar to those of Ménétrier's disease.

Duodenal polyps, found in 75% of patients,[99] tend to be smaller in number and size than those of the stomach.[100] Single or multiple gastrointestinal carcinomas were found in 8 of 55 patients.[51,99] Generalized vasculitis, most severe in the gastrointestinal tract, developed in one patient.[102]

Therapy consists primarily of nutritional supplementation. Antibiotics and steroids produced remission in some patients. Gastric and large bowel resections were rarely successful. Spontaneous recovery has been reported. Over half of the 55 cases have died of causes related to their disease.[99]

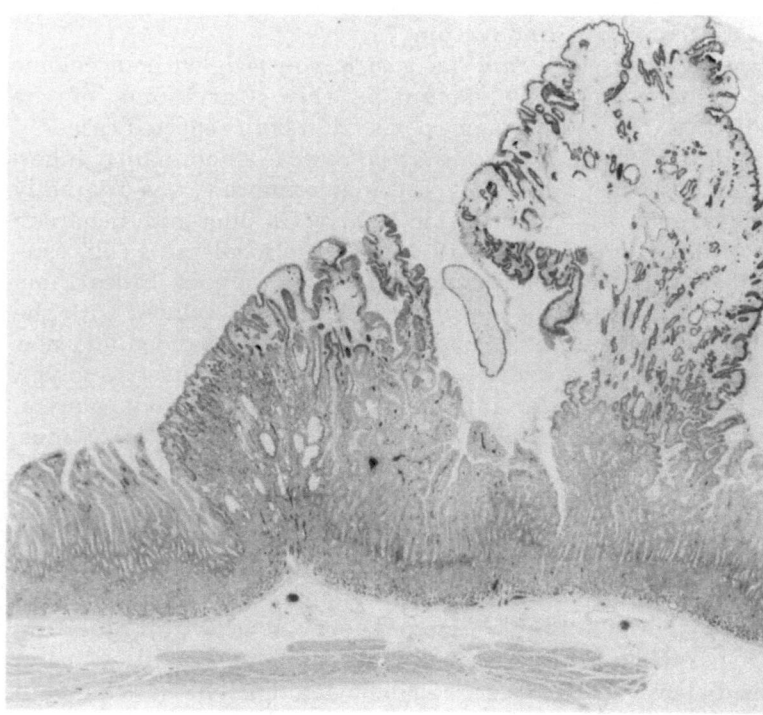

Figure 6-17. Cronkhite-Canada syndrome. Polyps are composed of elongated and cystic foveolae and of edematous stroma. Elongated foveolae are also seen in the mucosa between polyps. H&E, X20, reproduced at 85%.

Cowden's disease, a multiple hamartoma syndrome, is characterized by orocutaneous hamartomas, thyroid lesions, breast carcinoma, and gastrointestinal polyposis. Gastric lesions are less frequent than colonic ones, and are either hyperplastic polyps[103] or lymphoid aggregates.[104]

Peutz-Jeghers syndrome, as first observed by Peutz in a Dutch family in 1921 and subsequently described in detail by Jeghers[105] in 1949, is characterized by 1) hamartomatous polyps of the small intestine, colon, and/or stomach; 2) mucocutaneous pigmentation; and 3) a family history suggestive of a dominant inheritance pattern. Incomplete forms of the syndrome without family history and pigmentation, or pigmentation without polyps, also exist. Most polyps develop in the jejunum and ileum, and in decreasing order of frequency in colon, stomach, duodenum, and appendix.[106] The stomach is involved in 24%, and the duodenum in 11% of cases. Polyps are rarely as numerous as in adenomatosis coli, and even in familial cases, may be single.

Microscopically, lobules of mucinous glands are arranged around a smooth muscle core. Such entrapment of glands in smooth muscle should not be mistaken for invasive carcinoma. Cancer risk is estimated at 2%.[107] Such cancers have occurred in the duodenum and gastric antrum and rarely appear to develop within the polyps themselves.

Duodenal Polyps

Although polyps are rarer in the duodenum than in the stomach, it is noteworthy that approximately one-fifth of all small intestinal tumors are in the duodenum, which comprises less than one-tenth of the small intestine.[108] Forty-eight percent of all duodenal tumors are benign. In the proximal portion, most tumors are benign[109] as a result of the high proportion of Brunner's gland lesions. In the distal portion, malignant lesions are more common. Polyps are encountered in approximately 1% of duodenoscopic examinations[110] and are predominantly of neoplastic type. Among 19 histologically examined duodenal polyps, there were 8 adenomatous polyps, 6 villous adenomas, 2 Brunner's gland hyperplasias, 2 lipomas, and 1 carcinoid.

Duodenal Adenomatous Polyp

Duodenal adenomatous polyps are usually found incidentally. Occult and rarely massive bleeding is the most frequent symptom. These polyps seldom become large enough to produce obstruction, and intussusception is not a problem because of anatomic fixation of the duodenum. Most are less than 3 mm in diameter (Fig. 6-18). They may be single or multiple and are usually pedunculated. Most are found in the first portion of the duodenum. In Gardner's syndrome and familial polyposis, duodenal adenomatous polyps are numerous, often centered on folds, and may involve also the third portion of the duodenum.[111,112] Endoscopic or surgical polypectomy is suggested because of the danger of bleeding and malignant change. Dysplasia is commonly present in patients with polyposis syndromes, but the relatively low number of reports of duodenal cancer in familial polyposis suggests that the adenoma–cancer sequence requires a very long time in this location.[111] Nonetheless, carcinoma of the papilla of Vater showed residual adenoma in 18 of 22 cases examined.[113]

Duodenal Villous Adenoma

This is a rare lesion, and only 68 cases were found in the literature in 1981.[114] Most cases affect adults in the sixth and seventh decades. Symptoms in decreasing order of frequency are bleeding (27 to 49%), obstruction (24 to 40%), and jaundice (22%).[115] Jaundice is an ominous clinical sign, since 80% of jaundiced patients have coexisting carcinoma. Intussusception may complicate villous adenoma of the distal duodenum.[116] Radiographic studies yield a definite diag-

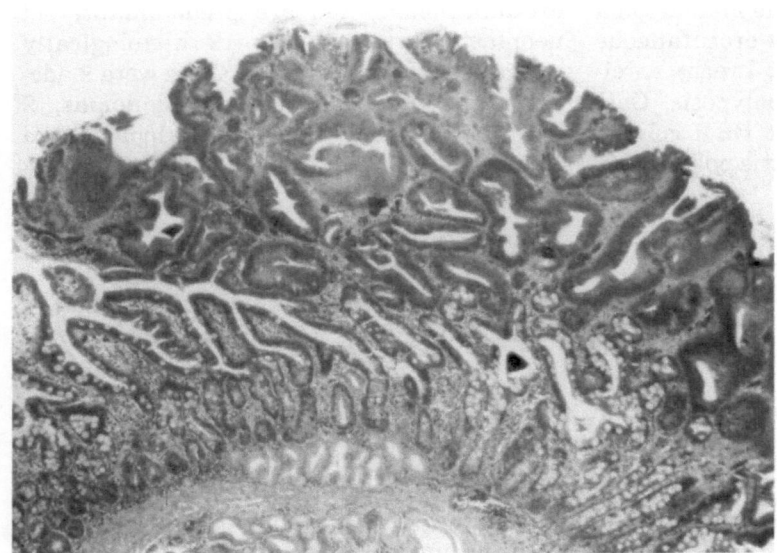

Figure 6-18. Adenomatous polyp of the duodenum. H&E, X40, reproduced at 85%.

nosis in approximately 33% of cases. Endoscopy, therefore, is the diagnostic method of choice.

Villous adenomas are more likely to be located in the proximal portion of the duodenum, but also occur in the third and fourth portions. In 20% of reported cases, the ampulla of Vater was involved. Most lesions are single, but multiplicity, in the absence of generalized polyposis, has been described.[114,117] Sizes vary from 1 to 9 cm in diameter.

Histologically, duodenal villous adenomas are composed of thin fibrovascular cores and crowded high columnar epithelium (Fig. 6-19). Some lesions present a mixed villous and glandular pattern. The epithelium is variable; it may be identical to that of the normal small intestinal mucosa and include absorptive cells, goblet cells, and Paneth cells, or show mucinous differentiation or cytoplasmic basophilia. Focal areas of nuclear stratification and hyperchromatism, increased mitotic activity, and loss of nuclear polarity are often present and represent signs of dysplasia (Fig. 6-20). Carcinoma is reportedly found in 35% of cases, but in 14% is only in situ.[117] This figure is significantly higher than the comparable 26% for colonic villous adenomas. Biopsies are often insuffi-

cient to determine whether invasive carcinoma is present or not. They should be multiple and sample the central portion of the lesion, since it is there that malignancy first develops. If secondary gland formation is seen in the intramucosal portion of the lesion, invasive carcinoma is likely to be present.[114] Positive-staining with anti-CEA antiserum at high dilutions was found in a large villous adenoma with cytologic atypia and coexisting invasive carcinoma, and may be an early indicator of malignancy.[117] Stromal changes are helpful: invasive carcinoma evokes a desmoplastic stromal response that can be recognized even in isolated tissue fragments, and differs from the loose lamina propria around adenomatous glands. Because of the uncertainties inherent in the biopsy diagnosis of villous adenomas, total removal is required, either by submucosal excision or by segmental resection.[114]

Duodenal Hyperplastic Polyp

No such polyps are recorded in reviews of duodenal polyps. An isolated report describes a 13-mm diameter hyperplastic polyp in the duodenal bulb composed of villi and crypts

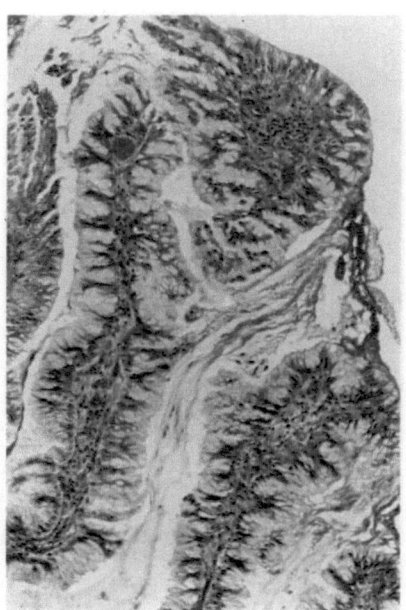

Figure 6-19. Villous adenoma of the duodenum. H&E, X100, reproduced at 70%.

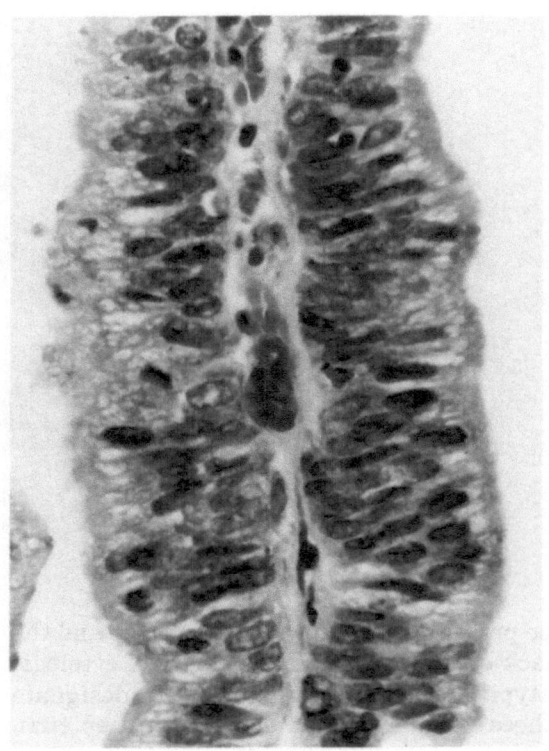

Figure 6-20. Villous adenoma with dysplasia. H&E, X250, reproduced at 60%.

lined by hyperplastic intestinal type epithelium.[118] A second endoscopically identical polyp composed of hyperplastic gastric type epithelium was designed as "metaplastic polyp."

Brunner's Gland Adenoma (Syn: Adenomatous Brunner's Gland Hyperplasia,[40] Brunneroma,[119] Hamartoma[120,121]

Feyrter[40] is generally credited with the first description and classification of Brunner's gland hyperplasia in 1934, and his category of adenomatous hyperplasia later became synonymous with adenoma. Tumors of Brunner's gland origin, however, were mentioned in the medical literature as early as 1835 and 1876 by Cruveilhier[122] and Salvioli,[123] respectively. The wide span of time between these dates attests to the rarity of the lesion. One hundred-seven cases were found in the medical literature in 1979,[124] and only few cases have been added since.[125,126]

Patients are usually in the fourth to sixth decade, although ages range from 22 to 76 years.[120] Most lesions are discovered incidentally by radiologic studies performed for unrelated conditions such as hiatal hernia and peptic ulcer disease.[121] Ulceration may cause blood loss and anemia. Large lesions occasionally cause obstruction or intussusception.[121] The duodenal bulb, in particular the posterior wall, is the most common site. Reported sizes vary from a few millimeters to 12 mm in diameter.[126] Brunner's gland adenomas are usually single and sessile, but may be pedunculated. Grossly, they appear mucoid and lobulated and sometimes show small, barely visible cysts.

Histologically, they are composed of lobules of acini, ducts that may be cystic, smooth muscle, and, in some cases, adipose tissue (Fig. 6-21). Eosinophils and lymphocytes may

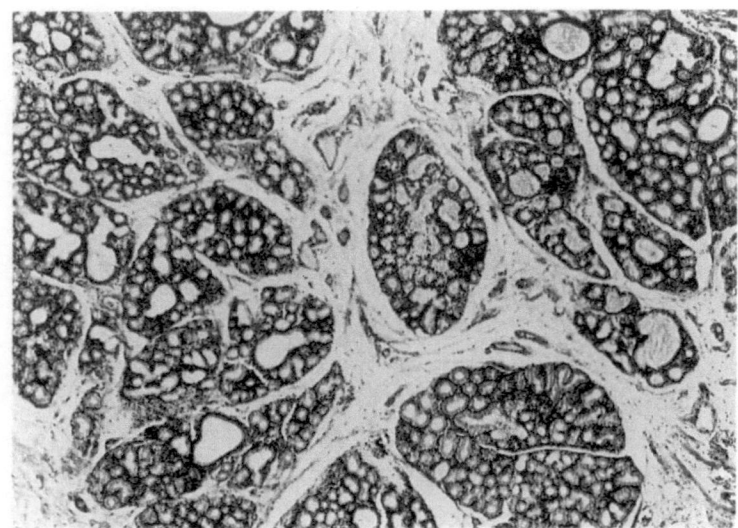

Figure 6-21. Brunner's gland adenoma. Courtesy of Dr. Weinberger, Lenox Hill Hospital, New York, New York. HPS, X250, reproduced at 60%.

be present. The admixture of tissues and the lack of encapsulation and rarity of cytologic atypia have led some authors to designate these lesions as hamartomas rather than adenomas.[120,121] Although overt malignancy has not been reported so far, one case showed severe atypia of ductal lining cells.[120] Diffusely cystic Brunner's gland lesions have also been referred to as mucoceles.[127]

Duodenal Hamartomatous Polyp

Isolated hamartomatous polyps of the duodenum in the absence of the Peutz-Jeghers syndrome are extremely rare, and only a single case was described in 1986.[128] A solitary 5-cm diameter pedunculated polyp was removed from the distal duodenum of a 23-year-old man. The histologic appearance was typical of a Peutz-Jeghers hamartomatous polyp. Upward radiating branches of muscularis mucosae were lined by normal small intestinal mucosa.

Duodenal Adenomyoma (Syn: Pancreatic Heterotopia)

These lesions are not neoplastic and represent one extreme of the spectrum of hetero-topic pancreas. Instead of all components of the pancreas (acini, ducts, and islets) only ductal elements are present and associated with proliferating bundles of smooth muscle. If located near the ampulla of Vater, biliary obstruction may result.[129]

References

1. Appelman HD: In: Pathology of the Esophagus, Stomach, and Duodenum. New York: Churchill Livingstone, 1984;104–115.
2. Komorowski RA, Caya JG, Greenen JE: The morphologic spectrum of large gastric folds: Utility of the snare biopsy. Gastrointest Endosc 1986;32:190–192.
3. Wolfe MM, Jensen RT: Zollinger-Ellison syndrome: Current concepts in diagnosis and management. N Engl J Med 1987;317:1200–1209.
4. Larsson LI: Pathology of the gastrin cell. Pathol Annu 1979;14(1):293–316.
5. Murphy TR, Goodsitt E, Morales H, et al: Peptic ulceration with associated endocrine tumors: Collective review and report of a case. Am J Surg 1960;100:764–778.
6. Stempien SJ, Heiskell CL, Goodman JR, et al: Hypertrophic secretory gastropathy: Analysis of 15 cases and a review of the literature. Am J Dig Dis 1964;9:471–493.

7. Lewin KJ, Yang K, Ulich T, et al: Primary gastrin cell hyperplasia. Am J Surg Pathol 1984;8:821–832.

8. Polak JM, Stagg B, Pearse AGE: Two types of Zollinger-Ellison syndrome: Immunofluorescent, cytochemical, and ultrastructural studies of the antral and pancreatic gastrin cells in different clinical states. Gut 1972; 3:501–512.

9. Wiesinga WM, Tytgat GN: Clinical recovery owing to target parietal cell failure in a patient with the Zollinger-Ellison syndrome. Gastroenterology 1977;73:1413–1417.

10. Case Records of the Massachusetts General Hospital: Case #41–78. N Engl J Med 1978; 299:878–885.

11. Ward MWN, Sarner M: The diagnosis of Ménétrier's disease. Post Grad Med J 1981;57: 562–565.

12. Ménétrier P: Des polyadenomes gastriques et leur rapport avec le cancer de l'estomac. Arch Physiol Norm Pathol 1888;1:32–55.

13. Simson JNL: Hyperplastic gastropathy. Br Med J 1985;291:1298–1299.

14. Chouraqui JP, Roy CC, Brochu P, et al: Ménétrier's disease in children: Report of a patient and review of 16 other cases. Gastroenterology 1981;80:1042–1047.

15. Engel JJ, Pierce W, Herst M, et al: Ménétrier's disease: Transient course in a recent immigrant during the puerperium. Am J Gastroenterol 1983;78:68–70.

16. Scharschmidt BF: The natural history of hypertrophic gastropathy (Ménétrier's disease): Report of a case with 16 year follow-up and review of 120 cases from the literature. Am J Med 1977;63:644–652.

17. Reese DF, Hodgson JR, Dockerty MB: Giant hypertrophy of the gastric mucosa (Ménétrier's disease): A correlation of the roentgenographic, pathologic, and clinical findings. Am J Roentgenol Radiol Ther Nucl Med 1962; 88:619–626.

18. Searcy RM, Malagelada JR: Ménétrier's disease and idiopathic hypertrophic gastropathy. Ann Intern Med 1984;100:565–570.

19. Frank WB, Kern F Jr: Ménétrier's disease: spontaneous metamorphosis of giant hypertrophy of the gastric mucosa to atrophic gastritis. Gastroenterology 1967;53:953–969.

20. Berenson MM, Sannella J: Ménétrier's disease: Serial morphological, secretory, and serologic observations. Gastroenterology 1977;70:257–263.

21. Miura S, Asakura H, Tsuchiya M: Lymphatic abnormalities in protein-losing enteropathy, especially in Ménétrier's disease. Angiology 1981;32:345–354.

22. Snider TG, Ochoa R, Williams JC: Ménétrier's disease: Animal model of human disease pre-Type II and type II ostertagiosis in cattle. Am J Pathol 1983;113:410–412.

23. Kondo M, Bamba T: Tissue plasminogen activator in the pathogenesis of protein losing gastroenteropathy. Gastroenterology 1976; 70:1045–1047.

24. Wijngaards G, Jespersen J: Fibrinolytic activity of the gastric mucosa in Ménétrier's disease. Eur J Clin Invest 1983;13:347–350.

25. Kelly DG, Miller LJ, Malagelada R, et al: Giant hypertrophic gastropathy (Ménétrier's disease): Pharmacologic effects on protein leakage and mucosal ultrastructure. Gastroenterology 1982;83:581–589.

26. Lam SK, Hui WK, Ho J, et al: Pachydermoperiostosis, hypertrophic gastropathy and peptic ulcer. Gastroenterology 1983;84:834–839.

27. Swindells SR, Simpson KH: Anorexia nervosa and gastric rugal hyperplasia. Br J Psych 1987;150:697–700.

28. Walker FB: Spontaneous remission in hypertrophic gastropathy (Ménétrier's disease). South Med J 1981;74:1273–1276.

29. Myerson RM: Cimetadine in hypertrophic protein losing gastropathy (Ménétrier's disease). Gastroenterology 1983;84:201–202.

30. Wood GM, Bates C: Intramucosal carcinoma of the gastric antrum complicating Ménétrier's disease. J Clin Pathol 1983;36:1071–1075.

31. Morson BC, Dawson IMP: In: Gastrointestinal Pathology, 2nd Edition. Oxford: Blackwell Scientific Publications, 1979:316.

32. Lechago J: The endocrine cells of the digestive tract: General concepts and historic perspective. Am J Surg Pathol 1987;11(Suppl 1):63–67.

33. Arnold R, Hulst MV, Neuhof CH, et al: Antral gastrin-producing G-cells and somatostatin-producing D-cells in different states of gastric acid secretion. Gut 1982;23:285–291.

34. Dayal Y, Wolfe HJ: G-cell hyperplasia in chronic hypercalcemia. An immunocytochemical and morphometric analysis. Am J Pathol 1984;116:391–397.

35. Creuzfeldt W, Arnold R, Creuzfeldt C, et al: Gastrin and G-cells in the antral mucosa of

patients with pernicious anemia, acromegaly, and hyperparathyroidism and in a Zollinger-Ellison tumour of the pancreas. Eur J Clin Invest 1971;1:461–479.

36. Patel HD, Parathasarathy TK: Antral G-cell hyperplasia. Am J Proctol Gastroenterol 1983;34:11–23.

37. Bordi C, Pilato FP, Bartelé A, et al: Expression of glycoprotein hormone alpha-subunit by endocrine cells of the oxyntic mucosa is associated with hypergastrinemia. Hum Pathol 1988;19:580–585.

38. Håkanson G, Böttcher G, Sundler F, et al: Activation and hyperplasia of gastrin and enterochromaffin-like cells in the stomach. Digestion 1986;35 (suppl 1):23–41.

39. Holle GE, Spann W, Eisenmenger W, et al: Diffuse somatostatin-immunoreactive D-cell hyperplasia in the stomach and duodenum. Gastroenterology 1986;91:733–739.

40. Feyrter F: Über Wucherungen der Brunnerschen Drüsen. Virchows Arch (Pathol Anat) 1934;293:509–526.

41. Stolte M, Schwabe H, Prestele H: Relationship between diseases of the pancreas and hyperplasia of Brunner's glands. Virchows Arch (Pathol Anat) 1981;394:75–87.

42. Buchanan EB: Nodular hyperplasia of Brunner's glands of the duodenum. Am J Surg 1961;101:253–257.

43. Franzin G, Musola R, Ghidini O, et al: Nodular hyperplasia of Brunner's glands. Gastrointest Endosc 1985;31:374–377.

44. Spellberg MA, Vucelic B: A case of Brunner's gland hyperplasia with diarrhea responsive to cimetadine. Am J Gastroenterol 1980;73:579–582.

45. Paimela H, Tallgren LG, Stenman S, et al: Multiple duodenal polyps in uremia: A little known clinical entity. Gut 1984;25:259–263.

46. Bentivegna S, Panagopoulos PG: Adenomatous gastric polyps. Am J Gastroenterol 1965;44:138–148.

47. Kamiya T, Morishita T, Asakura H, et al: Histoclinical long-standing follow-up study of hyperplastic polyps of the stomach. Am J Gastroenterol 1981;75:275–281.

48. Ming SC: The classification and significance of gastric polyps. In: Yardley JH, Morson BC, Abell MR (eds). The Gastrointestinal Tract. International Academy of Pathology Monograph. Baltimore: Williams and Wilkins, 1977:149–175.

49. Neimark S, Rogers AI: Gastric polyps: a review. Am J Gastroenterol 1982;77:585–587.

50. Snover DC: Benign epithelial polyps of the stomach. Pathol Annu 1985;20(1):302–329.

51. Amini AA, Stern DS, Chong TK: Endoscopic observation of large fundic gastric polyp prolapsing through the pylorus. Gastrointest Endosc 1982;28:117–118.

52. Gordon R, Laufer I, Kressler HY: Gastric polyps found on routine double-examination of the stomach. Radiology 1980;134:27–30.

53. Seifert E, Elster K: Gastric polypectomy. Am J Gastroenterol 1975;63:451–456.

54. Okada T, Nishizawa M: Magnifying observations of elevated lesions of the stomach based on magnifying fiberoptic endoscopy and dissecting microscopy. Endoscopy 1981;13:190–196.

55. Borrmann R: Geschwülste des Magens und Duodenums. In: Handbuch der speziellen Anatomie und Histologie. Henke F, Lubarsch O (eds). Berlin: Springer-Verlag, 1926; IV/1: p. 812–1052.

56. Ming S, Goldman H: Gastric polyps: a histogenetic classification and its relation to carcinoma. Cancer 1965;18:721–726.

57. Tomasulo J: Gastric polyps: histologic types and their relationship to gastric carcinoma. Cancer 1971;27:1346–1355.

58. Ming SC: Tumors of the esophagus and stomach. In: Atlas of Tumor Pathology, 2nd Series, Fasc 7. Washington DC: Armed Forces Institute of Pathology, 1973.

59. Elster K: Histologic classification of gastric polyps. In: Morson BC (ed). Current Topics in Pathology. New York: Springer-Verlag, 1976: 78–93.

60. Emmanoulidis A, Nicolopoulou-Stamati P, Merikas E: Esophagogastric polyp. Gastrointest Endosc 1985;31:55–56.

61. Sanchez MA, Font RG: Gastritis polyposa in a gastroenterostomy anastomosis. Am J Gastroenterol 1978;70:496–500.

62. Jablokow VR, Aranha GV, Reyes CV: Gastric stomal polypoid hyperplasia: report of four cases. J Surg Oncol 1982;19:106–108.

63. Buts J-P, Gosseye S, Claus D, et al: Solitary hyperplastic polyp of the stomach. Am J Dis Child 1981;135:846–847.

64. Dirschmid K, Walser J, Hügel H: Pseudomalignant erosion in hyperplastic gastric polyps. Cancer 1984;54:2290–2293.

65. Hattori T: Morphological range of hyperplastic polyps and carcinomas arising in hyperplastic polyps of the stomach. J Clin Pathol 1985;38:622–630.

66. Siurala M, Varis K, Wiljasalo M: Studies of patients with atrophic gastritis: A 10–15 yr follow up. Scand J Gastroenterol 1966;1:40–48.

67. Seifert E, Gail K. Weismüller J: Gastric polypectomy. Long-term results (survey of 23 centers in Germany). Endoscopy 1983;15:8–11.

68. Op den Orth JO, Dekker W: Gastric adenomas. Radiology 1981;141:289–293.

69. DeVita O, Bondi A, Euse-Bi V, et al: Simultaneous polypoid tumors of the stomach and duodenum with composite cell population (mucous, argyrophil, and lysozyme-containing cells): A case report. Am J Gastroenterol 1984;79:606–610.

70. Rubio CA, Cato Y: DNA profiles in mitotic cells from gastric adenomas. Am J Pathol 1988;130:485–488.

71. Burnett KR, Keyser B, Tamasulo J, et al: Giant gastric villous adenoma. Am J Gastroenterol 1980;74:363–368.

72. Wolk I: Villous tumors of the stomach. Arch Intern Med 1951;87:560–569.

73. Fieber SS, Boden RE: Polypoid villous adenoma of the stomach: A case report. Am J Gastroenterol 1977;68:286–289.

74. Tatsuta M, Okuda S, Tamura H, et al: Polyps in the acid-secreting area of the stomach. Gastrointest Endosc 1981;27:245–249.

75. Rohner HG: Drüsenkörperzysten des Magens. Erscheinungsbild und möglicher Enstehungsmechanismus. Leber Magen Darm 1977;7:62–64.

76. Eichenberger P, Hammer, B, Gloor F, et al: Gardner's syndrome with glandular cysts of the fundic mucosa. Endoscopy 1980;12:63–67.

77. Humphries TJ: Gastric glandular cysts: uncommon or unrecognized. Gastrointest Endosc 1982;28:251–252.

78. Burt RW, Berenson MM, Lee RG, et al: Upper gastrointestinal polyps in Gardner's syndrome. Gastroenterology 1984;80:295–301.

79. Irida M, Yao T, Watanabe H, et al: Fundic gland polyposis in patients without familial adenomatosis coli: its incidence and clinical features. Gastroenterology 1984;86:1437–1442.

80. Irida M, Yao T, Itoh H, et al: Natural history of fundic gland polyposis in patients with familial adenomatosis coli/Gardner's syndrome. Gastroenterology 1985;89:1021–1025.

81. Irida M, Yao T, Watanabe H, et al: Spontaneous disappearance of fundic gland polyposis: report of three cases. Gastroenterology 1980; 79:725–728.

82. Katz B, Tenembaum MM, Kreel I: Gastric hamartomatous polyps in the absence of familial polyposis: Report of two cases. Mt Sinai J Med 1982;49:426–429.

83. Ideda F, Senoue I, Hara M, et al: Gastric pseudopolyposis: A new clinical manifestation of type A gastritis. Am J Gastroenterol 1985;80:82–90.

84. Dinari G, Rosenbach Y: Generalized gastrointestinal juvenile polyposis and its treatment. Am J Proctol Gastroenterol Col Rect Surg 1983;34:5–8.

85. Watanabe A, Nagashima H, Motoi M, et al: Familial juvenile polyposis of the stomach. Gastroenterology 1979;77:148–151.

86. Sachatello CR, Hahn HL, Carrington CB: Juvenile gastrointestinal polyposis in a female infant: Report of a case and review of the literature of a recently recognized syndrome. Surgery 1974;75:107–114.

87. Erbe RW: Inherited gastrointestinal polyposis syndromes. N Engl J Med 1976;291: 1101–1104.

88. Beacham CH, Shields HM, Raffensperger EC, et al: Juvenile and adenomatous gastrointestinal polyposis. Dig Dis Sci 1978;23: 1137–1142.

89. Iida M, Yao T, Itoh H, et al: Natural history of gastric adenomas in patients with familial adenomatosis coli/Gardner's syndrome. Cancer 1988;61:605–611.

90. Watanabe H, Enjoji M, Yao T, et al: Gastric lesions in familial adenomatosis coli. Their incidence and histologic analysis. Hum Pathol 1978;9:269–283.

91. Ranzi T, Castagnone D, Velio P, et al: Gastric and duodenal polyps in familial polyposis coli. Gut 1981;22:363–367.

92. Nishiura M, Hirota T, Habashi M, et al: A clinical and histopathological study of gastric polyps in familial polyposis coli. Am J Gastroenterol 1984;79:98–103.

93. Dos Santos JG, deMagalhaes J: Familial gastric polyposis. A new entity. J Genet Hum 1980;28:293–297.

94. Gardner EJ, Richards RS: Multiple cutaneous and subcutaneous lesions occurring simultaneously with hereditary polyposis and osteomatosis. Am J Hum Genet 1953; 5:139–147.

95. Keshgegian AA, Enterline HT: Gardner's syndrome with duodenal adenomas, gastric adenomyoma and thyroid papillary-follicular adenocarcinoma. Dis Colon Rectum 1978; 21:255–260.

96. Burt RW, Berenson MM, Lee RS, et al: Upper gastrointestinal polyps in Gardner's syndrome. Gastroenterology 1984;86:295–301.

97. Sugihara K, Muto T, Kamiya J, et al: Gardner's syndrome associated with periampullary carcinoma and duodenal and gastric adenomatosis. Dis Colon Rectum 1982;25: 766–771.

98. Cronkhite LW, Canada WJ: Generalized gastrointestinal polyposis: An unusual syndrome of polyposis, pigmentation, alopecia, and onychotrophia. N Engl J Med 1955;252: 1011–1015.

99. Daniel ES, Ludwig SL, Lewin KJ, et al: The Cronkhite-Canada syndrome: An analysis of clinical and pathologic features and therapy in 55 patients. Medicine 1982;61:293–309.

100. Suzuki K, Uraoka M, Funatsu T, et al: Cronkhite-Canada syndrome. A case report and analytical review of 23 other cases reported in Japan. Gastroenterologia Jpn 1979;14: 442–449.

101. Kilcheski T, Kressel HY, Laufer I, Rogers D: The radiographic appearance of the stomach in Cronkhite-Canada syndrome. Radiology 1981;141:57–60.

102. Parsa C: Cronkhite-Canada syndrome associated with systemic vasculitis: an autopsy study. Hum Pathol 1982;13:758–760.

103. Weinstock JV, Kawanishi H: Gastrointestinal polyposis with orocutaneous hamartomas. Gastroenterology 1978;74:890–895.

104. Ortonne JP, Lambert R, Daudet J, et al: Involvement of the digestive tract in Cowden's disease. Int J Dermatol 1980;19:570–596.

105. Jeghers H, McKusick VA, Katz KH: Generalized intestinal polyposis and melanin spots of the oral mucosa, lips, and digits. N Engl J Med 1949;241:993–1031.

106. Bartholomew LG, Dahlin DC, Waugh JM: Intestinal polyposis associated with mucocutaneous melanin pigmentation (Peutz-Jeghers syndrome). Gastroenterology 1957; 32:434–451.

107. Reid JO: Intestinal carcinoma in the Peutz-Jeghers syndrome. JAMA 1974;229:833–834.

108. Hancock RJ: An eleven-year review of primary tumors of the small bowel including the duodenum. Can Med Assoc J 1970;105:1177–1179.

109. Stassa G, Klingensmith WC: Primary tumors of the duodenal bulb. Am J Roentgen 1969; 107:105–110.

110. Reddy RR, Schuman BM, Priest RJ: Duodenal polyps: Diagnosis and management. J Clin Gastroenterol 1981;3:139–145.

111. Sweeny BF, Anderson DS: Endoscopic removal of duodenal polyps in a patient with Gardner's syndrome. Dig Dis Sci 1982;27: 557–560.

112. Ranzi T, Castagnone D, Velio P, et al: Gastric and duodenal polyps in familial polyposis coli. Gut 1981;22:363–367.

113. Kozuka S, Tsubone M, Yamaguchi A, Hachisuka K: Adenomatous residue in cancerous papilla of Vater. Gut 1981;22:1031–1034.

114. Komorowski RA, Cohen EB: Villous tumors of the duodenum: A clinicopathologic study. Cancer 1981;47:1377–1386.

115. Everett GD, Shirazi S, Mitros F: Villous tumors of the duodenum. Am J Gastroenterol 1981;75:376–379.

116. Kalmar JA, Merritt CRB: Villous adenoma of the duodenum with intussusception. South Med J 1980;73:651–653.

117. Hasleton PS, Shah S, Buckley CH, Tweedle DEF: Ampullary carcinoma associated with multiple duodenal villous adenomas. Am J Gastroenterol 1980;73:418–422.

118. Franzin G, Novelli P, Fratton A: Hyperplastic and metaplastic polyps of the duodenum. Gastrointest Endosc 1983;29:140–142.

119. Farkas I, Patko A, Kovacs L, et al: The Brunneroma, the adenomatous hyperplasia of Brunner's glands. Acta Gastro-Enterol Belg 1980;63:179–186.

120. Zanetti G, Casada G: Brunner's gland hamartoma with incipient ductal malignancy. Report of a case. Tumori 1981;67:75–78.

121. Strutynsky IV, Posniak R, Mori K: Obstructing hamartoma of Brunner's gland of the duodenum. Dig Dis Sci 1982;27:279–282.

122. Cruveilhier J: Anatomic Patholgique du Corps Humain. Paris: JB Bailliere, 1835.

123. Salvioli G: Contributione alle studio ade-
     nomi losservatore. E Gazzetta Ital (Torino)
     1876;12:481–493.
124. Barnhart GR, Maull KI: Brunner's gland
     adenomas: Clinical presentation and surgi-
     cal management. South Med J 1979;72:
     1537–1539.
125. Hirschfeld J, Krebedunkel K, Schneider V:
     Kasuistischer Beitrag zu einem benignen
     Adenom der Brunner'schen Drüsen des Duo-
     denums. Chirurg 1979;50:732–734.
126. Plison B, Benisch B: Brunner's gland ade-
     noma of the duodenal bulb. Am J Gastroen-
     terol 1982;77:276–279.
127. Fisher JK: Mucocele of a Brunner gland.
     Radiology 1980;136:320.
128. Blott SJ, Hanks JB, Stone DD: Solitary
     hamartomatous polyp of the duodenum in
     the absence of familial polyposis. Am J Gas-
     troenterol 1986;81:993–994.
129. Bill K, Belber JP, Carson JW: Adenomyoma
     (pancreatic heterotopia) of the duodenum
     producing common bile duct obstruction.
     Gastrointest Endosc 1982;28:182–184.

CHAPTER 7

Carcinoma of the Stomach

Incidence

Carcinoma of the stomach was the leading cause of cancer death at the beginning of the century, but presently in the United States, ranks sixth among cancer deaths and third among malignant tumors of the gastrointestinal tract. The yearly death toll is approximately 14,000 (i.e., half the mortality of 1948).[1] The incidence of the disease has declined steadily over the last decades as reflected by the change in the age-adjusted death rates. The death rate in the United States was 10 men and 5 women per 100,000 population in 1965 as opposed to 6.8 and 3.2 in 1976.[2] For 1984, however, the comparable figures are higher as 8 per 100,000 men and 4 per 100,000 women died of gastric cancer.[3] The estimated number of new cases has also increased slightly, and was reported as 23,000 in 1979, 23,900 in 1981, 24,000 in 1982, and 24,600 in 1987.[3]

The incidence of carcinoma of the stomach, more than that of any other gastrointestinal malignancy, shows wide geographic differences.[2,4] The highest incidence rates are reported from Japan, where 88 men and 42 women per 100,000 population develop gastric cancer every year.[5] In Trinidad, gastric carcinoma is the most common cause of death from malignant disease.[6] China, Chile, Costa Rica, Yugoslavia, Finland, Hungary, Poland, and Czechoslovakia report unusually high incidences.[5,7] Recent statistics from France state an annual incidence rate of 15.2 men and 6.1 women per 100,000, representing a substantial decline in incidence for men, but less so for women.[8] Low rates are recorded in Africa, Thailand, India, the Philippines, Nicaragua, the Dominican Republic, and El Salvador.[5,7] The United States had the third lowest incidence rate among 18 countries in 1982, with 11.1 men and 5.1 women with newly diagnosed gastric cancer per 100,000 population[5] (see Table 7-1).

This national variation is somewhat paralleled by regional variations (Table 7-2). The Northeast and North Central areas of the United States have significantly higher incidence rates than the rest of the country. Blacks, American Indians, and native Hawaiians have higher rates than whites.[9]

Men outnumber women by a factor of 2 to 1 in the age group above 50, but not among young American adults less than 35 years of age, among whom the male to female ratio is reversed (1:1.3).[10] In the United States most young patients with gastric carcinoma belong to high-risk groups, such as Japanese and blacks.[11] A study from China reports a male to female ratio of 1:3.5 for patients less than 29 years old.[12] Apparently, the younger the age group studied, the greater the proportion of women. The youngest reported case of gastric carcinoma occurred in a 20-month-old girl.[13]

Table 7-1. International Variation of Stomach Cancer, Incidence Rates per 100,000 Population*

Country	Male	Female
Japan	88	42
China	56	21
Brazil	46	19
Colombia	46	27
Iceland	43	24
Yugoslavia	42	18
Spain	35	20
Finland	29	15
Czechoslovakia	28	13
Norway	20	10
Sweden	18	9
Denmark	17	9
New Zealand	17	8
Australia	14	7
Canada	12	5
United States – Connecticut	11	5
India	9	8
Senegal	4	2

*Modified from Møller Jensen[4] and Waterhouse et al.[5]

Table 7.2. Gastric Cancer: Average Age-Adjusted (1970 Standard) Annual Incidence Rates per 100,000 Population for Males Only, 1973–1977, by Race*

Location	Whites	Blacks	Other
Connecticut	14.3		
Detroit	14.1	20.5	
Iowa	10.1		
Atlanta	7.4	18.0	
New Orleans	9.8	29.0	
New Mexico	15.0		30.9 (American Indian)
Utah	10.1		
Seattle	11.4		
San Francisco/ Oakland	14.7	24.9	33.0 (Japanese)
Hawaii	15.6		51.4 (Hawaiian)
Puerto Rico			28.4 (Hispanic)

*Modified from Young et al.[9]

It should be emphasized that the observed decrease in incidence rates reflects the collective experience of a population as a whole, but affects different age groups differently: older individuals experience the same high risk, whereas young individuals display a much lower risk.[14] Migrants from high-risk countries maintain their high risk despite having moved to a low-risk country, whereas their descendants exhibit a lower risk.[15] Such observations suggest a major effect of environmental factors on gastric carcinogenesis.

Incidence rates also have to be considered in the context of the histologic type of gastric cancer. Carcinoma of the stomach is considered, by some, as two separate diseases: the intestinal type is most common in high-risk countries and sometimes referred to as the epidemic type, whereas the diffuse type, with similar incidence rates in most populations, is sometimes referred to as the endemic form. Populations with declining gastric cancer rates have shown a selective decrease of the intestinal type.[16] In young patients (i.e., those less than 40 years old) the diffuse type is most common.[17,18]

Etiology and Pathogenesis

Carcinoma of the stomach, like most human malignant tumors, is a multifactorial disease. No single cause is known, and among the multiple factors known to play an etiologic role, no single one is dominant or always identifiable.

Genetic Factors

A number of observations indicate that heredity is important in the development of carcinoma of the stomach, but the extent is probably limited and the exact mechanism remains unknown. Familial clustering of cases of gastric cancer was first reported in 1950.[19] In San Marino, a country with an unusually high incidence of gastric cancer, 25% of patients had first-degree relatives affected by the disease versus 5.6% of the controls.[20] In the United States, the comparable figure among 300 patients was only 4.3%.[21] In China, the risk of gastric cancer among blood relatives was reported to be 7.75 times greater than that among controls.[22] Some investigators could recognize familial factors only in cases of diffuse gastric carcinoma and not in the more common intestinal type. Analysis based on age and sex showed that familial factors were restricted to females, particularly young women.[18,23] Therefore, only in cases of a mother or a sister with diffuse gastric carcinoma should genetic predisposition be considered an important factor. Heredity probably plays a role in the rare cases of gastric carcinoma in patients with Gardner's syndrome[24] and Peutz-Jeghers syndrome.[25] Blood type A is linked to diffuse gastric cancer[26] especially in young patients.[18] Not surprisingly, a genetic predisposition was also shown for conditions etiologically related to gastric carcinoma, such as atrophic gastritis, intestinal metaplasia, and achlorhydria.[27] The latter two conditions occurred at an age significantly younger than that of controls. The association between gastritis and the diffuse type of gastric cancer is valid only for type A gastritis (gastritis of the fundus and corpus) and is significant only at the family level and not at the individual level. In individuals with diffuse carcinoma, gastritis and intestinal metaplasia occur no more frequently than in individuals of the same age in the general population.[28]

In experimental carcinogenesis, female gender protects against gastric cancer. This protection, however, seems to be mediated at least partially by hormonal and not exclusively by chromosomal factors. Male rats had the highest incidence; estrogen-treated male rats had a lower incidence, and female rats developed no cancer at all after treatment with the carcinogen N-methyl-N-nitro-N-nitrosoguanidine (MNNG).[29]

Simultaneous occurrence of gastric carcinoma in twins has been reported at least three times[30] but is not necessarily proof of genetic predisposition, since the occurrence could also be explained on the basis of common environmental factors.

Studies of the two genetically transmitted pepsinogen phenotypes (A, the more common phenotype, is present in 84.4% of white Americans, 85.4% of inhabitants of Liverpool, and 100% of 229 healthy Japanese so tested) have shown a nearly eightfold greater risk of contracting gastric cancer for phenotype A individuals as compared to phenotype B individuals.[31]

Carcinogens

Experimental Carcinogens

Gastric carcinogens have been the subject of more than 500 articles, mostly from Japan. The earlier literature on experimental carcinogens has been reviewed by Sugimura and Kawachi.[32] In rats, gastric carcinoma has been produced variously by submucosal injection of 3-methylcholanthrene,[33] by feeding of Aroclor 1254, a mixture of polychlorinated biphenyls (PCBs),[34] or by adding MNNG to their drinking water.[35] MNNG-induced carcinomas usually develop in the pyloric region, as do human tumors, but if ulceration (induced by freezing) coexists, tumors will develop at the ulcer site.[36] This enhancing effect of local injury, unlike in humans, was most marked in the rat duodenum. It has been suggested that regenerating intestinal epithelium is more susceptible to chemical carcinogenesis than gastric epithelium. While this is certainly not true for human duodenal ulcers, which practically never become malignant, this hypothesis is supported by the fact that most human gastric carcinomas, especially the intestinal type, develop against a background of atrophic gastritis with intestinal metaplasia. The latter change has been seen in conjunction with Aroclor-induced adenocarcinomas[34] but not in MNNG-induced carcinogenesis. MNNG, however, was found to produce other precancerous changes in the rat stomach, such as increased acid mucin secretion and dysplasia in the proliferating neck zone of hyperplastic foci.[37]

Gastrin, originally isolated as a factor stimulating gastric acid secretion, has been demonstrated to have a trophic effect on the gastrointestinal mucosa as well. Each of these two effects may influence carcinogenesis. Clinical observations suggest that hyperacidity protects the gastric mucosa from the development of carcinoma. The trophic effect of gastrin, on the other hand, is growth stimulating and may conceivably enhance the effects of carcinogens. The protective effect of gastrin-induced hyperacidity, which has been demonstrated in rats exposed to MNNG, results from the conversion of MNNG to the noncarcinogenic derivative N-methyl-N-nitrosoguanidine and nitrous oxide in acid medium.[38] An enhancing effect was demonstrated in the early stage of carcinogenesis.[35]

The influence of duodenal contents on gastric carcinogenesis was studied in rats receiving 3-methylcholanthrene.[33] Diversion of duodenal contents had no protective effects against the development of carcinoma. This negative finding is interesting for two reasons. First, reflux of duodenal contents is implicated in the pathogenesis of atrophic gastritis; atrophic gastritis in the genesis of intestinal metaplasia; and intestinal metaplasia in gastric carcinogenesis. However, there seems to be no direct carcinogenic or carcinogenesis-enhancing effect of duodenal contents. Second, the increased incidence of gastric carcinoma occurring after partial gastrectomy could possibly be related to exposure of the gastric remnant to duodenal secretions. This apparently is not so. Rather, vagotomy, gastroenterostomy per se, and increased serum gastrin are considered the main causal factors. For a more detailed discussion of gastric stump carcinoma, see page 175.

The significance of these animal models for human carcinogenesis is not entirely clear. The general biologic effects of PCBs in humans became well known in 1968, when widespread ingestion of rice oil contaminated with PCBs in Japan led to the epidemic of "Yusho" or "oil disease," characterized by eye discharge, swelling of eyelids, acne-like skin eruptions, skin pigmentation, and weakness.[39] PCBs were used from 1929 to the late 1970s in electrical systems, investment casting, and numerous commercial products, including carburators, copy paper, and microscope immersion oil.[34] So far, however, no human gastric cancers related to PCBs have been detected.

Nitrosamines

The marked and distinct national and regional differences in the incidence rates of gastric carcinoma stimulated investigations of the cause of these differences. In Chile, which ranks second in the world after Japan in gastric cancer mortality, three agricultural provinces located about 200 miles south of Santiago had a median rate of 50.1 per 100,000 in 1971, whereas both extremes of the country, where little or no agriculture exists, had less than one-half that risk.[40] Chile is also the only country in the world with natural deposits of nitrates and with a long tradition of using them in large amounts as fertilizers. Data concerning the use of nitrates were collected for the period 1945 to 1972 and showed a high correlation between death rates from gastric cancer and a cumulative per capita exposure index measured in kilograms of nitrogen. Residence in high-risk areas, especially before the age of 25, and occupation in agriculture increases the risk.[41] Only the intestinal type of gastric cancer, however, correlated with residency in a high-risk area in early life.

In China, where the overall age-adjusted death rate is 21 per 100,000 male and 16 per 100,000 female populations, countries in high-risk areas in the Northwest, the Qinghai, Ningxia, and Gansu provinces, have death rates three times greater than the national average.[22] These regional differences correlated with the levels of nitrate (NO_3) and nitrite (NO_2) in drinking water and vegetables, as well as with the levels of both compounds in the fasting saliva and gastric juice. Gastric cancer rates also paralleled the incidence of chronic gastritis and atrophic gastritis.

Table 7-3. Fasting Gastric Microenvironment in Normal Individuals and Those at High Risk for Gastric Cancer*

Microenvironmental Component	Normal	High Risk
Histology	Normal	Chronic atrophic gastritis
pH	Below 5	Above 5
Thiocyanate	Present	Present
Nitrate	Present	Present
Nitrite	Absent or minimal	Usually high
Bacteria	Sterile	Abundant
Trace elements	Present	Present

*From Correa et al.[42] Reproduced by permission, National Cancer Institute.

In Colombia, patients with atrophic gastritis from the high-risk cancer region of Narino were analyzed as to their fasting gastric microenvironment.[42] Among the seven parameters studied (Table 7-3), nitrites were usually high in high-risk patients. Significantly, there were also abundant bacteria and a high pH. The sequence of events in human nitrite carcinogenesis evolves as follows: Water or foods rich in nitrates are converted to the potentially harmful nitrites by the action of nitrate reductase-positive bacteria, which are allowed to proliferate at a gastric pH above 5. The high pH, of course, is the result of destruction of gastric acid-producing glands by chronic atrophic gastritis. Carcinogenic N-nitroso compounds are formed when amines and amides react with nitrite. Nitrosatable amines are generated by intestinal organisms, such as enterococci and micrococci, by deamination and decarboxylation of amino acids in gastric juice.[43] Catalysts for the formation of nitroso compounds and stimulators of physiologic importance include chloride, bromide, thiocyanate, and bacteria.[44] Thiocyanate is present in saliva, particularly in smokers. Vitamins C and E inhibit nitrosation. Most of the nitroso compounds are formed in vivo, but occasionally they may already be present in ingested food such as nitrite-cured

meats, some cheeses, fish, and beer.[44] The concentration of gastric N-nitroso compounds rises significantly with age and correlates with high pH, high concentration of nitrites, and growth of nitrate reductase-positive bacteria.[45]

There is, at present, considerable debate as to the potential carcinogenic effect of cimetadine. Cimetadine treatment can create an intragastric milieu resembling that of atrophic gastritis, namely, increases in nitrate-reducing and amine-producing bacteria and in nitrite and N-nitrosamine concentrations.[46-48] These effects were shown to be transient and revert to normal after cessation of short-term (1 g per day for 6 weeks) treatment. Patients on low-dose (0.4 g at night) maintenance therapy, however, exhibited persistent high nitrite and N-nitrosamine levels.[41] The real question is whether N-nitrosocimetadine, the end product of a chain of events, is carcinogenic to the stomach or not. No final answer is available. Neither rats nor dogs fed large doses of cimetadine developed gastric or other cancers.[42,43] On the other hand, the argument can be advanced that humans may differ in their reaction to N-nitrosocimetadine. This, however, is unlikely, since rats in particular have proven susceptible to nitrosocompound (MNNG)-induced gastric cancers. The 21 cases of gastric cancer reported in cimetadine-treated patients[49] may well have been present before therapy was begun. Large patient series with long follow-up times will be needed before a satisfying answer can be given.

Hydrocarbons

A role of hydrocarbons in human gastric carcinogenesis was suggested by Enterline in 1964[50] when a threefold excess of mortality from gastric cancer was found among U.S. coal miners in Pennsylvania. This finding was confirmed by later studies.[51] Elevated gastric cancer mortality has been the most consistent finding in coal miners other than accident and pneumoconiosis mortality. A recent case–control study in a coal mining region of Pennsylvania showed an excess risk only for foreign-born and eastern European miners and for women whose husbands were miners.[52] Coal mine dust may absorb polynuclear aromatic hydrocarbons that are then inhaled, cleared via the bronchial mucus and cilia, and finally swallowed. Within the pulmonary system some precarcinogens may be activated by oxidases, and swallowing may result in a greater concentration of carcinogens in the stomach than in the lung. This hypothesis can also explain the relatively lower mortality from lung cancer than stomach cancer in coal miners in Pennsylvania. This reciprocal relationship between lung and stomach cancer is further illustrated by the contrasting mortality rates in cigarette smokers.[53] Heavy smokers have a relatively lower risk of stomach cancer than light smokers. It is supposed that the impairment of the normal bronchial clearing mechanism in heavy smokers results in retention of inhaled carcinogens in the lung and a relatively low concentration of carcinogens in the stomach. By contrast, in light smokers there is no significant impairment of the bronchial clearing mechanisms and carcinogens are expelled and swallowed.

Dietary Factors

The importance of dietary factors in gastric carcinogenesis is threefold: 1) Carcinogens may be ingested with a particular diet; 2) carcinogens may be formed in the stomach with the help of precursors or cofactors present in the diet; and 3) the diet may contain factors that protect against potential carcinogens. Foods containing carcinogens account for the high gastric cancer mortality in Japan and Iceland, where large amounts of salted fish containing nitrosamine and smoked fish containing benz(a)pyrene, a hydrocarbon, are consumed.[54] Foods containing high levels of nitrates supply potential precursors for nitrosamines and are common in Chile and Colombia, as already mentioned. [40-42] In Colombian villages, the one food item that correlated most strongly with a high risk of gastric cancer was fava beans.[55] Dietary cofactors that may enhance or even be essential

for the nitrate–nitrite–nitrosamine conversion are arsenic and selenium.[56]

A high salt intake is found in most regions with a high gastric cancer mortality.[14] Salt may be considered a promoting factor by delaying emptying of a hypotonic gastric content and by damaging the gastric mucosa.[57] The observed geographic association between gastric cancer and stroke mortality has led to the so-called *salt hypothesis* as the common link between the two. In Belgium, a deliberate attempt to lower the salt intake of the population was associated with a decrease in gastric cancer and stroke mortality.[57] Japan, Korea, and Portugal, for instance, are countries with a high salt intake and a high prevalence of stroke and gastric cancer. More recently, the salt hypothesis has been challenged.[58] A study of multiple causes of death confirmed the concordance between gastric cancer and cerebrovascular disease, but showed the same degrees of concordance between pancreatic or lung cancer and cerebrovascular disease.

In Poland, regional differences in the incidence of gastric cancer coincided with differences in drinking water: mortality rates were lower in areas with hard water (with high magnesium, sulfate, and chloride content) than in areas with soft water.[59] In France, drinking of red wine was found to be a significant risk factor for gastric cancer, especially if combined with cigarette smoking.[60]

Foods with a protective effect against gastric cancer contain high levels of vitamins C and E, which inhibit the nitrosation process. Such foods include fresh fruits and vegetables, especially fresh green, leafy vegetables.

A dietary pattern that promotes gastric carcinogenesis can thus be summarized as follows:

1. Low intake of animal fat and protein.
2. High intake of complex carbohydrates.
3. High intake of salt.
4. High intake of nitrates.
5. Low intake of salads and fresh green, leafy vegetables.
6. Low intake of fresh fruits.

Occupational Factors

Coal miners have been cited previously as a risk group in our discussion of carcinogens (hydrocarbons). The risk for asbestos workers remains unclear. A twofold increase in the mortality for gastric cancer was recently detected in mining districts in South Africa, where crocidolite, a type of asbestos fiber, is mined.[61] No significant increase was found in any asbestos factory workers, insulators, shipyard workers, and asbestos miners in the United States. Elevated risks for gastric cancer in farmers and quarrymen may be related to exposure to elaiomycin, a product of soil bacteria known to be carcinogenic.[51,63] Exposure to synthetic abrasives in polishing pastes was found to carry an increased risk of gastric cancer, possibly related to silicon carbide.[64] Workers employed in the manufacturing of the product, as well as jewelry polishers using it, were affected.

Lifestyle

Diet, drinking habits, and smoking form parts of a lifestyle, and their respective roles have been discussed previously. Emotional and social factors have been implicated as the cause of cancer in general and gastric cancer in particular. In a series of 400 cancer patients, 72% were shown to have suffered the loss of a central relationship within a few months to 8 years before the onset of symptoms.[65] A significantly greater degree of change in lifestyle was found in a group of 14 gastric cancer patients when compared to normal controls and to colorectal cancer patients.[66] Thus, it appears that emotional stress may be a promoting factor in gastric cancer, more so than in other cancers.

Radiation

Radiation-related gastric carcinogenesis has been observed in two situations: 1) in Japanese survivors of the atomic bomb[67,68] and 2) in patients receiving radiotherapy for benign or malignant disease.[69-71]

The incidence of gastric cancer increased significantly 14 to 34 years after exposure to the atomic bomb in Nagasaki, with an excess incidence of 0.5 cases per 10,000 exposed persons.[67] Persons exposed at younger ages tend to be at greater risk than those exposed later in life. The minimal latency period for solid cancers is about 10 years, quite different from the much shorter interval for leukemia (2 years). The increased risk persists for many years, as reflected by the figure of 51% of radiation-related gastric cancer in Hiroshima and Nagasaki occurring 22 to 33 years after the explosion.[68]

Gastric carcinoma related to therapeutic radiation was first observed between 1950 and 1960 in patients who were given x-radiation as a therapy for peptic ulcer[69] and was subsequently also reported after irradiation for ankylosing spondylitis[70] and gastric lymphoma.[71,72] Although radiation carcinogenesis is well known as a phenomenon, its mechanism is still not fully understood. Whether radiation generates the essential oncogenic genetic changes, removes impediments to their function, or induces dormant malignant change is not clear. X-irradiation carcinogenesis is dependent on the age at exposure, the dose of radiation, and the site of radiation. The risk of radiation cancer is about one-third greater for women than for men.[67]

Gastrectomy

The role of partial gastrectomy in the genesis of carcinoma developing in the gastric remnant is discussed in Chapter 5, and gastric stump cancer is described in detail under Advanced Carcinoma—Gross Appearance.

Precancerous Conditions and Epithelial Dysplasia in the Stomach

The knowledge that certain disease states of the stomach cause a predisposition to the development of gastric cancer is not new. Ménétrier in 1888 was concerned about the increased incidence of gastric cancer in patients with hyperplastic gastropathy.[73] Since then, there has been a growing list of case reports of carcinoma of the stomach complicating Ménétrier's disease,[74] but neither is the statistical risk known nor the condition frequent enough to account for a significant number of gastric cancer cases. A variety of other more common disease states have become known to predispose patients to gastric cancer, including chronic atrophic gastritis with or without intestinal metaplasia, adenoma, chronic ulcer, and gastric remnant after partial gastrectomy.[74,75] The evidence that links chronic atrophic gastritis to gastric cancer is manifold and has been discussed in Chapter 4. To summarize the main points of evidence: 1) There is a significant geographic relationship between areas of high frequency for gastric carcinoma and the incidence of chronic atrophic gastritis. 2) Most gastric cancers develop in stomachs with chronic atrophic gastritis. 3) The epithelial change most significantly correlated with carcinoma (i.e., intestinal metaplasia) develops almost exclusively in chronic atrophic gastritis. Among all precancerous conditions, chronic atrophic gastritis is most prevalent and therefore, numerically, the most important.

The malignant potential of adenomas has been discussed in Chapter 6. Although the potential for malignant change of adenomas is significant, the lesion is uncommon and plays only a small role in gastric carcinogenesis at large.

Gastric ulcer, in contrast, is common, but the incidence of carcinoma developing in it is low and probably no higher than 1%.[74] For a detailed discussion, see Chapter 5. Carcinoma developing in the gastric stump after partial gastrectomy is also discussed in this chapter.

The probability of cancer developing in any individual case is unpredictable. In terms of tissue changes, the determining factor appears to be the presence or absence of dysplasia. Recognition of dysplasia in the gastric mucosa is, therefore, of paramount importance, since it warns of the possibility of coexisting carcinoma and, even in the absence of the latter, may contribute to the management of the patient in terms of follow-up studies, early detection of cancer, and possible cancer prevention.[76] Gastric dysplasia, similar to uterine cervical dysplasia, denotes excessive abnormal proliferation of the gastric epithelium that is recognized microscopically on the basis of cellular atypia, abnormal maturation, and a disorganized mucosal architecture.[74-77]

Dysplasia may be associated with any of the above disease states, but in practice is most often encountered in association with chronic atrophic gastritis. Gastric epithelium, as it evolves toward malignancy, appears to progress through a sequence of changes identifiable as superficial gastritis, chronic atrophic gastritis, intestinal metaplasia, dysplasia, carcinoma in situ, and finally invasive carcinoma.[78] Dysplasia, however, may be seen in unaltered foveolar epithelium as well as in intestinal metaplasia.

Special techniques to measure DNA content and cell kinetics[79-80] as well as histochemical[81-83] and immunohistologic[84-88] methods have been successfully applied to the study of gastric dysplasia and will be discussed later; however, the routine pathologic diagnosis remains dependent on the recognition of light microscopic morphologic changes. The increased use of endoscopy and endoscopic biopsy in the 1970s yielded the necessary material for systematic investigation and led to a variety of morphologic grading systems, which are summarized in Table 7-4.[75,75,89-92]

A World Health Organization Expert Committee on Precancerous Changes of the Stomach convened in London in 1978 to define and subclassify dysplasia.[74,75] The three main criteria of cellular atypia, abnormal differentiation, and disorganization of mucosal architecture were defined in great detail.

Cellular atypia has the following features:

Table 7-4. Comparison of Different Grading Systems of Gastric Dysplasia*

	No atypia	Slight atypia	Borderline	Probable cancer	Cancer
Nagayo (1971)[89]	No atypia	Slight atypia	Borderline	Probable cancer	Cancer
Grundmann and Schlake (1979)[90]	Inflammatory	Mild dysplasia	Moderate dysplasia	Severe dysplasia	
Oehlert (1979)[79]		Grade I	Grade II	Grade III	
Ming (1979)[91]	Grade 1	Grade 2	Grade 3	Grade 4	
		Hyperplastic dysplasia		Adenomatous dysplasia	
Cuello et al. (1979)[92]	Mild	Severe	Mild	Severe	
Morson et al. (1980)[74]	Inflammatory regenerative	Mild dysplasia	Moderate dysplasia	Severe dysplasia	
		Hyperplasia		Dysplasia	
ISGGC (1982)	Simple	Atypical	Possible carcinoma		

Abbreviation: ISGGC, International Study Group of Gastric Cancer.* From Ming et al.[76] Reproduced by permission, JP Lippincott.

1. Hyperchromasia and dense distribution of elongated nuclei in tall columnar epithelia.
2. Irregular arrangement of nuclei leading to pseudostratification.
3. Increased nucleocytoplasmic ratio.
4. Nonuniformity of nuclei.
5. Disturbances of cellular polarity.

Abnormal differentiation is indicated by:

1. Decrease in the number of secretory granules in foveolar cells or of goblet cells.
2. Disappearance of maturing cells on the surface of the mucosa.
3. Atrophy or disappearance of normal pyloric or fundic glands leading to intestinal or pseudopyloric metaplasia.
4. Loss or irregular distribution of Paneth cells in areas of intestinal metaplasia.
5. Increase of the generative cell layer.

Disorganized mucosal architecture is characterized by:

1. Irregularities of tubules or glands.
2. Cystic dilatation of glands with or without irregular contour.
3. Diffuse or sporadic glandular heterotopia.

4. Irregularities of the muscularis mucosae and fibrosis or scarring at the base.
5. Loss of smoothness of the mucosal surface.

Grades of dysplasia are defined as follows:

Mild dysplasia. Atypical foveolar epithelium is seen in the upper half of elevated or eroded lesions. Slender and hyperchromatic nuclei are crowded, but show a normal position at the base of the cell (Fig. 7-1). Glandular cysts are usually present in the deeper layer of the mucosa. Intestinal metaplasia may be present.

Moderate dysplasia. Nuclei are not only hyperchromatic and crowded but piled up (pseudostratified) (Fig. 7-2). Mucin secretion or number of Paneth cells is decreased. Numerous cystically dilated and deformed glands are seen in the lower half of the lesion. Atypical epithelia do not occupy the full thickness of the mucosa, leaving pyloric or pseudopyloric glands at the base (Fig. 7-3).

Severe dysplasia. The most important feature is severe cellular atypia. Severe dysplasia in intestinal metaplasia shows deficiency in goblet cells and Paneth cells. Arrangement of nuclei is dense and stratified, some nuclei reaching the luminal surface of the

Figure 7-1. Mild dysplasia of foveo-lar epithelium. Nuclei are crowded, enlarged, and hyperchromatic, but polarity is maintained. H&E, X100.

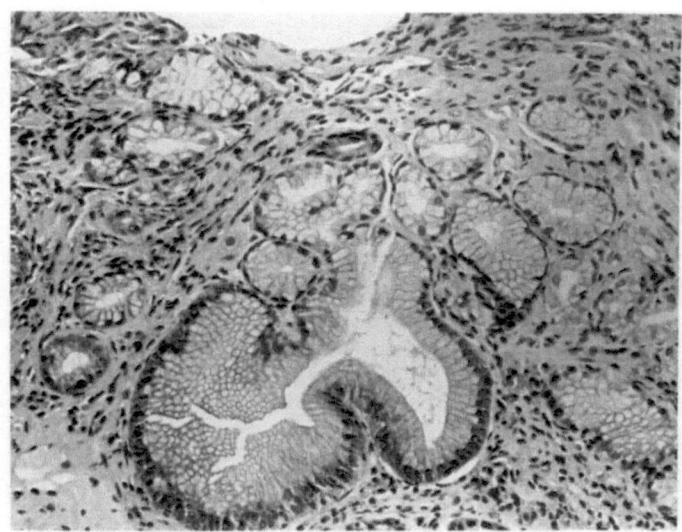

Figure 7-2. Moderate dysplasia of intestinalized epithelium. Nuclei are crowded, enlarged, and hyperchro-matic as in mild dysplasia, but, in addition, are focally stratified. H&E, X250, reproduced at 90%.

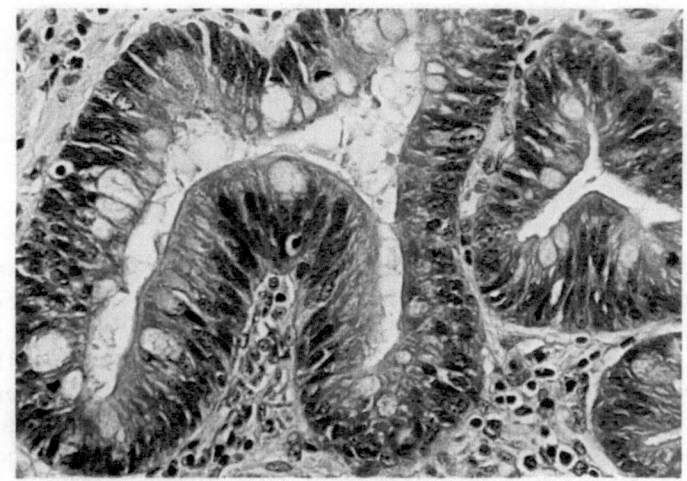

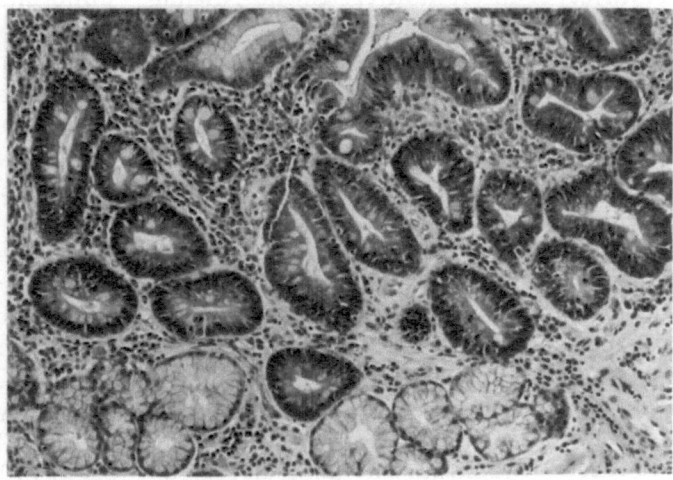

Figure 7-3. Moderate dysplasia of intestinalized epithelium. Only the upper mucosa is involved. Pyloric glands at the base are preserved. H&E, X100, reproduced at 90%.

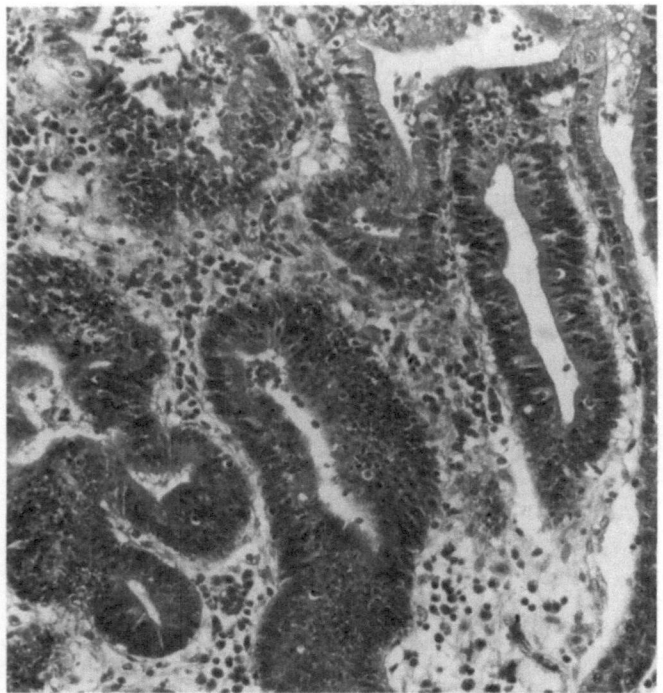

Figure 7-4. Severe dysplasia of intestinalized epithelium. Loss of nuclear polarity is characteristic. Some degree of maturation can be seen toward the surface. HPS, X160, reproduced at 85%.

epithelial cell. In contrast to preinvasive cancer, nuclei maintain some degree of uniformity (Fig. 7-4).

Morphometrical studies concluded that volume and surface densities of glands and epithelium, as well as arrangement and shape of nuclei and nuclear size, are especially good discriminators between the different degrees of dysplasia.[77]

A variety of different investigations, including a study of dysplasia in experimental carcinogenesis[93] and follow-up studies of patients with biopsy-proven dysplasia,[79,94] have shown that mild and moderate degrees are probably clinically insignificant and largely reactive in nature. Among 25 cases with dysplasia at the edge of a gastric ulcer, only one case of mild dysplasia progressed to moderate dysplasia, whereas 23 other cases of mild or moderate dysplasia either regressed within 1 to 74 months (15 cases) or showed no change (8 cases). Only one patient had severe dysplasia, which was no longer demonstrable on a repeat biopsy.[94] In another follow-up study of 46 cases of dysplasia, carcinoma developed

in 3 cases, each of which had severe dysplasia. Most of the cases with mild and moderate changes showed regression or became stationary the longer dysplasia persisted.[79] In gastrectomy specimens, only severe dysplasia shows a clear topographic relationship to cancer localization.[95]

The problem in the study of gastric dysplasia is twofold. First, there is the difficulty of uniformity of the diagnostic criteria, which is obvious from Table 7-4. Second, there is the sampling error in follow-up studies. Biopsies should be taken from a designated area to ensure that a later biopsy samples the same region, which may be extremely difficult. Problems are minimized if diagnosis and follow-up are handled by the same institution. A registry for the study of gastric dysplasia, created in 1985 under the auspices of the World Health Organization,[96] is presently collecting cases. (Cases should be sent to Dr. Si Chun Ming, Department of Pathology, Temple University School of Medicine, 3400 North Broad Street, Philadelphia, PA 19140, USA.) The stated purposes of the registry are 1) to study the natural history of gastric dysplasia, 2) to determine the incidence of malignant transformation in the dysplastic epithelium, 3) to determine the time trends and sequential changes in the transformation process, 4) to delineate the features of the dysplastic epithelium that are most relevant to malignant transformation, and 5) to develop guidelines for the management of gastric dysplasia.

Although the final answers to these questions will not be available for years, the practicing pathologist and clinician need some guidelines for the present time. Dysplasia diagnosed in a gastrectomy specimen with carcinoma or ulcer poses no therapeutic problem; dysplasia diagnosed in an endoscopic biopsy does. It has been recommended that mild dysplasia is "suitable for follow-up observations at long intervals."[75] The intervals of observation in cases of moderate dysplasia should be shorter (3 to 6 months). "Reexamination at relatively short intervals" is advised in patients with severe dysplasia. There is general agreement that severe dysplasia on its own is not an indication for surgical intervention.[73-75,96] Some of the difficulty in clinical management can be eliminated by being very conservative with the use of the word dysplasia. Since mild and moderate forms seem to be reversible in the majority of cases, the most recent classification of Ming[76] eliminates these categories altogether and recognizes only severe dysplasia as a significant form. His diagnostic criteria are as follows:

1. *Increased proliferation of cells.* In nonmetaplastic mucosa the growth region is expanded beyond the neck region, in metaplastic mucosa beyond the basal region. Immature cells and mitoses may be found throughout the entire length of the gland (Fig. 7-5).
2. *Abnormal morphology.* Cells are of abnormal size, shape, and orientation and are moderately to severely pleomorphic (Fig. 7-5). Mucus secretion is reduced. Nuclei are hyperchromatic and the cytoplasm is basophilic. The nucleocytoplasmic ratio is

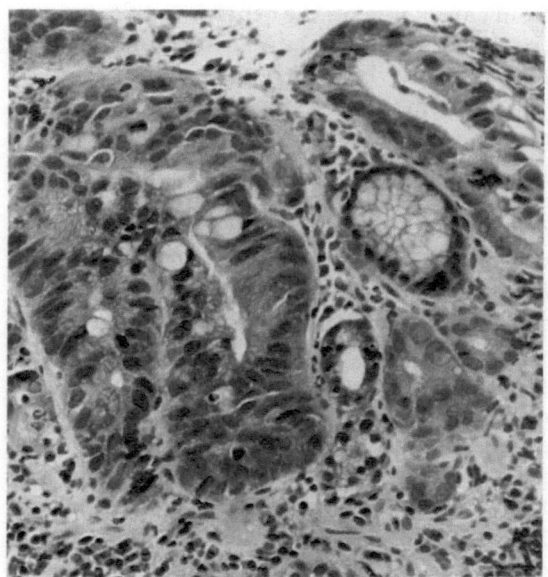

Figure 7-5. Severe dysplasia. Mitotic activity and nuclear pleomorphism persist to the very surface. There is no maturation. Normal foveolae are focally preserved. H&E, X250, reproduced at 65%.

increased. The location of the nucleus in the cytoplasm is random, and the normal polarity is lost, resulting in pseudostratification. Pseudostratification is less prominent in more pleomorphic glands. In metaplastic glands, goblet cells are few, and dysplastic changes affect primarily the absorptive cells.
3. *Architectural derangements of glands.* Cellular and glandular crowding, intraluminal folding, and glandular budding and branching are seen (Fig. 7-6). Papillary ingrowth may be present.
4. *Stromal changes.* There are no specific stromal changes, but lymphocytic and neutrophilic infiltrates are common.

Morphometric studies of gastric dysplasia, using automated image analysis techniques, have proved nuclear size to be the most important discriminating change, followed by nuclear variability and number of nuclei in the epithelium.[97]

Dysplasia must be differentiated from regenerative changes on the one hand and from carcinoma on the other hand. Regenerative changes such as cellular immaturity, cytoplasmic basophilia, nuclear hyperchromatism, and reduced mucus secretion resemble dysplastic changes. Distinct from dysplasia, however, regeneration produces cells of uniform size and shape, nuclei with orderly arrangement along the base or the center of the cell, and some degree of maturation toward the surface (Fig. 7-7). Regenerative changes of this type have been called *simple hyperplasia* by Ming.[76] Atypical regenerative changes have been called *atypical hyperplasia* and differ from simple hyperplasia by the appearance of slight loss of nuclear polarity, pseudostratification, and less maturation and differentiation. Inflammatory infiltrates are more pronounced in regeneration than in dysplasia.

The advantage of this working formulation for gastric dysplasia lies in its simplicity and the reduction of the various grades of dysplasia to a single severe form, which seems to be the only clinically relevant form. Milder grades are no longer called dysplasia, but are included in the categories of simple or atypical hyperplasia (i.e., regeneration). The problem of this grading system, as well as of all others, is the lack of a category "indefinite for dysplasia," a category that has proved helpful and relevant in determining the presence of dysplasia in ulcerative colitis. Confronted with a poorly oriented endoscopic biopsy, the most experienced pathologist may well be unable to decide whether atypia is reactive or premalignant. In such cases, it may be wiser to consider the changes indefinite rather than forcing them into categories of hyperplasia (regeneration) or dysplasia.

Severe dysplasia must be distinguished from carcinoma. Carcinoma, as distinct from dysplasia, is characterized by the appearance of pleomorphic cells with large nuclei (macronuclei). Abnormal mitotic figures are common. Evidence of invasion is often seen in the form of single cells trailing off a gland into the lamina propria (Fig. 7-8). Although carcinoma in situ would theoretically be the next stage of carcinogenesis following dysplasia, this is extremely difficult to recognize. We agree with those who favor the use of the term *intramucosal carcinoma* to include in situ lesions and invasive lesions that have broken through the basement membrane and invaded the lamina propria.[74] The type of carcinoma most often seen to develop in dysplasia is the intestinal type.[89,98]

The term *borderline lesion* or *group III lesion* was coined in Japan in 1971 to describe dysplasia of the protruded type.[89]

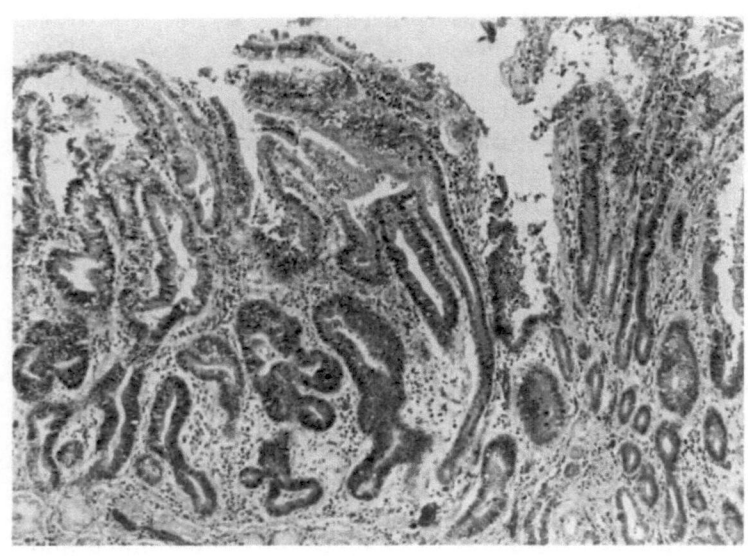

Figure 7-6. Severe dysplasia. In addition to cytologic atypia there is glandular budding, branching, and crowding. HPS, X63, reproduced at 75%.

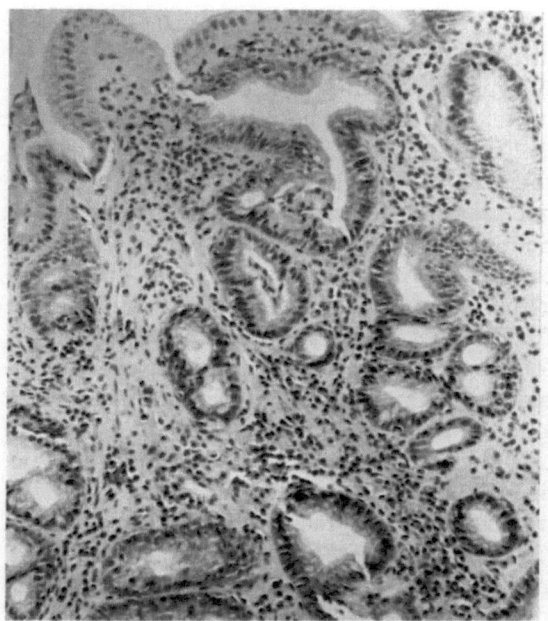

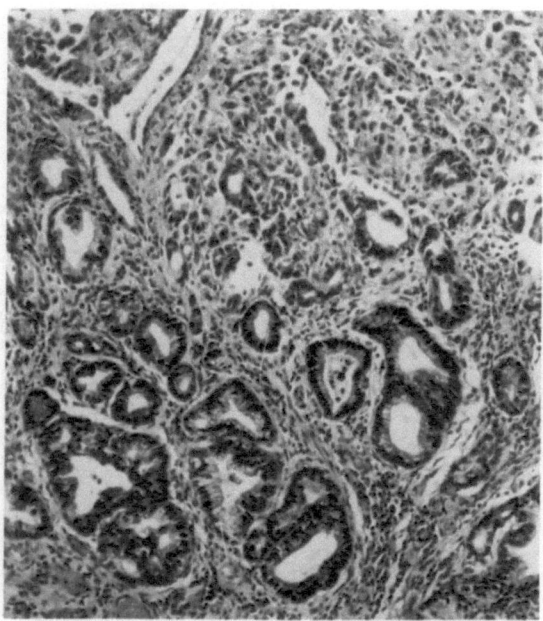

Figure 7-7. Atypia of repair. Although nuclei are enlarged and hyperchromatic, nuclear polarity is preserved and cellular maturation is seen toward the surface. H&E, X100.

Figure 7-8. Severe dysplasia with transition to carcinoma and focal invasion of lamina propria. H&E, X100, reproduced at 95%.

Other terms used in the literature include *atypical epithelial lesion of the stomach*[99] or *elevated dysplasia.*[100] To understand the term "group III," a short review of the Japanese reporting of gastric biopsy diagnoses is necessary. For purposes of standardization of histologic reporting, each finding is assigned to a group: group I, normal or benign lesions without atypia; group II, benign lesions with slight atypia; group III, borderline lesion; group IV, probably carcinoma; group V, definite carcinoma.[89] The main importance of borderline lesions resides in the high incidence (66%) of associated carcinoma.[99]

Borderline lesions are well demarcated, usually 1 to 2 cm in diameter—the largest reported case in Japan was 4 cm—and endoscopically visible. They have a characteristic appearance when examined with magnifying fiberoptic endoscopy or dissecting microscopy: The normal sulciolar surface pattern is in disarray and ditches are narrowed, areolae distended, and areolar borders hardened and angulated.[98] Histologically, normal or cysti-

cally dilated glands are seen at the bottom and crowded atypical glands toward the luminal aspect (Fig. 7-9). Cytologically, atypical epithelium is identical to adenomatous epithelium with varying degrees of superimposed atypia (i.e., dysplasia). The cystic glands consist of intestinalized metaplastic glands or hyperplastic pseudopyloric glands.

Cystically dilated glands, even in the absence of associated borderline lesions, are significantly correlated with the presence of dysplasia or early cancer, in the area of cystic dilatation as well as elsewhere in the stomach.[101] Finding cystic glands should prompt a careful sampling of the remaining gastric mucosa.

Autoradiography of borderline lesions has shown that the proliferative zone, normally restricted to the neck glands in the middle third of the mucosa, moves upward to involve the luminal third.[80] Mitoses are present at all levels. Atypical mitotic figures increase in frequency as dysplasia worsens.[100] Ultrastructurally, borderline lesions have shown

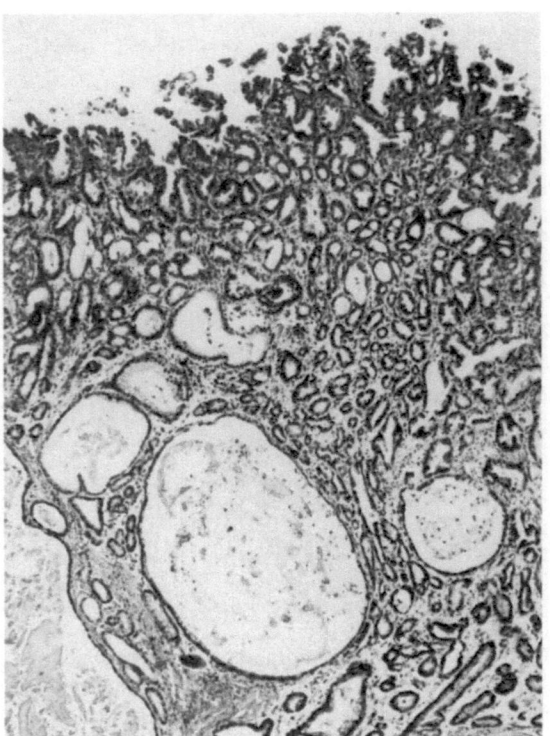

Figure 7-9. Borderline lesion or dysplasia of protruded type: dysplastic glands occupy the upper half, cystically dilated glands the lower half of the mucosa. H&E, X100.

signs of loss of differentiation, such as loss of rough endoplasmic reticulum, mucin granules, and cell polarity.[102] Frequently encountered luminal bulges and blebs may represent the first sign of expansive growth and malignant behavior.

Other techniques applied to the study of dysplasia involve mucin histochemistry, tumor markers, blood group antigens, secretory immunity, and flow cytometry.

Enzymatic staining characteristics of intestinalized gastric epithelium, with or without dysplasia, have been explored extensively in the hope of identifying the earliest precancerous change that antedates or coincides with histopathologically identifiable dysplasia.[81,82,103-107] The suspicion that intestinal metaplasia is not a uniform entity followed the observations of the close associa-

tion of gastric intestinal type cancer with intestinal metaplasia on the one hand and of the high frequency of intestinal metaplasia in healthy random population samples (20% in Finland)[103] on the other hand. It was further discovered that, even morphologically, not all intestinalized epithelium was alike. Some intestinalized glands showed a greater content of goblet cells and a loss of enterocytes with a well-developed brush border, APUD cells, and Paneth cells and was called "enterocolic, colonic, incomplete, or type II metaplasia" as opposed to the more common small intestinal, complete, or type I intestinal metaplasia.[82,103,104] These morphologic differences are paralleled by changes in mucus and enzyme production. In small intestinal or complete intestinal metaplasia, goblet cells contain neutral mucin and sialomucin and columnar cells contain no mucin.

In colonic or incomplete metaplasia, sulfated mucosubstances, stainable with Alcian blue at pH 1 and with high iron diamine, appear in goblet cells as well as in other epithelial cells.[81-83,103-107] Since the columnar mucous cells in incomplete intestinal metaplasia secrete a combination of neutral and sulfomucin, incomplete intestinal metaplasia can be further subdivided into two types, IIA with predominance of neutral mucosubstances, and IIB with predominance of sulfomucins,[81] also referred to as type III intestinal metaplasia.[104] Small intestinal-like enzymes, such as aminopeptidase, alkaline phosphatase, and disaccharidases, are no longer demonstrable. Different types of intestinal metaplasia often coexist in the same stomach and, with increasing age, the incomplete type decreases and the complete type increases in frequency, suggesting that incomplete metaplasia may mature with time toward complete metaplasia.[108]

Incomplete intestinal metaplasia has the greater precancerous significance, is often associated with histologically recognizable dysplasia, and is seen adjacent to 94% of carcinomas of the intestinal type.[82,83] When comparing the subtypes of incomplete intestinal metaplasia in gastrectomy specimens, only incomplete intestinal metaplasia with predominance of sulfomucins (type III) showed a statistically significant correlation with early[105] and advanced[106] gastric cancer. An attempt to use biopsy findings of intestinal metaplasia for predicting the risk of gastric carcinoma in the future was unsuccessful. Among 14 patients with type II intestinal metaplasia, and 14 patients with type III intestinal metaplasia, only one in each group developed carcinoma 10 and 11 years later.[104]

Nevertheless, an association between intestinal metaplasia and carcinoma is also suggested by the similarity of staining patterns for tumor markers. Tumor markers including tumor-derived colon-specific antigen (tCSA), carcinoembryonic antigen (CEA), alpha fetoprotein (AFP), pregnancy-specific S-glycoprotein 1 (SP1), human placental lactogen (HPL), human beta chorionic gonadotropin (β-hCG), transferrin (TF), and ferritin (FE) are commonly present in cells of adenocarcinoma as well as in cancer-associated intestinal metaplasia, but not in metaplastic cells of atrophic gastritis cases without cancer.[84] The presence of tCSA and SP1 is most closely linked to carcinoma. The significance of CEA staining remains unclear. On the one hand, the intensity of CEA staining paralleled the grade of dysplasia and the loss of normal gastric mucosubstances[108]; on the other hand, there was no difference in positivity of CEA staining in intestinal metaplasia with or without cancer.[84] Fetal antigens appear with increasing frequency in the epithelium of superficial gastritis, chronic atrophic gastritis, intestinal metaplasia, dysplasia, and carcinoma.[85] Monoclonal antibodies to gastric cancer-associated antigens react with dysplastic and adenomatous epithelium, but the number of positively staining cells is smaller in dysplastic and adenomatous epithelium than in cancer cells.[86]

Another biochemical marker that has been explored for possible use as an indicator for precancerous change are blood group antigens.[87,109] These occur not only on erythrocytes, but in many other tissues of the body in accordance with the blood type and secretor status of the individual. The secretor status depends on the presence of a secretor gene, which, independent from the blood group genes, controls the level of the H enzyme, the acceptor for A and B antigens in epithelial tissues.[109] Thus, in the normal mucosa of the more common secretor type, there is positive staining for ABH antigens in columnar cells of the surface epithelium and the pits. Normal nonsecretor mucosa, in contrast, stains for an I antigen, termed Ma. Gastric carcinomas in secretors commonly loose ABH antigens, either totally or regionally, and strongly express the I (Ma) antigen, which now behaves as a tumor-associated antigen. Anomalous expression of these antigens has also been found in gastric mucosa adjacent to carcinoma, in intestinal metaplasia, and in apparently normal mucosa of stomachs that showed intestinal metaplasia elsewhere. It is likely that the inappropriate blood group antigen expression in these diverse situations is not an indicator of cancer or precancer, but rather reflects an accelerated maturation process analogous to wound healing and increased hematopoiesis in hematologic disorders, in which anomalous expression of blood group antigens have also been observed.[109]

Changes in the expression of secretory immunity of gastric epithelium parallel cytologic changes of regeneration, intestinal metaplasia, dysplasia, and carcinoma.[88] Secretory component, immunoglobulin (Ig)A, and lysozyme are absent from normal gastric epithelium, except pyloric glands, which stain positive for lysozyme. In gastritis, the regenerative zone of the gastric mucosa (i.e., the mucous neck region) can be shown, by immunoperoxidase staining, to contain each of the three substances. Regenerating epithelium at the edges of peptic ulcers stains the same way. Positivity is most intense in intestinal metaplasia and dysplasia, more so for secretory component and IgA than for lysozyme. Well-differentiated intestinal type carcinoma, but not poorly differentiated types, as well as diffuse carcinoma stained as strongly positive as dysplastic epithelium. These findings further emphasize the close relationship of dysplasia and carcinoma, but are of no help in distinguishing regenerative atypia from precancerous atypia.

The most promising technique that may perhaps allow such a distinction in the future seems to be flow cytometry.[110] DNA patterns suspicious for malignancy (i.e., a high percentage of cells in the S phase and G_2+M phase and aneuploidy) were found in 6% of cases of severe chronic atrophic gastritis without histomorphologic evidence of precancer.

Gastric epithelial atypia following hepatic artery infusion chemotherapy probably has no precancerous significance and needs to be distinguished from premalignant dysplasia.[111,112] Hepatic arterial and celiac axis infusion, used in the treatment of metastatic and primary hepatic carcinoma, may be complicated by peptic ulceration and/or erosive gastroduodenitis. Associated cytologic changes of ulcer edges and nonulcerated mucosa have been misinterpreted as carcinoma.[111] Atypia is characterized by crowding and distortion of glands; pleomorphism, enlargement, and smudging of nuclei; and abundance of eosinophilic, granular, and finely vacuolated cytoplasm. The lamina propria is fibrotic and infiltrated with moderate numbers of small lymphocytes, neutrophils, and eosinophils. Capillaries in granulation tissue may be lined by atypical endothelium. Features that distinguish this reactive type of atypia from precancerous dysplasia include nuclear smudging, lower nucleocytoplasmic ratio, absence of mitotic activity, vacuolization of nuclei and cytoplasm, cytoplasmic eosinophilia rather than basophilia, and the presence of atypia in capillary endothelium. Impaired nucleic acid synthesis resulting from the antimitotic effects of chemotherapeutic agents has been implicated as the cause.

Early Gastric Cancer

Definition

Early gastric cancer, although originally described in Japan, is now recognized as a clinicopathologic entity worldwide, and the literature on the subject, here and abroad, abounds. For recent reviews, see the articles by Bogomoletz[113] and Fernando and Nakamura.[114]

The definition and macroscopic classification of early gastric cancer were agreed upon by endoscopists, pathologists, radiologists, and surgeons at a meeting of the Japanese Gastroenterological Society in 1962.[115] Japan, with its unusually high incidence of gastric cancer, began a mass screening program in 1960, using a photofluorographic barium meal examination followed by gastrocamera examination if any abnormality was found.[116] About 8% of the population over 40 years old in rural areas and 1% of the target population in large urban areas underwent this procedure, yielding a gastric cancer detection rate of 0.5%. This mass screening resulted in a significant decline in gastric cancer mortality and the accumulation of an enormous body of information that formed the basis of the recognition and classification of early gastric cancer.

Early gastric cancer is defined as a carcinoma limited to the mucosa and/or submucosa. The muscularis propria is not involved. Lymph node metastasis, blood vessel invasion, or large size do not preclude inclusion in this category. This entity, of course, existed before the creation of the term *early cancer*, and many cases are identical to what Stout called "superficial spreading carcinoma."[117] In addition to the latter, however, early cancer includes polypoid and ulcerated forms, which differ in appearance and growth pattern from Stout's superficial spreading carcinoma. The reason for incorporating these different morphologic types in one category lies in their similar behavior. The prognosis of gastric cancer, although dependent on multiple factors, is primarily determined by the depth of invasion. It is the depth of invasion, or rather the absence of deep invasion, that characterizes all forms of early gastric cancer. Thus, early gastric cancer is to be understood as a clinicopathologic entity with definite and easily recognizable diagnostic criteria and specific clinical implications. Although the overall prognosis of gastric cancer is dismal, with a 5-year survival rate of 12%,[118] that of early cancer is very good, and most 5-year survival rates reported from various parts of the world are between 82 and 100%.[115,119-122] In Japan, the 10-year actuarial survival rate for mucosal cancer was 100% and for submucosal cancer 95%.[123] Some of the lower 5-year survival rates of 70%[124] and 68%[125] from Germany and New York City are in part due to the high incidence of metachronous gastric and nongastric malignancies, the latter having a greater likelihood of being lethal than early gastric cancer.

It has been argued that the term *early* is misleading in that it suggests the cancer to be of recent origin and representing the initial phase in a continuum with ordinary gastric carcinoma.[126] This is a valid argument. Early cancer differs from ordinary gastric cancer in its greater tendency to grow laterally rather than vertically, a relationship somewhat akin to that of superficial spreading melanoma and nodular melanoma. Evidence for slow growth are the long intervals between the onset of symptoms and diagnosis[127] and between incomplete resection and clinical recurrence (6 years).[120] "Early" in early gastric cancer must be understood to mean "early enough" for cure.

Frequency of Early Gastric Cancer

The frequency with which early gastric cancer has been diagnosed has shown a steady increase over the past 20 years. The greatest increases are reported from Japan, where 3.7% of gastric cancers were "early" between 1958 and 1960 and 33.1% during 1967 and 1969, after mass screening had been introduced.[128] An unprecedented high rate of 43%

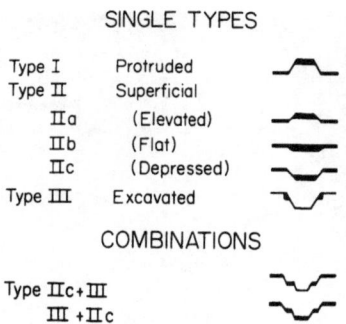

Figure 7-10. Classification of early gastric cancer.

was reported from the same institution in 1978.[129] Similar increases have occurred in the United States and Europe, but the numbers have been significantly lower. In the United States, incidences have been between 8.3 and 13%.[125,130-132] In our own series of gastrectomy specimens with cancer, early cancer accounted for 4.9% of cases during 1966 to 1973 and 8.8% during 1974 to 1981.[132] In Britain, the incidence was 0.5 and 10%, respectively, before and after the introduction of the endoscope.[133] Comparable figures from other countries are as follows: Australia, 20%[134]; West Germany, 16%[121]; Sweden, 15%[135]; Switzerland, 12%[136]; Italy, 9%[127]; and Scotland, 5%.[137] In China, where, like Japan, cancer of the stomach ranks first among cancer mortalities, early cancer quadrupled in frequency since fiberoptic endoscopy and periodic mass screening were introduced in 1973[122,138] and is now 9.3%.[139]

The incidence of early cancers in gastroscopies is low and was 0.1% among 2500 procedures between 1969 and 1979.[140]

Classification of Early Gastric Cancer

Three main types of early gastric cancer, three subtypes, and various combinations of these are generally recognized. These are macroscopic types identifiable by the endoscopist, radiologist, surgeon, and pathologist (Fig. 7-10). In the combination types, the more prominent type is designated first.

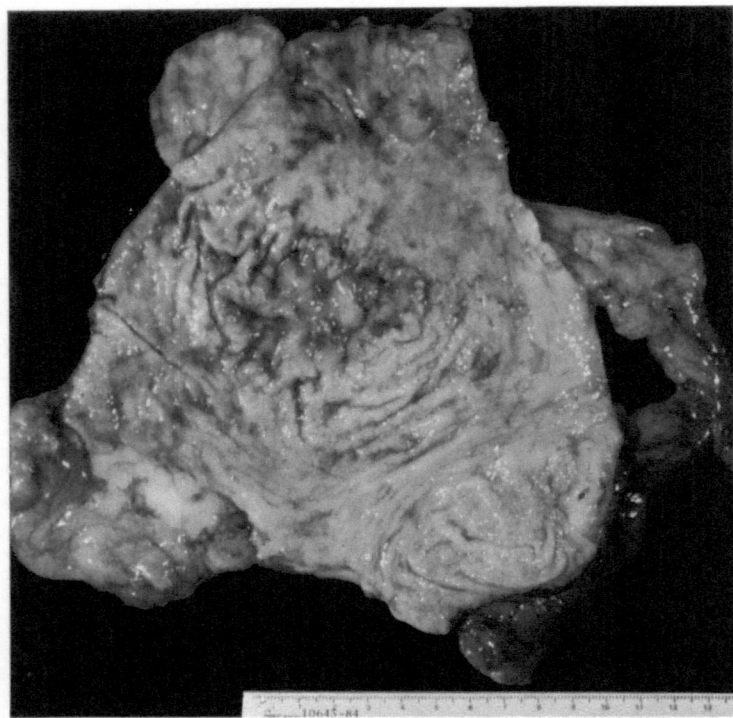

Figure 7-11. Early gastric cancer, Types III and IIC (excavated and depressed).

During the 20 years since its adoption in Japan, this classification has been proved easily reproducible and applicable worldwide. The only difficulties that arose were the differentiation of Types I and IIa and of Types IIc and III. Disagreements in classification, however, are of minor importance, since differences in prognosis among the different types are minor. Ulcerated types had a slightly more aggressive course than other types in one series.[138] The significance of the classification lies in the fact that it makes the observer aware of the multiplicity of possible appearances of the same clinicopathologic entity. Types IIc and III are often combined, and their distinction becomes irrelevant. Type I, the most elevated type of early cancer, may arise from an adenoma. Types IIc and III are ulcerated cancers that either form at the edge of a preexisting benign ulcer or, more often, represent secondarily ulcerated carcinomas (Fig. 7-11). It

has been suggested that gastric cancer develops first in the neck of glands, in the midportion of the mucosa, as a lateral bud without elevation or depression of the surface. Three directions of growth are possible, and each will result in a different type of early cancer; predominant upward growth results in Type IIa, horizontal growth in Type IIb, and downward growth with superficial erosion in Type IIc.[115]

Frequencies of these different macroscopic types have been relatively consistent in different parts of the world (i.e., Japan, Germany, the United States, and China).[116,119,121,130,138] Ulcerated types are definitely most frequent. In some Western series Type I is relatively more frequent, accounting for 29% of early cancers in the United States,[125] 30% in Italy,[127] and 36% in Scotland.[137] Whether this difference reflects a greater frequency of adenomas or easier endoscopic recognition of the elevated type is not clear. Type I early gastric cancer is relatively more common in older patients.[124]

Early gastric cancer is also classified according to extent into mucosal and submucosal cancer. The proportion of mucosal versus submucosal types has been variously reported between 0.37%[132] and 2%,[122,138] with the lower figures from countries with a low overall incidence of early cancer and the high figures from Japan and China.

Natural History of Early Gastric Cancer

It is not clear how long early cancer remains intramucosal and what determines the spread into the submucosa and progression to advanced cancer. What is known is that at least until a diameter of 3 mm is reached, all lesions remain intramucosal.[141] Unusually large sizes of intramucosal early cancer may be the result of collision of multiple small lesions, especially in the aged.[142] The largest intramucosal carcinoma had a diameter of 7.8 cm. Exceedingly slow tumor growth has been demonstrated in some Japanese and European patients who had biopsy-proven diagnoses of carcinoma, refused surgery, and were found to have early cancer restricted to the mucosa at gastrectomy up to 7 years later.[143,144] When submucosal invasion occurs, it usually is seen in an area where lymphoid aggregates disrupt the muscularis mucosae.[145] Tumor invasion follows the course of small blood vessels and may reach a size 3 to 10 times that within the mucosa, forming what has been appropriately termed an *expanded balloon*.[146] Submucosal invasion is more frequent in Type IIc cancers than in any other type.[119] The size of early cancer has been reported anywhere between 0.1 and 10 cm, with an average diameter of 2.7 cm.[125]

The frequency of lymph node metastasis correlates with the depth of invasion and growth pattern.[147,148] Early cancer restricted to the mucosa shows lymph node metastasis in 4.2% of cases and early cancer with submucosal invasion in 16.8%.[147] The particu-larly low incidence in the mucosal type may be explained by the rarity of lymph capillaries in the mucosa. In normal gastric mucosa as well as in patients with carcinoma and a variety of polypoid lesions, lymphatics are confined to the deep lamina propria adjacent to and within the muscularis mucosae.[147,149] In atrophic gastritis, however, in which the overall height of the mucosa is decreased, lymphatics may be found near the surface epithelium.[149] This difference may account for the fact that in early cancer, as opposed to advanced cancer, the intestinal type, arising in atrophic mucosa with easier access to lymphatics, carries a slightly worse prognosis than the diffuse type, which is usually not associated with atrophic gastritis.[150]

Three different histologic growth patterns can be recognized in early cancers.[148] The term *small mucosal type* is used for cancers less than 4 cm in diameter that are primarily mucosal and show only focal and shallow submucosal invasion. The term *superficial spreading type* is used for cancers with a diameter greater than 4 cm and with no or focal submucosal invasion (Fig. 7-12). It is the most common type. The term *Pentype*, for penetrating growth pattern, is used for cancers with a diameter of less than 4 cm that invade the submucosa broadly. If invasion is accompanied by complete destruction of the muscularis mucosae, the pattern is referred to as Pen A; if the muscularis mucosae is only fenestrated, as Pen B (Fig. 7-13). Lymph node metastasis is least frequent in the small mucosal type and most frequent in the Pen type, especially Pen A (25%). Blood vessel invasion is found only in the Pen type, again more often in subtype A than B (25% versus 14%). Ten-year survival was 90% in all types except for Pen A, which carried a 5-year survival of only 65%.[148] These differences are reflected in differences of cell nuclear DNA content as measured by microspectrophotometry.[151] The prognostically worst Pen A subtype showed widely scattered DNA values, identical to those found in advanced gastric cancer.

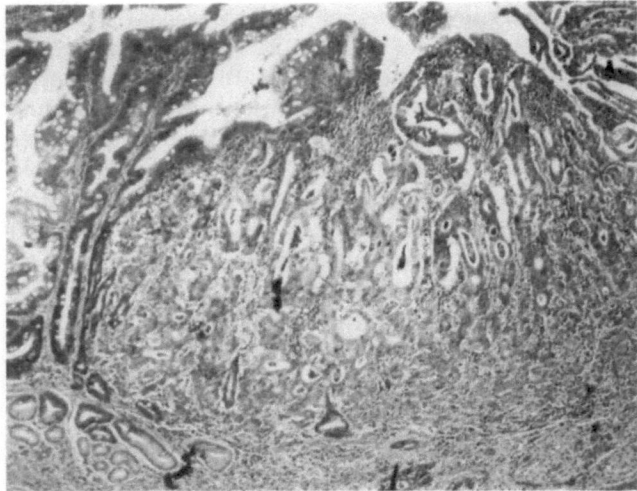

Figure 7-12. Early gastric cancer, mucosal type. Carcinoma is predominantly intramucosal and invades the muscularis mucosae only focally. Intestinal metaplasia is present at the edge. H&E, X40.

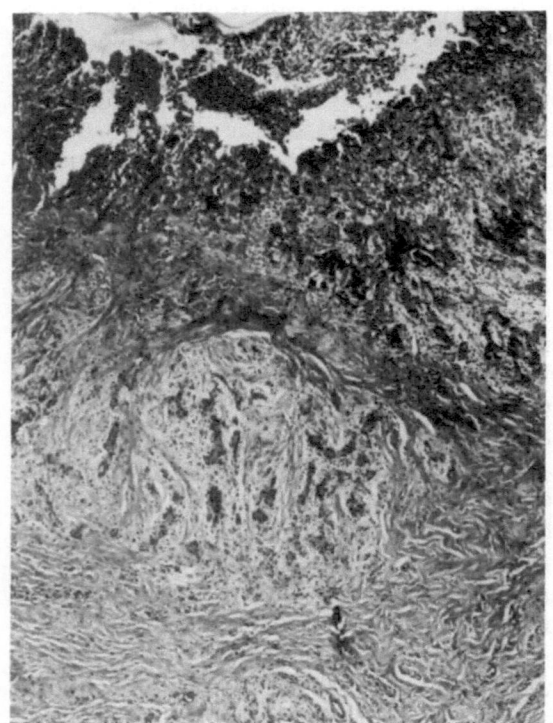

Figure 7-13. Early gastric cancer, penetrating growth pattern (Pen B). Carcinoma invades the submucosa. Submucosal fibrosis is prominent. H&E, X40.

Minute Gastric Cancer

Cancers with a maximum dimension of less than 5 mm have been called "minute gastric cancers" and account for 5.17% of early cancers in Japan.[141] Cancers measuring 5 to 10 mm have been referred to as "small gastric cancers" and are of equal frequency. The majority of minute cancers are associated with larger gastric cancers and only diagnosed intraoperatively, or by the pathologist examining the gastrectomy specimen. Most recently, minute cancers have been detected preoperatively by x-ray (15.5%) or by endoscopy and endoscopic biopsy (44.8%).[152,153]

Diagnosis of Early Gastric Cancer

In Japan, most patients with early gastric cancer are asymptomatic and identified through screening programs. In the United States, most patients are investigated because of symptoms indistinguishable from peptic ulcer or advanced gastric cancer.[125] Early gastric cancer is usually detected by the radiologist and endoscopist. The pathologist plays a confirmatory role. Using a double-contrast method (i.e., high-quality contrast media combined with air), the radiologist can demonstrate elevated lesions as small as 5 mm and depressed lesions as small as 10 mm.[114] Nonetheless, about half of early cancers may be missed,[125] and the diagnosis depends primarily on the endoscopist and an aggressive approach to biopsy.

Endoscopically, the gastric mucosa is screened for discoloration, irregularities, depressions, or elevations. Better definition of a suspicious area can be achieved with the endoscopic Congo red–methylene blue test, which will stain areas of acid secretion and intestinal metaplasia, but not carcinoma,[154] or by intraarterial injection of indigo carmine.[155] Most early carcinomas are located in the pyloric antrum and along the lesser curvature,[113] where visualization and biopsy are relatively easy. The cardia is the site of early cancer in only 5% as opposed to 31% of advanced cancers.[145] The lack of an increase in frequency of cardiac early cancers over a period of 13 years (1965 to 1978), in contrast to the marked increase in frequency of early cancers elsewhere in the stomach, reflects the difficulty in making the diagnosis in this area.

Biopsies should be multiple and designated clearly as to their site of origin. Ideally four or five biopsies should be taken[114] and include samples of the lesion as well as adjacent mucosa.[113]

The histopathologist must take care to recognize dysplasia and borderline lesions as distinctly different from early cancer, and if cancer is present, not to assure the surgeon or endoscopist that the cancer is "early." Even if the biopsy shows only intramucosal carcinoma, a definite diagnosis of early cancer can only be made after a detailed gross and microscopic examination of the resected stomach. Examination of a gastrectomy specimen should include photography of the opened, stretched-out stomach (Fig. 7-14) and sectioning of the entire lesion[114] (Fig. 7-15). The mucosa should be carefully examined for second or third lesions, since approximately 10% of early cancers are multicentric,[113] especially Types IIB and IIC.[141] After micro-

scopic examination, a diagram is useful to illustrate the extent of the carcinoma, which is usually greater than appreciated grossly. At times, islands of normal mucosa are completely surrounded by carcinoma. Such "sanctuary areas" may represent areas of spontaneous regression or simply reflect a peculiar uneven spread of the carcinoma.[113]

Microscopically, early carcinoma may either be of the intestinal type (Fig. 7-16) (63% in a Japanese series,[148] 55% in a European series[156]) or of the diffuse type (Figs. 7-17 and 7-18). Micronests of neoplastic, Grimelius-positive endocrine cells may be associated with the intestinal type.[157] DNA distribution patterns studied by cytophotometry are identical to those of advanced gastric cancer: most intestinal types are aneuploid and most diffuse types diploid.[158]

Intramucosal cysts are often seen in early cancers, in the tumoral as well as in the nontumoral mucosa (Fig. 7-19). Their presence should stimulate an especially careful examination of the gastric mucosa, even if cancer has not been suspected clinically.[159] Almost all cases with an intestinal pattern show some form of gastritis, especially chronic atrophic gastritis. The diffuse type is mostly associated with a mild or moderate superficial gastritis only.[156] Submucosal fibrosis may be present in mucosal or submucosal carcinoma, with or without ulceration, and is usually associated with the depressed macroscopic type[160] (see Fig. 7-13). Its presence should alert the pathologist to the possibility of deep invasion, that is, involvement of the muscularis propria, which was detected in 33% of cases with marked submucosal fibrosis.[148]

Treatment and Prognosis

Since early gastric cancer is a diagnosis made with certainty only after pathologic examination of a gastrectomy specimen, gastrectomy is the obvious mode of diagnosis as well as therapy. Endoscopic or endoscopic laser resections have been successfully per-

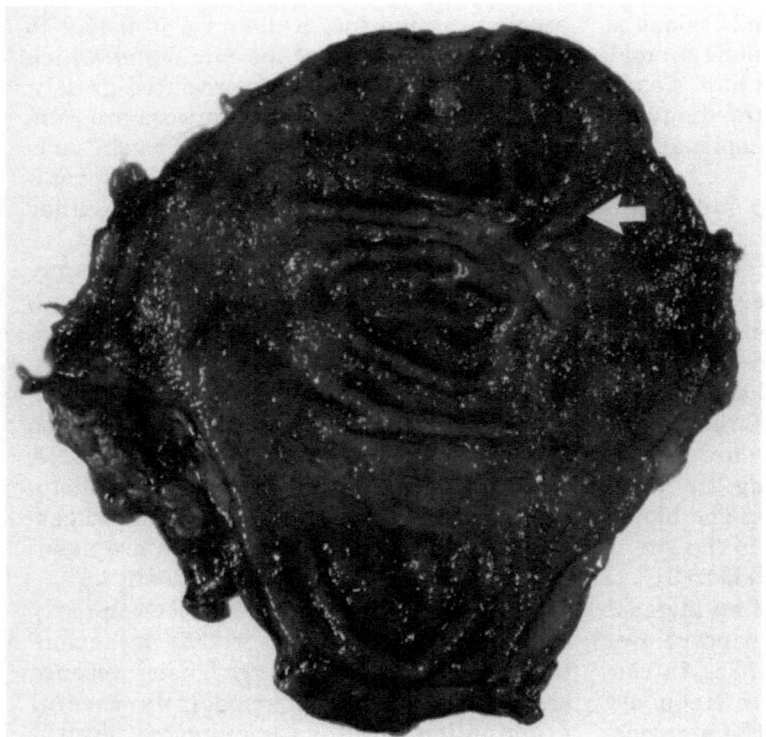

Figure 7-14. Early gastric cancer, Type IIa (superficial and elevated).

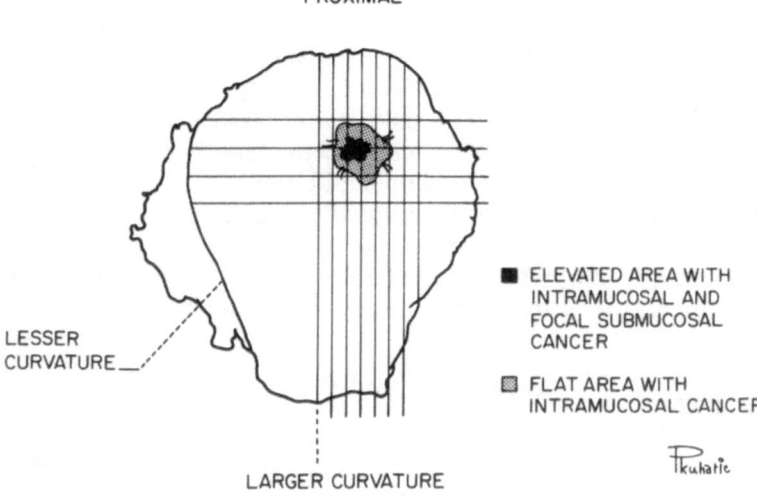

PROXIMAL

■ ELEVATED AREA WITH INTRAMUCOSAL AND FOCAL SUBMUCOSAL CANCER

▨ FLAT AREA WITH INTRAMUCOSAL CANCER

LESSER CURVATURE

LARGER CURVATURE

Figure 7-15. Diagram of sectioning of gastrectomy specimen shown in Fig. 14. Intramucosal carcinoma extends beyond the elevated central area.

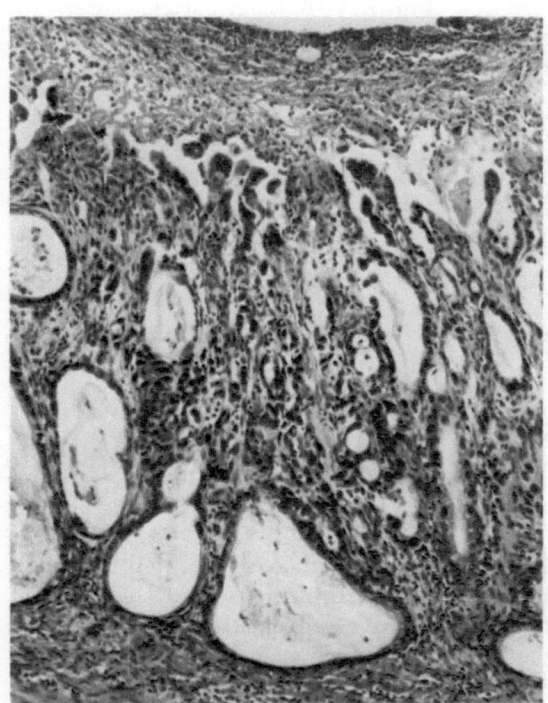

Figure 7-16. Early gastric cancer, intestinal type, ulcerated. Cysts are present at the base. H&E, X100, reproduced at 95%.
◄

formed on patients in whom a tentative diagnosis of early cancer was based on endoscopic biopsy findings, and who represented poor surgical risks.[161,162]

The overall good prognosis of early cancer has been discussed. The most important prognostic factors are depth of invasion and growth pattern. In Japan, 5-year survival

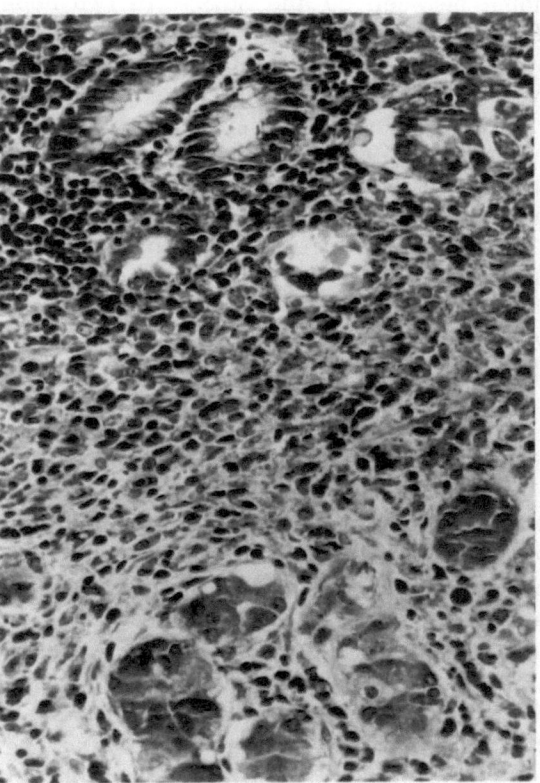

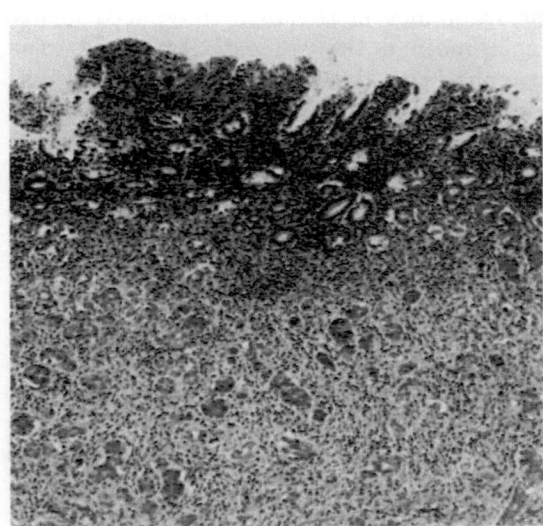

Figure 7-17. Early gastric cancer, diffuse type. Normal gastric glands are pushed apart by a diffuse infiltrate of single carcinoma cells. Superficial gastritis is present. HPS, X40, reproduced at 90%.

Figure 7-18. Higher-power magnification of Fig. 17. Carcinoma cells in the diffuse type of gastric cancer may resemble histiocytes. Mucin stains usually demonstrate focal intracytoplasmic mucin. HPS, X250, reproduced at 85%.

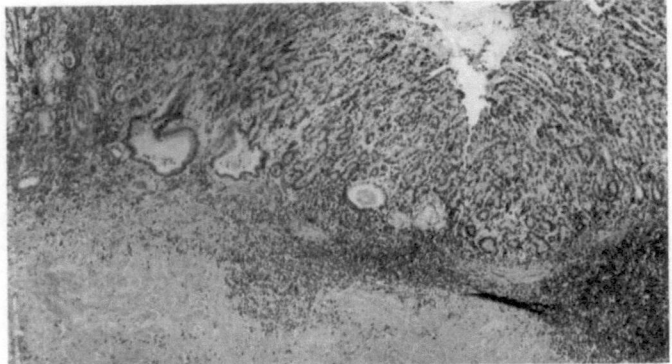

Figure 7-19. Early gastric cancer, intramucosal, with prominent intramucosal cysts. H&E, X25.

rates for mucosal carcinoma range between 90 and 100%, those for submucosal carcinoma between 80 and 85%.[120] In two non-Japanese studies, only 70% of patients survived 5 years.[125,156] The lowest survival was seen in patients with submucosal carcinomas of the penetrating type A, 45% of whom were dead in 10 years.[148] Lymph node metastasis does not significantly alter the outcome.

The cause of death in many nonsurvivors is unrelated to their early cancer. In two large Japanese series, only 7 and 11% of nonsurvivors with early cancer died of their original disease. In these patients liver metastases, carcinoma in the remnant stomach, bone metastases, and jejunal metastases were described in decreasing order of frequency.[120,148] Postgastrectomy survival times ranged from 1 to 12 years. Liver metastases usually occur within 3 years after the resection, but recurrent carcinoma in the stump may occur after a longer postoperative period. Whether late recurrences, such as 12 years after gastrectomy, represent second primary occurrences or recurrences is difficult to assess. The two features predictive of recurrence are tumor extending to the surgical margin of resection and the aggressive penetrating growth pattern Pen A.[148] Interestingly, the presence of lymph node metastasis in cases without these features had no prognostic significance.[120,148]

Advanced Gastric Cancer

Definition and Frequency

Advanced gastric cancer is defined as carcinoma extending into or beyond the muscularis propria. Its relative frequency among gastric carcinomas has decreased proportionately to the increase in the frequency of early cancer. This decrease, in our own experience, affects primarily invasive carcinomas restricted to the muscularis propria, whereas the frequency of the more advanced forms has remained the same.[132] Advanced cancer constitutes between 67 and 57% of gastric cancers in Japan[128,129] and between 92 and 87% of gastric cancers in the United States.[125,130-132]

Classification

Gastric carcinoma may be classified according to gross morphology, pattern of infiltration, extent, and histologic type. The earliest classification dates back to 1926, when Borrmann[163] classified gastric cancer into four groups based on gross morphology: I, polypoid; II, ulcerating; III, combined ulcerating and polypoid; and IV, infiltrating, noting that the prognosis was worst with infiltrating tumors (Fig. 7-20). Schindler,[164] the inventor of the first gastroscope, in 1941 distinguished a polypoid, plateau-like, ulcerating, and flat type. Ming[165] in 1977 intro-

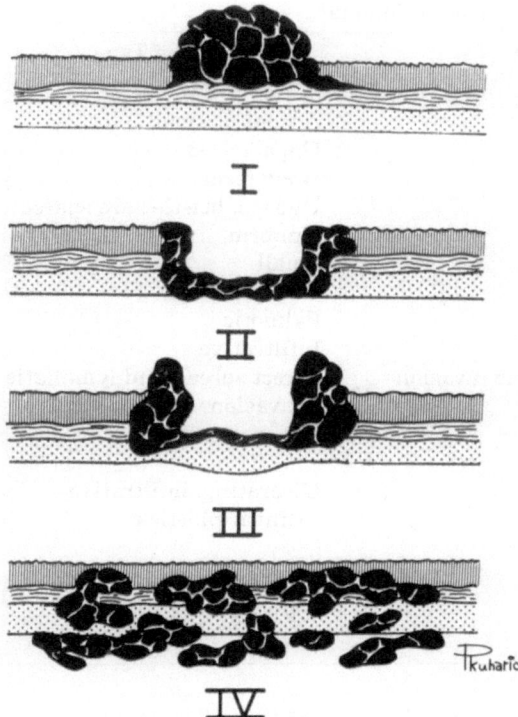

Figure 7-20. Borrmann classification of advanced gastric cancer: I, polypoid; II, ulcerating; III, combined ulcerating and polypoid; IV, infiltrating.

Table 7-5. American Joint Committee Stage Grouping of Carcinoma of the Stomach (1983): Surgical Evaluative (sTNM) or Postsurgical Pathologic Assessment (pTNM)*

Stage	TNM	Tumor Limited to
0	Tis, NO, MO	In situ, no invasion of lamina propria
I	T1, NO, MO	Mucosa, submucosa
II	T2, T3; NO; MO	Muscularis propria, subserosa, or serosa
III	T1–3; N1, N2; MO	Any invasion through serosa, with N1 or N2 nodes involved
	T4a; NO–N2; MO	Direct extension to immediately adjacent tissues or organs,[†] any nodal involvement up to N2
IV	T1–T3, T4a; N3; MO	Any invasion through serosa including direct extension to immediately adjacent tissues or organs,[†] with N3 nodes involved
	T4b; any N; MO	Direct extension to further contiguous organs,[‡] any nodes
	Any T, any N, M1	Distant metastasis (either site or nodes)

*From Curtis et al.[166] Reproduced by permission, Grune & Stratton.

[†]T4a = Tumor penetrates through the serosa and involves immediately adjacent tissues such as lesser omentum, perigastric fat, regional ligaments, greater omentum, transverse colon, spleen, esophagus, or duodenum (by way of intraluminal extension).

[‡]T4b = Tumor penetrates through the serosa and involves the liver, diaphragm, pancreas, abdominal wall, adrenal glands, kidney, retroperitoneum, small intestine, esophagus, or duodenum (by way of serosa).

duced a pathobiologic classification based on patterns of infiltrations and divided gastric cancer into an expanding type and an infiltrating type. The expanding type accounts for 67% of gastric cancers and is characterized by discrete tumor nodules, usually composed of well-differentiated glands. The infiltrative type is seen in 33% of gastric cancers and typically shows diffuse infiltration by individual tumor cells without gland formation.

The most frequently used and clinically most relevant classification is the TNM (T = tumor, N = lymph node metasis, M = distant metastasis) staging, formulated in 1978 by the American Joint Committee for Cancer Staging and End Results Reporting[166] (Table 7-5). Staging is based on pathologic and clinical findings and correlates better than any

other classification with prognosis. Staging based on computed tomographic findings may prevent unneeded, noncurative surgical exploration and was shown to compare well with the above staging system.[167]

The most widely used histologic classification of gastric carcinoma is that of Lauren, who subdivided adenocarcinoma into an intestinal and a diffuse type.[168] Synonyms for

Table 7-6. Lauren's Histologic Classification of Gastric Adenocarcinoma*

Characteristics	Intestinal Type	Diffuse Type
Pathologic		
Glandular lumina	Present and large	Absent or small
Cell polarization	Well polarized	Unpolarized
Apical surface of cell	Continued unbroken	Wavy form
Brush border	Well developed	Uneven, bristles are sparse
Cell Shape	Variable	Uniform
Size	Large	Small
Nuclei Mitosis	Often	Rare
Chromatin	Hyperchromatic	Pyknotic
Growth pattern	Expansive	Infiltrative
Mode of spread	Blood vessel and lymphatic invasion	Direct spread and lymphatic invasion
Intestinal metaplasia	Very common	Less common
Most common gross type	Polypoid, fungating	Ulcerating, infiltrative (linitis plastica)
Clinical		
Mean age (yr)	55	48
Male:female ratio	3:1	1:1
Frequency (%)	45–53	33–34

*Modified from Lauren,[168] Noda et al.,[169] and Antonioli.[170]

the latter are signet-ring and mucous cell type. The intestinal type resembles intestinal adenocarcinoma and is associated with chronic atrophic gastritis and intestinal metaplasia. It is the epidemic form of gastric cancer that is most common in countries with a high incidence of gastric cancer and decreases in frequency as the overall incidence of gastric cancer decreases. The diffuse type is typically, but not exclusively, a Borrmann group IV lesion with an infiltrating pattern, and its relative frequency increases as the incidence of gastric cancer decreases.

Lauren[168] categorized 53% of gastric adenocarcinomas as intestinal and 33% as diffuse. In Japan, equivalent figures are 45 and 34%.[169] Lauren's classification has been adopted worldwide[169,170] and has proved useful in clinicopathologic correlations as well as in epidemiologic studies. The main correlates are summarized in Table 7-6. Problems arise in individual cases, many of which defy rigid categorization. Lauren himself left a large number of tumors (14%) "unclassified."

Other classifications have attempted to introduce additional histologic types, such as the pylorocardiac type of adenocarcinoma described by Mulligan[171] and the nine subtypes of adenocarcinoma in Japan[172] (Table 7-7).

Clinical Presentation of Advanced Gastric Cancer

The majority of patients with advanced gastric cancer are men between the ages of 50 and 79 years. The male to female ratio is 2 to 1.[173] Patients younger than 35 years old comprise 2.2% of cases and differ from the older patients in their even sex distribution.[174] The onset of symptoms is insidious and the symptoms themselves are nonspecific, explaining why nearly one-quarter of all patients with newly diagnosed gastric cancer have inoperable lesions and are not even explored, and another quarter of those who are explored have nonresectable tumors.[175] A history of peptic ulcer disease is found in 22% of cases, abdominal pain in 66%, weight loss in 50%, nausea and vomiting in 32%, anorexia in 25%, dysphagia in 23%, and gastrointestinal bleeding in 23%.[173] A palpable mass is present in one-third and abdominal tenderness in one-fifth. Laboratory findings may show anemia (42%), hypoproteinemia (26%), abnormal liver function tests (26%), and positive stool guaiacs (40%).

Rarely, gastric carcinoma may present with paraneoplastic syndromes produced by abnormal secretory products of the tumor cells. Tumor antigen access may lead to raised plasma concentrations of immune complexes that cause microangiopathic hemolytic anemia, thrombocytopenia, renal insufficiency, and neurologic abnormalities.[176] Tumor antigen and carcinoembryonic antigen were identified in the glomeruli of patients with membranous nephropathy and the nephrotic syndrome.[177,178] Secretion of a growth-stimulating factor is postulated in cases presenting with acanthosis nigricans, that is, sudden eruption of filiform and papular pigmented lesions on skin and mucous membranes, especially the body folds, and around the mouth and anus.[179] Excessive granulocytosis has been ascribed to a colony-stimulating factor stimulating granulocytes in the bone marrow.[180] Severe hypoglycemia sensitive to diazoxide was reported in a case of gastric carcinoma with widespread metastasis. Impaired gluconeogenesis was postulated as a pathogenic mechanism.[181]

Diagnosis of Advanced Gastric Cancer

The diagnosis of advanced gastric cancer is made by radiography, endoscopy, biopsy, and cytology.[170,171,182] Determinations of cancer-associated enzymes and antigens in gastric juice or serum remain investigational tools, useful perhaps as screening devices in high-risk populations, but not as diagnostic modalities in individual cases.[183-188]

While conventional radiographic examinations may miss as many as 30% of biopsy-proven gastric carcinomas,[170,182] the use of double-contrast examination has reduced the error rate to 10%.[189] Computerized axial

Table 7-7. Japanese Histologic Classification of Gastric Carcinoma*

Type	Total[†]
Adenocarcinoma, well differentiated	63(50)
Adenocarcinoma, moderately differentiated	55(40)
Adenocarcinoma, poorly differentiated	66(37)
Adenocarcinoma, solid medullary	16(12)
Mucoid carcinoma, well differentiated	15(12)
Mucoid carcinoma, poorly differentiated	8(4)
Diffuse carcinoma, desmoplastic	27(16)
Diffuse carcinoma, signet ring	25(11)
Diffuse carcinoma, anaplastic	13(6)
Others	6(6)

*Modified from Ishii T, et al.[172] Reproduced by permission, John Wiley.
[†]Total number for both sexes, with number of male cases in parentheses.

tomographic (CAT) scanning has been successfully applied in preoperative staging[167] and is especially helpful in detecting infiltrative tumors, metastases,[190] and local tumor extension and in guiding percutaneous fine-needle aspiration biopsy.[191]

Fiberoptic endoscopy combined with biopsy and brush cytology is the most reliable diagnostic modality. Before the use of fiberoptics, endoscopy alone yielded findings "consistent with malignancy" in 75% of cases.[170] With the use of fiberoptics, the detection rate rose to 87%. Fiberoptic endoscopy and biopsy have yielded recent accuracy rates between 72 and 99.8%.[171,192-195] Percutaneous biopsy under ultrasound guidance has been successfully employed in patients unable to undergo gastroscopy.[196] Lower rates are reported for cancers arising in ulcers and for infiltrative cancers of the linitis plastica type than for exophytic lesions.[195,197] Seven biopsies are suggested for each lesion. The center as well as the tumor margins should be sampled, especially of ulcerated lesions, since as many as 56% of radiologically benign-appearing ulcers harbor a carcinoma. Deep tissues may be sampled by taking multiple biopsies from the same site, a procedure sometimes referred to as "digging." Biopsies should be cut at mul-

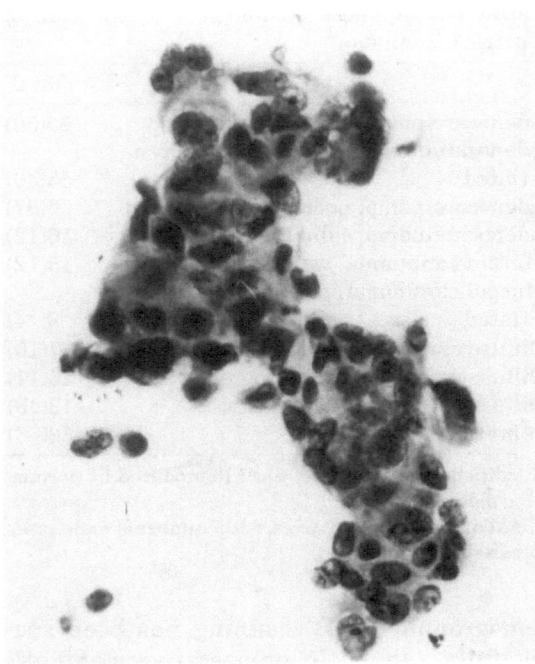

Figure 7-21. Cytology of gastric adenocarcinoma, intestinal type. There is marked cellular and nuclear pleomorphism, multinucleation, and overlapping of cells. Papanicolaou stain X400.

tiple levels. Six levels are routinely cut at the New York University Medical Center, three levels at most other centers. For a discussion of the histopathology of gastric cancer, see the section on microscopic appearance.

Cytologic techniques applicable to the diagnosis of gastric cancer include direct brushing of the lesion, direct vision lavage, and biopsy touch smear cytology.[198] Of these, brush cytology is the most widely accepted technique and has raised diagnostic yields of 72 to 74% after biopsy alone to cumulative yields of 88 and 91% after biopsy and brush cytology.[195,199] Brush cytology has proved especially useful in cancers associated with an ulcer.[200] The results of endoscopic gastric cytology, in experienced hands, may prove more accurate than those of endoscopic biopsy. A 98% accuracy in the cytologic diagnosis of gastric carcinoma, as compared to a 68.9% accuracy of biopsy, was reached during

a 3-year clinical trial period in Glasgow.[201] Significantly, there were no false-positive reports and in the 2% of cases that were false negative, the biopsy was negative as well. Although these results are impressive, the routine use of cytology in patients with radiographically and endoscopically visible advanced cancers is probably not warranted.[202] In cytologic preparations, the classic signs of cytologic atypia such as anisocytosis, anisonucleosis, abnormal nucleoli, and variation in nuclear chromasia increase in severity from benign toward malignant atypia, but have not proved reliable diagnostic criteria. Nuclear pleomorphism and mitotic figures are slightly more specific, but only abnormal mitotic figures, irregular multinucleation, and abnormal intercellular relationships are highly specific for carcinoma (Fig. 7-21). Abnormal intercellular relationships typical for carcinoma include loss of polarity and a cell distribution pattern, on the slide, characterized by the predominance of single rather than clustered atypical cells.[198]

Fine-needle aspiration biopsy under direct vision with a gastrofiberscope may prove helpful in diffusely infiltrative carcinomas that escape endoscopic biopsy and brush cytology diagnosis.[203]

In gastric carcinoma, there is a shift toward anaerobic metabolism in tumor tissue as well as in uninvolved mucosa, resulting in the appearance of enzymes in the gastric juice that are normally not present. Lactate dehydrogenase (LDH), L-lactate, D-lactate, and beta-glucuronidase have been identifiable in the gastric juice of most gastric cancer patients.[183,184] While false-negative results for LDH and beta-glucuronidase are rare, a false-positive result occurs in about 10% and is due to precancerous lesions or intestinal metaplasia.[184] Correlation with tumor size and depth of invasion has been shown for lactate and LDH levels.[183]

Plasma levels of carcinoembryonic antigen (CEA) have been shown to be significantly higher in patients with gastric cancer than in those with noncarcinomatous gastric disease.[188] The absolute CEA titer, however, is

Figure 7-22. Advanced gastric cancer, polypoid type.

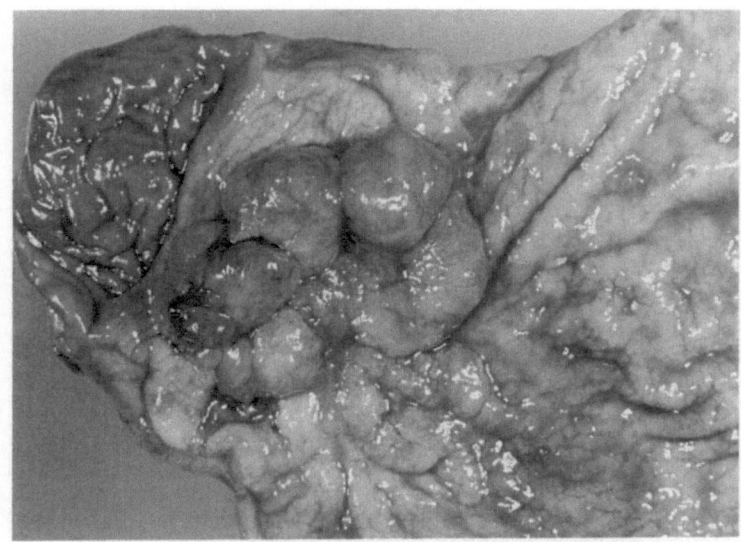

of no diagnostic value. Continuously rising postoperative CEA levels are indicative of tumor progression.

Alpha-fetoprotein (AFP), best known as a tumor marker for yolk sac tumors, teratomas, and hepatomas, is frequently demonstrable in the sera of gastric cancer patients. Especially high AFP levels may be indicative of gastric adenocarcinoma with a "hepatoid" differentiation.[187]

Low serum levels of pepsinogen 1[185] and positive serum levels for fetal sulfoglycoprotein antigen[186] have been used for mass screening for gastric cancer in high-risk populations.

Tetracycline-induced fluorescence, persisting for more than 24 hours, is a function of rapidly growing tissues and can be used to identify tumor tissue at any site. Fluorescence of the sediment of gastric aspirates has been demonstrated in 93% of gastric cancer patients.[204]

Gross Appearance of Advanced Gastric Cancer

Grossly, advanced gastric cancer may be exophytic and appear polypoid, fungating, or papillary (Figs. 7-22 and 7-23); ulcerated, flat or plaque-like; infiltrative, also referred to as

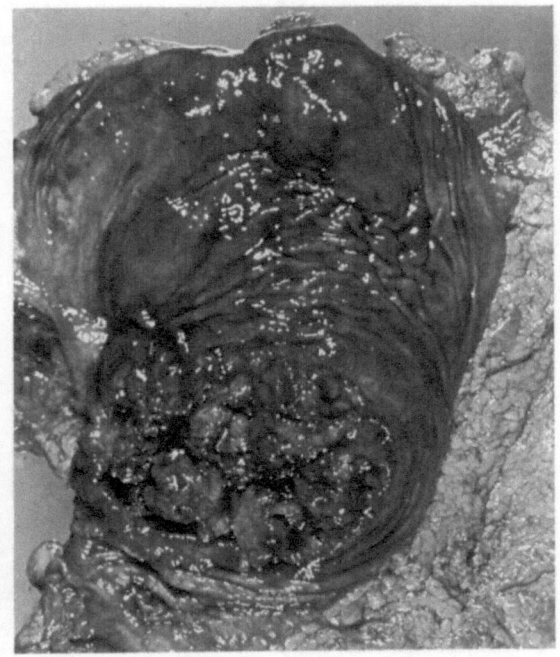

Figure 7-23. Advanced gastric cancer, fungating type.

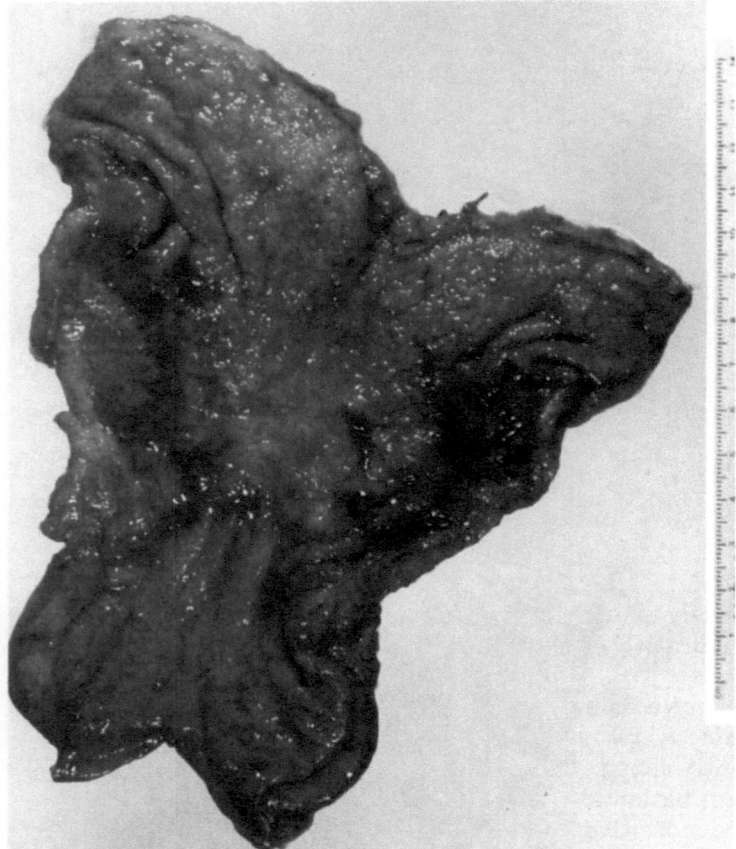

Figure 7-24. Advanced gastric cancer, infiltrative type (linitis plastica).

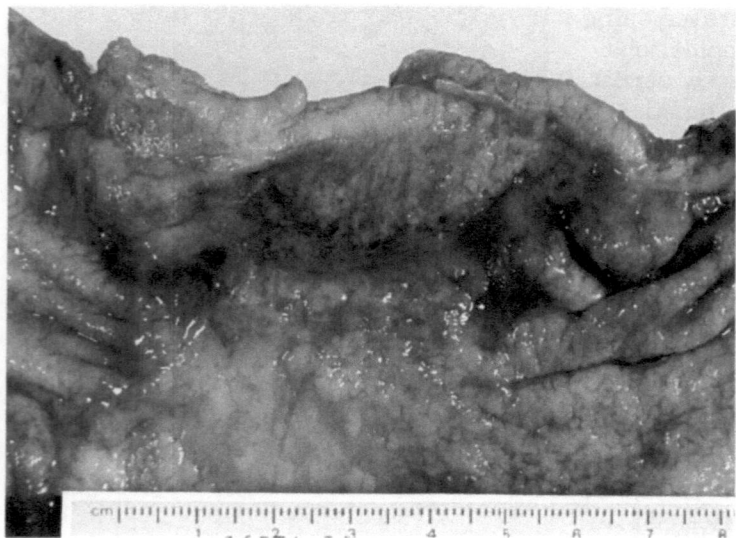

Figure 7-25. Advanced gastric cancer, infiltrative type (linitis plastica). The wall is diffusely thickened and stiff.

Figure 7-26. Advanced gastric cancer, combined ulcerative and infiltrative type.

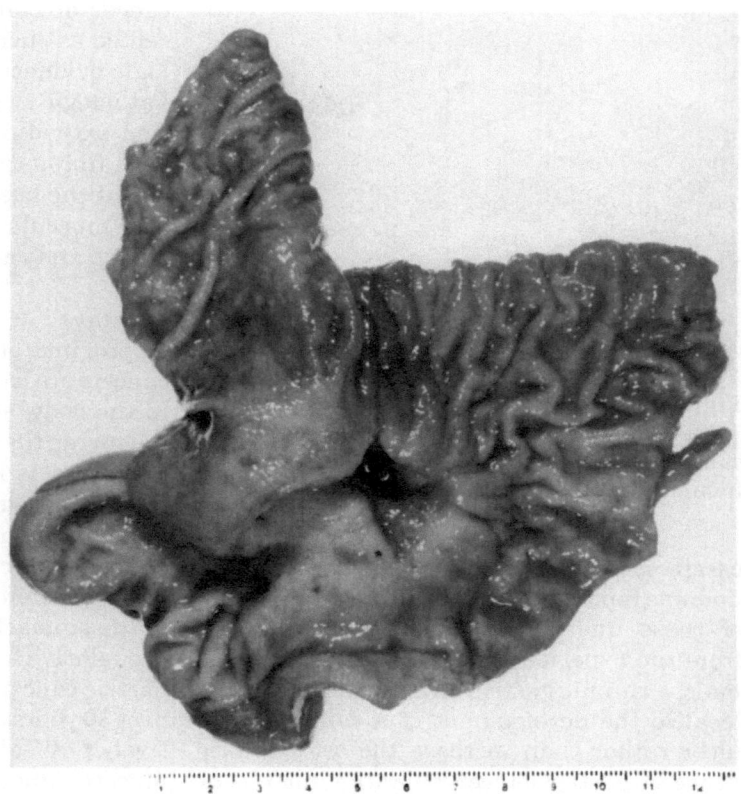

scirrhous carcinoma or linitis plastica (Figs. 7-24 and 7-25); or present a combination of any of these appearances (Fig. 7-26). The term *linitis plastica* dates back to 1859, when William Brinton described this supposedly inflammatory condition and saw a resemblance between the fibrous tissue on the cut surface and threads of woven linen (i.e., "linitis").[205]

Infiltrative cancers are characterized by diffuse thickening of the gastric wall (Fig. 7-27), loss of rugae, and frequently preserved surface mucosa. They are often extensive and may involve large parts of the stomach or even the entire stomach. In the latter case, the stomach is shrunken and stiff and referred to as "leather bottle" stomach.

The rarest macroscopic type is the pure polypoid one, the most frequent the ulcerated type.[206] Infiltrative cancers are now found with increasing frequency, reflecting the relative increase of the diffuse histologic

type, which most often, but not exclusively, produces this gross appearance. The relative frequency of polypoid carcinoma is around 7%, flat carcinoma 6%, ulcerated types between 25 and 65%, and linitis plastica between 10 and 26%.[165,206] Differences are due in part to the frequent occurrence of mixed forms that may be classified either as ulcerative or as infiltrative and in part to geographic differences. Exophytic tumors are histologically most often of the intestinal type, and ulcerative and infiltrative tumors more often of the diffuse type. Ulcerated cancers, in contradistinction to benign ulcers, have nodular margins and are surrounded by disrupted rugae, instead of the stellate converging rugal pattern seen around peptic ulcers (Fig. 7-28).

Malignant transformation of a benign peptic ulcer is rare and is estimated to occur in about 1% of cases.[74] The incidence of peptic ulcer-associated carcinomas among gastric

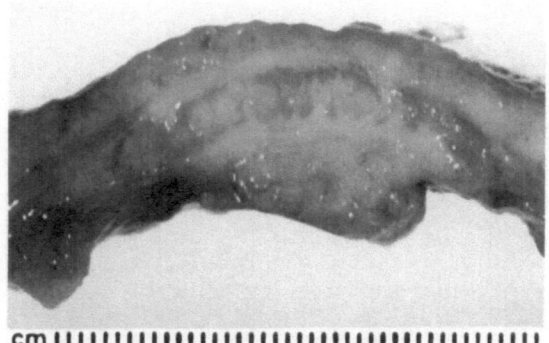

Figure 7-27. Linitis plastica. On cross section, white strands of tumor infiltrate the darker muscularis and penetrate into the subserosa. The luminal surface remains flat.

carcinomas in general, however, is higher and was reported as 3.1% of all cases and 6.9% of those undergoing operation.[207] Judging from the experience with experimental animals, a chronic gastric ulcer is more likely to localize the development of a tumor to the ulcer rather than increase the overall incidence of gastric cancer.[208] Malignant ulcers tend to be larger than benign ones (greater than 1 cm in diameter), but do not differ in site. The most common sites for benign as well as malignant ulcers are the lesser curvature and the prepyloric region.[209] Such ulcer-

cancer or cancer ex ulcero can only be accepted as such if there is clinical and pathologic evidence of previous peptic ulceration. Pathologic evidence includes peptic ulceration extending into the muscularis propria with fibrous scar tissue and granulation tissue at the base, fusion of muscularis propria and muscularis mucosae around the ulcer cavity, and carcinoma at the ulcer edge.[207]

Location

Approximately half (49 to 52%) of all gastric cancers are located in the pyloric antrum, 28% in the body, and 11% in both areas, with 9% occupying the entire stomach.[165,210] The lesser curvature is involved more commonly than the larger curvature, and the posterior wall more commonly than the anterior wall.[210] Location in the cardia, that is, in the proximal 3 to 4 cm of stomach (Fig. 7-29), and upper third of the stomach is increasingly common, and the relative frequency of such cancers among gastric cancers in general has doubled in the past 30 years and is now 27% and 39%, respectively.[206,210] Most gastric cancers arise near mucosal junctions along the lesser curvature: at the junction of antral and fundic type mucosa or antral and duodenal mucosa, or at the gastroesophageal junction.[211]

Location correlates with macroscopic types. Three-quarters of polypoid and ulcerated car-

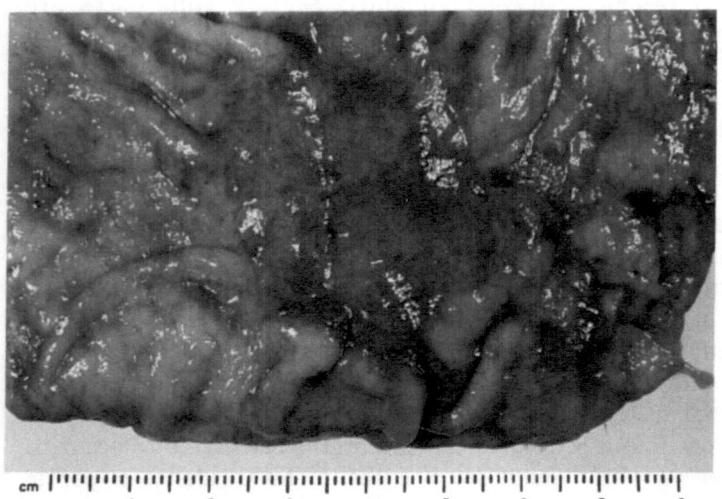

Figure 7-28. Advanced gastric cancer, ulcerative type. The margins are nodular and gastric rugae end abruptly.

cinomas are located in the pyloric antrum, whereas infiltrative or diffuse carcinomas occur with approximately equal frequency in both body and antrum, but in one-third of cases involve the entire stomach.[165]

Multiplicity of gastric carcinoma is rare in the U.S., but more frequent elsewhere. In Japan, in one study 47% of patients with advanced gastric cancer had multiple lesions.[212] Most multiple cancers were of the well-differentiated intestinal type and arose in stomachs with extensive intestinal metaplasia. Among older patients (mean age, 73 years), 13% of cancers were multiple, and of these almost one-third were intramucosal.[142]

Carcinoma of the Gastric Remnant

Carcinoma of the gastric remnant, also termed *stump carcinoma*, is defined as carcinoma developing in the remnant of the stomach when primary resection was carried out at least 5 years earlier for benign disease, ulcer, or other disease.[213] The first such case was described by Balfour[214] in 1922, and carcinoma of the gastric remnant has been the subject of numerous publications ever since. By 1978 there were an estimated 2000 cases in the world literature.[215] Whether or not gastrectomy per se is an independent risk factor is still debated. Reported incidence figures vary remarkably due to differences in methodology, length of follow-up time, and the population studied, and range from 0.4 to 8.7%.[216] The greatest rise in incidence begins 15 years after surgery,[217] and an increased risk persists for up to 26 to 37 years after gastrectomy.[218] The risk has been estimated to be increased three- to sixfold, more so after surgery for gastric than for duodenal ulcer.[219] The interval between gastric surgery and the diagnosis of gastric carcinoma may vary anywhere from 5 to 45 years. Intervals tend to be longer in older patients and in patients with a previous history of duodenal rather than gastric ulcer, or with gastrojejunostomy without gastrectomy rather than with gastrectomy.[220] Since the incidence of carcinoma of the stomach shows marked geographic variations, the true risk of developing carcinoma

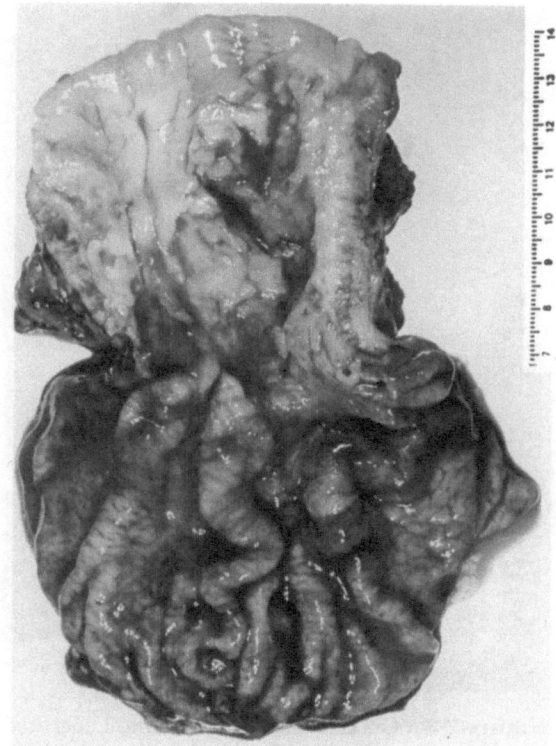

Figure 7-29. Carcinoma of the cardia, combined ulcerative and infiltrative type. Carcinoma extends into the esophagus.

in a gastric remnant has to be related to the gastric cancer risk of the local population. Such comparisons of observed and expected incidences in local populations using actuarial analysis have yielded no increased risk of gastric cancer in patients with partial gastrectomies.[213,215,221,222] Many of the benign pathologic conditions found in the postoperative stomach, such as chronic atrophic gastritis, present in 93% of cases,[223] intestinal metaplasia, present in 54% of cases,[224] and bile reflux account for a premalignant environment that by itself, without surgical intervention, increases the risk of cancer. Experimental gastric stump carcinomas in rats depend on the intensity of duodenogastric reflux, which, in turn, depends on the type of surgical procedure.[225] Gastroenterostomy without resection had the highest tumor incidence, followed in order of decreas-

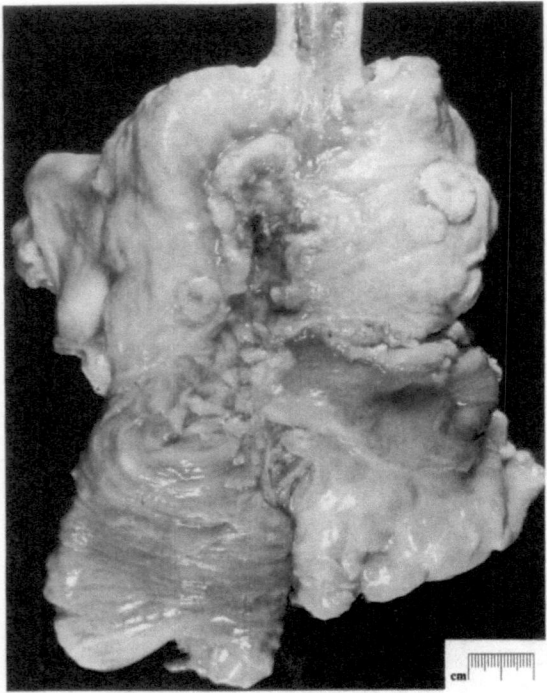

Figure 7-30. Gastric stump carcinoma. Ulcerated tumor nodules are located on the gastric side of the gastrojejunostomy as well as at a distance from the anastomosis in the gastric remnant.

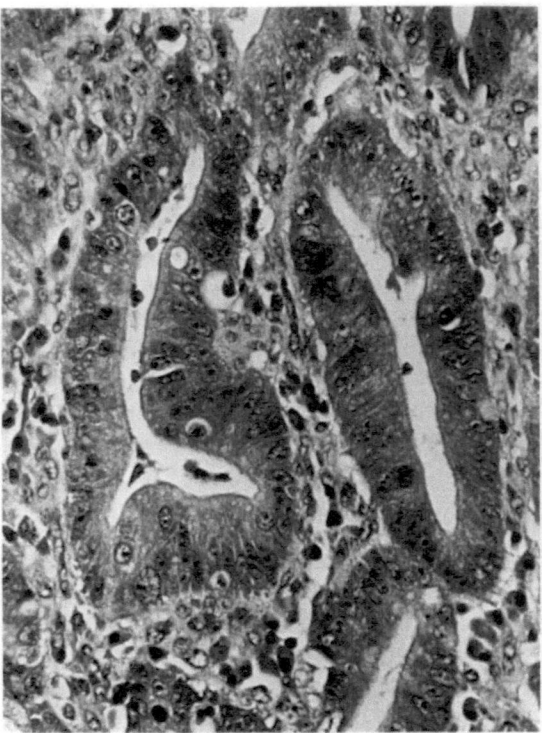

Figure 7-31. Adenocarcinoma, intestinal type, well differentiated. H&E, X250

ing frequency by Billroth II resection without Braun's (i.e., antecolic) anastomosis, Billroth II resection with Braun's anastomosis, and Billroth I resection. No tumors were found in gastric remnants following Billroth II resection with Rouxen-Y gastroenterostomy. Results in humans have been similar.[226]

Since the length of exposure to the putative carcinogen is 15 years or longer after partial gastrectomy and since many patients will die of other causes during this period, endoscopic screening of postgastrectomy patients is recommended only for patients less than 70 years of age who had gastric surgery 15 years or more previously and for patients less than 55 years old who had gastric surgery 10 years previously.[215]

The proportion of gastric cancers found in gastric remnants at least 5 years after surgery varies from 1.1 to 8.7%.[216] Most tumors (60%) are located directly at the gastrojejunal anastomosis, on the gastric side, 36% at the cardia, and the remainder elsewhere in the gastric remnant.[227] Grossly, gastric stump carcinoma most often presents as prominent mucosal folds with or without ulcerated tumor nodules at the stoma[228] (Fig. 7-30). Rarely, there is a polypoid mass or diffusely infiltrating tumor. Numerous cysts, up to 0.6 cm in diameter, are often recognized on the cut surface within the tumor as well as in the adjacent gastric, but not jejunal, mucosa and submucosa, and are an indication of coexistent gastritis cystica polyposa.[228]

Microscopic Appearance of Advanced Gastric Cancer

Microscopically, the vast majority of gastric carcinomas are adenocarcinomas. Unusual other types are described subsequently. As discussed under Classification, adenocarci-

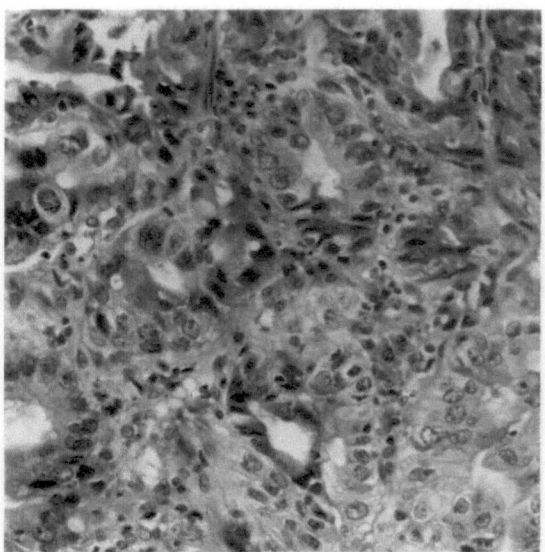

Figure 7-32. Adenocarcinoma, intestinal type, moderately differentiated. HPS X250, reproduced at 75%.

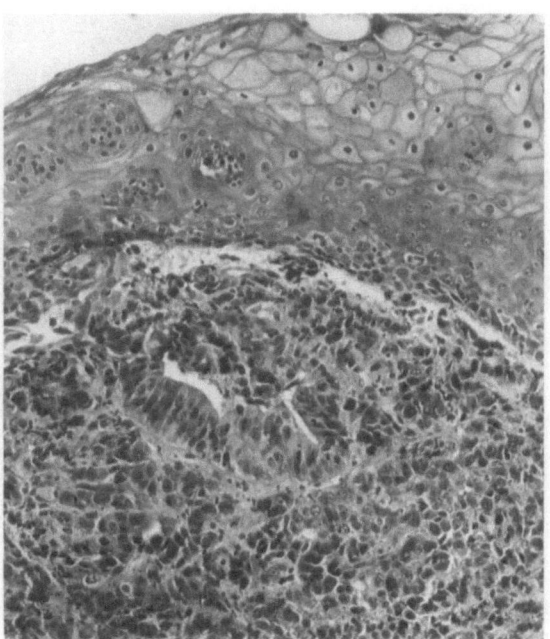

Figure 7-33. Adenocarcinoma, intestinal type, poorly differentiated, invading the esophagus. H&E, X100, reproduced at 85%.

nomas are now generally classified as intestinal or diffuse (Table 7-6, p. 168); a slightly different system is used in Japan (Table 7-7 p. 169).

The intestinal type is usually well differentiated, papillary, tubular, or glandular (Fig. 7-31) and infiltrates in a nodular fashion with a propensity for blood vessel invasion, even in the early stages. In less well-differentiated forms, tubules coalesce (Fig. 7-32), and in poorly differentiated areas there is a solid pattern (Fig. 7-33). Tumor cells resemble resorptive intestinal epithelium in well-differentiated intestinal type carcinoma and are columnar and relatively large, with well-defined cell borders and prominent basilar nuclei with macronucleoli (see Fig. 7-31). Nuclei are ovoid and show a relatively uniform long axis but a variable-length short axis, a feature helpful in the distinction of reactive from malignant change.[229] Cytologic atypism is paralleled by structural atypism. A back-to-back and net-like growth pattern is produced by interconnections of neoplastic glands, best appreciated by reconstruction of the three-dimensional microstructure from serial two-dimensional sections.[230] In less well-differentiated intestinal type adenocarcinoma, cells become more cuboidal and nuclei are located in the middle or luminal portion of the cytoplasm. In poorly differentiated forms, cells are polygonal and markedly pleomorphic. Increased structural atypism is expressed by progressive loss of inner connections and an increase in the number of separate parts.[230] Mucin production is restricted to luminal mucin stainable with periodic acid–Schiff (PAS) or mucicarmine. Paneth cells occur in well-differentiated adenocarcinomas.[231] Neuroendocrine cells may be intermixed. (For details, see section on special studies.) Intestinal metaplasia and chronic atrophic gastritis are almost invariably present in the adjacent nonneoplastic mucosa.

The diffuse type of gastric adenocarcinoma is always poorly differentiated and shows absent or abortive gland formation. As the name implies, it is characterized by a diffuse infiltrate of loosely anastomosing cords or singly scattered cells, often resembling mac-

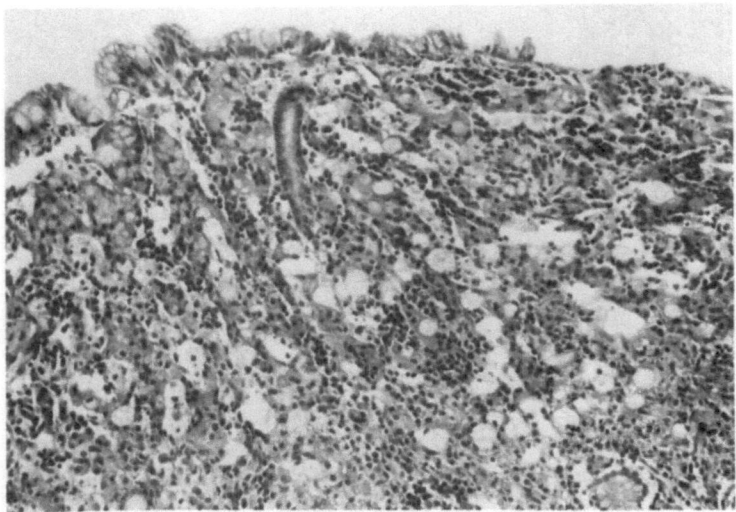

Figure 7-34. Adenocarcinoma, diffuse type. The surface epithelium and a few pyloric glands (lower right corner) are preserved. H&E, X60.

rophages (Figs. 7-17, 7-18, and 7-34). Cells are rounded and pale and may show intracytoplasmic vacuoles, which, if of sufficient size, push the nucleus toward one side, creat-

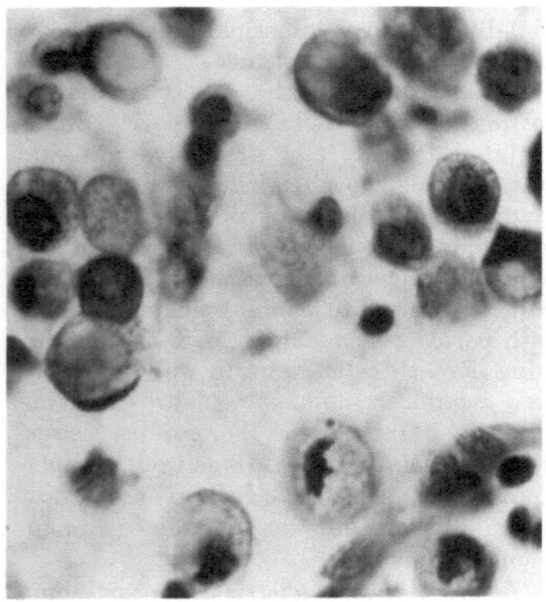

Figure 7-35. Signet-ring cells in diffuse type of gastric adenocarcinoma. The nucleus is pushed to the side by intracytoplasmic mucin. H&E, X500, reproduced at 80%.

ing the so-called "signet-ring cell" (Fig. 7-35). Cytoplasmic mucus stains variably with mucicarmine, PAS, or Alcian blue at pH 2.5. More often, however, the main cell type contains no cytoplasmic vacuoles but has rather amphophilic cytoplasm with poorly defined cell borders. The nucleus, in contradistinction to histiocytes, is enlarged and irregular with a nucleolus. The tumor spreads between preserved structures, pushes gastric pits apart, and dissects between submucosal collagen bundles and along blood vessels and intramural ganglia into the muscularis (Fig. 7-36). The surface epithelium may remain intact, and in mucosal biopsies the first indication that tumor is present may be the observation under the low-power objective of widely spaced pits. Preserved pits often show varying degrees of cytologic atypia, and a transition from mild to severe dysplasia and carcinoma can sometimes be demonstrated (see Fig. 7-8). In the submucosa and muscularis propria, tumor cells are often compressed and appear spindle shaped.

Signet-ring cells may be scattered among less characteristic cancer cells or constitute the main cell type. Diffuse type adenocarcinoma with a predominance (i.e., greater than 50%) of signet-ring cells has shown a recent increase in frequency and constituted 39% of

Figure 7-36. Adenocarcinoma, diffuse type, invading muscularis propria. H&E, X40, reproduced at 95%.

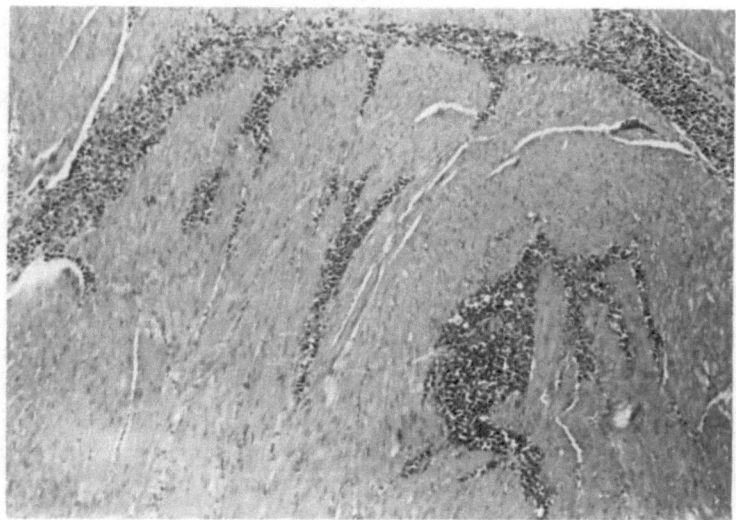

cases of gastric cancer in Boston between 1975 and 1978, as compared to only 9% between 1938 and 1942.[206] Pure signet-ring carcinomas are more frequent in women than in men.

A desmoplastic stromal reaction is often present, especially in the submucosa, and accounts for much of the increase in wall thickness. Fibrosis may be so marked as to mask the tumor infiltrate, which consists of widely scattered single spindle-shaped cells, distinguishable from fibroblasts only by their enlarged and irregular nucleus and occasionally vacuolated cytoplasm. Depending on the predominance of any of the above histologic features, diffuse type adenocarcinoma can be subclassified into desmoplastic, signet-ring, or anaplastic variants[172] (Fig. 7-37). Neuroendocrine cells may be intermixed. (For details, see section on special studies.)

The diffuse type of gastric adenocarcinoma, sometimes referred to simply as *poorly differentiated adenocarcinoma*, is relatively more common in areas with a low risk of gastric cancer[26] and has shown a recent increase in frequency, even in high-risk countries like Japan, concomitant with a decrease in well-differentiated (i.e., intestinal type) adenocarcinoma.[232]

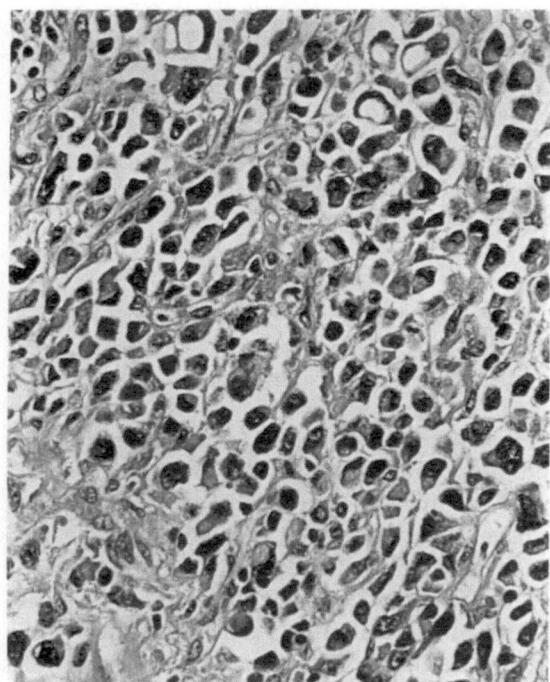

Figure 7-37. Adenocarcinoma, diffuse type, anaplastic variant. Only a few signet-ring cells are present. H&E, X250.

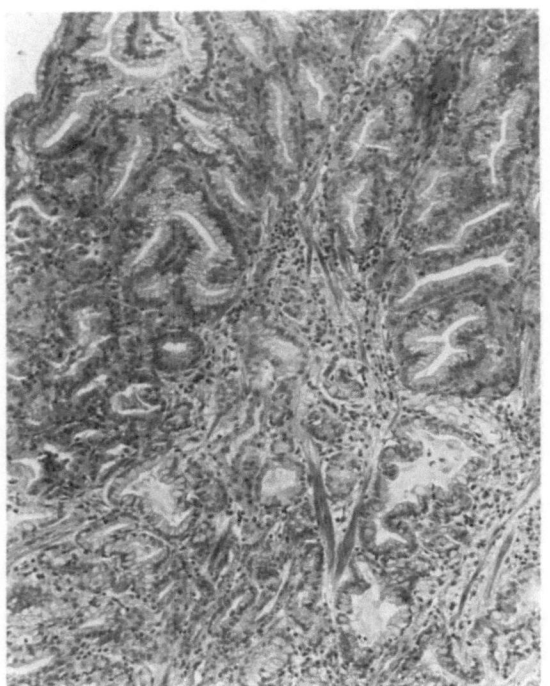

Figure 7-38. Adenocarcinoma, pylorocardiac gland cell type. Glands are well differentiated and composed of columnar cells with clear cytoplasm. HPS, X100, reproduced at 80%.

Mixed forms of adenocarcinoma, with a diffuse and intestinal type appearance, or unclassifiable carcinomas make up 10 to 20% of gastric carcinomas.[26,169]

Pylorocardiac gland cell carcinoma is a histologic type often included in the intestinal type or unclassified group. It supposedly arises from cardiac or pyloric glands, is especially common in the cardia, and accounted for 28% of gastric carcinomas in the series studied by Mulligan,[171] who introduced the term. The tumor presents microscopically as a well-differentiated, focally papillary adenocarcinoma composed of columnar cells with pale or clear cytoplasm (Fig. 7-38). Desquamated tumor cells may accumulate in gland lumina and adopt rounded shapes resembling signet-ring cells. Cytoplasmic mucin stains with PAS but rarely with mucicarmine. As in intestinal type adenocarcinoma, there is a great tendency for blood vessel invasion.

Special Features of Advanced Gastric Cancer

Histochemistry

Histochemistry is used to define mucin profiles and carbohydrate contents.[228,233,234] Histochemical methods to characterize gastric mucin types include staining with Alcian blue at pH 2.5 plus PAS (AB/PAS), to distinguish between acid and neutral mucins, and staining with high iron diamine plus Alcian blue at pH 2.5 (HID/AB), to demonstrate sulfated and nonsulfated (i.e., sialomucins) acid mucins.[228] Normal gastric mucin is neutral and stains AB−, PAS+, and HID−, AB−. Carcinomas usually produce varying amounts of neutral and acid mucins and varying proportions of the two types of acid mucins, that is, sialomucin (AB+) and sulfomucin (HID+).[228] Sulfomucins are demonstrated in 88% of cases and sialomucins in 17% of cases.[234] Signet-ring cells contain a variety of mucosubstances resembling those of normal pyloric glands, gastric surface epithelial cells, and small and large intestinal goblet cells.[233]

Lectin binding has been used to demonstrate differences in type and distribution of carbohydrates in mucins of gastric cancers relative to normal superficial epithelial cells.[235] Carbohydrate abnormalities are related to changes in blood group antigen expression, most often deletion of ABH antigens, or inappropriate expression of the ABH precursor antigen, I (Ma), in tumors from patients who are secretors of ABH antigens.[87,109] For further discussion, see page 157.

Immunohistochemistry

Immunohistochemistry may be applied to demonstrate the presence of tumor antigens,[236] most often CEA[237,238] or, rarely, AFP,[187] of immunoglobulins,[237] enzymes,[231,236,239] and hormones, primarily polypeptide hormones and amines.[236,238] The demonstration of CEA is of diagnostic importance in undifferentiated carcinomas that need to be distinguished from large cell lymphomas. In such cases, concomitant staining for cytokeratin, epithelial membrane antigen, and leukocyte common antigen should be employed. Positive staining for CEA is proof of epithelial differentiation; negative staining is highly unlikely in carcinomas, but some undifferentiated carcinomas show only weak equivocal staining.[237] Moderately well-differentiated adenocarcinomas show positive staining of cell membranes and luminal surfaces of neoplastic glands. Poorly differentiated carcinomas show cell membrane staining only. Secretory IgA is demonstrable in well-differentiated but not in poorly differentiated adenocarcinomas.[239]

Enzymes produced by gastric adenocarcinomas include lysozyme and protease inhibitors.[231,236,239] Tumor cells containing lysozyme have been seen in about one-third of gastric carcinomas, regardless of extent or histologic type.[240] Advanced cancers with lysozyme have a worse prognosis than those without. Lysozyme immunoreactivity combined with electron microscopy can be used as a marker for Paneth cells.[231] Protease inhibitors, such as α_1-antitrypsin (AAT), α_1-antichymotrypsin (ACT), and α_2-macroglobulin (AMG) have been demonstrated in varying proportions.[236] Frequency of positive staining differs for each enzyme and depends on the extent and histologic type of carcinoma. Advanced cancers and well-differentiated papillary and tubular carcinomas had the highest frequencies of positive staining, early cancers and signet-ring carcinomas the lowest. Well-differentiated adenocarcinomas with AAT carry a worse prognosis than those without. No such correlations apply to the other protease inhibitors.

Neuroendocrine cells can be demonstrated by silver stains in approximately 8% of gastric carcinomas and are more common in the diffuse type (17%) than in the intestinal type (2 to 5%),[238,241] and usually are present only in the primary tumor and not the metastases.[238] Adjacent nonneoplastic mucosa may show an increase as well. Argyrophil cells, stainable with the Grimelius stain, are more frequent than argentaffin cells, stainable with the Fontana stain. Polypeptide hormones identified by immunoperoxidase staining include somatostatin, serotonin, gastrin, glicentin, human gonadotropin, and a parathyroid hormone-like substance.[236,238,242,243] Beta-endorphine-like immunoreactivity has been found in tissue extracts of a moderately well-differentiated adenocarcinoma.[244] Estrogen and progesterone receptors have been recently identified in gastric cancers with varying frequencies, dependent on sex and age. Men more than 60 years of age have the highest incidence (50%), women older than 60 years the lowest (6%).[245] No correlation with intracytoplasmic estradiol is as yet discernible.[245,246]

Immunoperoxidase staining with anti-S100 protein has demonstrated Langerhans cells interspersed among tumor cells. In Stage III cancer, greater density of Langerhans cells correlated with longer survival.[247]

Electron Microscopy

Electron microscopically, intestinal type carcinoma is characterized by cuboidal or columnar cells with microvilli resembling those of intestinal epithelial cells. Microvilli face the glandular lumina, vary in length, and have a core of microfilaments that extend deep into the apical cytoplasm, forming long rootlets. Microtubules are occasionally seen in the deep cytoplasm. Lateral cell membranes show well-developed junctional complexes. The cytoplasm contains round mitochondria, scanty granular endoplasmic reticulum in the central and apical portions, a Golgi apparatus, lyzosomal dense bodies, and small, round, homogeneous mucous droplets. Nuclei are of variable shape and often scalloped.[248] Paneth cells, characterized by large, moderately electron-dense granules of 1 to 2 nm in diameter in the supranuclear cytoplasm, may be intermixed.[231]

Diffuse type carcinoma cells are round or polygonal, poorly cohesive, and form only occasional irregular microvilli on the free surface of the tumor cell. Cells have been classified into three types depending on the amount of intracellular mucin.[249] Type A cells contain few and small (0.3 to 0.4 nm) mucin granules of high electron density, abundant cell organelles, and a round, centrally located nucleus. Type B cells contain a moderate number of medium-sized (0.5 to 1 nm) mucin granules of moderate electron density, decreased organelles, and an elliptic eccentric nucleus. Type C cells are signet-ring cells filled with coalescing large (2 nm or more) mucin granules of low electron density, with extremely few organelles and a peripherally located crescent-shaped nucleus. Type A cells stain with PAS only, type B and C cells with PAS and/or Alcian blue at pH 2.5.[249] Most diffuse type adenocarcinomas are composed of a mixture of these three cells and show transitional forms. Cytoplasmic granules sometimes display a network-like internal structure resembling that of intestinal goblet cells.[248] Other ultrastructural features, however, are similar to those of gastric mucous neck cells and pyloric gland cells. Vacuolated granules probably reflect poor tissue preservation.

Intracytoplasmic lumina filled with mucin and surrounded by microvilli are present in intestinal as well as diffuse type adenocarcinomas.[248] An admixture of diffuse and intestinal type cells is found in the majority of carcinomas that are classified as signet-ring carcinomas by light microscopy.[233]

DNA Ploidy Patterns
DNA ploidy patterns observed in advanced gastric carcinomas include diploid, heteroploid, mixed diploid and heteroploid, and mixtures of two or more different heteroploid patterns.[250] Diploid patterns are most frequent and were seen in 68% of Japanese cases. The other patterns were far less common and accounted for 15, 13, and 4% of cases, respectively. Most diffusely infiltrative carcinomas are heteroploid.[251] DNA ploidy is a valid marker of a given tumor and remains constant in primary and recurrent carcinomas.[252]

The distribution patterns of ^{3}H-thymidine-labeled DNA synthesizing cells is highly variable from case to case as well as from area to area in the same case.[253] In intestinal type adenocarcinoma, labeled cells are scattered at random over the entire tumor tissue,

whereas in diffuse type carcinoma, labeling is absent from typical signet-ring cells and restricted to the smaller cells with less or no intracytoplasmic mucin.

Rare Types of Gastric Carcinoma

Mucoid or Mucinous Adenocarcinoma
Mucoid or mucinous adenocarcinoma is a rare, well-differentiated tumor with an indolent course.[254] The mean survival of six reported cases was 9 years. Mucin is characteristically extracellular and accumulates in large lakes surrounded by scanty columnar epithelium (Fig. 7-39). Granular calcifications resembling psammoma bodies may form within extracellular mucin and are recognizable by CT scan.[255]

Choriocarcinoma
Choriocarcinoma may occur either in association with adenocarcinoma or as a pure form. Of 44 cases published in 1982, most showed combined choriocarcinoma and adenocarcinoma.[256-258] Metastases, by contrast, are more commonly pure choriocarcinoma.[256] Retrodifferentiation or metaplasia of an adenocarcinoma is the most widely accepted histogenetic theory and explains the similarities in epidemiology and in age and sex distribution.[257] Pure choriocarcinoma, according to this postulate, is the result of complete replacement of the original adenocarcinoma.

Grossly, these tumors are usually large, polypoid and ulcerated, hemorrhagic, and spongy and may show extensive infarction. Microscopically, the characteristic areas show large bizarre cells with abundant eosinophilic cytoplasm and multinucleation, resembling syncytiotrophoblasts (Fig. 7-40). Mononuclear cytotrophoblast cells are usually seen as well. Rarely, associated embryonal carcinoma has been found.[259] The adenocarcinomatous element, if present, may be of the intestinal type and well, moderately, or poorly differentiated; mucinous; or of signet-ring type.[258] Immunohistochemically, the beta-subunit of human chorionic

Figure 7-39. Adenocarcinoma, mucinous or colloid type. Tumor cells float in lakes of extracellular mucin. HPS, X100.

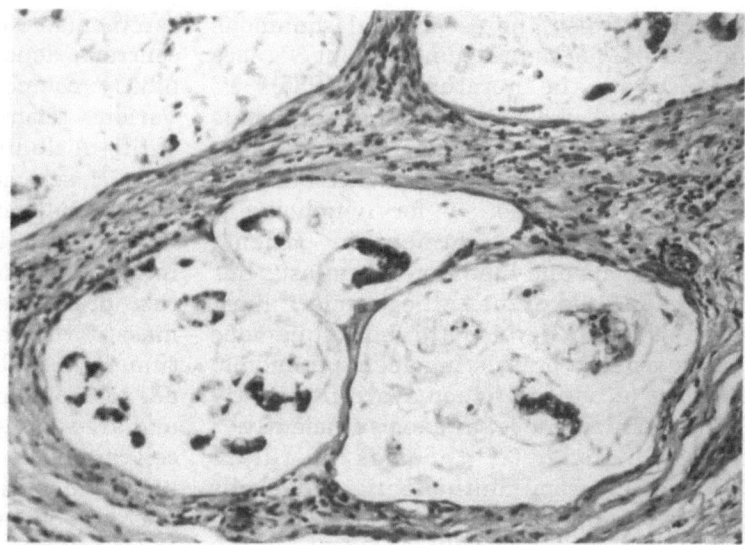

gonadotropin (hCG) can be localized to both types of trophoblast, predominantly the syncytiotrophoblast, but not to the adenocarcinoma. In the serum, high levels of hCG can be demonstrated before surgery and a decrease after gastrectomy.[258] Estrogen- and progesterone-related tissue responses (mammary ductal proliferation, lobular secretion, and endometrial stromal decidualization) have been documented, and production of these hormones by the choriocarcinoma has been suggested.[257]

Hepatoid Adenocarcinoma
Hepatoid adenocarcinoma is a rare type of gastric carcinoma composed of large polygonal cells with abundant eosinophilic cytoplasm and PAS-positive intracytoplasmic globules resembling hepatocellular carcinoma. Alpha-fetoprotein, α_1-antitrypsin, transferrin, albumin, and hCG have been demonstrated in tumor cells by immunohistochemistry.[187,260]

Squamous Cell Carcinoma
Squamous cell carcinoma, primary in the stomach, is an acceptable diagnosis only if there is no evidence of squamous cell carcinoma in other organs and if there is no con-

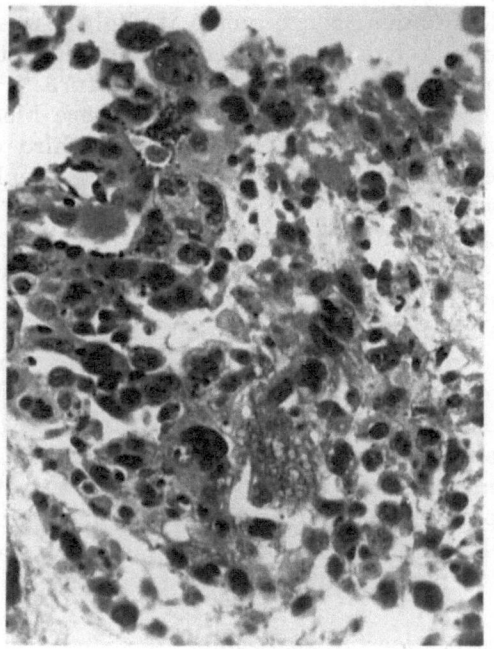

Figure 7-40. Choriocarcinoma. Large bizarre cells and multinucleation are characteristic. H&E, X400.

nection between the esophageal squamous mucosa and the gastric tumor. About 80 cases were found in the literature up to 1985.[261,262] Development from preexisting squamous metaplasia has been demonstrated in syphilitic gastritis,[263] after corrosive acid burns,[264] and after chemotherapy for lymphoma.[265] Cyclophosphamide treatment in patients with myeloma and lupus erythematosus has been implicated in the pathogenesis.[266] Most cases seem to develop through squamous metaplasia of a preexisting adenocarcinoma, and foci of adenocarcinoma are frequently found if the tumor is sampled sufficiently.[262] Other histogenetic theories postulate development from multipotential stem cells or ectopic squamous epithelial islands along the lesser curvature.[261]

Adenosquamous Carcinoma

Adenosquamous carcinoma is slightly more common than squamous cell carcinoma, with more than 100 cases in the literature.[267,268] There is a marked male predominance. Most tumors are located in the distal third of the stomach, are ulcerated, and are deeply invasive by the time they are discovered. If located in the proximal stomach, collision of esophageal squamous and gastric adenocarcinoma must be considered as a differential diagnosis.[269] In adenosquamous carcinoma of the stomach, squamous and glandular elements are intermingled. Single mucin-containing vacuolated cells may be seen within squamous islands. In a collision tumor, the two elements remain relatively separate. The glandular component may be well differentiated or poorly differentiated. Of 24 patients, none survived 5 years.[268]

Neuroendocrine Carcinoma

Scattered argyrophil and argentaffin neuroendocrine cells are found in 1.7 to 8% of ordinary gastric adenocarcinomas without features of carcinoid tumor.[238,270] In some of these, rare tumor cells show synchronous exocrine and endocrine differentiation, so-called *amphocrine cells*.[271] Such tumors should not be designated as neuroendocrine

carcinoma. Neuroendocrine carcinoma, by contrast, denotes a tumor that is predominantly composed of neuroendocrine cells. Various terms have been applied to this entity, including carcinoma with argyrophil cells,[270] scirrhous argyrophil carcinoma,[239] and oat cell carcinoma.[272]

Grossly, most cases presented as a diffusely infiltrative tumor, Borrmann Type IV.[239] One case presented with a fungating ulcerated mass of the cardia.[272] Microscopically, most tumors resemble the diffuse type of gastric adenocarcinoma, contain signet-ring cells, and are scirrhous. Rarely, they resemble oat cell carcinoma of the lung.[272] Argyrophil granules predominate, but argentaffin granules may be demonstrable as well. Immunocytochemically, gastrin, somatostatin, glucagon, serotonin, and parthyroid hormone-like substance have been identified in association with CEA, lysozyme, and hCG.[239,242] No hormonal syndrome has as yet been detected in 16 patients examined.[239] Electron microscopically, secretory granules are pleomorphic and highly osmophilic, varying in diameter from 240 to 480 nm.[239] One case resembling pulmonary oat cell carcinoma contained only few and small (80 to 110 nm) secretory granules.[272] Psammomatous calcification, described in argyrophil gastric carcinoma with glandular differentiation,[242] resembles somatostatinoma.

Parietal Cell Carcinoma

Parietal cell carcinoma has only been recently defined as a distinct tumor type.[273] Three such tumors described in 1984 presented as large transmural masses with an expanding growth pattern and involvement of gastric body and antrum. Microscopically, the tumor had a medullary pattern with tumor cells arranged in sheets and large clusters or in elongated cords and single files. Glandular differentiation was observed only focally. Individual tumor cells resembled parietal cells, were round or polygonal, rarely spindle shaped, and had clear cell margins and eosinophilic, faintly granular cytoplasm. Nuclei were round, ovoid, or slightly irregular and hypochromatic with small nucleoli and variable mitotic activity. Extensive necrosis was present. Mucin and Grimelius stains were negative, but PTAH and Luxol–fast blue, known to react with normal parietal cells as well as with other cells rich in mitochondria, stained the cytoplasm of many tumor cells. The adjacent foveolae and gastric glands were dysplastic.

Electron microscopically, tumor cells had a large number of round or oval mitochondria with numerous cristae extending completely across a clear or poorly dense matrix. Intracytoplasmic lumina with microvilli were seen. The cytoplasm contained tubulovesicles, Golgi complexes, and numerous lysosomes, but no secretory granules. Desmosomes were prominent. No basal lamina was formed.

Too few cases are known to allow prognostic evaluation. The paucity of lymph node metastases, absence of distant metastases, and expanding growth pattern seen in three cases suggest a malignant potential lower than that of other types of gastric carcinoma.

Carcinosarcoma

Carcinosarcoma is a malignant tumor composed of epithelial and mesenchymal elements. For years the question remained unanswered whether the mesenchymal element represented spindle cell carcinoma or true sarcoma. Recent ultrastructural and immunohistochemical studies favor the latter.[274,275]

There were slightly more than 30 case reports in the literature in 1985, the first one dating back to 1904.[276] Carcinosarcoma presents most often as a polypoid large mass in the pyloric area. Histologically, the carcinoma has been described as well-differentiated and tubulopapillary with anaplastic foci. The sarcoma is composed of spindle cells, sometimes with a myxoid matrix, and scattered bizarre giant cells. Carcinoma and sarcoma may be sharply demarcated from one another (collision tumor), intricately admixed without distinct separation of cell types (combination tumor), or mixed with preservation of differentiating features (composition tumor).[274]

Ultrastructurally, stromal cells show myogenic features and contain numerous microfilaments arranged into dense bodies along the plasma membrane, rare pinocytotic vesicles, and discontinuous basal lamina. Carcinoma cells show easily identifiable desmosomal attachments.[275]

Immunohistochemical staining for CEA is positive in carcinomatous areas and negative in the sarcoma. However, rare spindle to polygonal transitional cell types also stain positive, suggesting that these tumors are primarily carcinomas that have undergone gradual sarcomatous transformation, a sequence of events also proposed for esophageal carcinosarcoma.

A combination of carcinosarcoma and separate carcinoid tumor has been described.[274]

Spread of Advanced Gastric Carcinoma

Carcinoma of the stomach spreads by local extension into adjacent structures, by peritoneal dissemination, and by lymphatic and blood vessel invasion. As carcinoma spreads, first locally, then to distant sites, tumor doubling times shorten remarkably. The doubling time for early cancer is 577 to 3462 days, for advanced cancer 69 to 305 days, and for metastatic cancer 18 to 60 days.[277]

Local Extension

Local extension may lead to involvement of the esophagus, duodenum, lesser and larger omentum, mesocolon, small and large intestine, especially transverse colon, pancreas, and spleen.

The frequency of distal esophageal involvement depends on the location and stage of the gastric carcinoma and has been reported in 50 to 90% of resectable carcinomas of the corpus.[278] Involvement occurs either by direct submucosal spread (Fig. 7-41) or by embolization of intramural and periesophageal lymphatics. In most instances the tumor extends further than is evident from inspection of the gastrectomy specimen as a whole (Fig. 7-42).

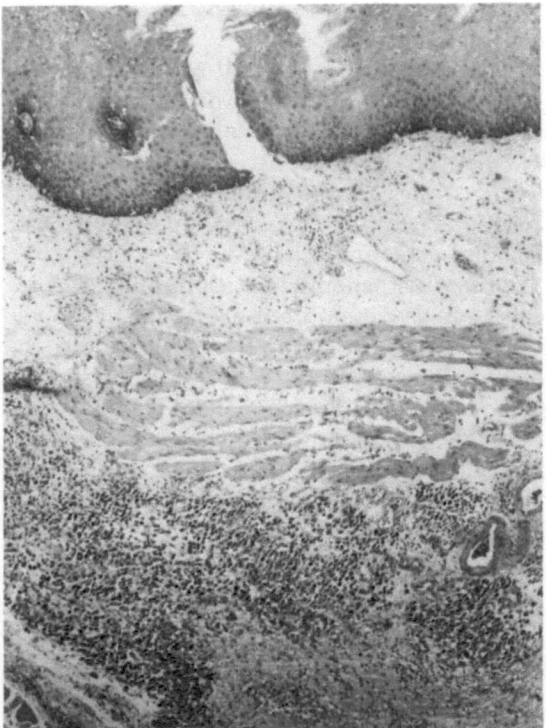

Figure 7-41. Submucosal extension of diffuse type of gastric adenocarcinoma into the esophagus. H&E, X40.

Continuous spread beyond the grossly recognized proximal tumor margin may reach a distance of 4 cm, and discontinuous spread a distance of 6 cm.

Recognition of tumor extension to the proximal surgical margin at the time of gastrectomy is important, since recurrence at the anastomotic line and fatal dehiscence are likely to occur unless additional esophageal tissue is resected.[279] Frozen sections, although not always accurate, are recommended to determine adequacy of esophageal resection. Frozen sections are inadequate in cases with skip submucosal lesions or invasion of periesophageal tissues, which may occur in the absence of submucosal and mucosal involvement.[278] Transpyloric extension into the duodenum can be demonstrated in about 20% of cases.[280]

Intramural spread of diffuse type adenocarcinoma (i.e., linitis plastica) into the entire small and large intestine is a rare event and occurs most likely by submucous lymphatic permeation.[281,282]

Larger curvature cancers may extend into the mesocolon and the transverse colon and produce gastrocolic fistulas (Fig. 7-43), or, rarely, a gastrojejunal fistula.[283,284] Direct extension into the pancreas or spleen is usually associated with large ulcerated carcinomas.

Peritoneal Dissemination

Peritoneal dissemination occurs in about one-quarter of patients with advanced gastric cancer,[169,285] most, if not all, of which exhibit serosal extension of the primary tumor (Fig. 7-44) with free intraperitoneal tumor cells and subsequent peritoneal implantation.[286] Implantation, according to scanning electron microscopic observations, is preceded by sloughing of mesothelial cells and exposure of submesothelial connective tissue, to which cancer cells adhere. Cancer cell proliferation results in a nodule, in well-differentiated adenocarcinoma (i.e., the intestinal type), and in an infiltrative desmoplastic lesion in poorly differentiated adenocarcinomas (i.e., the diffuse type).[285] The overall frequency of peritoneal dissemination appears to be the same for both types.[169]

Lymphatic Spread

Lymphatic spread in the form of lymph node metastases is evident at autopsy in about 85% of cases, regardless of histologic type.[287] In gastrectomy specimens, the incidence varies with the extent of the disease and the histologic type.[169] In intestinal type adenocarcinoma, lymph node metastases are present in 62% of cancers extending into the muscularis propria or subserosa and in 88% of cancers extending to the serosal surface. Interestingly, for the diffuse type of adenocarcinoma, comparable figures are lower (i.e., 30 and 71%), indicating a different biologic behavior.

Lymphatic networks are described in detail in Chapter 1 and illustrated in Fig. 7-45. To summarize the main points: Tumors of the cardiac region will metastasize to juxtacardiac nodes and superior gastric nodes along

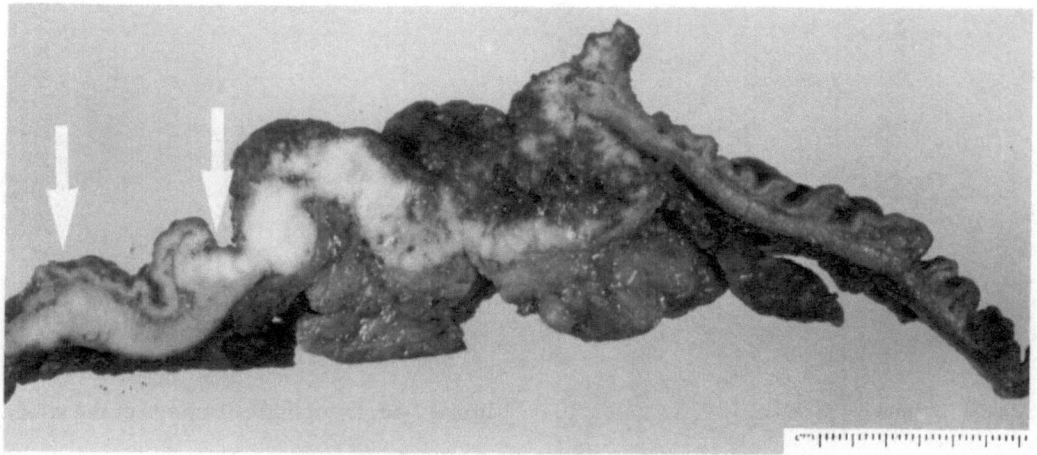

Figure 7-42. Intramural extension, continuous and discontinuous (*arrows*) of gastric carcinoma beyond the tumor visible on the mucosal surface.

the lesser curvature. Tumors in the upper half of the stomach around or near the larger curvature drain into lymph nodes along the splenic and gastroepiploic vessels along the larger curvature and to splenic hilar nodes. Tumors of the lower half of the stomach along or near the larger curvature drain into the gastroepiploic and peripyloric and into pancreaticoduodenal and superior mesenteric lymph nodes. Tumors of the gastric body and antrum along or near the lesser curvature drain into the superior gastric and supra-

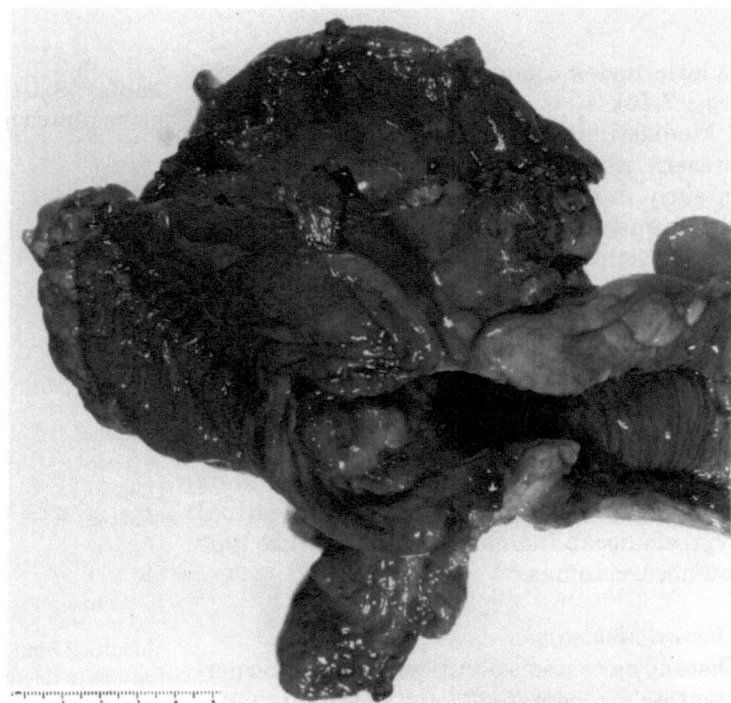

Figure 7-43. Gastrocolic fistula produced by gastric carcinoma of the larger curvature eroding into transverse colon.

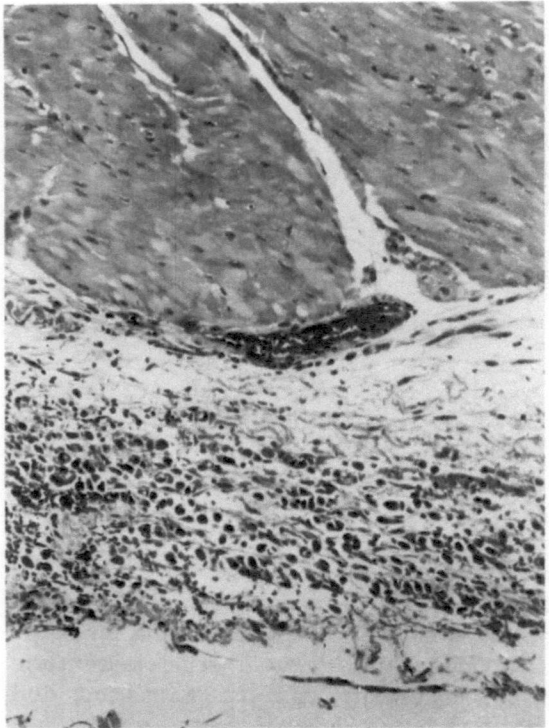

Figure 7-44. Serosal extension of diffuse type of gastric adenocarcinoma. The muscularis propria may remain intact. H&E, X40.

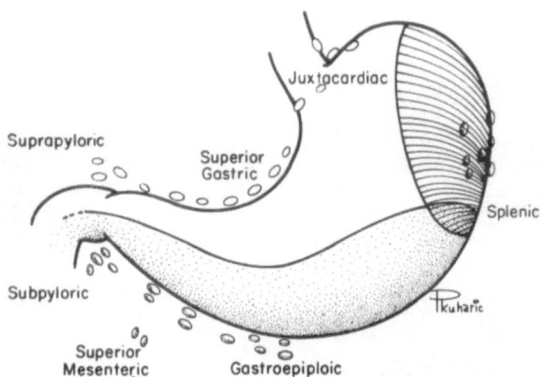

Figure 7-45. Lymphatic drainage of the stomach.

angitis carcinomatosa of lung[290] or breast[291] have been described in patients with the diffuse type of adenocarcinoma. Pulmonary involvement may become clinically manifest before the gastric cancer does. Distant metastases may affect virtually any organ in the body. Frequency of the most common sites according to histologic type from two countries with a high prevalence of gastric cancer, Chile and Japan, are summarized in Table 7-8. Differences in frequencies may reflect differ-

pyloric nodes along the lesser curvature[288] (Fig. 7-45).

Mediastinal lymph node involvement is present at autopsy in 30% of cases, more frequently in the intestinal type (33%) than in the diffuse type (21%),[169] and is often associated with and supposedly preceded by lymphatic spread to the lung.[289] Cases without concomitant lung involvement may be explained by retrograde tumor spread from the thoracic duct into bronchomediastinal lymphatic trunks or antegrade seeding from hepatic metastases.

Cervical lymph node metastases are rare, but were found at autopsy in 3% of intestinal type adenocarcinomas and 4% of diffuse type adenocarcinomas.[287]

Distant Metastasis
Distant metastasis occurs via lymphatic permeation or hematogenous spread. Lymph-

Table 7-8. Distant Metastases in Gastric Carcinoma (Autopsy Data)*

Site	Intestinal Type (%)	Diffuse Type (%)
Liver	60–78	30–38
Lung	33–46	43–52
Peritoneum	23–63	47–87
Pancreas	7–50	15–56
Adrenal	7–33	21–32
Ovary	7–9	19–28
Intestines	3–31	8–51
Kidney	3–16	11–21
Spleen	3–17	11–26
Heart	3–2	9–8
Muscle	3–2	6–4
Uterus	0–7	4–11
Skin	0–3	4–6
Thyroid	0–2	2–6

*Modified from Ishii et al.[172] and Duarte and Llanas.[287] Figures in the first row are from Chile, in the second row from Japan.

ences in the definition of metastasis, in classification, and perhaps in biologic behavior of gastric cancer in different populations.

Rare sites of distant spread include the urinary bladder, prostate, breast, brain, meninges, and bone.[171,287,292,293] Japanese statistics include frequencies of involvement of the gallbladder (9% versus 14%) the diaphragm (17% versus 38%), esophagus (12% versus 45%), pleura (20% versus 37%), and pericardium (3% versus 7%) for intestinal as compared to diffuse type adenocarcinoma.[171]

Metastatic gastric carcinoma to the ovary may present with bilateral firm and rapidly growing tumors characterized by diffuse infiltration of the stroma with carcinoma cells, some or all of which show intracellular mucin and appear as signet-ring cells. Krukenberg,[292] who described this condition in 1896 under the name of "fibrosarcoma ovarii mucocellulare carcinomatodes," believed it to be a primary sarcoma of the ovary. Schlagenhaufer[293] in 1902 was the first to recognize its epithelial nature and emhasized its metastatic origin from a primary gastric tumor. Subsequently, many authors used the term rather loosely to include any metastatic adenocarcinoma to the ovary until, in 1938, Novak and Gray[294] proposed restriction of the term *Krukenberg tumor* to metastatic carcinoma with diffuse infiltration of the ovaries, a definition which has been applied to most reviews ever since.[295] Krukenberg tumors account for 1 to 3% of ovarian tumors[296] and for 9% of cancers metastatic to the ovary.[297] They may be the first manifestation of gastric carcinoma and produce endocrine symptoms due to estrogen or androgen production by the hyperplastic ovarian stroma.[296] Metastases to other organs are usually present at the time of diagnosis, especially to the peritoneum, and less often to bones, producing replacement of the hematopoietic marrow and severe anemia.[296] The average duration from onset of symptoms to death is 7 months.

Rarely, occult gastric carcinoma, usually of the diffuse type, may present with widespread skeletal metastases,[298,299] progressive blindness due to leptomeningeal carcinomatosis,[300] or ureteral obstruction secondary to retroperitoneal metastases.[301] The extremely unlikely event of an occult gastric carcinoma metastasizing to a pituitary prolactinoma has been documented.[302]

Treatment

Treatment of advanced gastric cancer is primarily surgical, although chemotherapy, radiotherapy, and recently laser therapy have a role as well. Surgical resection is ideally curative, but palliative resection is still preferable over no surgery at all if curative resection is impossible.[303] Although the operability rate is 82%, the resectability rate is considerably lower (48%). Curative resection rates have been variously reported between 22.5 and 50%.[303-305] For curative resection, a 5-cm margin of normal tissue is suggested proximally and distally.[173]

For pathologists handling surgical specimens, it is important to understand the different types of resections encountered in gastric cancer surgery.[173] In general, curative resection means radical subtotal gastrectomy for lesions restricted to the distal two-thirds of the stomach, and total gastrectomy with splenectomy for lesions of the upper third.[306] Resections of tumors of the distal stomach include the greater and lesser omentum and lymph nodes along the hepatic artery and along the left gastric artery. If these lymph nodes appear involved, lymph nodes on the celiac axis and along the superior border of the pancreas and splenic artery may also be removed. If the tumor is located at the pylorus, lymph nodes along the superior mesenteric artery may be removed as well. A wedge of liver may be adherent to deeply penetrating tumors.

Tumors located in the greater curvature half of the anterior wall above the antrum, or in the posterior wall require splenectomy, removal of lymph nodes along the splenic artery and the superior border of the body and tail of the pancreas, and greater and lesser omentectomy. Lymph nodes on the celiac axis may be resected if lymph nodes along the splenic artery or lesser curvature are involved. The parietal peritoneum of the lesser sac over the pancreas may be removed if cancer penetrates the serosa. Caudal pancreatectomy is performed if cancer is adherent to the pancreas.

The transverse colon may be resected in tumors of the greater curvature and antrum that extend into the mesocolon.

Cancers of the fundus or cardioesophageal junction may be treated with a proximal gastric resection as long as a 5-cm margin is obtained.[173] Extended total gastrectomy with en bloc distal pancreatectomy and splenectomy has been suggested for cancers involving the middle one-third of the stomach.[307] Frozen section verification of tumor-free margins is recommended.

Intraoperative radiotherapy[308] or combined external radiation therapy and chemotherapy[309] have been found to improve survival in patients with incompletely resected cancers.

Laser therapy has been successfully applied as palliative treatment for advanced carcinoma of the cardia.[310]

Prognosis and Prognostic Factors of Advanced Gastric Cancer

The overall dismal prognosis of advanced gastric cancer (i.e., a 5-year survival rate of only 10 to 12%[118,303]) has changed little in the past decades despite the additional use of radiotherapy and chemotherapy and despite a decrease in operative mortality and an increase in the resectability rate over the past 50 years.[303] The curative resection rate now approaches 50%, and the 5-year survival rate of these patients has been reported between 20.5 and 42%.[173,175,303,305,311,312] Patients with nonresectable tumors who undergo biopsy and gastroenterostomy survive less than 6 months.[305] Those with palliative resections live longer. In a collected series of almost 20,000 cases from the literature, 6.5% such patients were alive after 5 years.[173]

A great number of clinical and pathologic parameters of possible prognostic significance have been studied. These include sex, age, duration of symptoms, stage, tumor location and size, gross and microscopic tumor types, endocrine immunoreactivity and pro-

tease activity of tumor cells,[236] desmoplasia, lymphatic and blood vessel invasion, lymphocytic infiltration, and reaction pattern of lymph nodes without cancer.[311,313] By multivariate analysis, stage and blood vessel invasion evolve as the most important prognostic factors.[311]

Stage

The most important prognostic factor is the extent of the disease. Five-year survival figures for Stage I are between 85 and 90%, for Stage II 52 to 55%, for Stage III 17 to 20%, and for Stage IV 3%. The mean survival in months is 109, 95, 41, and 6 for Stages I through IV, respectively.[313]

Sex and Age

Male gender and age of less than 40 years correlate with a worse prognosis than female gender and age of more than 40 years, but only because men and young patients tend to have more advanced disease than women and older patients, and because women, especially those less than 40 years of age, are more likely to have the more aggressive diffuse type of gastric carcinoma.[169] No statistically significant correlation of age and sex with prognosis is demonstrable after multivariate analysis.[311]

Duration of Symptoms

Patients with a long history of digestive symptoms have less invasive tumors and longer survival times than patients with a short history of digestive symptoms. Similarly, a short clinical history correlates with inoperability and nonresectability.[313]

Location

Antral tumors are associated with a better prognosis than those of the fundus or body (48.3% versus 39.2% and 36.3% versus 28.2% for 5- and 10-year survival, respectively).[311,313] Patients with tumors of the middle third of the stomach live longer than those with tumors of the proximal third. Location along the lesser curvature is a good prognostic factor.[313]

Size and Macroscopic Appearance

The prognostic value of either of these factors almost disappears when the influence of stage, blood vessel invasion, and desmoplasia is controlled. As isolated variables they correlate with 5-year survival as follows: for patients with tumors less than 3 cm in diameter, 58%; for patients with tumors between 3 and 6 cm, 49%; and for those with tumors greater than 6 cm, 35%.[311] Among the three macroscopic types of advanced gastric cancer the ulcerating type has the best prognosis, the polypoid or fungating type an intermediate prognosis, and the infiltrative type the poorest prognosis, with respective 5-year survival rates of 63 to 68, 59, and 27%.[311]

Microscopic Type

Although the main purpose of microscopic classifications is to distinguish tumor types of different behavior and although meaningful correlations between microscopic type and growth pattern and epidemiology have been shown, no significant correlation emerges with survival after multivariate analyses. The only significant correlation was found in Ming's classification between poorly differentiated carcinoma and a poor prognosis and well-differentiated tumors and a better prognosis.[311]

Immunoreactivity

In a study of gastric carcinoma in patients less than 40 years of age, tumors with endocrine immunoreactivity tended to be less advanced and associated with longer survival than those without endocrine immunoreactivity.[238] Well-differentiated adenocarcinomas with α_1-antitrypsin (AAT) immunoreactivity have worse prognoses than well-differentiated adenocarcinomas without AAT.[236]

Desmoplasia

A desmoplastic stromal reaction is significantly correlated with a poor prognosis. Five-year suvival rates for patients with tumors with and without desmoplasmia are 22 and 52%, respectively.[311]

Lymphocytic Reaction

Lymphocytic permeation is seen predominantly in tumors that produce little or no mucin and has no predictive prognostic value as an independent variable. Survival rates are higher for tumors with marked lymphocytic infiltration than for those with moderate and poor or absent lymphocytic infiltration after 5 years, but become less so after 10 years.[311]

DNA Ploidy

An aneuploid DNA pattern is more frequent in poorly differentiated (75%) than in well differentiated (36%) gastric adenocarcinomas and is associated with a poorer prognosis, both in early and in advanced cancers.[314] Heterogeneity of DNA ploidy in undifferentiated gastric carcinomas signals a particularly poor prognosis with a 100% incidence of lymph node metastasis.[315]

Lymphatic Invasion

The presence of lymphatic permeation is an important discriminating feature in tumors without lymph node metastases. Such cases behave clinically like those with nodal involvement and should be classified as N1 lesions (see Table 7-5).[311]

Blood Vessel Invasion

Venous invasion, present in about one-third of cases, worsens the prognosis significantly regardless of the stage of the disease.[312]

Lymph Nodes

The prognostic significance of nodal metastases is reflected in the prognostic importance of tumor stage. If metastatic tumor shows extracapsular spread, the prognosis worsens further and is comparable to that of tumors with extragastric involvement.[316] Lymphocytic depletion of lymph nodes without metastases is a prognostically unfavorable sign, especially if sinus histiocytosis is absent. Prognostically favorable signs include follicular hyperplasia and sinus histiocytosis.[311,317]

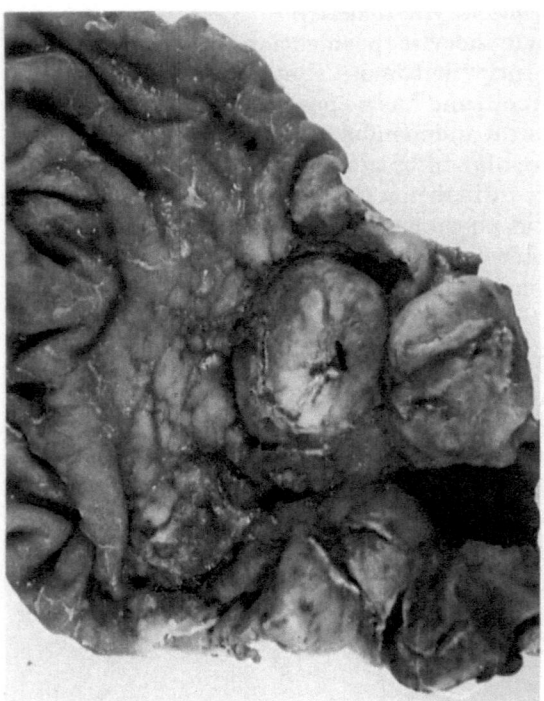

Figure 7-46. Gastric metastases of malignant melanoma. An ulcerated submucosal nodule is surrounded by cobblestoned mucosa, indicating submucosal spread that mimics linitis plastica.

Secondary Carcinoma of the Stomach

Secondary carcinomas of the stomach are either those that arise in neighboring structures and penetrate the gastric wall by direct extension or those that reach the stomach by lymphatic or blood vessel dissemination from distant sites. Among the former are carcinomas of the esophagus, pancreas, colon, liver, and rarely left kidney and left adrenal gland.[318]

Truly metastatic carcinomas of the stomach are rare and usually only discovered at autopsy. The incidence of gastric metastases among patients dying of known cancer has been reported between 1.2 and 1.7%.[319,320] The order of frequency with which types of carcinomas occur in the stomach has changed from melanoma, carcinoma of the breast, and germ cell tumors of the testis in 1952[318] to carcinoma of the lung, carcinoma of the breast, and melanoma in 1975,[320] reflecting the increase in the incidence of carcinoma of the lung in the last decades rather than a decrease in the other types of cancer. Also, metastases of carcinomas of the pancreas, thyroid, kidney, and ovary have, on occasion, been found in the stomach at autopsy.

The greater longevity of cancer patients and increased use and accuracy of gastroscopy and biopsy have resulted in an increasing detection rate of gastric metastases during life.[321-325] A wide range of metastatic tumors are now diagnosed endoscopically, including the above-named carcinomas as well as those of the mouth, parotid gland, and esophagus and testicular choriocarcinoma.[321-324]

Gastric metastases present as solitary or multiple submucosal or polypoid masses with ulcerated or intact surfaces (Fig. 7-46) or as linitis plastica.[320,326] The latter presentation is characteristic of metastatic lobular carcinoma of the breast, which is not as rare as one may think, since more than 60 such cases were found in the literature in 1980.[326] Microscopically, a diffuse infiltrate of relatively small cells, separating compressed but intact glands, is characteristic (Fig. 7-47). The relative frequencies with which these tumors are found in the stomach depend on their overall incidence and their particular pattern of metastatic spread. Carcinoma of the lung, although the most common source of gastric metastases, produces gastrointestinal metastases at autopsy in only 4.3% of cases,[327] whereas carcinoma of the breast does so in 15% of cases.[326]

Malignant melanoma is considered the most frequent tumor to metastasize to the gastrointestinal tract as a whole, with an incidence found at autopsy of 60%.[328] Metastases to the small bowel, however, are more frequent than those to the stomach, which occur in 10 to 26% of cases as compared to a 36% incidence of small intestinal involvement.[328] Gastric metastases are most common in the body and fundus and arise on the crest of normal rugae. Bleeding is the most common symptom. Widespread metastases to other organs are usually present at the

Figure 7-47. Gastric metastasis of lobular carcinoma of the breast. There is a diffuse infiltrate of rather small cells between the foveolae. PAS, X80.

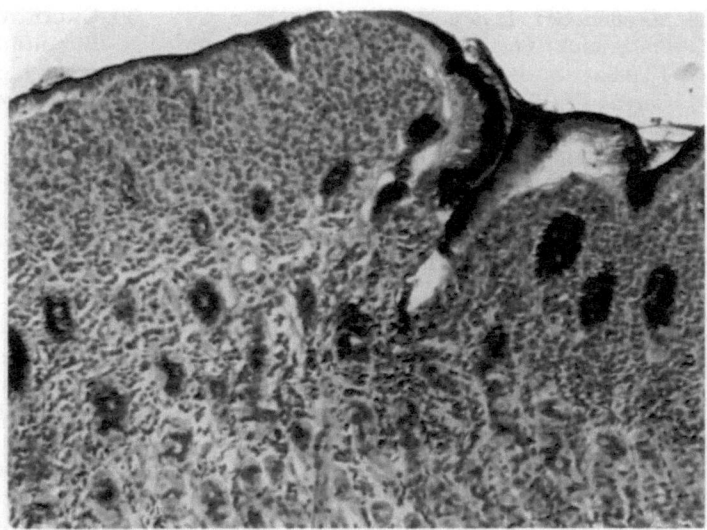

time of diagnosis. The interval between diagnoses of primary malignant melanoma and a gastric metastasis may be as long as 6 years.[328]

The incidence of gastric metastases in patients with esophageal carcinoma is about 6% at autopsy and 1.7% in surgical specimens.[329] Location in the lower third, size greater than 7 cm, and poor differentiation are features associated with gastric involvement by esophageal carcinoma. Only 10% of gastric metastases are discovered before surgery and only 41% before autopsy. Lymphatic permeation rather than blood vessel invasion accounts for the majority of lesions.

References

1. American Cancer Society: Cancer Facts and Figures, 1983. New York: American Cancer Society, 1983.
2. Segi M: Age-adjusted death rates for cancer for selected sites (A-classification) in 40 countries in 1976, Nagoya: Segi Institute of Cancer Epidemiology, 1981.
3. Silverberg E: Cancer statistics 1987. CA 1987;37:2–19.
4. Møller Jensen O: Trends in the incidence of stomach cancer in the five Nordic countries; in Magnus K (ed): Trends in Cancer Incidence. Washington: Hemisphere Publishing, 1982:127–142.
5. Waterhouse J, Muir C, Shanmugaratnam K, et al (eds): Cancer Incidence in Five Continents. Vol. IV (IARC Scientific Publications No. 42). Lyon: International Agency for Research on Cancer, 1982.
6. Naraynsingh V: Gastric carcinoma in the West Indies: a Trinidad study. Cancer 1985; 56:2117–2119.
7. Kawai K, Kizu M, Miyaoka T: Epidemiology and pathogenesis of gastric cancer. Front Gastrointest Res 1980;6:71–86.
8. Faivre J, Justrabo E, Hillon P, et al: Gastric carcinoma in Cote d'Or (France). A population-based study. Gastroenterology 1985;88: 1874–1979.
9. Young JL, Percy CL, Asire AJ: Surveillance, Epidemiology and End Results. Incidence and Mortality Data, 1973–1977. National Cancer Institute Monograph No. 57. Washington DC: U.S. Government Printing Office, 1981.
10. Blass RS, Miller TA, Copeland EM: Carcinoma of the stomach in the young adult. Surg Gynecol Obstet 1980;150:883–886.
11. Hansen RM, Hanson GA: Gastric carcinoma in young people. Am J Gastroenterol 1980; 1974:497–503.
12. Chen P-C, Wu C-S, Chang-Chien C-S, et al: Gastric carcinoma in young adults. J Formosan Med Assoc 1981;80:625–629.

13. Mahour GH, Isaacs H, Chang L: Primary malignant tumors of the stomach in children. J Pediatr Surg 1980;15:603–608.

14. Correa P: Clinical implications of recent developments in gastric cancer pathology and epidemiology. Semin Oncol 1985;12:2–10.

15. Haenszel WM: Cancer mortality and incidence among the foreign born in the United States. J Natl Cancer Inst 1961;26:37–132.

16. Munoz N, Connelly R: Time trends of intestinal and diffuse type of gastric cancer in the United States. Int J Cancer 1971;8:158–164.

17. Grabiec J, Owen D: Carcinoma of the stomach in young persons. Cancer 1985;56:388–396.

18. Mecklin J-P, Nordling S, Saario I: Carcinoma of the stomach and its heredity in young patients. Scand J Gastroenterol 1988;23:307–311.

19. Woolf CM, Gardner EJ: Carcinoma of gastrointestinal tract in Utah family. J Hered 1950;41:273–276.

20. Jackson CE, Brownlee RW, Schuman BM, et al: Observations on gastric cancer in San Marino. Cancer 1980;45:599–602.

21. Cruze K, Clarke JS, El Farra S: Familial aspects of gastric adenocarcinoma. Am J Dig Dis 1961;6:7–10.

22. Xu G-W: Gastric cancer in China: A review. J R Soc Med 1981;74:210–212.

23. Lehtola J: Familial behaviour of gastric carcinoma. Ann Clin Res 1981;13:144–148.

24. Coffey RJ, Knight CD, van Heerden JA, et al: Gastric adenocarcinoma complicating Gardner's syndrome in a North American woman. Gastroenterology 1985;88:1263–1266.

25. Halbert RE: Peutz-Jeghers syndrome with metastasizing gastric adenocarcinoma. Report of a case. Arch Pathol Lab Med 1982;106:517–520.

26. Correa P, Sasano N, Stemmermann GN, Hanszel W: Pathology of gastric carcinoma in Japanese populations: Comparison between Miyagi prefecture, Japan, and Hawaii. J Natl Cancer Inst 1973;51:1449–1459.

27. Ihamoki T, Sipponen P: Familial characteristics of gastric carcinoma. Ann Clin Res 1981;13:149–150.

28. Varis K: Family behaviour of chronic gastritis. Ann Clin Res 1981;13:125–129.

29. Furukawa H, Iwanaga T, Koyama H, et al: Effect of sex hormones on the experimental induction of cancer in rat stomach—a preliminary study. Digestion 1982;23:151–155.

30. Cwern M, Garcia RL, Davidson MI, et al: Simultaneous occurrence of gastric carcinoma in identical twins. Am J Gastroenterol 1981;75:41–47.

31. Ellis A, Hughes S, McConnell RB: Gastric neoplasms and pepsinogen phenotypes. Br J Cancer 1982;46:289–290.

32. Sugimura T, Kawachi T: Experimental stomach cancer. Methods Cancer Res 1973;7:245–308.

33. Wieman TJ, Max MH, Voyles CR, et al: Diversion of duodenal contents. Its effect on the production of experimental gastric cancer. Arch Surg 1980;115:959–961.

34. Morgan RW, Ward JM, Hartmen PE: Aroclor 1254-induced intestinal metaplasia and adenocarcinoma in the glandular stomach of F344 rats. Cancer Res 1981;41:5052–5059.

35. Tahara E, Shimamoto F, Toniyama K, et al: Enhanced effect of gastrin on rat stomach carcinogenesis induced by N-methyl-N-nitro-N-nitrosoguanidine. Cancer Res 1982;42:1781–1787.

36. Takahashi M, Shirai T, Fukushima S, et al: Ulcer formation and associated tumor production in multiple sites within the stomach and duodenum of rats treated with N-methyl-N-nitro-N-nitrosoguanidine. J Natl Cancer Inst 1981;67:473–477.

37. Tsiftsis D, Jass JR, Filipe MI, et al: Altered patterns of mucin secretion in precancerous lesions induced in the glandular part of the rat stomach by the carcinogen N-methyl-N-nitro-N-nitrosoguanidine. Invest Cell Pathol 1980;3:399–408.

38. Deveney CW, Freeman H, Way LW: Experimental gastric carcinogenesis in the rat. Effects of hypergastrinemia and acid secretion. Am J Surg 1980;139:49–54.

39. Kuratsuhe M, Yoshimura T, Matsuzaka J, et al: Epidemiologic study on yosho, a poisoning caused by ingestion of rice oil contaminated with a commercial brand of polychlorinated biphenyls. Environ Health Perspect 1972;1:119–128.

40. Armijo R, Coulson AH: Epidemiology of stomach cancer in Chile—the role of nitrogen fertilizers. Int J Epidemiol 1975;4:301–309.

41. Armijo R, Orellana M, Medina E, et al: Epidemiology of gastric cancer in Chile: I—case control study. Int J Epidemiol 1981;10:53–62.

42. Correa P, Cuello C, Gordillo G, et al: The gastric microenvironment in populations at high

risk to stomach cancer. Natl Cancer Inst Monogr 1979;53:167–170.

43. Drasar BS, Hill MJ: Metabolism of nitrogen compounds, in Human Intestinal Flora. London: Academic Press, 1974:72–102.

44. Reed PI, Haines K, Smith PLR, et al: Gastric juice N-nitrosamines in health and gastroduodenal disease. Lancet 1981; Sept 12: 550–553.

45. Schmähl D, Habs M: Carcinogenicity of N-nitroso compounds. Oncology 1980;37:237–242.

46. Stockbrugger RW, Cotton PB, Eugenider N, et al: Intragastric nitrites, nitrosamines, and bacterial overgrowth during cimetidine treatment. Gut 1982;23:1048–1054.

47. Brimblecombe RW, Duncan WAM, Duran GJ, et al: Characterization and development of cimetidine as a histamine H_2-receptor antagonist. Gastroenterology 1978;74:339–347.

48. Crean GP, Leslie GB, Roe FJC: Cimetidine and gastric cancer: Negative studies in dogs. Lancet 1979; Oct 13:797–798.

49. Reed PI, Haines K, Walters CL, et al: Cimetidine, nitrosation and carcinogenicity. Lancet 1981; Dec 5:1281–1282.

50. Enterline PE: Mortality rates among coal miners. Am J Pub Health 1964;54:758–768.

51. Ames R: Gastric cancer in coal miners: Some hypotheses for investigation. J Soc Occup Med 1982;32:73–81.

52. Weinberg GB, Kuller LH, Stehr PA: A case-control study of stomach cancer in a coal mining region of Pennsylvania. Cancer 1985;56: 703–713.

53. Meyer MB, Luk GD, Sotelo JM, et al: Hypothesis: The role of the lung in stomach carcinogenesis. Am Rev Respir Dis 1980;121: 887–892.

54. Berg J: Diet, in Fraumeni J (ed): Persons at High Risk of Cancer. New York: Academic Press, 1975:201–224.

55. Correa P, Cuello C, Fajardo LF, et al: Diet and gastric cancer: Nutrition survey in a high risk area. J Natl Cancer Inst 1983;70:673–678.

56. Armijo R, Gonzales A, Orellana M, et al: Epidemiology of gastric cancer in Chile: II – nitrate exposures and stomach cancer frequency. Int J Epidemiol 1981;10:57–62.

57. Joossens JV, Geboers J: Nutrition and gastric cancer. Nutr Cancer 1981;2:250–261.

58. Whelton PK, Goldblatt P: An investigation of the relationship between stomach cancer and cerebrovascular disease. Am J Epidemiol 1982;115:418–427.

59. Zemla B: A possible association between quality of drinking water and stomach cancer incidence among native and immigrant populations of a selected industrial city. Neoplasma 1980;27:55–61.

60. Hoey J, Montvernay C, Lambert R: Wine and tobacco: Risk factors for gastric cancer in France. Am J Epidemiol 1981;113:668–673.

61. Botha JL, Irwig LM, Stebel PM: Excess mortality from stomach cancer, lung cancer, and asbestosis and/or mesothelioma in crocidolite mining districts in South Africa. Am J Epidemiol 1986;123:30–40.

62. Morgan RW, Foliart DE, Wong O: Asbestos and gastrointestinal cancer. West J Med 1985;143:60–65.

63. Kraus AS, Levin ML, Gerhardt PR: A study of occupational associations with gastric cancer. Am J Pub Health 1957;47:961–970.

64. Järvholm B, Lillienberg L, Axelson O: The risk of digestive cancer in workers using synthetic abrasive products. J Occup Med 1982; 24:562–563.

65. LeShan L: You Can Fight for Your Life: Emotional Factors in the Causation of Cancer. New York: M Evans, 1977.

66. Lehrer S: Life change and gastric cancer. Psychosom Med 1980;42:499–502.

67. Kohn HI, Fry RJM: Radiation carcinogenesis. N Engl J Med 1984;310:504–510.

68. Wakabayashi T, Kato H, Ikeda T, et al: Studies of the mortality of A-bomb survivors. Report 7. Part III. Incidence of cancer in 1959–1978, based on the Tumor Registry, Nagasaki. Radiat Res 1983;93:112–146.

69. Scott RK, Holman WP, Sinckh ES: X-ray irradiation and conservative surgery with chronic duodenal ulcer. J Fac Radiol (London) 1953;5:42–47.

70. Brown WMC, Doll R: Mortality from cancer and other causes after radiotherapy for ankylosing spondylitis. Br Med J 1965;2:1327–1332.

71. Sellin J, Levin B, Reckard C, et al: Gastric adenocarcinoma following gastric lymphoma. Cancer 1980;45:996–1000.

72. Brumback RA, Gerber JE, Hicks DG, et al: Adenocarcinoma of the stomach following irradiation and chemotherapy for lymphoma in young patients. Cancer 1984;54:994–998.

73. Ménétrier P: Des polyadenomes gastriques et

de leurs rapport avec le cancer de l'estomac. Arch Physiol Norm Pathol 1888;1:32–55.

74. Morson BC, Sobin LH, Grundmann E, et al: Precancerous conditions and epithelial dysplasia in the stomach. J Clin Pathol 1980; 33:711–721.

75. Nagayo T: Dysplasia of the gastric mucosa and its relation to the precancerous state. Gann 1981;72:813–823.

76. Ming S-C, Bajtai A, Correa P, et al: Gastric dysplasia. Significance and pathologic criteria. Cancer 1984;54:1794–1801.

77. Tosi P, Luzi P, Baak JPA, et al: Gastric dysplasia: A stereological and morphometrical assessment. J Pathol 1987;152:83–94.

78. Correa P, Cuello C, Dugue E, et al: Gastric cancer in Columbia. III. Natural history of precursor lesions. J Natl Cancer Inst 1976; 57:1027–1035.

79. Oehlert W, Keller P, Henke M, et al: Gastric mucosal dysplasia: What is its clinical significance? Front Gastrointest Res 1979;4:173–182.

80. Hattori T: Histological and autoradiographic study on development of group III lesion (dysplasia grade III) in the stomach. Pathol Res Pract 1985;180:36–44.

81. Jass JR, Filipe MI: The mucin profiles of normal gastric mucosa, intestinal metaplasia and its variants, and gastric carcinoma. Histochem J 1981;13:931–939.

82. Iida F, Kusama J: Gastric carcinoma and intestinal metaplasia. Significances of types of intestinal metaplasia upon development of gastric carcinoma. Cancer 1982;50:2854–2858.

83. Lei D-N, Yu J-Y: Types of mucosal metaplasia in relation to the histogenesis of gastric carcinoma. Arch Pathol Lab Med 1984;108:220–224.

84. Skinner JM, Whitehead R: Tumor markers in carcinoma and premalignant states of the stomach in humans. Eur J Cancer Clin Oncol 1982;18:227–235.

85. Higgins PJ, Correa P, Cuello C, et al: Fetal antigens in the precursor stages of gastric cancer. Oncology 1984;41:73–76.

86. Stranignoni D, Coola R: Distribution of tumor-associated antigens in gastric lesions as detected by two monoclonal antibodies on tissue sections. Cancer Detect Prev 1985;8:193–206.

87. Kapadia A, Feizi T, Jewell D, et al: Immunocytochemical studies of blood group A H I, and i antigens in gastric mucosae of infants with normal gastric histology and of patients with gastric carcinoma and chronic benign peptic ulceration. J Clin Pathol 1981;34:320–337.

88. Isaacson P: Immunoperoxidase study of the secretory immunoglobulin system and lysozyme in normal and diseased gastric mucosa. Gut 1982;23:578–588.

89. Nagayo T: Histological diagnosis of biopsied gastric mucosae with special reference to that of borderline lesions. Gann 1971;11:245–256.

90. Grundmann E, Schlake W: Histology of possible precancerous stages in stomach, in Herfarth CH, Schlag P (eds): Gastric Cancer. Berlin: Springer-Verlag, 1979:72–82.

91. Ming S-C: Dysplasia of gastric epithelium. Front Gastrointest Res 1979;4:164–172.

92. Cuello C, Correa P, Zarama G, et al: Histopathology of gastric dysplasia: Correlations with gastric juice chemistry. Am J Surg Pathol 1979;3:491–500.

93. Kunze E, Schauer A, Eder M, Seefeldt C: Early sequential lesions during development of experimental gastric cancer with a special reference to dysplasia. J Cancer Res Clin Oncol 1979;95:247–264.

94. Farini R, Farinati F, Leandro G, et al: Gastric epithelial dysplasia in relapsing and non-relapsing gastric ulcer. Am J Gastroenterol 1982;77:844–853.

95. Meister H, Holubarsch CH, Haferkamp O, et al: Gastritis, intestinal metaplasia, and dysplasia versus benign ulcer in stomach and duodenum and gastric carcinoma. A histotopographical study. Pathol Res Pract 1979; 164:259–269.

96. Newsletter of the Gastrointestinal Pathology Club 1985;3(2):20–27.

97. Jarvis LR, Whitehead R: Morphometric analysis of gastric dysplasia. J Pathol 1985;147:133–138.

98. Nishizawa M, Okada T: Magnified observations of ulcerated borderline lesions (adenoma) of the stomach based on dissecting microscopy and magnifying fiberoptic endoscopy. Endoscopy 1981;13:234–237.

99. Hirono M, Shimura K, Nagami K, et al: Macroscopic demonstration of atypical epithelial lesion of the stomach by the leucine aminopeptidase-alkaline phosphatase double staining method. Gann 1981;72:331–332.

100. Rubio CA, Hirota T, Habashi T: Atypical

mitoses in elevated dysplasias of the stomach. Pathol Res Pract 1985;180:372– 376.

101. Rubio CA, Kato Y, Sugano H: The intramucosal cysts of the stomach in Japanese subjects having focal (elevated) dysplasia. Gann 1983;74:391–397.

102. Riemann JF, Schmidt H, Hermanek P: On the ultrastructure of the gastric "borderline lesion." J Cancer Res Clin Oncol 1983;105: 285–291.

103. Sipponen P: Intestinal metaplasia and gastric carcinoma. Ann Clin Res 1981;13:139–143.

104. Bramesar KCR, Sanders DSA, Hopwood D: Limited value of type III intestinal metaplasia in predicting risk of gastric carcinoma. J Clin Pathol 1987;40:1287–1290.

105. Turani H, Lurie B, Chaimoff C, et al: The diagnostic significance of sulfated acid mucin content in gastric intestinal metaplasia with early gastric cancer. Am J Gastroenterol 1986;81:343–345.

106. Huang C-B, Xu J, Huang J-F, et al: Sulphomucin colonic type intestinal metaplasia and carcinoma of the stomach. Cancer 1986;57: 1370–1375.

107. Matsukura N, Suzuki K, Kawachi T, et al: Distribution of marker enzymes and mucin in intestinal metaplasia in human stomach and relation of complete and incomplete types of intestinal metaplasia to minute gastric carcinomas. J Natl Cancer Inst 1980; 65:231–236.

108. Wurster K, Rapp W: Histological and immunohistological studies on gastric mucosa. I. The presence of CEA in dysplastic surface epithelium. Pathol Res Pract 1979;164: 270–281.

109. Feizi T: Blood group antigens and gastric cancer. Med Biol 1982;60:7–11.

110. Weiss H, Wildner GP, Gütz H-J, et al: DNA distribution patterns of preneoplastic cells and their interpretation. Stomach and cervix uteri. Oncology 1981;38:210–218.

111. Weidner N, Smith J, LaVanway JM: Peptic ulceration with marked epithelial atypia following hepatic arterial infusion chemotherapy. Am J Surg Pathol 1983;7:261–268.

112. Jewell LD, Fields AL, Murray CJW, et al: Erosive gastroduodenitis with marked epithelial atypia following hepatic arterial infusion chemotherapy. Am J Gastroenterol 1985;80:421–424.

113. Bogomoletz WV: Early gastric cancer. Am J Surg Pathol 1984;8:381–391.

114. Fernando SSE, Nakamura K: Japanese technique of early gastric cancer diagnosis. Am J Gastroenterol 1986;81:757–764.

115. Murakami T: Early cancer of the stomach. World J Surg 1979;3:685–692.

116. Morrissey JF: Mass screening for gastric cancer. Gastrointest Endosc 1982;28:112–113.

117. Stout AP: Tumors of the stomach, in Atlas of Tumor Pathology, Section VI, Fascicle 21. Washington DC: Armed Forces Institute of Pathology, 1953.

118. Cancer statistics 1983. CA 1983;33:9–25.

119. Sowa M, Ohkita H, Nitta M, et al: Evaluation of clinicopathological analysis of the early gastric cancer. World J Surg 1981;5:717–720.

120. Matsusaka T, Kodama Y, Soejima K, et al: Recurrence in early gastric cancer. A pathologic evaluation. Cancer 1980;46:168–172.

121. Gebhardt C, Husemann B, Hermanek P, et al: Clinical aspects and therapy of early gastric cancer. World J Surg 1981;5:721–724.

122. Tong-Hua L, Ming-Chang C: Carcinome gastrique primitif. Analyse clinicopathologique de 50 cas. J Chir (Paris) 1982;119:105–113.

123. Takasugi T, Hirota T, Sasagawa M, et al: Actuarial survival rate of early gastric cancer. Stomach Intestine 1977;12:933.

124. Rösch W: Das Magenfrühkarzinom – spezielle geriatrische Probleme. Akt Gerontol 1981;11:57–59.

125. Green PHR, O'Toole KM, Weinberg LM, et al: Early gastric cancer. Gastroenterology 1981; 81:247–256.

126. Haubrich WS: "Early" gastric cancer. Gastrointest Endosc 1979;25:77–78.

127. Alampi G, Bazzocchi F, Briccoli A, et al: Considerazioni su 50 casi di early gastric cancer. Min Chir 1980;35:891–894.

128. Kawai K: Diagnosis of early gastric cancer. Endoscopy 1971;1:23–27.

129. Kawai K: Brief communication on early gastric cancer in Japan. ESGE News Lett 1978; 2:13–14.

130. Yoshiaki I, Blackstone MO, Riddell RH, et al: The endoscopic diagnosis of early gastric cancer. Gastrointest Endosc 1979;25:96–100.

131. Goldstein F, Kline TS, Kline IK, et al: Early gastric cancer in a United States hospital. Am J Gastroenterol 1983;78:715–719.

132. Rotterdam H, Zietz C: Changing incidence of early gastric cancer (abst). Lab Invest 1983; 48:72A.

133. Evans DMD, Craven JL, Murphy F, et al: Comparison of early gastric cancer in Britain and Japan. Gut 1978;19:1–9.

134. Fevre DI, Green PHR, Barratt PJ, et al: Review of five cases of early gastric carcinoma. Gut 1976;17:41–47.

135. Ohman U, Emas S, Rubio C: Relation between early and advanced cancer. Am J Surg 1980;140:351–355.

136. Caduff B, Rüedi TH, Hartmann G, et al: Magenkarzinom-Fründiagnose: Realität oder Illusion? Schweiz Med Wschr 1982;112:526–528.

137. Busuttil A, Webb JN: Early carcinoma of the stomach. J R Coll Surg Edinburgh 1981;26:322–327.

138. Tonghua L, Minzhang C: Early gastric carcinoma. Clinicopathologic analysis of 50 cases. Chin Med J 1981;94:345–354.

139. Guangbi Y, Shuzong L, Buyue X: Clinical and endoscopic study of early gastric cancer. Report of 15 cases and review of Chinese literature. Aust NZ J Med 1982;12:284–286.

140. Eckstam EE: Early gastric cancer: report of 5 cases. Gastrointest Endosc 1981;27:174–175.

141. Oohara T, Tohma H, Takezoe K, et al: Minute gastric cancers less than 5 mm in diameter. Cancer 1982;50:801–810.

142. Esaki Y, Hirokawa K, Yamashiro M: Multiple gastric cancers in the aged with special reference to intramucosal cancers. Cancer 1987;59:560–565.

143. Tsukuma H, Mishima T, Oshima A: Prospective study of "early gastric cancer." Int J Cancer 1983;31:421–426.

144. Eckhardt VF, Willems D, Kanzler G, et al: Eighty months persistence of poorly differentiated early gastric cancer. Gastroenterology 1984;87:719–724.

145. Kobayashi S: Diagnosis of early gastric cancer of the upper stomach. Gastroenterol Endosc (Jpn) 1981;23:1108–1114.

146. Sakuma A, Ouchi A, Sugawara T, et al: Histologic infiltrating pattern of gastric microcarcinoma by means of serial sections. Cancer 1985;55:1087–1092.

147. Lehnert T, Erlandson RA, Decosse JJ: Lymph and blood capillaries of the human gastric mucosa. A morphologic basis for metastasis in early gastric carcinoma. Gastroenterology 1985;89:939–950.

148. Kodama Y, Inokuchi K, Soejima K, et al: Growth patterns and prognosis in early gastric carcinoma. Cancer 1983;51:320–326.

149. Owen DA: Normal histology of the stomach. Am J Surg Pathol 1986;10:48–61.

150. Miwak: Advances in treatment of stomach carcinoma in Japan, in Hirayana T (ed): Epidemiology of Stomach Cancer: Key Questions and Answers. Tokyo: WHO-CC Monograph, 1977:109.

151. Inokuchi K, Kodama Y, Sasaki O, et al: Differentiation of growth patterns of early gastric carcinoma determined by cytophotometric DNA analysis. Cancer 1983;51:1138–1141.

152. Oohara T, Aono G, Ukawa S, et al: Clinical diagnosis of minute gastric cancer less than 5 mm in diameter. Cancer 1984;53:162–165.

153. Iishi H, Tatsuta M, Okuda S: Endoscopic diagnosis of minute gastric cancer of less than 5 mm in diameter. Cancer 1985;56:655–659.

154. Tatsuta M, Okuda S, Tamura H, et al: Endoscopic diagnosis of early gastric cancer by the endoscopic Congo red-methylene blue test. Cancer 1982;50:2956–2960.

155. Ikeda K, Sannohe V, Araki S, et al: Intraarterial dye method with vasomotors (PIAD method) applied for the endoscopic diagnosis of gastric cancer and the side effects of indigo carmine. Endoscopy 1982;14:119–123.

156. Elster K, Carson W, Wild A, et al: Evaluation of histological classification in early gastric cancer. Endoscopy 1979;3:203–206.

157. Ambe K, Mori M, Enjoji M: Early gastric carcinoma with multiple endocrine cell micronests. Am J Surg Pathol 1987;11:310–315.

158. Czerniak B, Herz F, Koss LG: DNA distribution patterns in early gastric carcinoma. Cancer 1987;59:113–117.

159. Rubio CA, Ohman U: The intramucosal cysts of the stomach. Acta Pathol Microbiol Immunol Scand (A) 1982;90:363–366.

160. Lin C-C, Taki K, Kuwabara N, et al: The significance of submucosal fibrosis in mucosal carcinoma of the stomach. J Formosan Med Assoc 1981;90:93–103.

161. Rösch W, Frühmorgen P: Endoscopic treatment of precanceroses and early gastric carcinoma. Endoscopy 1980;12:109–113.

162. Sakita T, Koyama S, Ishii M, et al: Early cancer of the stomach treated successfully with an endoscopic neodymium-YAG laser. Am J Gastroenterol 1981;76:441–445.

163. Borrmann R: Geschwülste des Magens und Duodenums, in Henke F, Lubarsch O (eds): Handbuch der speziellen pathologischen

Anatomie und Histologie, Vol 4. Berlin: Julius Springer, 1926:812.

164. Schindler R, Steiner PF, Smith WM, et al: Classification of gastric carcinoma. Surg Gynecol Obstet 1941;73:30–39.

165. Ming SC: Gastric carcinoma. A pathobiologic classification. Cancer 1977;39:2475–2485.

166. Curtis RE, Kennedy BJ, Myers MH, et al: Evaluation of AJC cancer staging using the SEER population. Semin Oncol 1985;12: 21–31.

167. Moss AA, Schnyder P, Marks W, et al: Gastric adenocarcinoma: A comparison of the accuracy and economics of staging by computed tomography and surgery. Gastroenterology 1981;80:45–50.

168. Lauren P: The two histologic main types of gastric carcinoma: diffuse and so-called intestinal-type carcinoma. Acta Pathol Microbiol Scand 1965;64:31–49.

169. Noda S, Soejima K, Inokuchi K: Clinicopathological analysis of the intestinal type and diffuse type of gastric carcinoma. Jpn J Surg 1980;10:277–283.

170. Antonioli DA: Current concepts in carcinoma of the stomach, in Appelman HD (ed): Pathology of the Esophagus, Stomach, and Duodenum. New York: Churchill Livingstone, 1984.

171. Mulligan RM: Histogenesis and biologic behavior of gastric carcinoma, in Sommers SC, (ed): Pathology Decennial 1966–1975. New York: Appleton-Century-Crofts, 1975: 31–102.

172. Ishii T, Ikegami N, Hosoda Y, et al: The biological behaviour of gastric cancer. J Pathol 1981;134:97–115.

173. Weed TE, Nuessle W, Ochsner A: Carcinoma of the stomach. Why are we failing to improve survival? Ann Surg 1981;193:407–412.

174. Tso PL, Bringaze WL, Dauterive AH, et al: Gastric carcinoma in the young. Cancer 1987;59:1362–1365.

175. Douglass HO, Nova HR: Gastric adenocarcinoma–management of the primary disease. Semin Oncol 1985;12:32–45.

176. Zimmerman SE, Smith FP, Philips TM, et al: Gastric carcinoma and thrombotic thrombocytopenic purpura: association with plasma immune complex concentrations. Br Med J 1982;284:1432–1434.

177. Pascal RR, Slovin SF: Tumor directed antibody and carcinoembryonic antigen in the glomeruli of a patient with gastric carcinoma. Hum Pathol 1980;11:679–682.

178. Wakashin M, Wakashin Y, Iesato K, et al: Association of gastric cancer and nephrotic syndrome. An immunologic study in three patients. Gastroenterology 1980;78:749–756.

179. Andreev VC, Boyanov L, Tsankov N: Generalized acanthosis nigricans. Dermatologica 1981;163:19–24.

180. Obara TO, Ito Y, Kodama T, et al: A case of gastric carcinoma associated with excessive granulocytosis. Cancer 1985;56:782–788.

181. Tamburrano G, Tamburrano S, Natoli C, et al: Gastric carcinoma associated with severe hypoglycemia sensitive to diazoxide. Diabete Metab (Paris) 1979;5:287–291.

182. Bralow SP: Diagnosis and staging of esophageal and gastric cancer. Cancer 1982;50: 2566–2570.

183. Armstrong CP, Dent DM, Berman P, et al: The relationship between gastric carcinoma and gastric juice lactate (L&D) and lactate dehydrogenase. Am J Gastroenterol 1984;79: 675–678.

184. Williams GT, Rogers K: Elevated gastric juice enzymes–a marker for increased gastric cancer risk. Clin Oncol 1984;10:319–323.

185. Nomura AMYk, Stemmermann GN, Samloff IM: Serum pepsinogen I as a predictor of stomach cancer. Ann Intern Med 1980;93: 537–540.

186. Häkkinen IPT, Heinonen R, Inberg MV, et al: Clinicopathological study of gastric cancers and precancerous states detected by fetal sulfoglycoprotein antigen screening. Cancer Res 1980;40:4308–4312.

187. Ishikura H, Fukasawa Y, Ogasawara K, et al: An AFP-producing gastric carcinoma with features of hepatic differentiation. A case report. Cancer 1985;56:840–848.

188. Dittrich C, Havelec L, Breyer S, et al: Carcinoembryonic (CEA) plasma level determination in the management of gastric cancer patients. Cancer Detect Prev 1985;8:181–188.

189. Keto P, Suoranta H, Ihamäki T, et al: Double contrast examination of the stomach compared with endoscopy. Acta Radiol Diagn (Stockh) 1979;20(5):762–768.

190. Li DKB, Burhenne HJ: Computed tomography of the stomach and duodenum: A review. Am J Gastroenterol 1983;78:36–41.

191. Freeny PC, Marks WM: Adenocarcinoma of the gastroesophageal junction: Barium and CT examination. AJR 1982;138:1077–1084.

192. Shi Z-R, Cai D-I: Endoscopic diagnosis of gas-

tric cancer: An analysis of 872 cases in China. Gastrointest Endosc 1985;31:191–193.

193. Llanos O, Guzman S, Duarte I: Accuracy of the first endoscopic procedure in the differential diagnosis of gastric lesions. Ann Surg 1982;193:224–226.

194. Rösch W: Wandel gastroenterologischer Krankheitsbilder durch die Endoskopie. Z Gastroenterol 1982;20:257–262.

195. Gupta JP, Jain AK, Agrawal BK, et al: Gastroscopic cytology and biopsies in diagnosis of gastric malignancies. J Surg Oncol 1983;22:62–64.

196. Carrera GF, Mascatello VJ, Holm H, et al: Ultrasonically guided percutaneous biopsy of gastric lesions. Wisc Med J 1979;78:28–29.

197. Graham DY, Schwartz JT, Cain D, et al: Prospective evaluation of biopsy number in the diagnosis of esophageal and gastric carcinoma. Gastroenterology 1982;82:228–231.

198. Young J, Hughes HE, Hole DJ: Morphological characteristics and distribution patterns of epithelial cells in the cytological diagnosis of gastric cancer. J Clin Pathol 1982;35:585–590.

199. Shanghai Gastrointestinal Endoscopy Cooperative Group, People's Republic of China: Value of biopsy and brush cytology in the diagnosis of gastric cancer. Gut 1982;23:774–776.

200. Lightdale CJ, Sherlock P: The diagnosis and treatment of gastric malignancies. Front Gastrointest Res 1980;6:138–147.

201. Young JA, Hughes HE: Three year trial of endoscopic cytology of the stomach and duodenum. Gut 1980;21:241–243.

202. Hanson JT, Thoreson C, Morrissey JF: Brush cytology in the diagnosis of upper gastrointestinal malignancy. Gastrointest Endosc 1980;26:33–35.

203. Iishi H, Yanamoto R, Tatsuto M, et al: Evaluation of fine-needle aspiration biopsy under direct vision gastrofiberscopy in diagnosis of diffusely infiltrative carcinoma of the stomach. Cancer 1986;57:1365–1369.

204. Gupta S, Annamma ML, Gupta S: Tetracycline fluorescence in gastric malignancy. Am J Gastroenterol 1979;30:17–18.

205. Brinton W: The Diseases of the Stomach. London: H Renshaw, 1859:310.

206. Antonioli DA, Goldman H: Changes in the location and type of gastric adenocarcinoma. Cancer 1982;50:775–781.

207. Haukland HH, Johnson JA, Eide JT: Carcinoma diagnosed in excised gastric ulcers. Acta Chir Scand 1981;147:439–443.

208. Wong J, Ong GB: Gastric carcinoma developing in chronic gastric ulcer in the rat treated with N-methyl-N-nitro-N-nitrosoguanidine. J Surg Res 1980;29:445–450.

209. Mountford RA, Brown P, Salmon PR, et al: Gastric cancer detection in gastric ulcer disease. Gut 1980;21:9–17.

210. Paterson M, Easton DF, Corbishley M, et al: Changing distribution of adenocarcinoma of the stomach. Br J Surg 1987;74:481–482.

211. Evans OMD, Cleary BK: The sites of origin of gastric cancers and ulcers in relation to mucosal junctions and the lesser curvature. Invest Cell Pathol 1979;2:97–117.

212. Yamagiwa H, Yoshimura H, Matsuzaki O, et al: Pathological study of multiple gastric carcinoma. Acta Pathol Jpn 1980;30:421–426.

213. Welvaart K, Warnsinck HM: The incidence of carcinoma of the gastric remnant. J Surg Oncol 1982;21:104–106.

214. Balfour DC: Factors influencing the life expectancy of patients operated on for gastric ulcers. Ann Surg 1922;76:405–408.

215. Morgenstern L, Nicholls JC: Commentary in stump cancer following gastric surgery. World J Surg 1979;3:731–736.

216. Clark CG, Fresini A, Gledhill T: Cancer following gastric surgery. Br J Surg 1985;72:591–594.

217. Klarfeld J, Resnick G: Gastric remnant carcinoma. Cancer 1979;44:1129–1133.

218. Peitsch W, Becker H-D: Frequency and prognosis of gastric stump cancer. Front Gastrointest Res 1979;5:170–177.

219. Nicholls JC: Stump cancer following gastric surgery. World J Surg 1979;3:731–736.

220. Papachristou DN, Agnanti N, Fortner JG: Gastric carcinoma after treatment of ulcer. Am J Surg 1980;139:193–196.

221. Schafer LW, Larson DE, Melton J, et al: The risk of gastric carcinoma after surgical treatment for benign ulcer disease. N Engl J Med 1983;309:1210–1213.

222. Sandler RS, Johnson MD, Holland KL: Risk of stomach cancer after gastric surgery for benign conditions. Dig Dis Sci 1984;29:703–708.

223. Graem N, Fischer AB, Hastrup N, et al: Mucosal changes of the Billroth II resected stomach. Acta Pathol Microbiol Scand (A) 1981;89:227–234.

224. Öst A, Ewerth S, Hellers G: Intestinal metaplasia in the gastric remnant following resection for benign ulcer disease. Acta Chir Scand (Suppl) 1980;500:23–27.

225. Langhans P, Heger RA, Hohenstein J, et al: Gastric stump carcinoma–new aspects deduced from experimental results. Scand J Gastroenterol 1981;16(Suppl 67):161–164.

226. Dahm K, Eichfuss HP, Koch W: Cancer of the gastric stump after Billroth II resection. Front Gastrointest Res 1979;5:164–169.

227. Rakovec S, Kovic M: Predisposition of the resected stomach for malignancy. World J Surg 1981;5:725–727.

228. Bogolometz WV, Potet F, Barge J, et al: Pathological features and mucin histochemistry of primary gastric stump carcinoma associated with gastritis cystica polyposa. Am J Surg Pathol 1985;9:401–410.

229. Takeda M, Gomi K, Lewis PL, et al: Two histologic types of early gastric carcinoma and their cytologic presentation. Acta Cytol 1981;25:229–236.

230. Takahashi T, Iwama N: Three-dimensional microstructures of gastrointestinal tumors. Pathol Annu 1985;20(1):419–440.

231. Heitz PU, Wegmann W: Identification of neoplastic Paneth cells in an adenocarcinoma of the stomach using lysozyme as a marker and electronmicroscopy. Virchows Arch (A) Pathol Anat Histopathol 1980;386:107–116.

232. Kato Y, Kitagawa T, Nakamura K, et al: Changes in the histologic types of gastric carcinoma in Japan. Cancer 1981;48:2084–2087.

233. Tatematsu M, Furihata C, Katsuyama T, et al: Gastric and intestinal phenotypic expressions of human signet ring cell carcinomas revealed by their biochemistry, mucin histochemistry, and ultrastructure. Cancer Res 1986;46:4866–4872.

234. Montero C, Segura DI: Retrospective histochemical study of mucosubstances in adenocarcinomas of the gastrointestinal tract. Histopathology 1980;4:281–291.

235. Bur M, Franklin WA: Lectin binding to human gastric adenocarcinomas and adjacent tissues. Am J Pathol 1985;119:279–287.

236. Tahara E, Ito H, Taniyama K, et al: Alpha$_1$-antitrypsin, alpha$_1$-antichymotrypsin, and alpha$_2$-macroglobulin in human gastric carcinomas. Hum Pathol 1984;15:957–964.

237. Ejeckam GC, Huang SN, McCaughey WTE, et al: Immunohistopathologic study on carcinoembryonic antigen (CEA)-like material and immunoglobulin A in gastric malignancies. Cancer 1979;44:1606–1614.

238. Radi MJ, Fenoglio-Preiser CM, Key CR, et al: Gastric carcinoma in the young: A clinicopathological and immunohistochemical study. Am J Gastroenterol 1986;81:747–755.

239. Tahara E, Ito H, Nakagani K, et al: Scirrhous argyrophil cell carcinoma of the stomach with multiple production of polypeptide hormones, amine, CEA, lysozyme, and HCG. Cancer 1982;49:1904–1915.

240. Tahara E, Ito H, Shimamoto F, et al: Lysozyme in human gastric carcinoma. A retrospective immunohistochemical study. Histopathology 1982;6:409–421.

241. Proks C, Feit V: Gastric carcinomas with argyrophil and argentaffin cells. Virchows Arch [Cell Pathol] 1982;395:201–206.

242. Murayama H, Kamio A, Imai T, et al: Gastric carcinoma with psammomatous calcification. Cancer 1982;49:78–79.

243. Hisao I, Yokozaki H, Hata J, et al: Glicentin-containing cells in intestinal metaplasia, adenoma, and carcinoma of the stomach. Virchows Arch (A) Pathol Anat Histopathol 1984;404:17–29.

244. Tari A, Miyachi Y, Hide M, et al: Beta-endorphin-like immunoreactivity and somatostatin-like immunoreactivity in normal gastric mucosa, muscle layer, and adenocarcinoma. Gastroenterology 1985;88:670–674.

245. Nishi K, Tokunaga A, Shimizu Y, et al: Immunohistochemical study of intracellular estradiol in human gastric cancer. Cancer 1987;59:1328–1332.

246. Tokunaga A, Nishi K, Matsukura N, et al: Estrogen and progesterone receptors in gastric cancer. Cancer 1986;57:1376–1379.

247. Tsujitani S, Furukawa T, Tamada R, et al: Langerhans cells and prognosis in patients with gastric carcinoma. Cancer 1987;59:501–505.

248. Nevalainen TJ, Järvi OH: Ultrastructure of intestinal and diffuse type gastric carcinoma. J Pathol 1977;22:129–136.

249. Yamashiro K, Suzuki H, Nagayo T: Electron microscopic study of signet-ring cells in diffuse carcinoma of the human stomach. Virchows Arch (A) Pathol Anat Histopathol 1977;374:275–284.

250. Hattori T, Hosokawa Y, Fukuda M, et al: Analysis of DNA ploidy patterns of gastric carcinomas in Japanese. Cancer 1984;54:1591–1597.

251. Hattori T, Hosokawa Y, Sugihara H, et al: DNA content of diffusely infiltrative carcinomas in the stomach. Pathol Res Pract 1985;180:615–618.

252. Korenaga D, Haraguchi M, Okamura T, et al: Consistency of DNA ploidy between primary and recurrent gastric carcinomas. Cancer Res 1986;46:1544–1546.

253. Sasaki K, Takahashi M, Ogino T, et al: An autoradiographic study on the labeling index of biopsy specimens from gastric cancers. Cancer 1984;54:1307–1309.

254. Brander WL, Needham PRG, Morgan AD: Indolent mucoid carcinoma of stomach. J Clin Pathol 1974;27:536–541.

255. Libson E, Bloom RA, Blank P, et al: Calcified mucinous adenocarcinoma of the stomach–the CT appearances. Comput Radiol 1985;9:255–258.

256. Saigo PE, Birgatti DJ, Sternberg S, et al: Primary gastric choriocarcinoma. Am J Surg Pathol 1981;5:333–342.

257. Wurzl J, Brooks JJ: Primary gastric choriocarcinoma. Cancer 1981;48:2756–2761.

258. Mari H, Soeda O, Kamano T, et al: Choriocarcinomatous change with immunocytochemically HCG-positive cells in the gastric carcinoma of the males. Virchows Arch (A) Pathol Anat Histopathol 1982;396:141–153.

259. Garcia RL, Ghali VS: Gastric choriocarcinoma and yolk sac tumor in a man: Observations about its possible origin. Hum Pathol 1985;16:955–958.

260. Kodama T, Kameya T, Hirota T, et al: Production of alpha-fetoprotein, normal serum proteins, and human chorionic gonadotropin in stomach cancer. Cancer 1981;48:1647–1655.

261. Bonnheim DC, Sarac OK, Fett W: Primary squamous cell carcinoma of the stomach. Am J Gastroenterol 1985;80:91–94.

262. Mari M, Iwashita A, Enjoji M: Squamous cell carcinoma of the stomach: Report of three cases. Am J Gastroenterol 1986;81:339–342.

263. Vaughan WP, Strauss FHH, Paloyan D: Squamous carcinoma of the stomach after luetic linitis plastica. Gastroenterology 1977;72:945–948.

264. Eaton H, Tennekoon GE: Squamous carcinoma of the stomach following corrosive burns. Br J Surg 1972;59:382–387.

265. Callery CD, Sanders MM, Pratt S, et al: Squamous cell carcinoma of the stomach: A study of four patients with common histogenesis. J Surg Oncol 1985;29:166–172.

266. McLoughlin GA, Cave-Bigley GJ, Tagore L, et al: Cyclophosphamide and pure squamous cell carcinoma of the stomach. Br Med J 1980;280:524–525.

267. Aoki Y, Tabuse K, Wada M, et al: Primary adenosquamous carcinoma of the stomach: Experiences of 11 cases and its clinical analyses. Gastroenterol Jpn 1978;13:140–145.

268. Mari M, Iwashita A, Enjoji M: Adenosquamous carcinoma of the stomach: A clinicopathologic analysis of 28 cases. Cancer 1986;57:333–339.

269. Spagnolo DV, Heenan PJ: Collision carcinoma at the esophagogastric junction. Cancer 1980;46:2702–2708.

270. Prade M, Bara J, Gadenne C, et al: Gastric carcinoma with argyrophilic cells: Light microscopic, electronmicroscopic, and immunochemical study. Hum Pathol 1982;13:588–592.

271. Chejfec G, Capella C, Solcia E, et al: Amphicrine cells, dysplasia, and neoplasia. Cancer 1985;56:2683–2690.

272. Eimoto T, Hayakawa H: Oat cell carcinoma of the stomach. Pathol Res Pract 1980;168:229–236.

273. Capella C, Frigerio B, Cornaggia M, et al: Gastric parietal cell carcinoma–a newly recognized entity: Light microscopic and ultrastructural features. Histopathology 1984;8:8131–824.

274. Bansal M, Kaneko M, Gordon RE: Carcinosarcoma and separate carcinoid tumor of the stomach. Cancer 1982;50:1876–1881.

275. Hanada M, Nakano K, Ii Y, et al: Carcinosarcoma of the stomach. Acta Pathol Jpn 1985;35:951–959.

276. Queckenstedt HHG: Über Karzinosarkome. Leipzig, 1904 (reference from Bansal et al.[274])

277. Kohli Y, Kawai K, Fujita S: Analytical studies on growth of human gastric cancer. J Clin Gastroenterol 1981;3:129–133.

278. Papachristou DN, Karas M, Fortner JG: Anastomotic recurrence in the esophagus complicating gastrectomy for adenocarcinoma of the stomach. Br J Surg 1979;66:609–612.

279. Keighley MRB, Moore J, Lee JR, et al: Preoperative frozen section and cytology to assess proximal invasion in gastro-esophageal carcinoma. Br J Surg 1981;68:73–74.

280. Menuck L: Transpyloric extension of gastric carcinoma. Dig Dis 1978;23:269–274.

281. Harper TG, Sperling HV, Easler RE: Linitis

plastica involving the entire gastrointestinal tract. J Clin Gastroenterol 1982;6:29–33.

282. Flatau E, Resnitzky P, Griehkan A, et al: Linitis plastica infiltrating the entire gut. Am J Gastroenterol 1982;77:559–560.

283. Mallaiah L, Fruchter G, Brozinsky S, et al: Malignant gastrocolic fistula. Case report and review of the literature. Am J Gastroenterol Colon Rect Surg 1980;31:12–17.

284. Shoji S, Soeno T, Takahashi T: Case of spontaneous gastrojejunal fistula due to gastric cancer. Am J Gastroenterol 1981;75:218–221.

285. Kiyasu Y, Kanestima S, Koga S: Morphogenesis of peritoneal metastasis in human gastric cancer. Cancer Res 1981;41:1236–1239.

286. Iitsuka Y, Kaneshima S, Tanida O, et al: Intraperitoneal free cancer cells and their viability in gastric cancer. Cancer 1979;40:1476–1480.

287. Duarte I, Llanas O: Patterns of metastases in intestinal and diffuse types of carcinoma of the stomach. Hum Pathol 1981;12:237–242.

288. del Regato JA, Spjut HJ: Cancer, Diagnosis, Treatment, and Prognosis, 5th ed. St. Louis: CV Mosby, 1977

289. Libson E, Bloom RA, Halpern I, et al: Mediastinal lymph node metastases from gastrointestinal carcinoma. Cancer 1987;59:1490–1493.

290. Tesar PJ, Goy J, Maynard J: Lymphangitis carcinomatosa. Med J Austral 1981;1:80–81.

291. Bardram L, Jensen NB, Pedersen T: Breast tumour. An unusual manifestation of a carcinoma of the stomach. Acta Chir Scand 1982;148:389–392.

292. Krukenberg F: Über das Fibrosarcoma Ovarii Mucocellulare (carcinomatoides). Arch Gynaekol 1896;50:287–295.

293. Schlagenhaufer F: Über das metastatische Ovarialkarzinom nach Krebs des Magens, Darmes und anderer Bauchorgane. Monatsschr Geburtshilfe Gynaekol 1902;15:485–494.

294. Novak C, Gray LA: Krukenberg tumor of the ovary: Clinical and pathological study of 21 cases. Surg Gynecol Obstet 1938;66:157–165.

295. Woodruff JD, Novak ER: Krukenberg tumor: A study of 48 cases from the ovarian tumor registry. Obstet Gynecol 1960;15:351–360.

296. Metz SA, Karnei RF, Veach SR, et al: Krukenberg carcinoma of the ovary with bone marrow involvement. Obstet Gynecol 1980;55:99–104.

297. Karsh J: Secondary malignant disease of the ovaries. Am J Obstet Gynecol 1951;61:154–160.

298. Carstens SA, Resnick D: Diffuse sclerotic skeletal metastases as an initial feature of gastric carcinoma. Arch Intern Med 1980;140:1666–1688.

299. Uchida T, Shikata T, Shimizu S-I, et al: Gonadotropin and alkaline phosphatase producing occult gastric carcinoma with widespread metastasis of generalized bone. Cancer 1981;48:140–150.

300. McCrary JA, Patrinely JR, Font RL: Progressive blindness caused by metastatic occult signet-ring cell gastric carcinoma. Arch Ophthalmol 1986;104:410–413.

301. Oesterwitz H, Bick C: Ureteral obstruction as primary manifestation of metastasizing gastric carcinoma. Int Urol Nephrol 1981;13:123–126.

302. von Seters AP, Bots GT AM, van Dulken H, et al: Metastasis of an occult gastric carcinoma suggesting growth of a prolactinoma during bromocriptine therapy: A case report with a review of the literature. Neurosurgery 1985;16:813–817.

303. Bizer LS: Adenocarcinoma of the stomach: Current results of treatment. Cancer 1983;51:743–745.

304. Du Pont JB, Lee JR, Burton GR, et al: Adenocarcinoma of the stomach: Review of 1497 cases. Cancer 1978;41:941–947.

305. Yap P, Pantangco E, Yap A, et al: Surgical management of gastric carcinoma. Am J Surg 1982;143:284–287.

306. ReMine WH: Indications and contraindications for surgery in gastric carcinoma. World J Surg 1979;6:709–714.

307. Shiu MH, Papachristou DN, Kosloff C, et al: Selection of operative procedures for adenocarcinoma of the midstomach. Ann Surg 1980;192:730–737.

308. Tobe T, Hikasa Y, Matsuda S, et al: Treatment of gastric cancer with combined surgery and intraoperative radiotherapy. World J Surg 1979;3:715–719.

309. Gastrointestinal Tumor Study Group: A comparison of combination chemotherapy and combined modality therapy for locally advanced gastric carcinoma. Cancer 1982;49:1771–1777.

310. Fleischer D, Sivak MU: Endoscopic Nd:YAG laser therapy as palliative treatment for advanced adenocarcinoma of the cardia. Gastroenterology 1984;87:815–820.

311. Ribero MM, Seixas M, Simones MS: Prognosis of gastric carcinoma. The preeminance of staging and the futility of histological classification. Dig Dis Pathol 1988; in press.

312. Nielsen J, Aagaard J, Toftgaard C: Gastric cancer with special reference to prognostic factors. Acta Chir Scand 1985;151: 49–55.

313. Ziliotto A, Kunzle JE, de Souza A, et al: Evolutive and prognostic aspects in gastric cancer. Analysis of 189 cases. Cancer 1987; 59:811–817.

314. Danova M, Riccardi A, Mazzini G, et al: Flow cytometric analysis of paraffin-embedded material in human gastric cancer. Analy & Quant Cytol Histol 1988;10:200–206.

315. Haraguchi M, Okamura T, Korenaga D, et al: Heterogeneity of DNA ploidy in patients with undifferentiated carcinomas of the stomach. Cancer 1987;59:922–924.

316. Zacho Z, Fischermann K, Sørensen BL: Prognostic role of breach of lymph node capsule in nodal metastases from gastric carcinoma. Acta Chir Scand 1963;125:365–369.

317. Riegrova D, Jansa P: Prognostic significance of reactive changes in regional lymph nodes in gastric and mammary carcinomas. Neoplasia 1982;29:481–486.

318. Willis RA: The Spread of Tumours in the Human Body. London: Butterworth, 1952: 216–217.

319. Berge T, Lundberg S: Cancer in Malmö, 1958–1969. An autopsy study. Acta Pathol Microbiol Scand (Suppl) 1977;260:1–235.

320. Menuck LS, Amberg JR: Metastatic disease involving the stomach. Am J Dig Dis 1974; 20:903–913.

321. Kibsgaard K: Gastric metastases from mucoepidermoid parotid tumor. Endoscopic diagnosis. Gastrointest Endosc 1979;25:106–107.

322. Sandler RS, Sartar B, Bozymski EM: Endoscopic appearance of cancer metastatic to the stomach. J Clin Gastroenterol 1981;3(suppl 1):35–37.

323. Fleck RM, Schade RR, Kowai CD, et al: Testicular choriocarcinoma with metastasis to gastric mucosa. Gastrointest Endosc 1984; 30:188–189.

324. Tawney S, Berger HW, Jayamanne DS, et al: Bronchogenic carcinoma with symptomatic metastasis to the stomach: A case report. Mt Sinai J Med 1982;49:338–340.

325. Sullivan WG, Cabot EB, Donohue RE: Metastatic renal cell carcinoma to stomach. Urology 1980;15:375–378.

326. Cormier WJ, Gaffey TA, Welch JS, et al: Linitis plastica caused by metastatic lobular carcinoma of the breast. Mayo Clin Proc 1980; 55:747–753.

327. Ochsner A, DeBakey M: Significance of metastasis in primary carcinomas of the lungs: Report of two cases with unusual site of metastasis. J Thorac Surg 1942;11:357–387.

328. Morini S, Bassi O, Colavolpe V: Malignant melanoma metastatic to the stomach. Endoscopic diagnosis and findings. Endoscopy 1980;12:86–89.

329. Saito T, Iizuka T, Kato H, et al: Esophageal carcinoma metastatic to the stomach. A clinicopathologic study of 35 cases. Cancer 1985; 56:2235–2241.

CHAPTER 8

Carcinoma of the Duodenum

Incidence

Primary duodenal carcinoma is rare, and only approximately 700 cases had been reported in the literature by 1974 (i.e., within the two centuries following the first description in 1746).[1] The files of the Mayo Clinic contained 104 cases for the 40-year period from 1937 to 1977,[2] yielding an incidence of 2 to 3 cases per year. In the New York Hospital–Cornell Medical Center, only 32 cases were found in 38 years.[3] The incidence at autopsy is between 0.019 and 0.5%.[3] The proportion of duodenal carcinomas among gastrointestinal carcinomas is 0.35%.[4] Interestingly, however, the duodenum is the preferential site of origin of small intestinal carcinomas, 33 to 45% of which arise there, according to data collected between 1937 and 1963.[5] More recent reviews of small intestinal carcinomas yield still higher incidences of 48 and 54%.[6,7] As Jefferson[8] said in 1916, "Inch for inch the duodenum is more liable to cancer than the rest of the small intestine." Carcinoma accounts for 70 to 80% of all duodenal malignant tumors; the remainder includes lymphoma, leiomyosarcoma, and carcinoid tumor.[1]

Etiology and Pathogenesis

Much less is known about the etiology and pathogenesis of duodenal carcinoma than that of gastric and colonic carcinoma. The importance of hereditary factors is exemplified by the high frequency of duodenal carcinoma in patients with familial adenomatous polyposis coli and Gardner's syndrome, an estimated 4 and 12% of whom develop carcinoma of the duodenum in the course of their illness.[9] At least 44 cases of duodenal carcinoma have been reported in familial adenomatous polyposis coli, and 3 to 6% of patients with duodenal cancer have Gardner's syndrome.[1,2] Most of the cancers associated with these familial syndromes are located in the periampullary region, but occasional bulbar location has been reported.[10] Periampullary duodenal carcinoma has also been described in association with von Recklinghausen's disease,[11] with Torre's syndrome,[1] and in two brothers.[12] It is noteworthy that duodenal carcinoma in the setting of hereditary disposition is almost exclusively periampullary in location, whereas in the general population 50 to 60% of duodenal carcinomas arise in other segments.[1-3]

Patients with celiac sprue (gluten-sensitive enteropathy) have an increased risk of developing intestinal lymphoma and gastrointestinal carcinoma. Duodenal carcinomas, however, are rare and only three cases were reported by 1986.[13,14]

There is no association between duodenal carcinoma and duodenal ulcer, but rare reports of carcinoma developing in the duodenal stump after gastroenterostomy for peptic ulcer disease have appeared in the literature.[15]

How frequently duodenal cancer develops de novo and how frequently within a preexisting adenoma is not known. What is known, however, is that many duodenal adenomas show severe dysplasia and carcinoma in situ and a number of invasive carcinomas, especially those developing in polyposis syndromes, show residual benign neoplastic glands at the edge, indicating that in some cases the pathogenesis of duodenal carcinoma is similar to the adenoma–carcinoma sequence observed in the colon.

Clinical Presentation

Duodenal carcinoma shows in some series a male predominance,[1] but in others a slight female predominance.[3,5] Ages at the time of diagnosis vary between 15 and 85 years, but mostly the disease appears in the fifth and sixth decades.[1-3,5,11] Patients in the younger age groups usually have a polyposis syndrome. Presenting symptoms include, in order of decreasing frequency, pain, anemia, obstruction, weight loss, anorexia, jaundice, melena, fever, hematemesis, and, rarely, a palpable mass.[2] Melena appears to be an ominous sign, since none of such patients in one series survived 5 years.[2] Rarely, patients may present with cutaneous manifestations, that is, the appearance of large numbers of seborrheic keratoses (sign of Leser-Trélat), which had been described previously in association with other intestinal malignancies.[16] It has been speculated that increased levels of epidermal growth factor, normally localized in Brunner's glands, may be the cause.

Diagnosis

Because of the nonspecific nature of most of the symptoms mentioned previously, carcinoma of the duodenum is usually diagnosed late in its course.[17] Periampullary tumors are an exception to this rule, since they produce obstructive jaundice relatively early.[18,19]

Diagnostic modalities most often used include radiology, endoscopy, and biopsy.

Upper gastrointestinal barium contrast studies have the greatest diagnostic yield, and accuracy rates of 61 to 100% have been reported.[2,3,17] Radiologically, carcinomas may produce duodenal constriction, obstruction, ulceration, mucosal derangement, polypoid or other filling defects, gastric or proximal duodenal dilatation, and duodenal rigidity.[3] Endoscopy is less frequently applied and visualization of the distal duodenum cannot always be achieved.[2] The diagnostic accuracy of duodenoscopy in tumors within the range of the instrument, however, is high (i.e., 79%).[20]

Accuracy of biopsy diagnoses has been reported as 85%.[20] False-negative diagnoses account for the 15% error rate and involve the differential diagnosis of adenoma and carcinoma, which may indeed be most difficult in small and superficial biopsy specimens.

Pathology

Gross Appearance

Duodenal carcinomas are usually single. Synchronous duodenal and jejunal carcinoma[21] and duodenal carcinoma and gangliocytic paraganglioma[22] have been described, and such carcinomas are mostly located distal to the ampulla of Vater (50 to 56%).[2,5] According to site of origin, duodenal carcinomas are designated as supraampullary, periampullary, and imfraampullary. Authors generally agree on the relative rarity of proximal or supraampullary duodenal carcinomas, the proportion of which is 7 to 18%,[3,5] but figures for periampullary tumors show greater variation (32 to 65%),[3,5] reflecting the difficulty of distinguishing duodenal carcinomas in this location from carcinomas arising in the pancreas, ampulla, or common duct. The duodenum is the least frequent site of origin among malignant tumors of the periampullary region, accounting for 9 to 12% of these tumors.[18,19] The pancreas is the site of origin in 34 to 47%, the ampulla in 37 to 40%, and the common duct in 7 to 12%. To distinguish a periampullary duodenal carcinoma from any of the above requires meticulous dissec-

Figure 8-1. Adenocarcinoma of the duodenum with papillary surface growth. HPS, X100, reproduced at 85%.

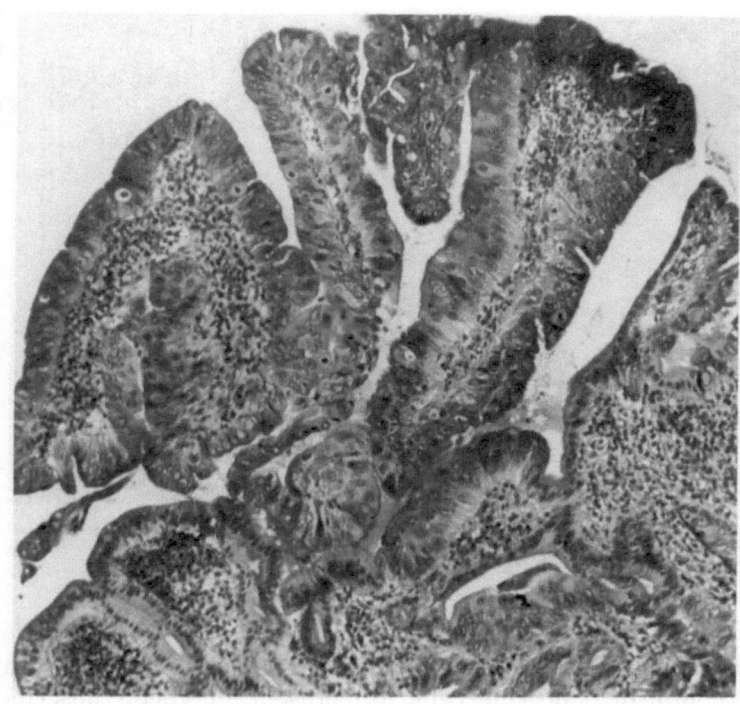

tion of the ampulla, common duct, and pancreas. Although this may be impossible, especially if the tumor is advanced, the attempt is justified because of prognostic implications. Patients with duodenal carcinoma have a significantly better 5-year survival rate than those with carcinoma of the pancreas (50% versus 29%).[19] Differences in survival rates for duodenal versus ampullary carcinoma are less consistent, perhaps because of the greater difficulty in distinguishing between these two tumors. There was no difference in one series[19] and a rather marked difference – one 5-year survivor among 12 patients with periampullary duodenal carcinoma as compared to 5 of 12 with ampullary carcinoma – in another series.[23] Mucin staining may be helpful since duodenal carcinomas contain predominantly non-sulfated mucins and ampullary carcinomas sulfomucins.[23]

Macroscopically, duodenal carcinoma presents most often as a cauliflower-like polypoid mass that is friable and prone to bleeding. Less frequently, duodenal carcinoma produces diffuse mural thickening and constriction or a localized, indurated, sessile lesion.[5]

Light Microscopy

Histologically, the vast majority of duodenal carcinomas are adenocarcinomas. The few exceptions are mentioned below. Adenocarcinomas are usually well or moderately differentiated. Of 91 tumors, 13% were grade 1, 46% grade 2, 21% grade 3, and 15% grade 4.[2] Papillary differentiation is commonly seen, especially on the surface (Fig. 8-1). Small biopsy specimens that fail to include the invasive base of the lesion are easily misdiagnosed as papillary or villous adenoma.[20] Any duodenal papillary neoplasm with dysplasia, therefore, should raise the suspicion of carcinoma. The invasive portion shows crowded intestinal type glands (Fig. 8-2). Varying amounts of mucin are usually present intracellularly as well as extracellularly. Poorly differentiated carcinomas may contain signet-ring cells and need to be distinguished from gastric signet-ring cell carcinoma extending into the proxi-

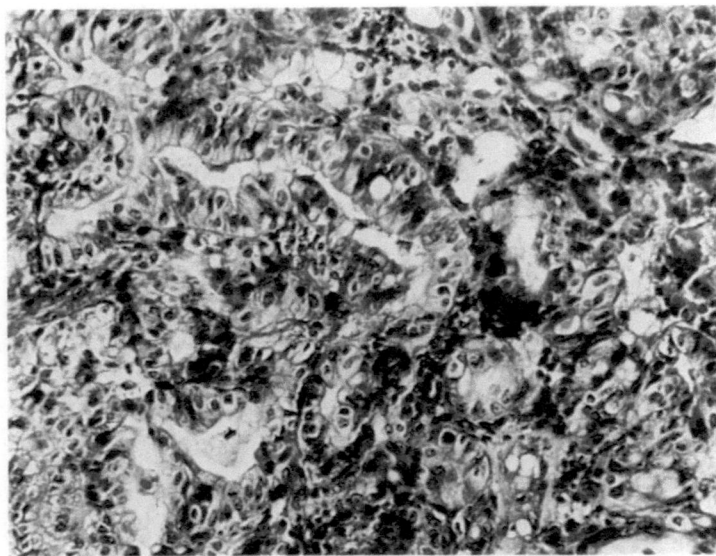

Figure 8-2. Adenocarcinoma of the duodenum. Invasive irregular glands are obvious in deeper areas. HPS, X160, reproduced at 90%.

mal duodenum. Scattered argyrophil and argentaffin endocrine cells are present in 50% of otherwise ordinary duodenal adenocarcinomas.[24] Some of these cells have shown immunoreactivity for serotonin, somatostatin, neurotension, big gastrin, and peptide YY. Carcinoembryonic antigen can be demonstrated histochemically in 75 to 100% of tumor cells.[20] Staining is moderate along the glycocalyceal borders, stronger along the cell membranes and within the cytoplasm, and strongest in luminal mucus. Cytoplasmic and membrane staining is stronger in poorly differentiated tumors than in well-differentiated tumors. Glycocalyceal staining for carcinoembryonic antigen is of little diagnostic help, since it is present in normal, adenomatous, and carcinomatous cells, whereas strong cytoplasmic staining was found only in carcinomas.[20]

Rare types of primary duodenal carcinoma, encountered as one or two case reports in the literature, include small cell neuroendocrine carcinoma[25] resembling pulmonary oat cell carcinoma (see Chapter 9), choriocarcinoma,[26] carcinoma arising in heterotopic pancreas,[27] and Brunner's gland adenocarcinoma.[28]

Extragenital choriocarcinoma has also been described in other gastrointestinal sites such as esophagus, stomach, and small intestine and must always be distinguished from metastatic gonadal choriocarcinoma. Duodenal choriocarcinoma, furthermore, may represent local extension of a retroperitoneal primary tumor.[29] The only documented primary duodenal choriocarcinoma found in 1986 involved a 29-year-old woman who, at autopsy, was found to have a choriocarcinoma 4 cm in diameter in the third portion of the duodenum. There were tumor emboli in the brain, but no evidence of tumor elsewhere. In contrast to primary gastric choriocarcinoma, which is usually associated with a poorly differentiated adenocarcinoma, the duodenal counterpart showed no such dual differentiation. Tumor cells stained positive for chorionic gonadotropin and human lactogen.[26]

Heterotopic pancreatic tissue is found relatively frequently in the wall of the duodenum; however, carcinoma developing in these lesions is extremely rare. No cancer was found in a series of 212 cases.[30] One case of giant cell carcinoma arising in heterotopic pancreas has been reported.[28]

Prognosis

The crude overall 5-year survival of patients with duodenal adenocarcinoma has been reported as 17.5%.[5] Resectability rates have been reported between 48 and 71%.[2,3,5] Five-year survival rates for patients undergoing potentially curative procedures (i.e., either pancreaticoduodenectomy or segmental duodenal resection) differ according to the criteria applied for resectability. In series with low resectability rates, 44 to 69% of patients survived 5 or more years.[2,3] In the series with the high resectability rate of 71%, only one-quarter of patients lived for 5 years.[5] At the time of surgery, two-thirds of patients already have metastases, mainly to regional lymph nodes and rarely to the liver. Spread to contiguous organs is more common than distant metastasis.

Factors of prognostic significance include the site of origin, the nodal status, the histologic grade, and surgical management.[2] Periampullary carcinomas, perhaps because they produce obstructive jaundice early in their course, carry a 5-year survival rate of 32%, twice that of tumors located elsewhere in the

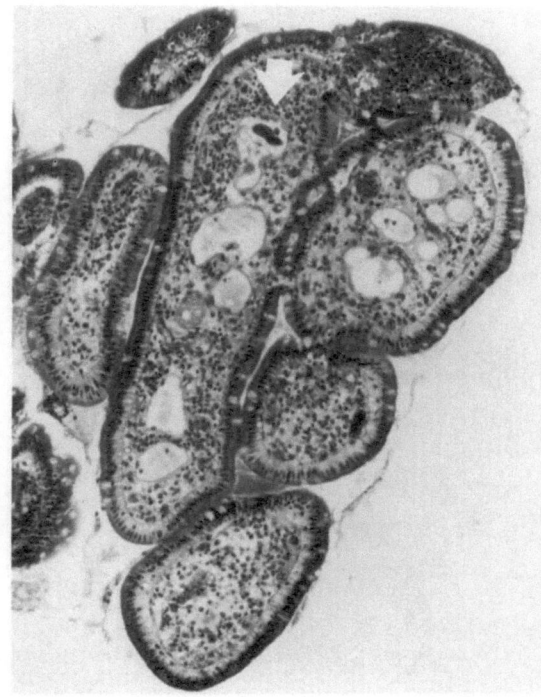

Figure 8-3. Lymphangiosis carcinomatosa. Lymphatics are distended and some (*arrow*) contain tumor cells. The source was carcinoma of the stomach. H&E, X100, reproduced at 80%.

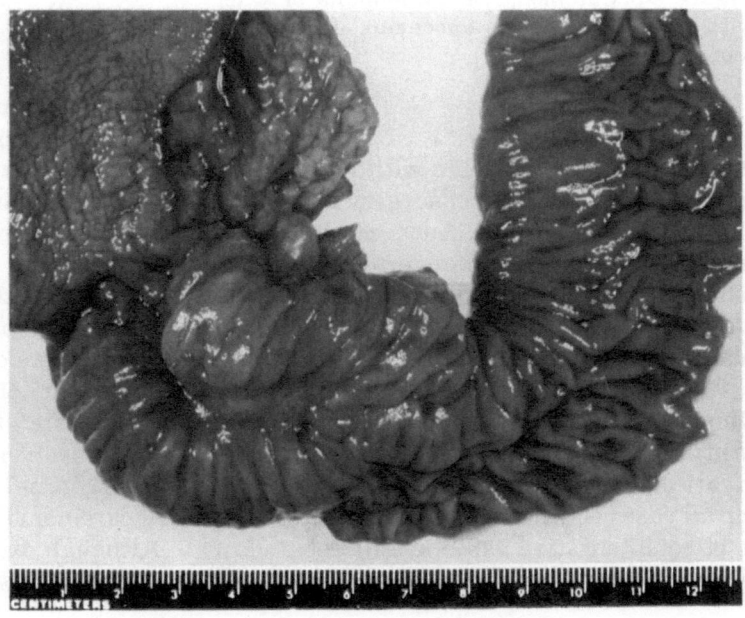

Figure 8-4. Carcinoma of the pancreas with extension into the first portion of the duodenum producing ulceration and stenosis.

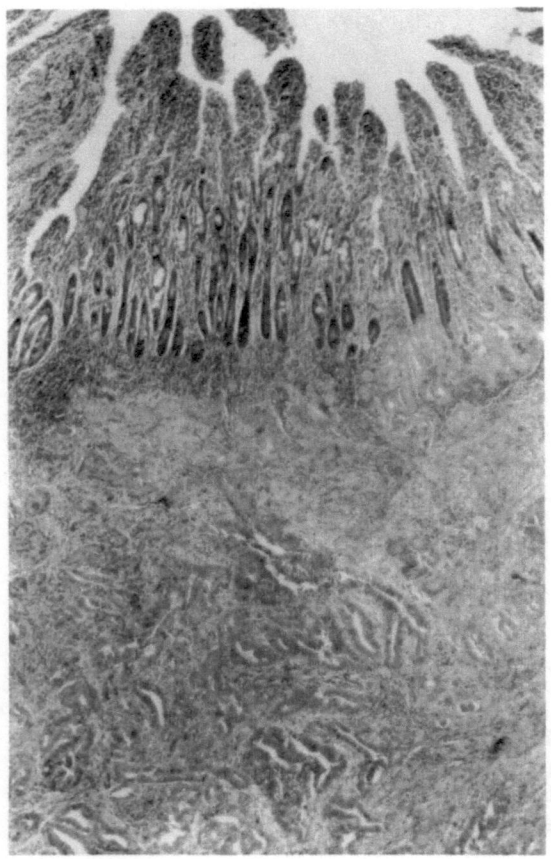

Figure 8-5. Carcinoma of the ampulla of Vater with extension into the duodenum. H&E, X40, reproduced at 95%.

Secondary Tumors

The duodenum may be involved with secondary tumors either by direct extension of cancers arising in neighboring organs or via lymphatic or hematogenous metastatic spread from distant sites. In a series of 13 secondary duodenal tumors, 7 represented direct extension and 6 distant metastases.[30] The most common secondary tumors of the former type are carcinomas arising in the stomach, pancreas, biliary tract, right colon, and right kidney.[32] Gastric carcinoma shows histologic evidence of transpyloric extension in 20% of cases.[33] Clinically, duodenal involvement by gastric cancer is rarely evident. If discovered, however, the diagnosis may save the patient from unnecessary surgery. A rare type of secondary duodenal involvement is lymphangiosis carcinomatosa, in which dilated mucosal lymphatics contain carcinoma cells (Fig. 8-3). Endoscopically, the mucosa appears white.[34] Pancreatic carcinoma shows endoscopic evidence of duodenal involvement in 17% of cases, either in the form of atypical ulcerations with or without associated stenosis (Fig. 8-4) or in the form of polypoid lesions.[35] Biopsy was positive in two-thirds of such cases. Carcinoma of the ampulla of Vater frequently extends into the duodenum (Fig. 8-5) and may be difficult to distinguish from primary duodenal carcinoma unless meticulous dissection discloses the site of origin. Carcinomas of the right colon may reach the duodenum either via lymphatic drainage to the central mesenteric lymph nodes surrounding the third portion of the duodenum or across a short fascial plane that attaches the hepatic flexure of the colon to the lower part of the descending duodenum.[36] Direct extension of metastatic tumor in retroperitoneal lymph nodes has been demonstrated to account for secondary duodenal involvement by testicular, uterine, ovarian, renal cell, and cervical squamous cell carcinoma.[30,37]

Although distant metastasis to the duodenum is less frequent than direct extension,

duodenum.[2] Most patients with lymph node metastases at the time of surgery die within the following 5 years, but occasionally a patient has survived longer. None of 15 patients with a poorly differentiated adenocarcinoma lived for 5 years, whereas 54% of patients with well-differentiated tumors did.

The importance of surgical management is illustrated by the decreased operative mortality in recent years.[2] Whether or not pancreaticoduodenectomy is the best treatment for all cases or whether segmental resection is of equal curative value is still debated in the surgical literature.[2,5,17]

the duodenum is the most commonly seeded segment of the gastrointestinal tract.[38] Its relatively fixed position may offer circulating tumor cells greater opportunity to settle and multiply. By far the most frequent tumor to metastasize to the duodenum is malignant melanoma, which accounts for almost half of all metastases, followed by carcinomas of the lung, breast, and ovary.[38]

References

1. Lillemoe K, Imbembo AL: Malignant neoplasms of the duodenum. Surg Gynecol Obstet 1980;150:822–826.
2. Joesting DR, Beart RW, van Heerden JA, et al: Improving survival in adenocarcinoma of the duodenum. Am J Surg 1981;141:228–231.
3. Cortese AF, Cornell GN: Carcinoma of the duodenum. Cancer 1972;29:1010–1015.
4. Iovine VM, Tsangaris N: Primary carcinoma of the duodenum. Am Surg 1961;27:744–750.
5. Spira IA, Ghazi A, Wolff WI: Primary adenocarcinoma of the duodenum. Cancer 1977;39:1721–1726.
6. Lanzafame RJ, Long JE, Hinshaw JR: Primary cancer of the small bowel. NY State J Med 1982;8:1325–1329.
7. Mittal VK, Bodzin JH: Primary malignant tumors of the small intestine. Am J Surg 1980;140:396–399.
8. Jefferson G: Carcinoma of the suprapapillary duodenum causally associated with preexisting simple ulcer. Br J Surg 1916;4:209–226.
9. Haggitt RC, Reid BJ: Hereditary gastrointestinal polyposis syndromes. Am J Surg Pathol 1986;10:871–887.
10. Itoh H, Iida M, Kuroiwa S, et al: Gardner's syndrome associated with carcinoma of the duodenal bulb: Report of a case. Am J Gastroenterol 1985;80:248–250.
11. McGlinchey JJ, Snater GJ, Haggani MT: Primary adenocarcinoma of the duodenum associated with cutaneous neurofibromatosis (von Recklinghausen's disease). Postgrad Med J 1982;58:115–116.
12. Kukleta JF, Altorfer J, Akovbiantz A: Jugendliches Duodenalkarzinom bei zwei Brüdern. Schweiz Rundschau Med (PRAXIS) 1982;71:920–923.
13. Javier J, Lukie B: Duodenal adenocarcinoma complicating celiac sprue. Dig Dis Sci 1980;25:150–153.
14. Levine ML, Dorf BS, Bank S: Adenocarcinoma of the duodenum in a patient with nontropical sprue. Am J Gastroenterol 1986;81:800–802.
15. Lipper S, Graves GV Jr: Villous adenocarcinoma arising in the bypassed duodenum 18 years after a Billroth II subtotal gastrectomy: Report of a case and review of the literature. Am J Gastroenterol 1985;80:174–176.
16. Curry SS, King LE: The sign of Leser-Trélat. Report of a case with adenocarcinoma of the duodenum. Arch Dermatol 1980;116:1059–1060.
17. Gaddy M, Max MH: Carcinoma of the duodenum. South Med J 1985;78:150–152.
18. Jones BA, Langer B, Taylor BR, et al: Periampullary tumors: Which ones should be resected. Am J Surg 1985;149:46–51.
19. Kellum JM, Clark J, Miller HH: Pancreatoduodenectomy for resectable malignant periampullary tumors. Surg Gynecol Obstet 1983;157:362–365.
20. Blackman E, Nash SV: Diagnosis of duodenal and ampullary epithelial neoplasms by endoscopic biopsy: A clinicopathologic and immunohistochemical study. Hum Pathol 1985;16:901–910.
21. Swift AC, Smith GT, Douglas DL: Dual primary adenocarcinoma of the duodenum and jejunum in a patient with previous colonic cancers. Postgrad Med J 1980;56:871–874.
22. Anders KH, Glasgow BJ, Lewin KJ: Gangliocytic paraganglioma associated with duodenal adenocarcinoma. Arch Pathol Lab Med 1987;11:49–52.
23. Connolly MM, Dawson PJ: Carcinoma of the ampulla of Vater: Classification and prognosis (abstr). Lab Invest 1987;56:15A.
24. Iwafuchi M, Watanabe H, Ishihara N, et al: Neoplastic endocrine cells in carcinomas of the small intestine: Histochemical and immunohistochemical studies of 24 tumors. Hum Pathol 1987;18:185–194.
25. Swanson PE, Dykoski D, Wick MR, et al: Primary duodenal small-cell neuroendocrine carcinoma with production of vasoactive intestinal polypeptide. Arch Pathol Lab Med 1986;110:317–320.
26. Matthews TH, Haton GH, Christopherson WM: Primary duodenal choriocarcinoma. Arch Pathol Lab Med 1986;110:550–552.

27. Gonzalez V, Michel J, Montano A, et al: Giant cell carcinoma in heterotopic pancreas localized in the duodenum. Am J Proctol Gastroenterol Colon Rectal Surg 1983;9:12–22.

28. Shorrock K, Haldane JS, Kershan MJ, et al: Obstructive jaundice secondary to carcinoma arising in Brunner's glands. J R Soc Med 1986;79:173–174.

29. Engel JM, Deitch EA, Risch J: Extragenital choriocarcinoma in the duodenum. Am J Radiol 1979;133-933-935.

30. Dolan RV, ReMine WH, Dockerty MB: The fate of heterotopic pancreas tissue. Arch Surg 1974;109:762–765.

31. Lämmli J, Bühler H, Bosseckert H, et al: Metastasen im Duodenum. Schweiz Rundschau Med (PRAXIS) 1982;71:1054–1057.

32. Veen HF, Oscarson JEA, Malt RA: Alien cancers of the duodenum. Surg Gynecol Obstet 1976;143:39–42.

33. Menuck L: Transpyloric extension of gastric carcinoma. Dig Dis 1978;23:269–274.

34. Cronstedt JI, Kalczynski J, Jonsson NGE: Involvement of the duodenum by gastric carcinoma. Gastrointest Endosc 1982;28:44–45.

35. Bonetti A, Deyhle P, Dolder M, et al: Häufigkeit und Art der Manifestation eines Pankreaskarzinoms im Duodenum. Schweiz Rundschau Med (PRAXIS) 1982;71:1058–1059.

36. Diamond RT, Greenberg HM, Boult IF: Direct metastatic spread of right colonic adenocarcinoma to duodenum—barium and computed tomographic findings. Gastrointest Radiol 1981;6:339–341.

37. Gurian L, Ireland K, Petty W, et al: Carcinoma of the cervix involving the duodenum: Case report and review of the literature. J Clin Gastroenterol 1981;3:291–294.

38. Willis RA: The Spread of Tumors in the Human Body, ed 2. London: Butterworths, 1952:212.

CHAPTER 9

Carcinoid (Neuroendocrine) Tumors

Nomenclature

The nomenclature of carcinoid tumors in general and of gastrointestinal carcinoid tumors in particular has undergone periodic changes reflecting changing concepts of their origin, histologic spectrum, natural history, and embryologic derivation.[1] It is certain that at the time of this writing not all that there is to know about these tumors is known, and therefore, the nomenclature is bound to undergo additional changes in the future.

The term *carcinoid*, or rather its German counterpart "Karzinoid," was first used by Oberndorfer in 1907 when he described carcinoma-like tumors of the small intestine.[2] The term later became broadened to include histologically similar tumors in other organs. Originally considered benign, it soon became evident that some such tumors behave in a malignant fashion, and the distinction between benign and malignant carcinoid tumors was made.[1] Today, all carcinoid tumors are regarded as potentially malignant, low-grade cancers, the behavior of which is determined by the site of origin, the tumor size, and the degree of differentiation.[1]

The variable staining with silver salts led to the distinction of argentaffin and argyrophil tumors (argentaffin tumors stain directly with silver salts, whereas argyrophil tumors require the addition of a reducing agent). Foregut carcinoids, that is, those originating in the esophagus, stomach, duodenum, pancreas, and bronchus, are generally argyrophil and have, at times, been designated "argyrophil cell carcinoids."[3]

The term *APUDoma* reflects the discovery of Pearse[4] that carcinoid tumors share with other endocrine neoplasms the ability of amine precursor uptake and decarboxylation. This APUD concept, initially understood only as a common metabolic pathway, was later expanded to denote a common neuroectodermal embryologic origin.[1,5] It soon became evident, however, that different APUDomas are derived from different germ layers, and carcinoid tumors of the gut have been rather convincingly shown to be of endodermal origin.[6]

In the more recent literature the term *neuroendocrine tumor* seems to gain acceptance.[7-9] It emphasizes the common cell of origin of all carcinoid tumors, regardless of degree of differentiation and inclusive of the least differentiated form, traditionally called oat cell carcinoma. Although the concept of the common neural crest origin of the diffuse endocrine system is no longer tenable, the prefix *neuro-* is appropriate if restricted to mean a common program of synthesis of peptides, amines, neuron-specific enolase,[10] and certain antigens shared by the diffuse endocrine cells and neurons.[11] In this sense, tumors as diverse as medullary carcinomas of the thyroid, pheochromocytomas, pituitary adenomas, islet cell tumors, and gastrointestinal carcinoids are neuroendocrine tumors.

Table 9-1. Endocrine Cells, Polypeptide Hormones, and Tumors of the Gastroduodenal Area*

Cell Type	Localization	Secretory Product	Tumor
ECL	Stomach: body	? Histamine ? Hydroxytryptophan	Functional or nonfunctional carcinoid
EC	Stomach: body, antrum	Serotonin, histamine	Carcinoid
G	Stomach: antrum; Duodenum	Gastrin	Gastrinoma
G	Stomach: antrum	ACTH-like peptide	?
D	Stomach: body, antrum; Duodenum	Somatostatin, ? Vasoactive intestinal polypeptide	Somatostatinoma
I	Duodenum	Cholecystokinin	?
k	Duodenum	Gastric inhibitory polypeptide	?
Mo	Duodenum	Motilin	?
N	Stomach; Duodenum	Neurotension	?
S	Duodenum	Secretin	?
?PP	? Duodenum	Pancreatic polypeptide	?

*Modified from Lewin,[19] with permission.

The World Health Organization has suggested that the term *carcinoid* be retained for and restricted to neuroendocrine neoplasms showing a characteristic histologic pattern and arising in the pancreas, gastrointestinal tract, thymus, bronchus, urogenital tract, uterine cervix, and other sites and that the neuroendocrine tumors of the thyroid, adrenal medulla, and pituitary gland be excluded from this designation.[12]

The advent of radioimmunoassay and immunohistology offered means of demonstrating and measuring the secretory products of carcinoid tumors. In the gastroduodenal area, carcinoid tumors that are functional are frequently named after their secretory product, such as gastrinoma,[13,14] or somatostatinoma.[15,16] Using such terms, one must keep in mind that most if not all functioning tumors, depending on the sensitivity of the method available, produce one or more secretory products, although one usually predominates, and that even those tumors that are clinically nonfunctional may produce small amounts of peptide hormone or amine that are only detectable histochemically.[1]

Some carcinoids, especially gastrin-producing tumors, are named after their presumed cell of origin, such as G-cell carcinoid[17] (G for gastrin producing). The same reservations apply as stated previously for gastrinoma.

Pathogenesis

Endocrine cells of the human gastrointestinal tract were first described by Kulchitzky in 1897,[18] and the Kulchitzky cell is generally considered the cell of origin of carcinoid tumors. Certain types of endocrine cells may give rise to specific endocrine tumors with specific secretory products. These are enumerated in Table 9-1. Enterochromaffin-like (ECL) cells constitute the major endocrine cell type of the body of the stomach, and the gastrin-producing G cells the major endocrine cell type of the antrum.[19,20] As is obvious from the number of question marks in Table 9-1, many uncertainties still exist and much needs to be learned. While tumors with a unidirectional differentiation, such as gastrinoma, can easily be traced back to one particular cell of origin, this is not possible in the majority of gastroduodenal carcinoids, which are clinically silent and which, histochemically, are nonfunctional or multidirec-

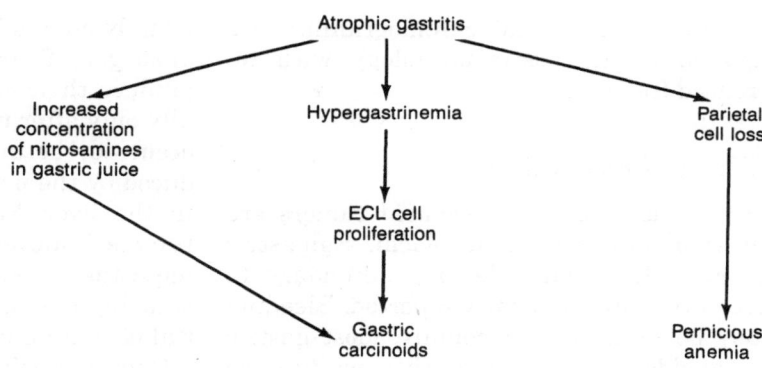

Figure 9-1. Presumed pathogenesis of gastric carcinoids (nonantral, ECL-cell type). From Wilander,[27] with permission.

tional in differentiation. Such carcinoids are thought to arise from a less-differentiated precursor cell. Anatomic studies on the turnover of normal intestinal mucosal cells have shown that the crypt base cell gives rise to both exocrine and endocrine epithelial cells.[21] These findings explain the existence of mixed glandular and endocrine cell tumors, which are mainly found in the appendix[1] but occasionally also in the stomach.[22,23]

The exact mechanism that triggers neoplastic proliferation is not known, but hereditary factors and certain local microenvironmental features may play a role. The association of carcinoid tumors with the hereditary syndromes of von Recklinghausen's neurofibromatosis[24] and multiple endocrine neoplasia (MEN)I[25] indicates the importance of genetic factors, at least in some cases.

The unexpectedly frequent association of gastric carcinoid tumors, especially nonantral carcinoids, with chronic atrophic gastritis and achlorhydria with or without concurrent pernicious anemia[20,26-28] suggests a causal relationship. Among 123 patients with pernicious anemia, endoscopic screening detected carcinoid tumors in 5 patients, an incidence of 4%, and biopsies showed endocrine cell hyperplasia in one-third.[26] Of all gastric carcinoids, up to 66% develop in achlorhydric stomachs.[28] Achlorhydria produces hypergastrinemia, and gastrin has been shown to have a trophic effect on gastric ECL cells.[29,30] This stimulation coupled with the carcinogenic effect of nitrosamines, which are found in increased concentrations as gas-

tric acid decreases, is thought to play a major role in the pathogenesis of nonantral gastric carcinoids of the argyrophil ECL-cell type (Fig. 9-1). This hypothesis would also explain the occurrence of diffuse ECL-cell hyperplasia and the multiplicity of tumors found in some of the reported cases,[20,31] as well as the absence of reports of gastric carcinoids in patients with antral resection.[32]

Gastric Carcinoid Tumors

Incidence

Gastric carcinoid tumors are relatively rare, representing only 0.3% of all gastric neoplasms and 2 to 6% of all gastrointestinal carcinoids.[33,34] There is a high incidence of second malignancies in patients with gastrointestinal carcinoids, variously reported as 11%[33] and 20%.[35]

The first report by Askanazy of a gastric carcinoid appeared in the German literature in 1923.[36] By 1975, 155 cases had appeared in the literature.[37] This rarity seems more apparent than real considering the frequency with which gastric carcinoids are misdiagnosed as carcinomas. Ten previously undiagnosed carcinoid tumors were discovered in a retrospective study of 140 gastric carcinomas, yielding an error rate of 7%.[38] Atypical variants of carcinoid tumors[39] in particular may easily be mistaken for carcinomas. Such errors will be diminished in the future as reliable, commercially available markers for endocrine cells and tumors, such as neuron-specific enolase[10] and chromogranin,[40] are applied in diagnostic pathology with increased frequency.

Clinical Presentation

Symptoms of gastric carcinoid tumors are those of any gastric neoplasm. Epigastric pain, melena, and bleeding secondary to ulceration are frequently reported. Bleeding may be massive. Hormonally, most gastric carcinoids are silent (i.e., they produce no amines and polypeptides or amounts too small to cause symptoms).[1] The carcinoid syndrome of diarrhea, flushing, cardiac lesions, and asthma-like attacks was seen in only 5 of 79 cases[28] and is often typical in that flushing is characterized by lobster-red splotches with sharp serpentine margins over the face, neck, and upper extremities, rather than the more diffuse cyanotic discoloration seen in the carcinoid syndrome of midgut carcinoids. Flushing tends to last longer and is elicited by eating, ethanol consumption, and emotional stress and is accompanied by lacrimation and itching of the flushed area. Symptoms are caused by 5-hydroxytryptophan rather than 5-hydroxytraptamine (serotonin) and by large amounts of histamine.[1,37] Flushing attacks can be prevented by histamine antagonists.[41]

Rare gastric carcinoid tumors are gastrinomas and associated with the Zollinger-Ellison syndrome, which is characterized by gastric hypersecretion, intractable peptic ulceration, and diarrhea and steatorrhea or, in 25% of cases, produces only mild symptoms of chronic diarrhea and steatorrhea.[1] In approximately one-quarter of cases, gastrinoma is part of MEN type I and other endocrine symptoms will be present. Rarely, gastric carcinoid tumors may secrete adrenocorticotropic hormone (ACTH) and clinically present as Cushing's syndrome.[42]

Diagnosis

Since the majority of gastric carcinoids are endocrinologically silent, the diagnosis is usually not made clinically but at autopsy or at surgery. Even functional carcinoid tumors produce their characteristic symptoms usually only after metastatic dissemination has occurred, because vasoactive amines produced by the primary tumor are inactivated in the liver. Functioning gastrin-secreting tumors, however, may be small and without metastases and yet produce symptoms, presumably due to the high physiologic potential of small quantities of hormone.[1]

Neuron-specific enolase, a marker of neuroendocrine cells and neurons of all organs, has been shown to be elevated in the serum in patients with neuroendocrine tumors with metastases or a heavy tumor burden.[10] A positive radioimmunoassay, however, only signifies the presence of a neuroendocrine tumor but does not allow determination of its type and origin.

Small polypoid carcinoids are now detected with increased frequency by fiberoptic endoscopy. They present as small, usually multiple and less than 1 cm in diameter, sessile reddish polyps with a small ulceration on top. Although endoscopically these polypoid carcinoids are usually thought to be benign gastric polyps, the correct diagnosis can be made histologically.[9,24]

Pathology

Gross Pathology

In the older literature, gastric carcinoid tumors were reported to be most commonly found in the antrum, and to be single.[43] In the newer literature, body or fundus are cited as the most common location[44] and multiplicity of lesions is reported frequently.[9,24,25,37] It is uncertain whether these differences represent true changes in biologic behavior. More likely, they reflect the greater detection rate of fiberoptic gastroscopy and greater diagnostic accuracy of the pathologist utilizing immunohistochemical stains. Most of the carcinoid tumors that are multiple are of the ECL-cell argyrophil type, occur in the body of the stomach, and are associated with diffuse or nodular endocrine

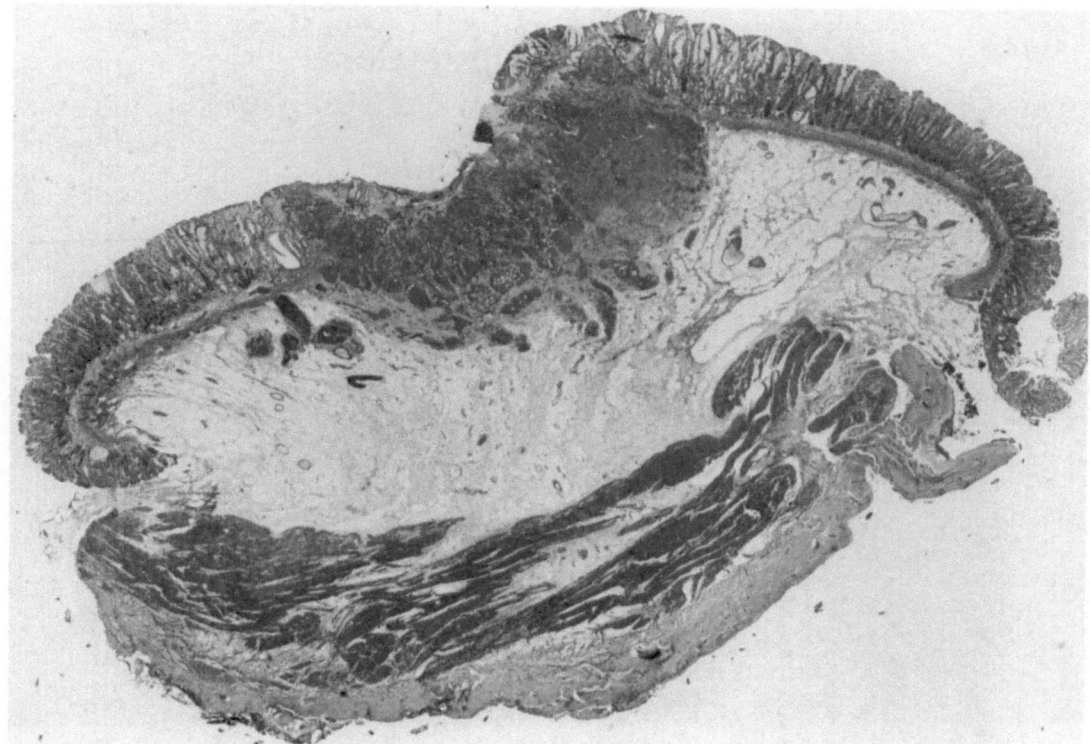

Figure 9-2. Carcinoid tumor of the stomach. Central ulceration is present. Tumor involves mucosa and parts of the submucosa. H&E, X4, reproduced at 95%.

cell hyperplasia.[20,27,44] Sizes vary from a few millimeters to 12 cm or more. Small tumors are polypoid, nodular umbilicated lesions with a smooth surface and central ulceration (Fig. 9-2). The cut surface is frequently yellow, but at times rather tan or gray.[34]

Light Microscopy

Histologically, the typical gastric carcinoid is composed of uniform, relatively small round to polygonal cells arranged in trabeculae, nests, ribbons, and occasionally glands infiltrating normal glands, smooth muscle, or submucosal collagen bundles (Fig. 9-3). Acinar structures may show luminal mucin. Squamous metaplasia has been observed. Spindle-shaped tumor cells may be mistaken for mesenchymal cells.[1] Cellular pleomorph-

ism is mild and mitotic figures are inapparent. Nuclei are uniform and round to oval and have finely stippled chromatin (Fig. 9-4). No information is available on the nuclear DNA patterns of gastric carcinoids. Of 22 intestinal carcinoids, however, 21 were found to be diploid.[45] Some gastric carcinoid tumors exhibit atypical cytologic and histologic patterns that may be difficult to distinguish from ordinary carcinoma[25] (see below). Intracytoplasmic granules, the hallmark of carcinoid tumors, are not visible in routine stains. Methods of visualization are formaldehyde-induced fluorescence, silver stains, immunoperoxidase stains, and electron microscopy. The stroma is often abundant and hyalinized and may show ossification.[37] Mast cells have been reported to be increased in the stroma as well as in the adjacent basal gastric glands.[46]

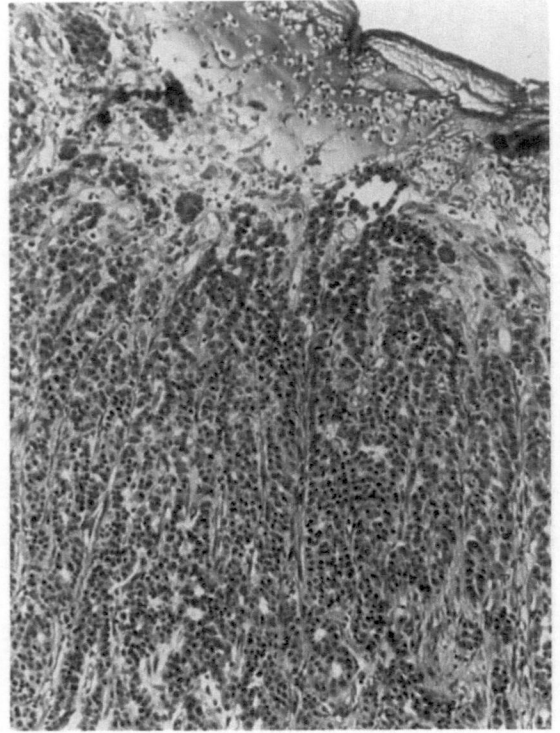

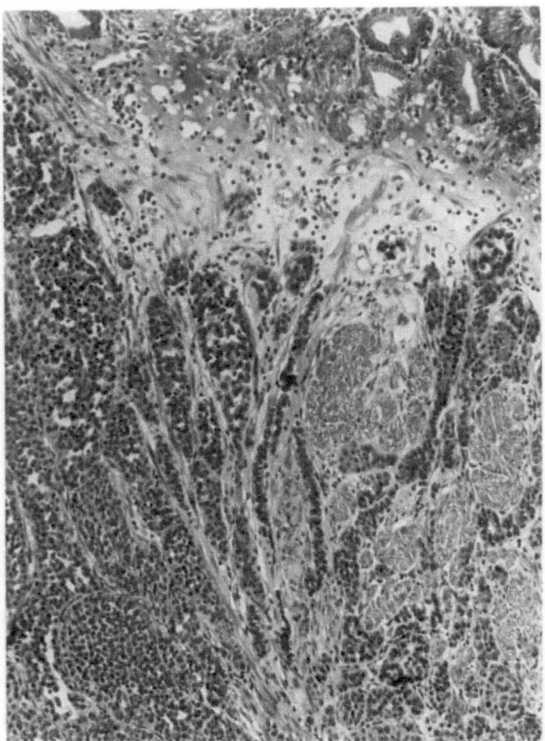

Figure 9-3. Carcinoid tumor of the stomach. H&E, X100, reproduced at 70%. **A.** Trabecular growth pattern adjacent to the ulcerated surface.

B. Nesting and glandular pattern in the deeper part invading the muscularis mucosae.

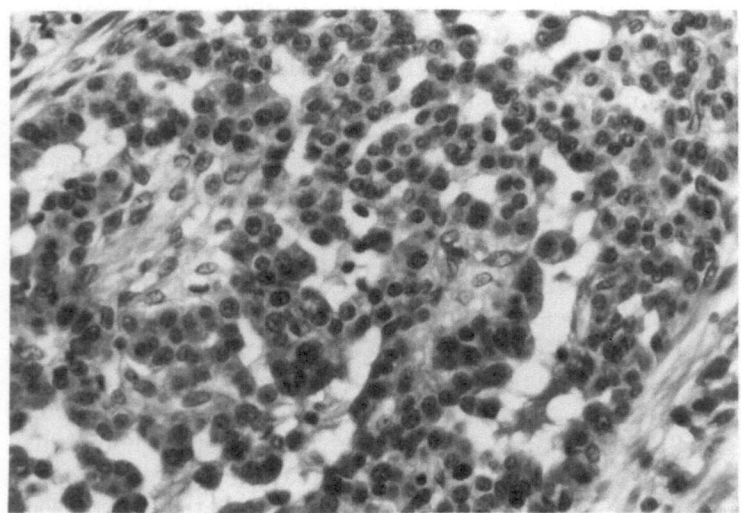

Figure 9-4. Carcinoid tumor of stomach. Nuclei are uniform and round. H&E, X250, reproduced at 85%.

Silver Stains and Immunoreactivity

Gastric carcinoid tumors are of foregut derivation and therefore characteristically argyrophil, that is, they bind silver ions after the addition of a reducing agent (argentaffin cells, in contrast, do not require a reducing agent) (Fig. 9-5). Argyrophil stains such as Sevier-Munger, Grimelius, Pascual, and Churukian-Schenk differ slightly in their sensitivity, and the latter has proved most reliable in demonstrating carcinoid granules.[47] With this most sensitive technique, even those gastric carcinoid tumors that failed to react with the other argyrophil stains were shown to contain cytoplasmic granules. Although generally considered argentaffin negative, some gastric carcinoids are positive with the Fontana-Masson argentaffin reaction. There is no correlation between silver staining characteristics and the histologic grade of the tumor.

The chemical basis of argyrophil staining methods is unknown, but acid sialoglycopeptides with one to four glycoside bonds may play a role. It is important to remember that a variety of other intracytoplasmic substances are argyrophilic and may be mistaken for endocrine granules. These substances include lipofuscin, mucin, and glycogen.[11] Distinctive features of argyrophil endocrine granules are their tendency to cluster at one side of the cell and their relatively even size. It is also important to remember that argyrophilic endocrine granules are not diagnostic of carcinoid tumors per se, but are also found in other neuroendocrine tumors such as pituitary adenomas, pheochromocytomas, and medullary thyroid carcinomas.[11]

Among the many immunohistochemical stains applied to carcinoid tumors, the two most consistently positive are those for neuron-specific enolase[10] and for chromogranin.[40] Neuron-specific enolase is the major enzyme of glycolysis and present in all thus far identified peptide- or amine-containing endocrine cells, as well as in neurons and peripheral nerves and nerves of the gut wall.

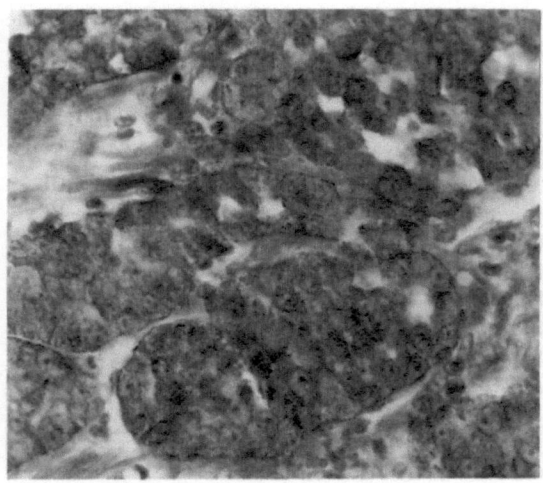

Figure 9-5. Carcinoid tumor of stomach. Cytoplasmic granules are typically argyrophil. Grimelius, X400, reproduced at 66%.

It serves as a marker of all neuroendocrine tumors, including carcinoid tumors, neuroblastomas, medullary thyroid carcinomas, melanomas, and pheochromocytomas. Its staining is positive regardless of the histologic grade, hormonal activity, or type of secretory product. Radioimmunoassay has been employed to demonstrate increased levels in tumor tissue and increased serum levels in metastatic disease. Serum levels of neuron-specific enolase correlate with tumor burden and can be used to monitor postoperative patients.

Chromogranin is a protein first detected in the adrenal medulla and later shown to occur also in the endocrine cells of the gut.[40] Its function is not clear, but is thought to involve stabilization of complexes within neuroendocrine granules. It represents the most recently detected marker for carcinoid tumors, and like neuron-specific enolase is not specific for gastrointestinal tumors.

Most gastric carcinoid tumors are nonfunctional, but immunoreactivity to a variety of biogenic amines and polypeptide hormones can be demonstrated in some of them despite the lack of endocrine symptoms. This dis-

Table 9-2. Proteins, Amines, and Polypeptide Hormones Identified by Immunohistochemistry in Gastric Carcinoid Tumors

Secretory Product	Occurrence	Reference
Neuron-specific enolase	Always	10
Chromogranin	Always	40
Gastrin	Sometimes	49
5-Hydroxytryptophan	Sometimes	37
Histamine	Sometimes	37
Serotonin	Rarely	48
Noradrenalin	Rarely	48
Adrenalin	Rarely	48
Adrenocorticotropic hormone	Rarely	50
α-Melanotropin	Rarely	52
Neurotensin	Rarely	51
α₁-Antitrypsin	Rarely	54
Peptide YY	Rarely	53

crepancy can be explained by the production of biologically inactive products, rapid degradation, or intermittent release of biologically active products, and lack of recognition of subtle clinical symptomatology.[11] Immunoreactivity for a given substance is rarely uniform within a tumor and may change over the course of the disease in recurring or metastatic lesions. Usually tumors express the hormonal profile of their precursor cells, but ectopic hormones do occur. It is advisable to stain each gastric carcinoid tumor with a variety of histochemical stains, if available, including those for hydroxytryptophan, histamine, serotonin, gastrin, and ACTH.

Hydroxytryptophan and histamine have been demonstrated in gastric and duodenal carcinoid tumors associated with the atypical carcinoid syndrome described previously.[1,37] 5-hydroxytryptamine (serotonin) is usually not produced by gastric carcinoids, but was demonstrated in one case in conjunction with noradrenalin and adrenalin.[48] Gastrin is present in gastrinomas, most of which arise in the pancreas and duodenum, but some of which originate in the gastric antrum as well as in such unusual primary sites as mesentery and liver.[49] Some gastri-

nomas are multihormonal and also produce adrenocorticotropin-like peptides, which may give rise to Cushing's syndrome,[50] and neurotensin, which may be demonstrable in the serum even before clinical symptoms are manifest.[51] Alpha-melanotropin-like peptides have been identified in normal human gastrin cells[52] and are likely, if sought, to be discovered in G-cell carcinoids.

Peptide YY, a gut hormone with molecular structure and biologic activity similar to that of pancreatic polypeptide (inhibition of jejunal and colonic motility, intestinal vasoconstriction, inhibition of pancreatic exocrine and gastric acid secretion, and reduction of interdigestive gastric contractile activity), has been identified immunohistochemically in 1 of 13 gastric carcinoid tumors as well as in other intestinal carcinoid tumors, all but one of which were argyrophil.[53] Normally, endocrine cells with immunoreactivity for peptide YY are confined to the small and large intestine, but in the one case of gastric carcinoid positive for peptide YY, adjacent nonneoplastic endocrine cells were also positive, suggesting that the tumor arose from ectopic endocrine cells rather than that the tumor produced an ectopic hormone.

Alpha-1-antitrypsin immunoreactivity has been demonstrated in human islet cells in gastric and intestinal mucosal cells and in argyrophil gastric carcinoid tumors that were negative pancreatic and gastric homones.[54] Cytoplasmic granules were periodic acid-Schiff (PAS) positive due to the glycoprotein nature of alpha-1-antitrypsin.

Monoamine oxidase activity can be measured in tumor homogenates and was found to be significantly higher in foregut carcinoids than in midgut carcinoids. Conversely, elevated levels of diamine oxidase activity are typical for midgut carcinoids. Such tests may be helpful in determining an unknown primary site from a metastatic lesion.[55]

Table 9-2 summarizes the proteins, amines, and polypeptide hormones that have so far been identified histochemically in gastric carcinoid tumors. Since carcinoid tumors in general often produce ectopic hormones, the list is likely to grow.

Electron Microscopy

The hallmark of neuroendocrine tumors of any type and localization is the presence of neuroendocrine granules, which are present ultrastructurally even in those cases that are neither argyrophil nor argentaffin and show no immunoreactivity for any of the known biogenic amines or polypeptide hormones. Neuroendocrine granules usually resemble their normal mucosal counterparts, but may show heterogeneity of granule size, shape, and electron density.[1] Less well-differentiated carcinoid tumors show increasingly sparse and immature granules.

Neuroendocrine granules are composed of an electron-dense core surrounded by a halo and a limiting membrane. Granules are usually clustered near one pole of the cell, a feature that is helpful in differentiating poorly formed granules from lysosomes (Fig. 9-6).

Rare carcinoid tumors of the antropyloric region contain intracellular fibrillary bodies.[56] These are composed of wavy, sometimes branching filaments 100 Å thick that form parallel bundles, whorls, or concentric rings. Electron-dense secretory granules are usually seen within the fibrillary bodies. Extracellular fibrils with ultrastructural and staining characteristics of amyloid may be seen in rare carcinoid tumors of the gastric body or antrum.[56]

Prognosis

Gastric carcinoid tumors are intermediate in behavior between the more aggressive small intestinal and colonic carcinoids and the indolent appendiceal carcinoids.[43] The incidence of metastasis at the time of diagnosis is 17% as compared to 35% for small intestinal carcinoids and 2.9% for appendiceal carcinoids. Regional lymph node metastasis is still compatible with cure. Only one of nine patients with gastric carcinoid tumors died of metastatic disease after 21 months. The primary tumor measured 10 cm and liver

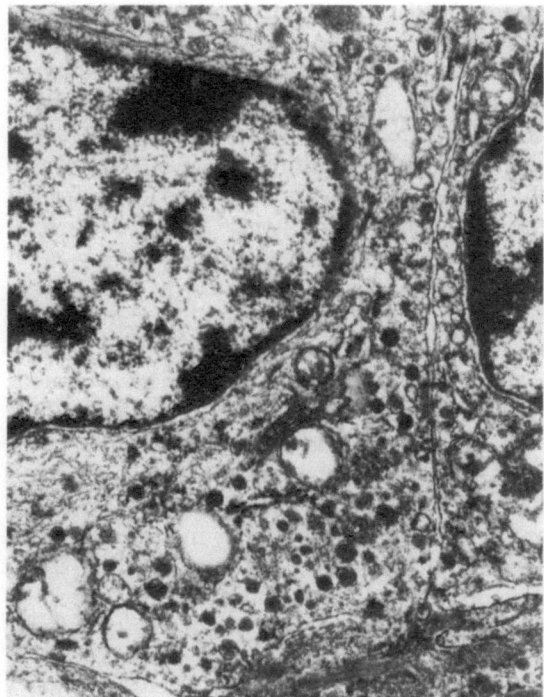

Figure 9-6. Electron micrograph of gastric carcinoid. Neuroendocrine granules are clustered near one pole of the tumor cell. X5000, reproduced at 95%.

metastases were present. Patients with carcinoid tumors less than 2 cm in diameter are usually cured by local excision or partial gastric resection.

Special Types of Gastric Carcinoid Tumors

ECL-Cell Carcinoids

ECL-cell carcinoids are derived from enterochromaffin-like cells, the major gastrin-dependent endocrine cell of the body of the stomach. ECL-cell carcinoids, therefore, always arise in the body. They are usually multiple, small polypoid lesions, often associated with ECL-cell hyperplasia and so-called "microcarcinoids" (i.e., microscopic nests of ECL cells). They are the major type of carcinoid tumor that arises in chronic atrophic gastritis and pernicious anemia.[25-28,31]

Argyrophilia and nests and cords of bland cuboidal cells are seen histologically. Poly-peptide hormones are usually not demonstra-ble, but 5-hydroxytryptophan and histamine are frequently secreted and, if present in sufficiently large amounts, can give rise to the atypical carcinoid syndrome (see Clinical Presentation). Cytoplasmic granules have an average diameter of 200 nm and may be of two types: the predominant type has a fairly dense core, often eccentrically placed,[27] an electron-lucent halo, and a limiting mem-brane; the less frequent type has a denser core and no halo.[31]

In spite of the bland histologic appearance and small size of most ECL-cell carcinoid tumors, invasion into the muscularis propria or serosa and lymph node metastasis have been described.[26,31] Total removal of these lesions is therefore mandatory, by endoscopy if possible, otherwise by laparotomy.[26] Their long-term behavior is not yet known.

Gastrinomas
Gastrinomas of the stomach are much rarer than gastrinomas of the pancreas and duode-num. They are derived from G cells, which, in the stomach, are strictly confined to the antropyloric region. Gastric gastrinomas, therefore, arise only in the distal stomach, where they have been described as small (1 to 2 cm in diameter) polypoid lesions that, despite their size, may already have metasta-sized to the liver at the time of diagnosis.[49] The histology, histochemistry, and ultrastuc-ture of gastrinomas are discussed under Duo-denal Carcinoids.

Gastric Atypical Carcinoid and Neuroendocrine Carcinoma
Gastric atypical carcinoid and neuroendo-crine carcinoma (i.e., moderately and poorly differentiated carcinoid tumors) comprises a spectrum of neuroendocrine tumors with varying degrees of differentiation that has long been recognized in the lung.[57,58] Whether we refer to these as carcinoid, atypi-cal carcinoid,[39] and oat cell carcinoma,[59] or well differentiated, moderately differenti-ated, and poorly differentiated carcinoid[1] or

as neuroendocrinoma[7] and neuroendocrine carcinoma[8,58] is less relevant than the prog-nostic importance of these variations in dif-ferentiation, especially in comparison with ordinary carcinoma with which these tumors are frequently confused. The 5-year survival rate of 10 patients with atypical gastric carci-noids, for example, was 70% as compared to 15% for patients with gastric carcinoma of the same extent.[38]

Atypical Carcinoid Tumor
Atypical carcinoid tumor is intermediate in differentiation between the typical carcinoid and the poorly differentiated carcinoid or neuroendocrine carcinoma. The true fre-quency of this lesion is unknown since many seem to be misdiagnosed as adenocarci-noma.[39] Features that distinguish atypical carcinoids from adenocarcinoma include the characteristic pattern of interlacing trabe-culae (which, although poorly developed or absent in some areas, remains recognizable in other areas), ultrastructural evidence of neuroendocrine granules (present in all cases so far studied[39]), and argyrophilia (present in 9 of 14 cases reported).[38,39] Variable amounts of mucin may be present and should not be taken as evidence of adenocarcinoma. From the limited number of cases available, it seems that mixed forms of carcinoid and adenocarcinoma behave as carcinoids, as long as the carcinoid pattern predominates.[38]

Cytologically, atypical carcinoids show more cellular pleomorphism than typical carcinoids and large nuclei. Mitotic activity was inapparent in atypical carcinoid tumors with a long survival.[38] Some cases reported under the designation of "atypical carcinoid" showed many mitoses, necrosis, and wide-spread disease and should instead be classi-fied as poorly differentiated carcinoids.[39]

Gastric Neuroendocrine Carcinoma
Gastric neuroendocrine carcinoma was first described in 1976 from Japan under the name oat cell carcinoma to stress the histologic, histogenetic, and prognostic similarities to the pulmonary counterpart. Subsequently reported cases appeared in the literature

under the designation of neuroendocrine carcinoma,[8] atypical carcinoid,[37] and extrapulmonary oat cell carcinoma.[59] The stomach is a rare primary site, not only in contrast to the lung but also in comparison to other parts of the gastrointestinal tract such as the esophagus, where oat cell carcinoma has been reported with greater frequency.[1,59] In Japan, 4 oat cell carcinomas were found in a review of 2000 gastric carcinomas.[60]

There is no preferred location within the stomach. Most cases presented with large, ulcerated masses with complete transmural penetration and regional and/or distant metastases. Survival ranged from 1 to 16 months.[8]

Histologically, the tumor resembles oat cell carcinoma of the lung and is composed of small cells packed into solid nests, sometimes with an organoid pattern. Large and intermediate-sized cells with vesicular nuclei, spindle cells, rare giant cells, and glandular arrangements have been described. Rare tumors are mixed and show dual differentiation into adenocarcinoma and poorly differentiated carcinoid.[59] Argyrophil granules were demonstrated in some cases.[39,57] ACTH and calcitonin production has been described in esophageal oat cell carcinomas, but not thus far in gastric tumors.[1] Vanillylmandelic acid and 5-hydroxy-3-indole-acetic acid was present in large amounts in tumor extracts in two cases.[7]

Neuroendocrine granules were present in small numbers in all tumors examined ultrastructurally.[37,59] Sizes varied from 80 to 250 nm. Filaments resembling cytokeratin and intracytoplasmic lumina are sometimes recognized.

The prognosis is dismal. Of 11 patients with documented disease, 9 died within a year with metastases to lymph nodes, liver, and pancreas. Two patients were alive 2 and 5 years after surgery.[37,59]

Mixed (Composite) Carcinoid Tumors
Mixed (composite) carcinoid tumors, regardless of their degree of differentiation, may be mixed with glandular and even squamous elements. Most of these arise in the appendix, where they have been described under a variety of names such as goblet cell carcinoid, adenocarcinoid, or mucinous carcinoid. In the stomach, scattered argyrophil cells are found in 3.1% of all carcinoma and in 7% of carcinomas of the diffuse type.[22] Tumors should only be classified as mixed, however, if there is a significant proportion of both elements. Scirrhous carcinomas show a diffuse admixture of argyrophil cells in more than one-quarter of cases and stain with antisera to gastrin, somatostatin, glucagon, serotonin, carcinoembryonic antigen, human chorionic gonadotropin, lysozyme, and acid mucin.[61] No hormonal syndrome was encountered in these cases.

Truly composite carcinomas with approximately equal volumes of carcinoid tumor and adenocarcinomas are rare in the stomach, and only few cases have been reported.[21,62,63] Among eight such composite tumors of the gastrointestinal tract, only one was located in the stomach.[62] The carcinoid part was negative for argyrophil and argentaffin granules, but showed immunocytochemical evidence of serotonin production. Ultrastructurally, the same tumor cell may contain neuroendocrine granules and mucin globules.[63] A rare type of mixed carcinoid–adenocarcinoma was described in Japan.[21] The tumor showed a uniform tubular growth pattern, and silver staining demonstrated the main component to be argentaffin cells and the lesser component argyrophil and mucin-producing columnar cells. There was abundant fibrous stroma. The tumor was located primarily submucosally, the overlying mucosa either remaining normal or ulcerated. The muscularis propria was infiltrated, but there was no evidence of nodal or distant metastases. No follow-up is available.

Duodenal Carcinoid Tumors
Incidence

Duodenal carcinoid tumors are still rarer than gastric carcinoid tumors and constitute

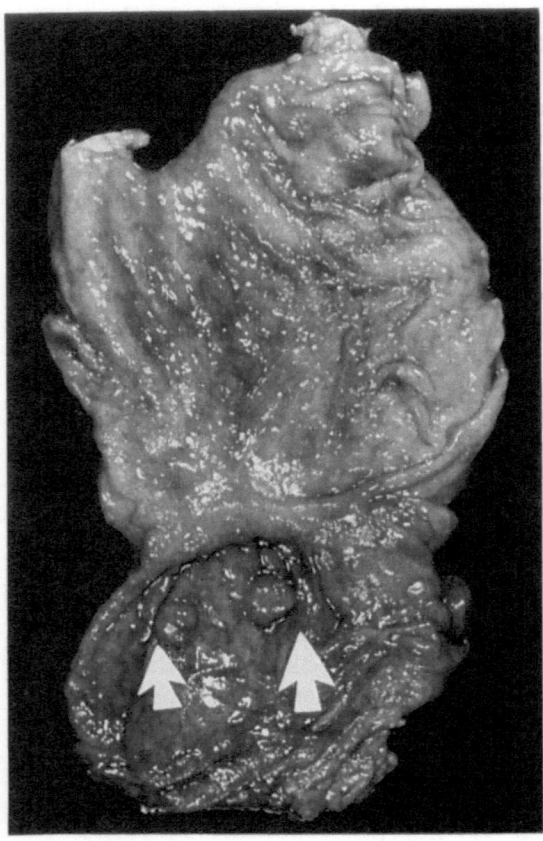

Figure 9-7. Duodenal carcinoids. Two sessile poly-poid lesions are present near the pylorus.

between 1 and 1.5% of all gastrointestinal carcinoids.[34,43] The proportion of carcinoid tumors among all duodenal malignancies is 1.6%.[43] Thirteen percent of patients with the Zollinger-Ellison syndrome have a duodenal gastrinoma, either alone or combined with pancreatic tumors.[64] Patients with von Reck-linghausen's disease have an unusual predis-position for developing duodenal carcinoids, especially in the region of the papilla of Vater. Fifteen such cases were collected in the literature in 1986,[65] but the overall inci-dence is not known.

Clinical Presentation

In contrast to the nonspecific symptoms of most gastric carcinoid tumors, those in the duodenum more often produce a rather spe-cific complex of symptoms. Approximately one-half of all patients present with endo-crine symptoms, one-third with mechanical obstruction, and some with bleeding or pain.[65] Obstructive jaundice may be the first sign of ampullary lesions.[43] In a series of 12 cases of duodenal carcinoids, 2 were detected incidentally.[65]

Four types of endocrinologically mediated syndromes may occur: the Zollinger-Ellison syndrome, the carcinoid syndrome, the gluca-gonoma syndrome, and the somatostatinoma syndrome.[65] The Zollinger-Ellison syndrome presents with peptic ulcer disease and hyper-gastrinemia, which may be due to either one or multiple gastrinomas (90%) or G-cell hyperplasia (10%). In 13% of cases a duodenal gastrinoma is found.[64] One-third to one-half of patients with duodenal gastrinoma is found.[64] One-third to one-half of patients with duodenal carcinoid tumors develop Zol-linger-Ellison syndrome.[65,66] Not all carci-noid tumors that produce immunoreactive gastrin, however, are associated with the syn-drome.[17] In such cases, either the amount of gastrin is too small or, more likely, the form of gastrin is an ineffective precursor mole-cule. Rare cases of Zollinger-Ellison syn-drome also have Cushing's syndrome, either due to a pituitary adenoma occurring in patients with MEN I or due to ACTH produc-tion by the gastrinoma.[50]

The carcinoid syndrome accompanying rare cases of duodenal carcinoid is atypical and resembles that seen in patients with gastric carcinoids (see above). It is due to elevated serum levels of 5-hydroxytryptophan and histamine rather than serotonin.

Glucagon-secreting carcinoid tumors have been described to present with a necrolytic migratory erythematous skin rash, anemia, and angular stomatitis with or without ac-companying diabetes mellitus.[67] Most gluca-gonomas arise in the pancreas, but occasion-ally they may originate in the duodenum.[68]

The somatostatinoma syndrome, charac-terized by diabetes mellitus, diarrhea, stea-torrhea, hypochlorhydria or achlorhydria, weight loss, cholelithiasis, and anemia, develops in patients with pancreatic tumors

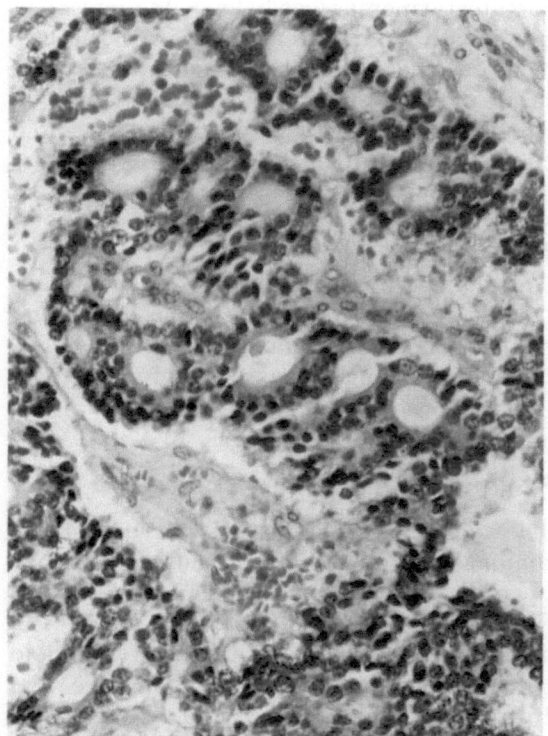

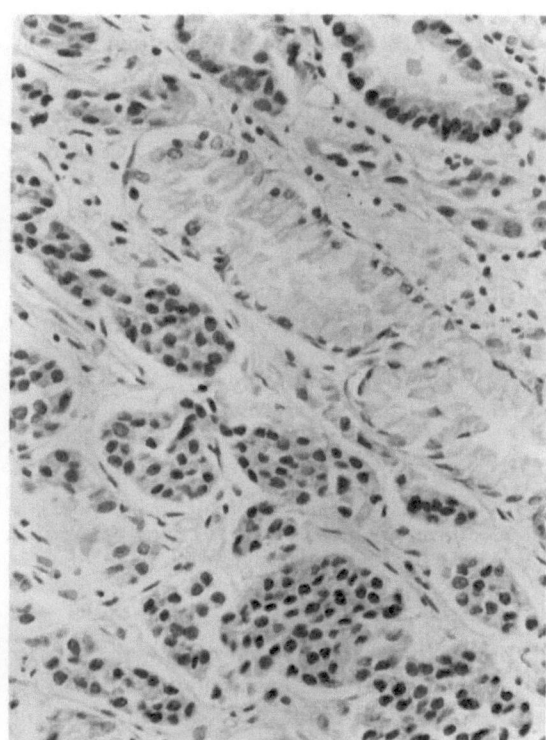

Figure 9-8. Metastatic carcinoid tumor in the liver. Note acinar pattern. The primary tumor was not detected until autopsy (see Fig. 9-9). H&E, X250, reproduced at 63%.

Figure 9-9. Duodenal carcinoid. This tumor, 6 mm in diameter, was the only primary found at autopsy in the case demonstrated in Fig. 9-8. H&E, X100, reproduced at 63%.

composed entirely or predominantly of somatostatin-producing D cells.[15,16] Although a number of somatostatinomas of duodenal origin have been described, none of these was associated with the above clinical features. Perhaps the hormone secreted was a biologically less active form, or perhaps duodenal tumors become symptomatic earlier than pancreatic tumors because of obstructive jaundice and bleeding.[15,16,23]

One percent of duodenal carcinoid tumors secrete insulin and present with episodes of hypoglycemia, either occurring spontaneously or induced by prolonged fasting.[69]

Pathology

Gross Pathology

Duodenal carcinoid tumors have a predilection for the first and second portions, especially the periampullary area.[65] They may be single or multiple and are usually small (less than 2 cm in diameter) submucosal sessile or pedunculated lesions (Fig. 9-7). The cut surface is yellow or tan. Lymph node metastases were present in one-quarter of such small lesions.[63]

Light Microscopy

Histologically, tumor cells grow in nests, ribbons, anastomosing trabeculae, or tubular structures, in decreasing order of frequency. Usually several growth patterns coexist within the same tumor, and metastases may differ in pattern from that of the primary tumor (Figs. 9-8 and 9-9). Tumor cells are polygonal with finely granulated eosinophilic cytoplasm that may be vacuolated. Nuclei are sometimes conspicuously polarized. Mitoses are rare and significant nuclear

Table 9-.3. Proteins, Polypeptide Hormones, and Amines Identified by Immunohistochemistry in Duodenal Carcinoid Tumors

Secretory Product	Occurrence	Reference
NSE	Always	10
Chromogranin	Always	40
Gastrin	Often	62,63
Somatostatin	Often	15,63
Progastrin	Rarely	68
Calcitonin	Rarely	63
Insulin	Rarely	67
Glucagon	Rarely	66
ACTH	Rarely	24,50
Serotonin	Rarely	24
VIP	Rarely	63
PP	Rarely	64

Abbreviations: NSE, neuron-specific enolase; ACTH, adrenocorticotropic hormone; VIP, vasoactive intestinal polypeptide; PP, pancreatic polypeptide.

atypia is uncommon, except for rare poorly differentiated tumors (see below). The fibrous stroma is delicate and well vascularized and usually not hyalinized. Psammoma bodies are characteristically present in somatostatin-producing carcinoid tumors. Concentric calcifications form primarily within glandular lumina from secretory products[16] or intracellularly.[67] Psammoma body formation is not exclusive for duodenal somatostatinomas but has been observed in 8% of carcinoid tumors of the gastroeteropancreatic axis, especially in those of the pancreas, small intestine, and appendix, in decreasing order of frequency.[67]

Silver Stains and Immunoreactivity
Duodenal carcinoid tumors are of foregut derivation, and most contain argyrophil granules.[47] Rarely, argentaffin cells are intermixed.[65] They are positive for neuron-specific enolase and chromogranin.[10,40] Secretory products identified by immunohistochemistry are summarized in Table 9-3. Immunoreactive gastrin and somatostatin are the two most frequently encountered polypeptide hormones[65] and, if present in the majority of cells, the tumors are termed gastrinomas or

somatostatinomas (see below). As mentioned previously, immunoreactivity in tissue sections does not always correspond with serum levels or with endocrine clinical manifestations.[1] The majority of duodenal carcinoid tumors are multihormonal, although one hormone usually predominates.

Electron Microscopy
Neuroendocrine granules are present in all lesions. Most granules are similar in size and shape to those of normal gastrin-producing G cells and somatostatin-producing D cells (see below).

Prognosis

The incidence of metastasis at the time of diagnosis of duodenal carcinoid tumor has been variously reported as 16%[43] and 33%.[65] Such data are based on small numbers of cases and include special types of carcinoid tumors described below. Lymph node and liver metastases have occurred in tumors less than 1 cm in diameter,[65] as proved by one of our cases (Figs. 9-8 and 9-9). Especially if multiple, carcinoid tumors only a few millimeters in size may have spread already to regional lymph nodes. No long-term follow-up data are available.

Special Types of Duodenal Carcinoid Tumors

Gastrinoma
Gastrinomas are carcinoid tumors that are predominantly or entirely composed of gastrin-producing G cells, identified as much by immunohistochemistry[65] and/or the demonstration of elevated serum gastrin levels that revert to normal after removal of the tumor.[11] Hypergastrinemia in itself is not diagnostic of gastrinoma, since it is present in a variety of other conditions such as pernicious anemia, atrophic gastritis, gastric ulcers, daily use of antacids, anticholinergics, or histamine H_2-receptor antagonists, renal failure, retained excluded antrum, pyloric stenosis, antral G-cell hyperplasia,

and short bowel syndrome.[11] The most common primary site of gastrinoma is the pancreas; however, 13% of gastrinomas arise in the duodenum, mostly in the second portion, and of these, half are associated with gastrinomas elsewhere.[64] In a series of 12 duodenal carcinoid tumors, 5 were gastrinomas and 4 developed the Zollinger-Ellison syndrome.[65] Gastrinomas, even those are endocrinologically symptomatic, may be only a few millimeters in diameter and difficult to find endoscopically and surgically even when metastasis is already manifest.[49] Endoscopically excised lesions are often mistaken for a common polyp.[9,11]

Histologically, duodenal gastrinomas present as mucosal or submucosal infiltrative lesions composed of orderly, uniform, cuboidal cells with oval nuclei arranged in clusters, glands, and festoons[10,17] (Fig. 9-10). The close resemblance to normal islet cells led to the histologic classification of some of these lesions as islet cell adenomas.[11] Amyloid is sometimes present in the stroma.[17]

Silver staining is variable. Argyrophilia is more common than positive argentaffin staining,[65] but several tumors stained with neither technique, suggesting that at times hormone is released so quickly that little or no granule storage occurs.[9,13]

In addition to gastrin, some gastrinomas have been shown to produce the hexapeptide progastrin.[70] The most common second hormone demonstrable immunohistochemically is somatostatin, which was present in four of five cases studied accordingly. Thirty percent of gastrinomas contain ACTH-like immunoreactivity, and some of these may actually produce enough ACTH to give rise to Cushing's syndrome.[50] ACTH cannot be regarded as an ectopic hormone, since ACTH-like as well as alpha-melanotropin-like peptides have been localized in a subpopulation of cytoplasmic granules of normal gastrin cells.[52]

Electron microscopy shows membrane-bound secretory granules with flocculant contents similar in size and shape to those of normal G cells.[13,65] Irregularly shaped angu-

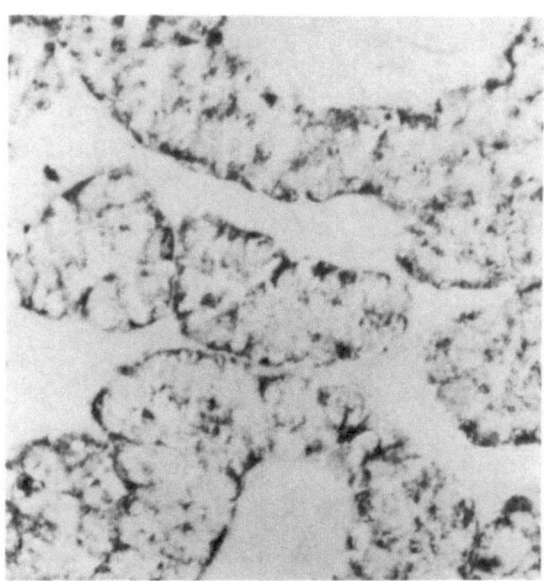

Figure 9-10. Duodenal gastrinoma. Immunoperoxidase stain for gastrin outlines clusters, glands, and festoons of tumor cells. Immunoperoxidase, X250, reproduced at 90%. (Courtesy of Dr. Enrico Solcia, University of Pavia, Italy.)

lar, dense granules of variable size are sometimes also seen[13] especially in gastrinomas immunoreactive for ACTH and alpha-melanotropin.[52] No ultrastructural findings are available for those gastrinomas that lacked endocrine granules on silver staining.[9,10] One gastrinoma associated with local amyloid deposition showed nonbranching, rigid amyloid fibrils in the stroma and cytoplasm of tumor cells.[17]

Gastrinomas are potentially metastasizing, slow-growing, malignant neoplasms. Although disseminated metastatic disease to lymph nodes, liver, spleen, bone, mediastinum, and skin has been described,[1] patients have been reported alive with tumor many years after the initial diagnosis[9] and rarely die from metastasis.[66] Recent surgical cure rates for patients with gastrinoma and the Zollinger-Ellison syndrome have been variously reported between 16 and 39%. The main problem for the surgeon is not resection itself, but localizing the primary tumor. The

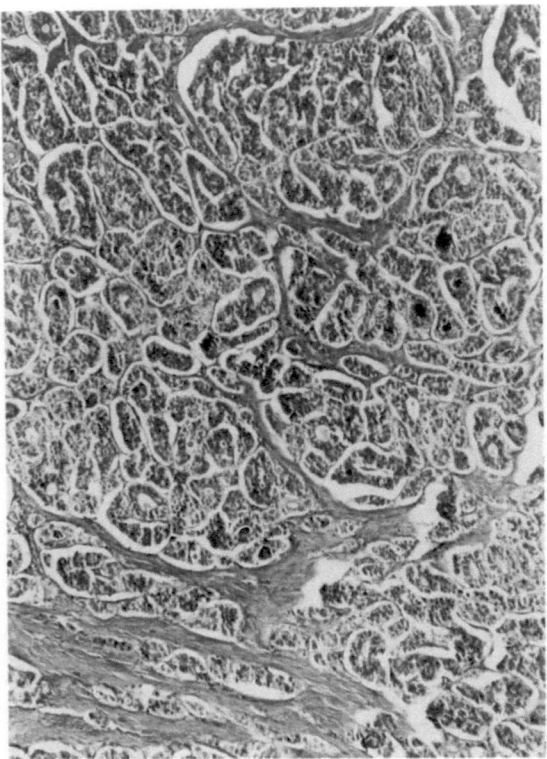

Figure 9-11. Somatostatinoma. The growth pattern is primarily glandular and may be confused with adenocarcinoma. Orderly arrangement, lack of cellular pleomorphism, and psammoma bodies (*arrow*) are characteristic of somatostatinoma. H&E, X100, reproduced at 57%. (Courtesy of Dr. Dayal, New England Medical Center, Boston.)

incidence of occult gastrinoma is 20 to 30% and tends to be less for extrapancreatic than pancreatic gastrinomas.[49]

In 1970 an estimated 60% of gastrinomas had evidence of lymph node or liver metastases at the time of initial exploration.[49] With earlier diagnosis this figure decreased to less than 30% by 1984.[71] These data, collected from gastrinomas at all sites, appear worse than those available for duodenal gastrinomas alone. Among eight duodenal gastrinomas in the recent literature, only one had evidence of lymph node metastasis at the time of diagnosis.[10,11,17,65] Two other cases were reported alive with lymph node metas-

tases 4 years after endoscopic removal of a polypoid duodenal gastrinoma.[9]

Somatostatinoma

Although somatostatin-containing cells may be present in up to one-third of clinically nonfunctioning gastrointestinal carcinoids, somatostatinomas (i.e., carcinoid tumors with a dominant or pure population of somatostatin-containing cells) are rare. Most are located in the pancreas. They arise from the somatostatin-producing D cell or from an undifferentiated precursor cell. In 6 of 12 duodenal carcinoid tumors somatostatin was the predominant secretory product, identified as the only hormone in one case and in association with gastrin in two cases, vasointestinal polypeptide and calcitonin in one case each, and vasointestinal polypeptide and calcitonin in one case.[65] Somatostatinomas in patients with von Recklinghausen's neurofibromatosis are mostly pure (i.e., they produce somatostatin only), whereas similar tumors unassociated with neurofibromatosis are more frequently multihormonal.[24] Detection of a pure somatostatinoma, therefore, should alert one to the possibility of coexistent von Recklinghausen's disease. The somatostatin syndrome of diabetes mellitus, steatorrhea, and cholelithiasis develops frequently in patients with pancreatic tumors but rarely in those with duodenal tumors.[24] Rather, the diagnosis depends on the immunohistochemical identification of somatostatin in the majority of tumor cells, its immunochemical identification in tumor extract, and/or the demonstration of elevated plasma levels. Hypersomatostatinemia may be induced by combined injection of calcium and pentagastrin.[15]

Most duodenal somatostatinomas arise in the vicinity of the ampulla and cause jaundice early, perhaps accounting for the fact that few reach sufficient size to develop the somatostatinoma syndrome.[24] Tumors vary from 0.5 to 4 cm in diameter and, in contrast to gastrinoma, are always single.[15,16,24] They produce an exophytic mass and ulceration of the duodenal mucosa. There is usually deep

Figure 9-12. Somatostatinoma. Note psammoma bodies in glandular lamina. H&E, X250, reproduced at 80%. (Courtesy of Dr. Dayal, New England Medical Center, Boston.)

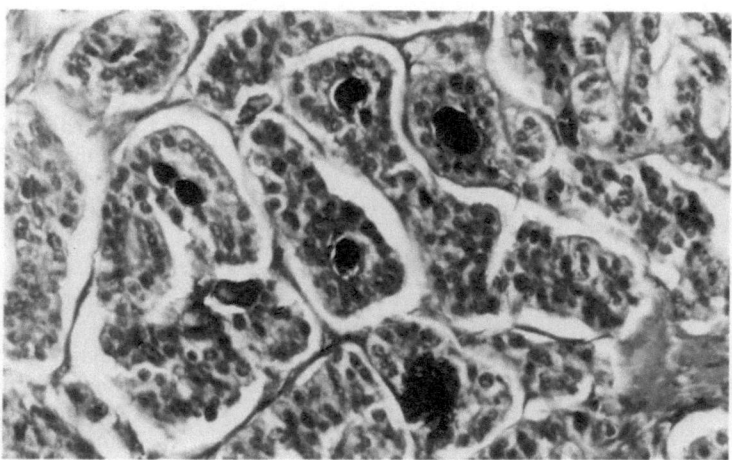

intramural infiltration and lymph node metastasis if lesions are 2 cm in diameter or larger.[24]

Histologically, a mixed architectural pattern with trabecular and glandular areas is found (Fig. 9-11). The glandular element usually predominates and may be mistaken for adenocarcinoma, although the uniformity of the single layered cuboidal epithelium with its granular, pale, eosinophilic cytoplasm and the lack of nuclear atypia and mitotic activity distinguish somatostatinoma from carcinoma. Luminal borders in glandular areas may show diastase-resistent PAS positivity.[24] Psammoma bodies, intensely immunoreactive for somatostatin, may be found within glandular lumina (Fig. 9-12). In the duodenum they are characteristic of somatostatinoma, but their absence does not preclude such a diagnosis.[15,24] Psammoma bodies have also been found in carcinoid tumors elsewhere, especially insulin-producing islet cell tumors of the pancreas and clinically silent carcinoid tumors of stomach, small intestine, colon, and appendix.[72]

Silver staining is consistently negative for argentaffin granules and variably positive for argyrophil granules. Tumors exhibit immunoreactivity for neuron-specific enolase, for chromogranin, and, by definition, for somatostatin. There may be additional positive staining for gastrin, calcitonin, vasoactive intestinal polypeptide, and rarely serotonin and ACTH.[23,65]

Electron microscopy has demonstrated numerous round, moderately electron-dense, membrane-bound secretory granules with an average diameter of 400 nm and preferential localization of somatostatin reactivity in the electron-dense cores[23] (Fig. 9-13). Sometimes two distinct populations of granules, 800 and 275 nm in diameter, are seen, the smaller ones denser than the larger ones, with immunoreactivity for somatostatin in both.[16]

Most somatostatinomas are deeply invasive when discovered. Follow-up data are scanty. One patient with a tumor 4 cm in diameter and regional lymph node metastases was alive and well and without evidence of tumor 5 years later.[16]

Duodenal Neuroendocrine Carcinoma
The duodenum is an extremely rare primary site for neuroendocrine carcinoma. A single case was found in the English literature in 1986.[73] The patient presented with liver metastases, and no primary lesion was discovered during the 6-week survival. At autopsy, a small ulcerated submucosal primary tumor was found in the periampullary region of the duodenum. Histologically, the tumor had an organoid pattern and was composed of small oval and spindle-shaped cells with sparse cytoplasm. There was extensive necrosis. Sil-

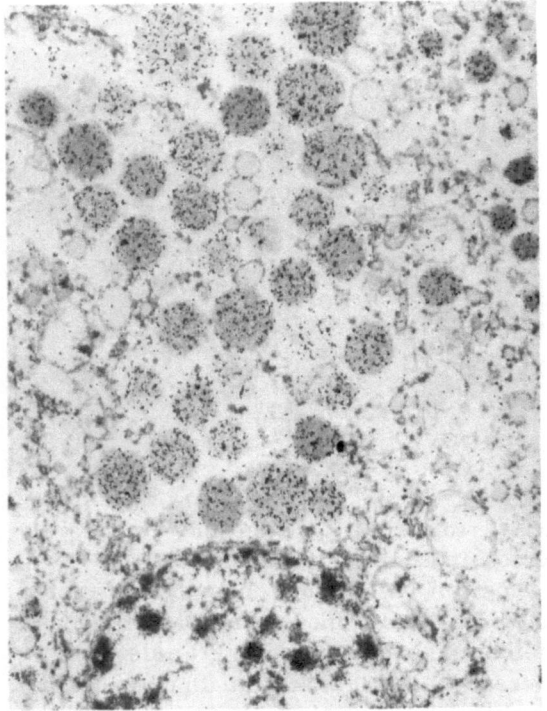

Figure 9-13. Somatostatinoma. Electron micrograph shows numerous moderately dense secretory granules with somatostatin reactivity. X16,126, reproduced at 56%. (Courtesy of Dr. Dayal, New England Medical Center, Boston.)

ver stains were negative, but stains for neuron-specific enolase, chromogranin, and vasoactive intestinal polypeptide were positive. Neuroendocrine granules were seen by electron microscopy. No endocrine symptoms were recognized.

References

1. Lewin KJ, Ulich T, Yang K, et al: The endocrine cells of the gastrointestinal tract. II. Tumors. Pathol Annu 1986;21:181–215.
2. Oberndorfer S: Karzinoide Tumoren des Dünndarms. Z Pathol (Frankfurt) 1907;1:426–432.
3. Soga J, Tazawa K, Wada K, et al: Argyrophil cell carcinoid of the stomach – a light and electronmicroscopic observation. Acta Pathol Jpn 1972;22:541–553.
4. Pearse AGE: The APUD cell concept and its implications in pathology. Pathol Annu 1974; 9:27–41.
5. Pearse AGE, Polak JM: Endocrine tumors of neural crest origin. Neurolophomas, apudomas and the APUD concept. Med Biol 1974; 52:3–18.
6. LeDouarin NM: The embryological origin of the endocrine cells associated with the digestive tract, in Bloom SR (ed): Gut Hormones. Edinburgh: Churchill Livingstone, 1978:49–56.
7. Cheifec G, Gould VE: Malignant gastric neuroendocrinomas. Ultrastructural and biochemical characterization of their secretory function. Hum Pathol 1977;8:433–440.
8. Gould VE, Jao W, Chejifec G, et al: Neuroendocrine carcinomas of the gastrointestinal tract. Semin Diagn Pathol 1984;1:13–18.
9. DeSchryver-Kecskemeti K, Clouse RE, Kraus FT: Surgical pathology of gastric and duodenal neuroendocrine tumors masquerading clinically as common polyps. Semin Diagn Pathol 1984;1:5–12.
10. Simpson S, Vinik AI, Marangos PJ, et al: Immunohistochemical localization of neuron-specific enolase in gastroenteropancreatic neuroendocrine tumors. Cancer 1984;54:1364–1369.
11. DeLellis RA, Dayal Y, Wolfe HJ: Carcinoid tumors. Changing concepts and new perspectives. Am J Surg Pathol 1984;8:295–300.
12. Williams ED, Siebenmann RE, Sobin LH: Histological Typing of Endocrine Tumors. International classification of tumors, no. 23. Geneva: World Health Organization, 1980.
13. Solcia E, Capella C, Buffa R, et al: Pathology of the Zollinger-Ellison syndrome. Prog Surg Pathol 1980;1:119–133.
14. Gilhool W: Endoscopic diagnosis and removal of a duodenal wall gastrinoma. Am J Gastroenterol 1984;79:679–683.
15. Somers G, Pipeleers-Marichal M, Gepts W, et al: A case of duodenal somatostatinoma: Diagnostic usefulness of calcium-pentagastrin test. Gastroenterology 1983;85:1192–1197.
16. Dayal Y, Doos WG, O'Brien MJ, et al: Psammomatous somatostatinomas of the duodenum. Am J Surg Pathol 1983;7:653–665.
17. Lee WM, Silva F, Price JB: Gastrin-secreting tumor of the duodenum (G-cell apudoma) associated with secondary biliary cirrhosis. Cancer 1982;49:2596–2601.

18. Kulchitzky N: Zur Frage über den Bau des Darmkanals. Arch Mikrosk Anat 1897;49:7–35.

19. Lewin KJ: The endocrine cells of the gastrointestinal tract. I. The normal endocrine cells and their hyperplasias. Pathol Annu 1986;21 (part 1):1–28.

20. Müller J, Kirchner T, Müller-Hermelink HK: Gastric endocrine cell hyperplasia and carcinoid tumors in atrophic gastritis type A. Am J Surg Pathol 1987;11:909–917.

21. Lebland CP, Cheng H: Identification of stem cells of the small intestine of the mouse, in Cairnie AB, Lala PK, Osmond DG (eds): Stem Cells of Renewing Cell Population. New York: Academic Press, 1976:7–31.

22. Soga J, Tazawa K, Aizawa O, et al: Argentaffin cell adenocarcinoma of the stomach. An atypical carcinoid? Cancer 1971;28:999–1003.

23. Kubo T, Watanabe H: Neoplastic argentaffin cells in gastric intestinal carcinomas. Cancer 1971;27:447–454.

24. Dayal Y, Tallberg KA, Nunnemacher G, et al: Duodenal carcinoids in patients with and without neurofibromatosis. Am J Surg Pathol 1986;10:348–357.

25. Alberti-Flor JJ, Halter S, Dunn GD: Multiple gastric carcinoids in a patient with a history of primary hyperparathyroidism. Am J Gastroenterol 1985;80:531–534.

26. Borch K, Renvall H, Liedberg G: Gastric endocrine cell hyperplasia and carcinoid tumors in pernicious anemia. Gastroenterology 1985; 88:638–648.

27. Wilander E: Achylia and the development of gastric carcinoids. Virchows Arch (Pathol Anat) 1981;394:151–160.

28. Solcia E, Capella C, Sessa F, et al: Gastric carcinoids and related endocrine growths. Digestion 1986;35(suppl 1):3–22.

29. Mendelsohn G, De La Monte S, Dunn JL, et al: Gastric carcinoid tumors, endocrine cell hyperplasia, and associated intestinal metaplasia. Cancer 1987;60:1022–1031.

30. Bordi C, Costa A, Missale G: ECL cell proliferation and gastrin levels. Gastroenterology 1975;68:205–206.

31. Goldman H, French S, Burbige E: Kulchitsky cell hyperplasia and multiple metastasizing carcinoids of the stomach. Cancer 1981;47: 2620–2626.

32. Bardi C: Nonantral gastric carcinoids and hypergastrinemia. Arch Surg 1981;116:1238.

33. Godwin JD: Carcinoid tumors: An analysis of 2837 cases. Cancer 1975;36:560–569.

34. Thompson GB, von Heerden JA, Martin JU, et al: Carcinoid tumors of the gastrointestinal tract: Presentation, management, and prognosis. Surgery 1985;98:1054–1062.

35. Jager R, Polk HC Jr: Carcinoid apudomas. Curr Probl Cancer 1977;1:1–53.

36. Askanazy M: Zur Pathogenese der Magenkrebse und über ihren gelegentlichen Ursprung aus angeborenen epithelialen Keimen in der Magenwand. Dtsch Med Wochenschr 1923;49:3–6.

37. Feldman AJ, Weinberg M, Raess D, et al: Gastric carcinoid tumor. Arch Surg 1981;116: 118–121.

38. Rogers LW, Murphy RC: Gastric carcinoid and gastric carcinoma, morphological correlates of survival. Am J Surg Pathol 1979;3: 195–202.

39. Sweeney EC, McDonnell L: Atypical gastric carcinoids. Histopathology 1980;4:215–224.

40. Facer P, Bishop AE, Wilson LBS, et al: Chromogranin: a newly recognized marker for endocrine cells of the human gastrointestinal tract. Gastroenterology 1985;89:1366–1373.

41. Oates JA: The carcinoid syndrome. N Engl J Med 1986;315:702–704.

42. Hirata Y, Sakamoto N, Yamamoto H, et al: Gastric carcinoid with ectopic production of ACTH and B-MSH. Cancer 1976;37:377–385.

43. Postlethwait RW: Gastrointestinal carcinoid tumors: A review. Postgrad Med 1966;40:445–454.

44. Cheifac G, Falkmer S, Askensten U, et al: Neuroendocrine tumors of the gastrointestinal tract. Path Res Pract 1988;183:143–154.

45. Cohn G, Erhardt K, Cedermark B, et al: DNA distribution pattern in intestinal carcinoid tumors. World J Surg 1986;10:548–554.

46. Aubock L: Intraepithelial mast cells in the human gastric mucosa in a case of microcarcinoidosis. Acta Morphol Acad Sci Hung 1980; 28:59–69.

47. Smith DM Jr, Haggitt RC: A comparative study of generic stains for carcinoid secretory granules. Am J Surg Pathol 1983;7:61–68.

48. Bader LV, Lykke WJ, Hinterberger H: Multiple biogenic amine-secreting carcinoid tumors of the stomach: A case report. Pathology 1977; 9:353–358.

49. Thompson NW, Vinik AI, Eckhause FE, et al:

Extrapancreatic gastrinomas. Surgery 1985;
98:1113–1120.

50. Maton PN, Gardner JD, Jansen RT: Cushing's
    syndrome in patients with the Zollinger-Elli-
    son syndrome. N Engl J Med 1986;315:1–5.

51. Theodorsson-Norheim E, Oberg K, Rosell S, et
    al: Neurotensin like immunoreactivity in
    plasma and tumor tissue from patients with
    endocrine tumors of the pancreas and gut.
    Gastroenterology 1983;85:881–889.

52. Larsson L-I: Adrenocorticotropin-like and β-
    melanotropin-like peptides in a subpopulation
    of human gastrin cell granules: Bioassay,
    immunoassay, and immunocytochemical evi-
    dence. Proc Natl Acad Sci USA 1981;78:
    2990–2994.

53. Iwafuchi M, Watanabe H, Ishihara N, et al:
    Peptide YY immunoreactive cells in gastroin-
    testinal carcinoids: immunohistochemical and
    ultrastructural studies of 60 tumors. Hum
    Pathol 1986;17:291–296.

54. Ray MB, Geboes K, Callea F, et al: Alpha-1-
    antitrypsin immunoreactivity in gastric carci-
    noid. Histopathology 1982;6:289– 297.

55. Feldman JM: Monoamine and diamine oxidase
    activity in the diagnosis of carcinoid tumors.
    Cancer 1985;56:2855–2860.

56. Wilander E, Westermark P, Grimelius L:
    Intracellular and extracellular fibrillar struc-
    tures in gastroduodenal endocrine tumors.
    Ultrastruct Pathol 1980;1:49–54.

57. Bensch KG, Corrin B, Pariente R, et al: Oat
    cell carcinoma of the lung: Its origin and rela-
    tionship to bronchial carcinoid. Cancer 1968;
    22:1163–1172.

58. Gould VE, Linnoila RI, Memoli VA, et al: Neu-
    roendocrine cells and neuroendocrine neo-
    plasms of the lung. Pathol Annu 1983;18(part
    1):287–330.

59. Ibrahim MBN, Briggs JC, Corbishley CM:
    Extrapulmonary oat cell carcinoma. Cancer
    1984;54:1645–1661.

60. Matsusaka T, Watanabe H, Enjoi M: Oat cell
    carcinoma of the stomach. Fukvoka Igaku
    Zashi 1976;67:65–73.

61. Tohara E, Ito H, Nakagami K, et al: Scirrhous
    argyrophil cell carcinoma of the stomach with

multiple production of polypeptide hormones,
amine, CEA, lysozyme, and HCG. Cancer
1982;49:1904–1915.

62. Klappenbach RS, Kurman RJ, Sinclair CF, et
    al: Composite carcinoma-carcinoid tumors of
    the gastrointestinal tract. Am J Clin Pathol
    1985;84:137–143.

63. Ali MH, Davidson A, Azzopardi JG: Composite
    gastric carcinoid and adenocarcinoma. Histo-
    pathology 1984;8:529–536.

64. Hofmann JW, Fox PS, Wilson SD: Duodenal
    wall tumors and the Zollinger-Ellison syn-
    drome: Surgical management. Arch Surg
    1973;107:334–339.

65. Stamm B, Hedinger CE, Saremaslani P: Duo-
    denal and ampullary carcinoid tumors. Vir-
    chows Arch (Pathol Anat) 1986;408:475–489.

66. Woodtli W, Gemsenjäger E, Hatz PU, et al:
    Endokrine Tumoren (APUDome) des Duode-
    nums-eine kooperative Studie. Schweiz Rund-
    schau Med 1982;71:1045–1053.

67. Stevens FM, Flanagan RW, O'Gorman D, et al:
    Glucagonoma syndrome demonstrating giant
    duodenal villi. Gut 1984;25:784–791.

68. Roggli VL, Judge DM, McGavran MH: Duo-
    denal glucagonoma: A case report. Hum
    Pathol 1979;10:350–353.

69. Miyazaki K, Funakoshi A, Nishihara S, et al:
    Aberrant insulinoma in the duodenum. Gas-
    troenterology 1986;90:1280–1285.

70. Pauwels S, Desmond H, Dimaline R, et al:
    Identification of progastrin in gastrinomas of
    antrum and duodenum by a novel radioim-
    munoassay. J Clin Invest 1986;77:376–381.

71. Stabile BE, Passaro E Jr: Benign and malig-
    nant gastrinoma. Am J Surg 1984;149:144–
    150.

72. Greider MH, DeSchryver-Kecskemeti K,
    Kraus FT: Psammoma bodies in endocrine
    tumors of the gastroentero-pancreatic axis: A
    rather common occurrence. Semin Diag Pathol
    1984;1:19–29.

73. Swanson PE, Dykoski D, Wick MR, et al:
    Primary duodenal small-cell neuroendocrine
    carcinoma with production of vasoactive intes-
    tinal polypeptide. Arch Pathol Lab Med 1986;
    110:317–320.

CHAPTER 10

Reactive and Neoplastic Lymphoid Lesions

Involvement of the gastrointestinal tract by malignant lymphoma is a common phenomenon judging from autopsy series. Two large autopsy series, which used the older classification, reported 40 to 82% of reticulum cell sarcomas, 42 to 52% of lymphosarcomas, and 13 to 20% of cases of Hodgkin's disease to have at least microscopic evidence of gastrointestinal involvement at the time of death.[1,2] The lower figures are from a series in which only stomach involvement was considered.[1] Most such involvement was late in the disease and often incidental.

Gastrointestinal involvement by lymphoma is divided into primary and secondary cases. Lymphomas are considered primary if the predominant lesion and/or symptoms traced to lymphoma are in the gastrointestinal tract and secondary if the initial diagnosis is from other sites.[3,4] Secondary involvement by lymphoma in the sense of a major lesion of clinical significance is about half as common as primary lymphoma.

Although the classification of types of lymphoma is discussed later, it should be noted that primary Hodgkin's disease of the gastrointestinal tract is exceedingly rare. Most such cases have been reported in the early literature and for the most part probably represent mistaken classification due to finding Reed-Sternberg-like cells in a setting of large cell pleomorphic lymphoma. For this reason, unless otherwise specified, herein we will discuss only non-Hodgkin's lymphoma. The stomach is by far the most common

Table 10-1. Site of Extranodal Non-Hodgkin's Lymphoma*

Site	Percentage	Range (%)
Stomach	23.8	21.7–25.3
Waldeyer's ring	10.9	8.9–14.1
Skin	10.7	7.8–13.6
Small bowel	9.7	7.8–11.8
Soft tissue	7.0	4.5–8.7
Colon–rectum	6.8	5.8–8.8
Bone	4.4	3.2–5.1
Major salivary glands	4.2	3.8–4.9

*Average of three series totaling 4356 cases. Adapted from Platz[5] with permission of the publisher.

site of primary extranodal non-Hodgkin's lymphoma (Table 10-1).

Within the gastrointestinal tract, well over one-half of cases of extranodal lymphoma are gastric, with a smaller number from the small intestine, colon, and esophagus in that order; esophageal primary lymphomas are exceedingly rare.[6]

Primary gastric lymphomas constitute only a minor fraction of the total malignancy burden of that organ. The Surveillance, Epidemiology, and End-Results (SEER) Program data of the National Cancer Institute from 1973 to 1977 reported 423 cases of primary gastric lymphoma among 9589 gastric malignancies, an incidence of 4.4%.[7] Figures from the hospital of one of the authors (H.T.E.) are higher (6.4%), perhaps indicating some bias induced by referral patterns. At

Table 10-2. Lymphoid Lesions of the Stomach*

Chronic gastritis
Chronic gastritis with follicular hyperplasia
Chronic ulcer with mild lymphoid reaction
Pseudolymphomas
  Common inflammatory type
    With focal lymphoma
  Nodular lymphoid hyperplasia
  Angiofollicular lymphoid hyperplasia
Lymphoma, primary or secondary
Leukemia, secondary

*Adapted from Brooks and Enterline,[9] with permission of the publisher.

the same hospital, gastric lymphoma was twice as common as gastric leiomyosarcoma. Although primary lymphomas form a higher percentage of the total primary malignancy burden in the small bowel, the total number of cases, as mentioned, is smaller than that of gastric origin. The bulk of the intestinal cases are distal to the area that concerns us here. Primary lymphomas of the duodenum are reported to constitute only 0.6 to 4% of all gastrointestinal lymphomas.[5,8]

In addition to true lymphomas, pseudo-lymphomatous mass lesions occur in the stomach. These total 5 to 15% of all gastric lymphoid lesions.[9] Rare cases of other tumors, such as plasmacytomas and chloromas, are encountered. Certain undifferentiated or very poorly differentiated carcinomas remain a problem in differential diagnosis. The range of lymphoid gastric lesions is listed in Table 10-2.

Pseudolymphoma

The recognition that certain lymphoid tumor-like conditions of the stomach were reactive in nature is credited to Smith and Helwig,[10] who presented a paper on the subject of malignant lymphoma of the stomach at the annual meeting of the American Association of Pathologists and Bacteriologists in 1958. They stated, "It is possible that some of the localized lesions that appear malignant but behave in a benign fashion are indeed hyper-plastic lesions. . . ." In a later seminar, Helwig cited criteria for differentiation from lymphoma that included a polymorphous cellular infiltrate, the presence of reaction centers, and a fibroblastic reaction.[11] Jacobs[12] used these criteria to separate out a group of 12 cases of pseudolymphoma from their series of lymphoid gastric infiltrates. None of these died of lymphoma. After the publication of this study, the concept of pseudolymphoma became accepted and the sometimes difficult problem of differentiating benign and malignant lymphoid gastric lesions became an additional task for the surgical pathologist.

Differential Diagnosis of Lymphoma and Pseudolymphoma

Pseudolymphomas, taken en masse, show some clinical and gross features that on average differ from those of true lymphoma. There is sufficient overlap so that the diagnosis still rests firmly on histologic findings aided to some extent by immunocytologic study. However, these features are worth reviewing. The area is well discussed by Platz.[5]

Pain, weight loss, vomiting, and anemia are common to both lymphoma and pseudolymphoma. The findings that are somewhat more helpful in pointing to one or the other diagnosis are listed in Table 10-3, which has been modified from Platz' review. As can be seen, none is diagnostic.

Of these findings, the usual short duration of symptoms in gastric lymphoma and the usual history of present or past peptic ulcer in gastric pseudolymphoma are perhaps the most discriminatory and have been commented on by many authors.

Radiologic examination usually reveals an ulcer, a mass, or both. It is difficult on purely radiologic grounds to pinpoint an accurate diagnosis, in particular the distinction from carcinoma. Endoscopy is chiefly useful in conducting biopsies. Biopsy specimens, if uncrushed and rapidly fixed, may be diagnostic of diffuse histiocytic lymphomas, occasionally those of the poorly differentiated lymphocytic type. It must be stressed that a

Table 10-3. Comparison of Certain Signs and Symptoms of Lymphoma and Pseudolymphoma*

	Lymphoma		Pseudolymphoma	
	Median	Range	Median	Range
Male/female	1.6	1.1–2.8	2.5	1–3.5
Age	59 yr	15–88 yr	52	18–76
Symptom duration	3 mo	1–36 mo	12 mo	4–60 mo
Systemic symptoms	8%	6–30%	–	–
Ulcer history	–	32–39%	–	67–70%
Mass	27%	14–47%	–	8–12%
Achlorhydria	–	59–76%	–	27%
Blood in stools	–	81%	–	36%

*Modified from Platz[5] with permission of the publisher.

normal biopsy, or one showing clearly reactive lymphoid mucosal aggregates, cannot be relied on to rule out lymphoma or to diagnose gastric pseudolymphoma. Such changes are common at the periphery or, at times, superficial to lymphomatous infiltrates. Frequently, resection is necessary to supply sufficient material for accurate diagnosis.

Site

Both lymphoma and pseudolymphoma are more common in the distal stomach, but either may be proximal. Pseudolymphoma has been reported from the duodenum, but is very rare at that site.[13]

Size

Gastric pseudolymphomas tend to be smaller than gastric lymphomas. In contrast to gastric pseudolymphomas, true lymphomas less than 5 cm in maximum dimension are very rare. However, many cases of gastric pseudolymphoma exceed this figure (Fig. 10-1).

Gross

The gross lesion of gastric pseudolymphoma tends to present as a diffuse thickening, with cobblestoning of the mucosa and usually with a prominent area of ulceration. However, it may be a massive lesion. The ulcers tend to be sharp edged, in contrast to the rolled-edge ulcerations seen in gastric lymphoma or carcinoma[5] (Fig. 10-2). Gastric

lymphoma usually presents as a plaque, often with multiple ulcerations, but may also appear as a localized mass, as an exaggeration of the rugal folds, or, rarely, as a polyp (Figs. 10-3 and 10-4). The depth of invasion is not discriminatory, since many gastric pseudolymphomas extend to the serosa or even to adjacent organs such as the omentum or pancreas.

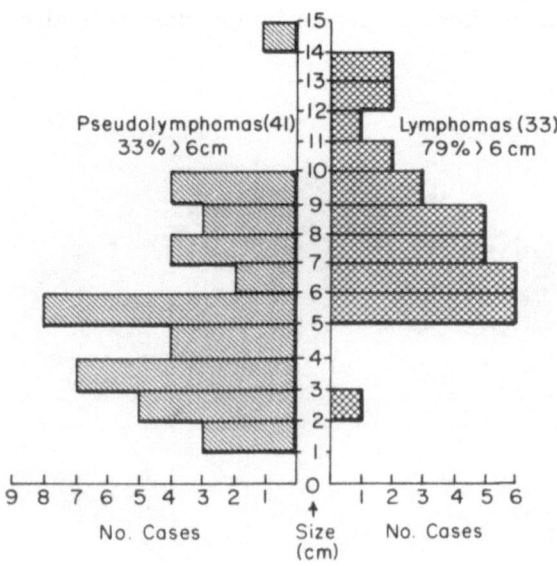

Figure 10-1. Size of gastric lymphomas and pseudolymphomas. From Brooks and Enterline,[9] with permission.

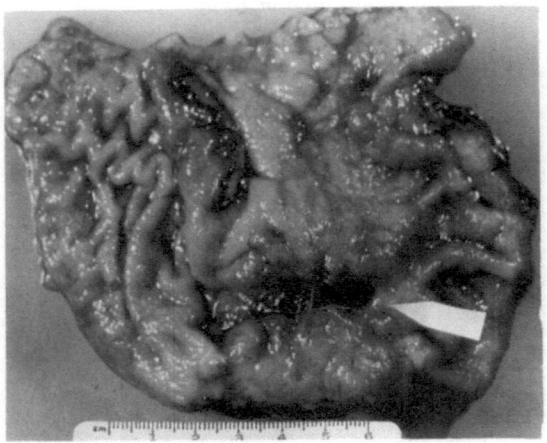

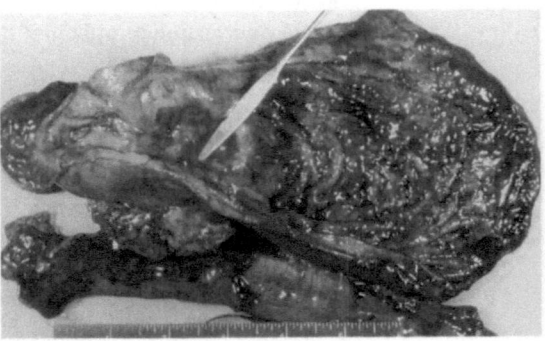

Figure 10-4. Diffuse lymphocytic lymphoma of the stomach. Note large antral mass with extension through the serosa.

Figure 10-2. Gastric pseudolymphoma. There is an extensive ill-defined mass with ulceration. Note the presence of a chronic gastric ulcer (*arrow*). This case also contained a focus of poorly differentiated lymphocytic lymphoma.

Associated Lesions

The gastric mucosa very commonly shows ulceration. The ulcers, especially in gastric lymphoma, may be multiple and are, strictly speaking, not peptic. Typical chronic peptic ulceration is a feature of most gastric pseudolymphomas (80% in one series[9]); however, about 20% of gastric lymphomas will also

show peptic ulceration.[14] Chronic gastritis is very common in both lesions. Brooks and Enterline[9,14] found chronic gastritis to be present in 60% of cases of gastric pseudolymphoma and 77% of cases of gastric lymphoma. It has been suggested that chronic gastritis tends to be more severe and extensive in gastric lymphoma, thus explaining the higher incidence of achlorhydria in that tumor.[5] According to the presence or absence and type of associated lesion, gastric pseudolymphoma may also be subdivided into 1) a nodular type that presents as a nodular elevation without ulceration and corresponds to submucosal lymphoid hperplasia, 2) an ulcerative type that is associated with deep ulceration and extensive fibrosis, and 3) an erosive type that shows superficial ulceration and lymphoid hyperplasia in the lamina propria and submucosa.[15]

Histology of Gastric Pseudolymphoma

Brooks and Enterline[9] divided the gastric pseudolymphomas into three types; the common inflammatory type and two very rare types. The first of the rare types is nodular lymphoid hyperplasia, identical to that described by Ranchod and co-workers.[13] In the only case encountered in our series, the stomach contained numerous nodulations caused by infiltration of lymphocytes in the

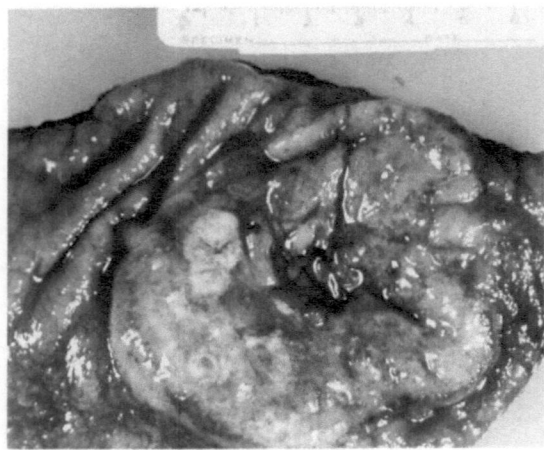

Figure 10-3. Diffuse histocytic lymphoma of the stomach. Note large ulcerated plaque.

mucosa and submucosa. These infiltrates contained widely scattered germinal centers showing good polarization (Fig. 10-5).

The other rare type is identical to the angiofollicular hyperplasia seen more typically elesewhere[16] (Fig. 10-6). We are aware of only three cases involving the stomach.[9,17] This type is the exception to the rule that lymph nodes are never involved in pseudolymphoma. The remaining comments refer to the "usual" type of gastric pseudolymphoma.

Most chronic gastric ulcers will show some lymphocytic response, often with accompanying germinal centers. These cases usually present no problem, and we will not discuss them further except to state that the line of division between the clear reactions to ulceration and pseudolymphoma is a subjective one and gives strength to the argument that pseudolymphoma represents an exaggerated response to antigens gaining access to the tissues via the ulceration. The "true" pseudolymphomas may be divided into relatively superficial infiltrates and those that involve the entire wall. The more superficial types present as a prominent band of lymphocytic infiltrate subtended by fibrosis, which involves the muscularis propria. The deeper forms, as stated, may involve the entire gastric wall or extend beyond it (Fig. 10-7).

Cellular Features of Gastric Pseudolymphoma

In gastric pseudolymphoma the predominant cell is a small, round, well-differentiated lymphocyte. Small cleaved lymphocytes are restricted to germinal centers. A variable number of plasma cells, eosinophils, and scattered immunoblasts may also be present. The latter, however, should not be in sheets, which would raise a question of accompanying focal lymphoma. The infiltrate tends to fade gradually into adjacent fibromuscular tissue and dissects and spreads muscle cells rather than destroying them. The accompanying fibrosis may rarely be restricted to the chronic peptic ulcer usually present. For the most part, however, fibrosis is also

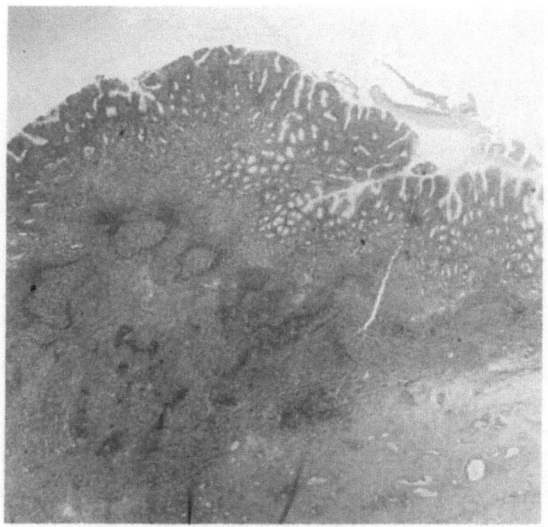

A

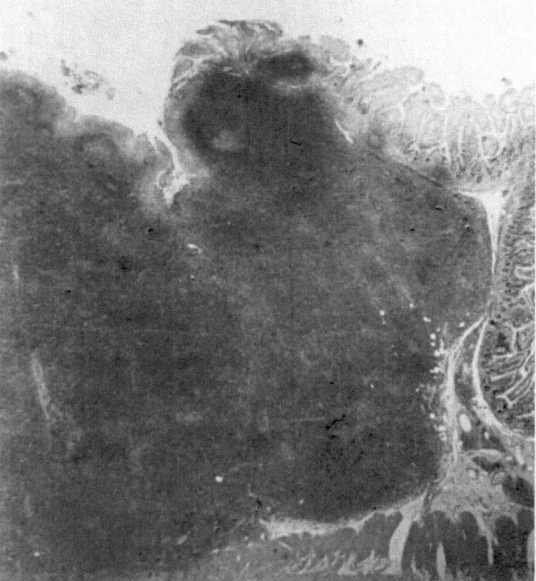

B

Figure 10-5. Nodular lymphoid hyperplasia of the stomach and small intestine. **A.** A nonulcerated, nonfibrotic lesion with polarized germinal centers in the mucosa and submucosa of the stomach. **B.** One of many large lymphoid nodules with germinal centers of the small intestine. From Brooks and Enterline,[9] with permission.

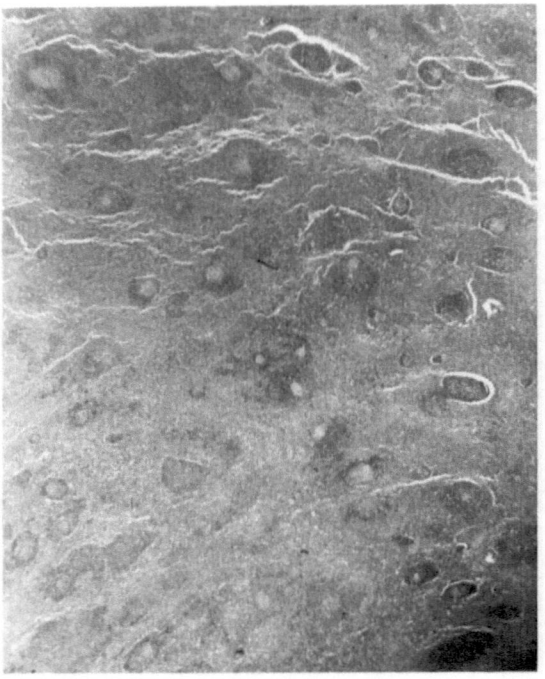

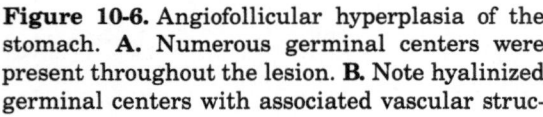

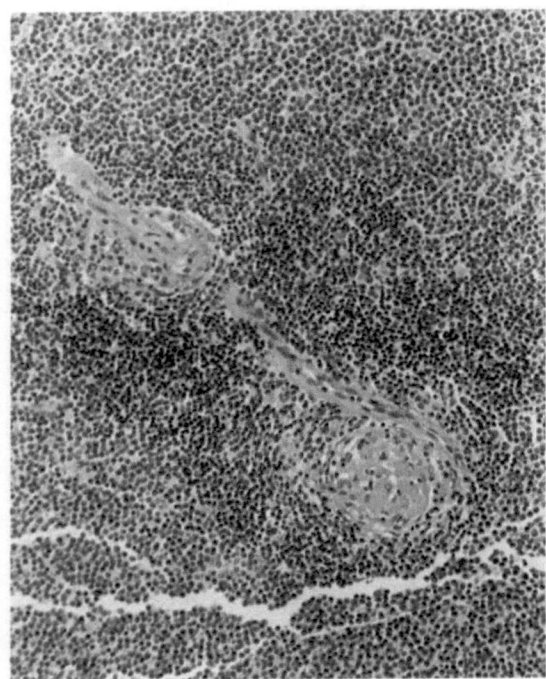

A   B

Figure 10-6. Angiofollicular hyperplasia of the stomach. **A.** Numerous germinal centers were present throughout the lesion. **B.** Note hyalinized germinal centers with associated vascular struc-tures in a background of lymphocytes and plasma cells. From Brooks and Enterline,[9] with permission.

present, forming bands that divide the infiltrate into cellular areas[5,9] (Fig. 10-8). This finding contrasts with the band-like fibrosis that often subtends gastric lymphoma. The mitotic index in gastric pseudolymphoma is low, which does not, however, differentiate this lesion from well and poorly differentiated lymphocytic lymphoma. A rare mitosis outside of germinal centers should not be construed as proof of malignancy.[18]

The sine qua non of gastric pseudolymphoma is the presence of germinal centers within the lesion as opposed to their presence in the periphery. Such germinal centers may be prominent or their identification may require searching of several slides. Lymphoid aggregates should not be confused with true germinal centers. At times germinal centers may be difficult to recognize. Hyjek and Kel-enyi[19] point out that follicles may enlarge but show progressively smaller germinal centers, which become crowded out by lymphocytes and finally disappear, whereupon their recognition depends on being outlined by reticulin fibers with appropriate staining. Platz[20] describes certain cases that he considered probably gastric pseudolymphoma despite the absence of centers (i.e., cases in which a patchy infiltrate in a pattern of fibrosis consistent with gastric pseudolymphoma was present). Although Platz accepts such cases, he agrees, as do most investigators, that the presence of germinal centers is the most reliable differentiating feature. We would reemphasize that a reactive lymphoid pattern may be seen at the periphery of lymphoma and, therefore, that superficial germinal centers or indeed those at the margin of the

Figure 10-7. Gastric pseudolymphoma. Note ulcer on luminal side. Lymphoid nodules extend through the entire gastric wall into fat. Note germinal center in lower right corner. X40, reproduced at 65%.

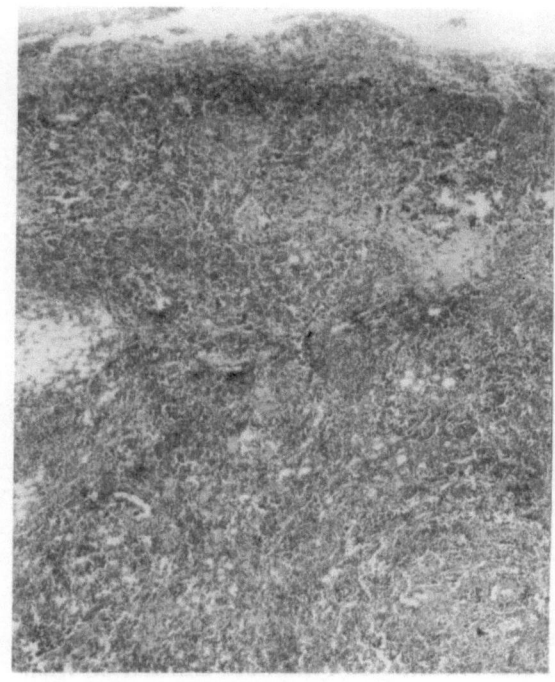

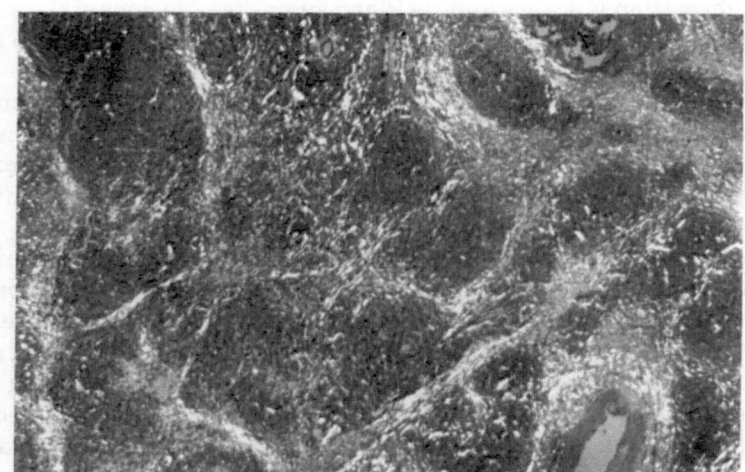

Figure 10-8. Gastric pseudolymphoma. Typical pattern of fibrosis seen on polarization. Collagen bands separate the infiltrate (dark areas) into large aggregates. From Brooks and Enterline,[9] with permission.

lesion, even if beneath it, should not be taken as proof of benignancy. In the study by Brooks and Enterline,[9] such deep centers subtending lymphomas but not within the actual neoplasm were seen in some cases (Fig. 10-9).

Recently, immunocytochemistry has been used as an aid in the differentiation of gastric lymphoma and gastric pseudolymphoma. The latter is usually polyclonal for globulins and light chains.[18] The immunologic problem

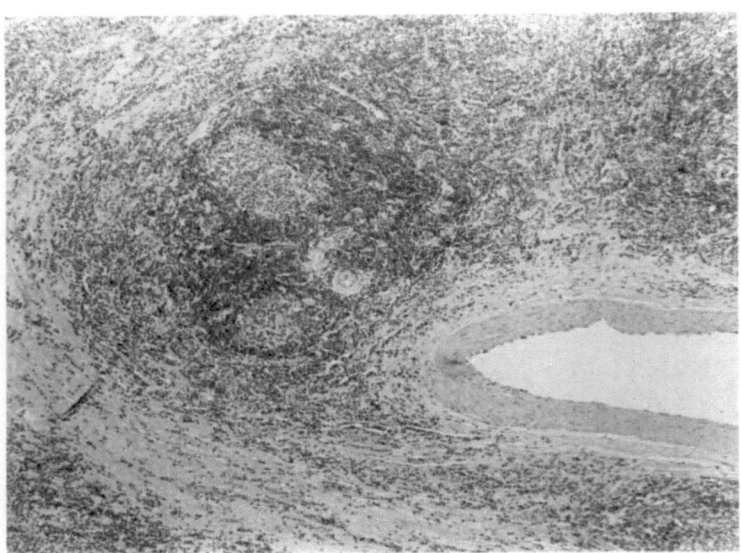

Figure 10-9. Gastric pseudo-lymphoma. Note deep germinal centers associated with a blood vessel. From Brooks and Enterline,[9] with permission.

is complicated by certain reports of mono-clonal staining in lymphoid infiltrates with germinal centers.[21-23] It is uncertain how these cases are to be regarded. The follow-up information is scanty and, as Platz[5] suggests, some of these lesions may be unrecognized well-differentiated lymphocytic lymphomas or mantle zone lymphomas. Galton and co-workers[24] have stated that monoclonality is not synonymous with malignancy, although the risk of transformation to a malignant clone with such cells is much higher than with polyclonal cells. Thus, although demon-stration of a basic polyclonal infiltrate may be taken as strong supportive evidence of benignancy, interpretation of monoclonal lesions must be made with caution until the situation is clarified. The various histologic features of gastric pseudolymphoma and gas-tric lymphoma are compared in Table 10-4. Finally, it should be recalled that small biopsy samples may show some crush artifact and lead to misinterpretation of a case as poorly differentiated lymphocytic lymphoma. In cases predominantly consisting of well-differentiated lymphocytes, we favor abso-lute peripheral lymphocyte counts to aid in the diagnosis to differentiate such dubious cases from chronic lymphatic leukemia.

Relationship of Pseudolymphoma to Lymphoma

In reviewing case material on lymphoid lesions of the stomach, Brooks and Enterline[9] became aware of five cases of what appeared to be typical pseudolymphomas in which focal lesions meeting the criteria of malig-nant lymphoma were present. In each of these the predominant infiltrate was composed of small, well-differentiated lymphocytes and the infiltrate was prominent, transmural, and accompanied by germinal centers plus significant fibrosis and evidence of benign ulceration. In each the area of lymphoma was both focal and superficial. Four were in men in the seventh or eighth decade of life. Four cases consisted of sheets of atypical cells diagnostic of "diffuse histiocytic" lymphoma, the fifth of nodular and diffuse, poorly differentiated lymphocytic lymphoma. The size of these lesions varied from 3 to 7 cm in diameter and that of the malignant foci from 0.9 to 2.5 cm (Fig. 10-10). One patient was lost to follow-up, three remained well for 5 to 10 years after resection, and one—the patient with the largest area of lymphoma—died of disseminated lymphoma 4 years after resec-tion. A similar case of diffuse histiocytic

Table 10-4. Differential Diagnosis of Gastric Pseudolymphoma (GPL) and Gastric Lymphoma (GL)*

Parameter	GPL	GL	Qualifying comment*
Lymphocyte nuclear size	Small	Mostly large, some small	Only WDL, PDL, CLL to be excluded
Nuclear morphology	Round	Elongated + cleaved small lymphocytes	PDL excluded (WDL, CLL to be excluded)
Germinal centers (intralesional)	Present	Absent	WDL + PDL + CLL excluded; some GL have these below lymphoma; GL may be focal in GPL
Peripheral blood lymphocytosis	Absent	Absent	CLL excluded
Polymorphic infiltrate	Always present	Rarely prominent	Aside from MLH, eosinophils plasma cells can be found in GL. Only small percentage of cells in GPL
Mitotic index	Low	Usually high	GPL, WDL, PDL essentially equal
Granulation base of ulcer	Usually present	Usually absent	Lymphocytic lymphomas often nonulcerated
Fibrosis	Intralesional	Below lesion	Pattern statistically significant
Depth of invasion	Mucosa to serosa	Mucosa to serosa	Nondiscriminating
Necrosis	Absent	Often present	Individual cell necrosis seen in many lymphomas
Vascular invasion	Absent	Common	
Muscular lymphoid aggregates	Present	Present	Cytology important
Tumor size	Usually small	Usually large	Considerable overlap
Lymph node status	Negative (with one exception)	Positive or negative	Angiofollicular lymphoid hyperplasia may involve lymph nodes

Abbreviations: WDL, well-differentiated lymphocytic lymphoma; PDL, poorly differentiated lymphocytic lymphoma; CLL, chronic lymphocytic leukemia; MLH, mixed lymphocytic histiocytic lymphoma.
*Adapted from Brooks and Enterline,[9] with permission of the publisher.

lymphoma has been documented by Murayama and co-workers,[25] who reported knowledge of at least 10 similar cases in the Japanese literature. In their case the major reactive lesion was polyclonal, but the lymphomatous focus was negative for globulins and for lysozyme. A case was also reported by Wolf and Spjut.[26] Dragosics and co-workers[27] reported that 3 of their 16 cases of gastric pseudolymphoma contained focal lymphoma. This finding is similar to those of Brooks and Enterline,[9] who found five such lymphomas in 15 cases of gastric pseudolymphoma. The increasing number of such reports raises the question of the prelymphomatous nature of gastric pseudolymphoma. This is not surprising considering the well-accepted role of reactive massive lymphoid hyperplasia in other organs as a seedbed for lymphoma as, for instance, the relationship of primary lymphoma of the thyroid to background chronic thyroiditis. The frequency of such an occurrence remains to be evaluated. From the practical point of view, it indicates a need

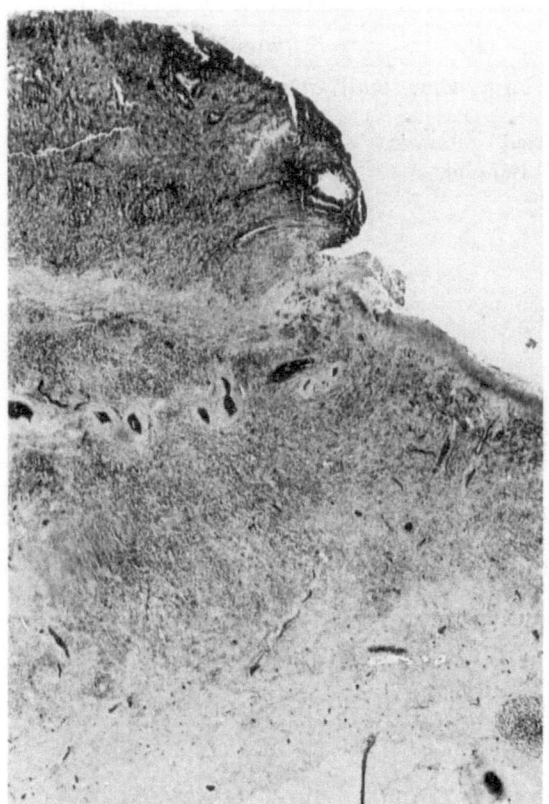

A

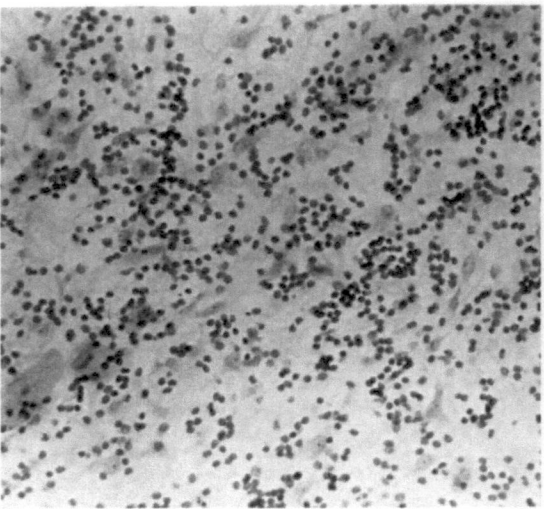

C

Figure 10-10. Focal lymphoma in gastric pseudo-lymphoma. **A.** A large fibrotic transmural pseudo-lymphoma was present adjacent to a benign ulcer. X10. **B.** A sheet-like infiltrate of large cell "histio-cytic" lymphoma is seen in the mucosa. X300, reproduced at 90%. **C.** A benign infiltrate of lymphocytes, plasma cells, and eosinophils composes most of the lesion. X300, reproduced at 90%. From Brooks and Enterline,[9] with permission.

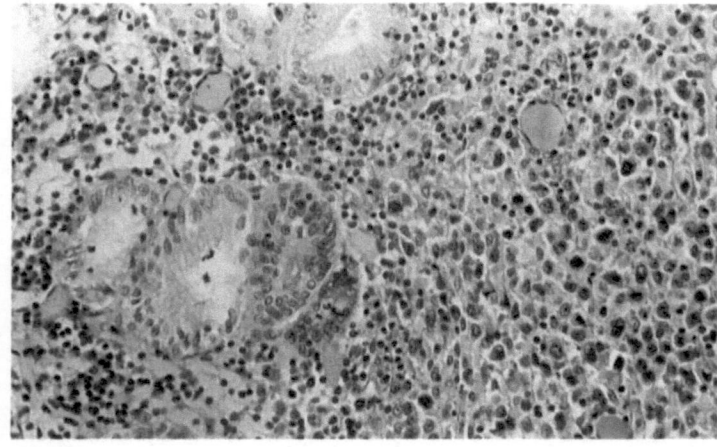

B

for careful sampling through multiple sectioning in cases of gastric pseudolymphoma even if the initial sections clearly indicate a reactive process.

Malignant Lymphoma

Duodenal Lymphoma

As indicated previously, primary duodenal lymphomas are rare. The majority of intestinal lymphomas occur more distally. Some cases of immunoproliferative small intestinal disease (IPSID) may involve the duodenal –jejunal junctional area, although more typically are distal to the duodenum. The most complete review of the non-IPSID-related lymphomas of the duodenum is that by Najem and co-workers.[28] They found 95 cases in the English literature, but do not comment on histologic types. Of interest is their report that the male/female ratio is higher for duodenal lymphoma than for lesions elsewhere in the gastrointestinal tract, approximately 2 to 1, and that the average patient age is distinctly younger (40 years) than for similar tumors of the stomach. The symptoms were dependent on the site, degree of obstruction, and rapidity of growth, with obstructive symptoms of vomiting, postprandial pain, or symptoms secondary to ulcerations, such as melena and anemia. Jaundice was present in those cases involving the periampullary area. Most were not resectable. Of those with some follow-up, a 2-year survival rate of 41% was noted. Nearly all of the survivors had received radiation therapy with or without surgical resection.

Gastric Lymphoma

Hodgkin's Disease
As mentioned previously, Hodgkin's disease of the gastrointestinal tract is usually only secondary. It does occur as a primary lesion, though very rarely, with an occasional case reported in large series.[29,30,31]

Non-Hodgkin's Lymphoma
The clinical presentation and gross features of gastric lymphoma have been discussed in the section covering the differential diagnosis of pseudolymphoma from lymphoma. Although radiologic diagnosis is improving, most cases are still usually considered to be carcinoma or ulcer prior to biopsy, cytology, or resection. Diffuse involvement, especially if showing umbilicated nodulations, is considered fairly diagnostic by the radiologist. Unfortunately, this presentation is not common.[14]

Role of Cytology and Biopsy

Before the introduction of fiberoptic endoscopy, biopsy- or resection-confirmed cytologic diagnostic accuracy ranged from 27 to 64%. This accuracy has improved to 70 to 80% since that time.[5] Carbé-Fiol and Vilardell[32] reported that with direct guidance brushing of lesions, the diagnosis of malignancy was made in 13 of 15 cases of lymphoma and a diagnosis of lymphoma in 11 of the 15 cases. Cytology plus biopsy in the same series resulted in a 93% accuracy level as compared with older results in their institution of a 41% diagnosis of malignancy among cases of lymphoma. Although such results may only be obtainable by those with considerable skill and experience, clearly the flexible gastroscope has been an extremely useful instrument in obtaining diagnostic material. Problems certainly exist. The accuracy of cytologic diagnosis is less with the small cell lymphocytic forms of lymphoma than with the large cell types. Cabré-Fiol and Vilardell[32] point out that lymphomas may not necessarily involve the mucosal surface or that large amounts of necrotic material from ulcerating lesions may dilute and obscure the cell population. In addition, sampling may be problematic where there is a considerable reactive lymphoid infiltrate overlying a lymphoma. Errors may also occur in differentiating lymphoma from very poorly differentiated carcinoma. These errors will be

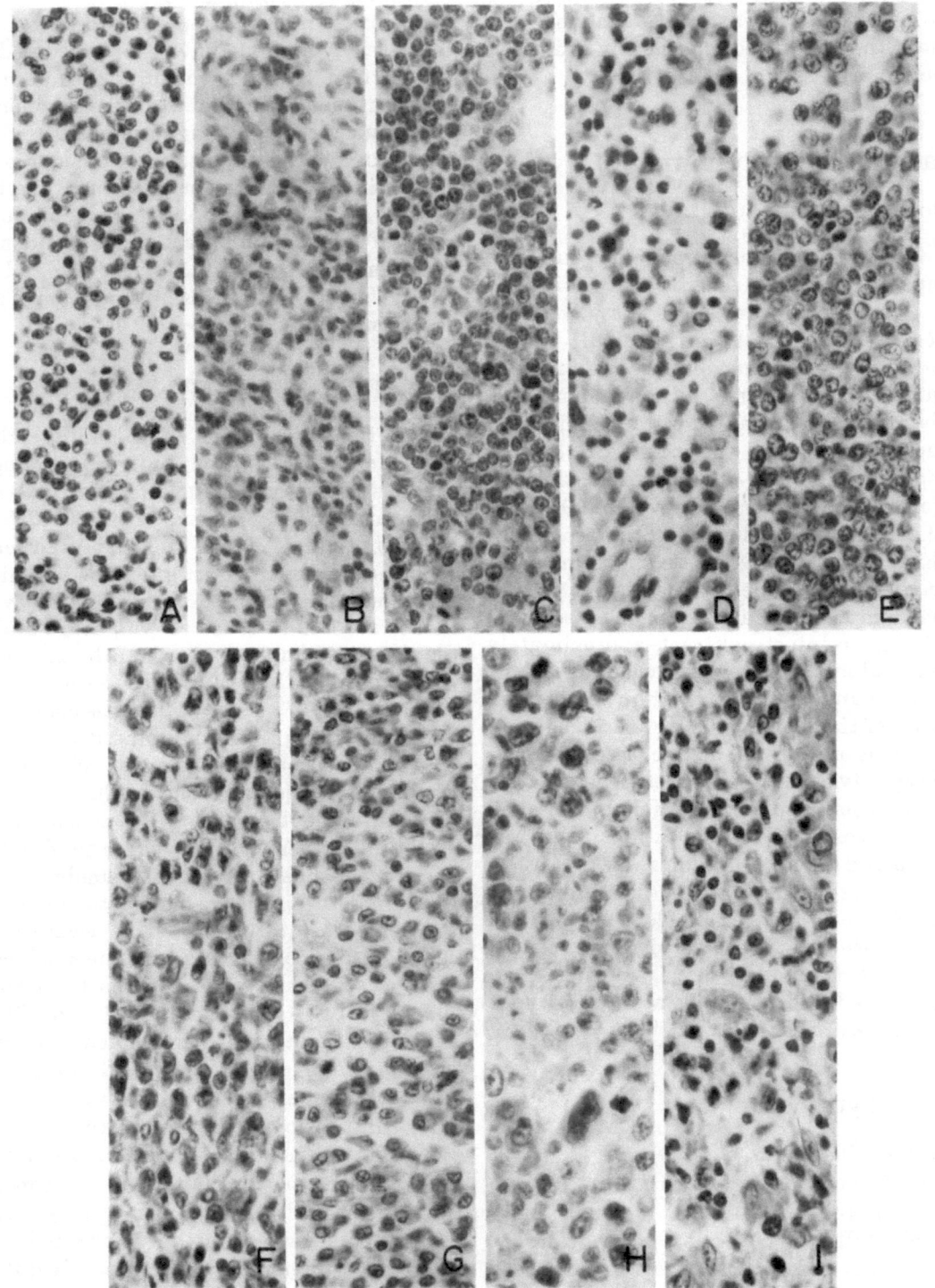

reduced as cytologists become less reliant on the Papanicolau stain as the only stain applied. Immunologic B- and T-cell markers and the recently commercially available monoclonal antileukocyte common antigen T-200 have been shown to be useful at the cytologic level.[33] Initial experience along these lines in the cytology laboratory of the hospital of one of the authors (H.T.E.) has been encouraging.[34]

The accuracy of endoscopic biopsies has also improved, now ranging from 52 to 88%.[5] Such endoscopically obtained biopsy specimens are also useful in the staging of lymphomas. Solidoro and co-workers[35] reported that 15% of nodal and 19% of extranodal extragastric lymphomas involved the stomach. We would repeat the cautions noted in the discussion of gastric pseudolymphoma, namely, that a negative biopsy or a biopsy showing only reactive infiltrate does not rule out lymphoma. The distinction on biopsy, even full-thickness biopsy, of pseudolymphoma and lymphocytic lymphomas may be difficult or impossible in the better-differentiated forms. We believe that the large cell lymphomas can be diagnosed with considerable accuracy by the experienced pathologist. Again, the stains for mucin may be helpful in differentiating carcinoma and lymphoma. Multiple biopsies are preferred and the endoscopist must attempt to avoid extremely superficial biopsies, to avoid crushing, and especially to avoid drying and delay in fixation of biopsy material.

Histologic Types

The histologic types of gastric non-Hodgkin's lymphoma include the full range of types seen in nodal non-Hodgkin's lymphoma. It has been stated, however, that the accepted histologic classifications of nodal lymphoma are difficult to apply to malignant lymphoma of mucosa-associated lymphoid tissue.[36] Immunocytochemical studies, discussed in detail below, have shown that the great majority of gastric lymphomas are of B-cell type,[36-38] but T-cell lymphoma also occurs.[36] The light microscopic appearance of types of gastric lymphoma are demonstrated in Figs. 10-11A through 10-11I. There are striking differences in the relative frequency of the various types of lymphoma in the stomach as compared to lymphoma at large (Tables 10-5 and 10-6). In the Rappaport classification (Table 10-5), the percentage of nodular gastric lymphomas is markedly less and that of diffuse large cell histiocytic lymphomas much higher than that of lymphomas in general. Using the working formulation division (Table 10-6), a much smaller percentage falls into the low-grade malignancy group. Also of note is that lymphomas showing plasmacytoid features are much more commonly seen among the gastric lymphoma group. These may present as small cell lymphocytic lymphomas with plasmacytoid differentiation or as large cell "immunoblastic" lymphomas with abundant amphophilic cytoplasm. In a series in which one of the authors was involved,[9] 78% of the cases were histiocytic diffuse by the Rappaport classification and 38% showed features of immunoblastic sarcoma. We were struck by the degree of histologic variation from area to area. In five cases, foci of poorly differentiated lymphocytic lymphoma were seen in predominantly histiocytic lymphomas. Other cases showed focal mixed lymphocytic–histiocytic lym-

---

◄

Figure 10-11. Histology of gastric lymphomas. **A.** Well-differentiated lymphocytic lymphoma (WDL); **B.** poorly differentiated lymphocytic lymphoma (PDL); **C.** lymphoblastic lymphoma (LB); **D.** mixed lymphocytic–histiocytic lymphoma (MHL); **E.** histiocytic lymphoma, large noncleaved type (HL, LNC); **F.** histiocytic lymphoma, large cleaved type (HL, LCC); **G.** histiocytic lymphoma, immunoblastic type (HL, IBL); **H.** histiocytic lymphoma, pleomorphic type (HL, PLEO); **I.** malignant lymphoma with high content of epithelioid histiocytes (Lennert's lymphoma). H&E, X400, reproduced at 85%.

Table 10-5. Comparison of Gastric Non-Hodgkin's Lymphoma to All Non-Hodgkin's Lymphoma (Rappaport System)

Characteristics	Platz[5] (Compilation of Series): Percent Gastric Lymphomas	Dragosics et al[27]: Percent Gastric Lymphomas	NHL PCP*: Percent All Lymphomas
Nodular			
Well-differentiated			
lymphocytic	3	–	–
Poorly differentiated			
lymphocytic	3	1.9	18.7
Mixed	2	1.0	8.1
Histiocytic	3	–	1.7
Nodular + diffuse	–	2.0	–
Total nodular	11	4.9	28.5
Diffuse			
Well-differentiated			
lymphocytic	8	11.4	4.1
Poorly differentiated			
lymphocytic	12	15.2	9.3
Mixed	8	16.2	4.5
Histiocytic	44	40	28.4
Lymphoblastic	1	–	8.4
Undifferentiated	2	9.5	2.1
Unclassified	2	2.7	14.7
Total diffuse	89	95	71.5

*Non-Hodgkin's Lymphoma Pathologic Classification Project.[39]

phomas or several subtypes of histiocytic lymphoma. In some cases submucosal sheets of immunoblastic histiocytic lymphoma with high degrees of plasmacytoid differentiation were associated with nodules of nonimmunoblastic or pleomorphic histiocytic lymphoma. These variations were quite discrete and indeed in several cases suggested a relationship similar to that of the plasma cell infiltrates of IPSID to the large cell lymphomas seen in that disease, although in the stomach the plasmacytoid cells were obviously malignant. These might be considered composite tumors; however, we thought it more likely that they represented the development of clones within the original tumor. Although the significance of this finding is not clear, it does emphasize the danger of classification based on meager biopsy material. Platz[5] points out the rarity of well-differentiated

small cell gastric lymphoma and cautions that the presence of a higher percentage of such cases in a series may, in reality, represent misdiagnosis of pseudolymphomas.

Immunologic Studies

Immunohistochemical techniques have added greatly to our understanding of lymphomas in general. The information available on gastric lymphomas in this area remains sketchy, although the results of such studies are now being reported with increasing frequency. The use of antibodies to common leukocyte antigen, cytokeratin, and carcinoembryonic antigen aids in the distinction of lymphomatoid lesions from certain very poorly differentiated carcinomas[40] (Fig. 10-12). Techniques to demonstrate the subsets of surface and intracytoplasmic glob-

Table 10-6. Comparison of Gastric Non-Hodgkin's Lymphoma to All Non-Hodgkin's Lymphoma

Characteristics	Dragosics et al[27] (%)	NHL PCP* (%)
Low-grade malignancy		
Small lymphocytic	10.5	3.6
(consistent with CLL or plasmacytoid)		
Follicular small cleaved	1.9	22.5
Follicular mixed	1.9	7.7
Intermediate malignancy		
Follicular large cell	–	3.8
Diffuse small cleaved	10.5	6.9
Diffuse mixed	21.9	6.7
Diffuse large cell	26.6	19.7
High-grade malignancy		
Immunoblastic	11.4	7.9
Lymphoblastic	–	4.2
Small noncleaved	10.5	5.0
Other + unclassified	4.8	12.0
Total	100	100

*Non-Hodgkin's Lymphoma Pathologic Classification Project.[39]

ulin and of the kappa and lambda light chains have been useful in demonstrating the B-cell origin of most gastric lymphomas[38] and monoclonality or lack thereof. Some B-cell lymphomas show no staining for light chains but only for pan-B antigens. Rare gastric lymphomas (2 of 86) express T-cell markers.[38]

The demonstration of monoclonality, of course, strongly supports the diagnosis of malignancy, although with certain provisos noted previously in the discussion of pseudolymphomas. Both techniques using frozen section material and paraffin-embedded tissue have been employed. The frozen section techniques avoid the problems of loss or alteration of antigenicity secondary to fixation, but are unavailable as a rule in any retrospective study. The problems involved are detailed by Platz[5] and by Warnke and Rouse.[40] In gastric lymphomas, at least with fixed material, more than half the cases in most series are negative by these techniques or show so few positive cells that interpretation is hazardous. Such negativity should

not necessarily be interpreted as due to null cells or T cells, since they may represent artifacts of fixation. A further problem is infiltration of tumor by nonneoplastic cells, either lymphocytes or histiocytes. While we do not propose to give here a detailed analysis of the results (for which see Platz[5]), it seems agreed that the gastric lymphomas are most commonly of B-cell origin with a few of proven T-cell origin.[42] T-cell markers have not been as well studied. Most investigators believe that the incidence of true histiocytic tumors, at least in the stomach, is low, although this frequency is debated (see below). The most consistently positive staining appears to be in the small cell plasmacytoid tumors and the most frequently negative, at least in paraffin sections, the small cleaved cell lymphomas (i.e., nonplasmacytoid poorly differentiated lymphocytic lymphoma).[27] Immunoglobulin (Ig)A, IgG, IgM, and IgD have all been reported in gastric lymphoma of the B-cell type, IgM with the greatest frequency. The lambda light chain has been the most common in most series, but not in all.

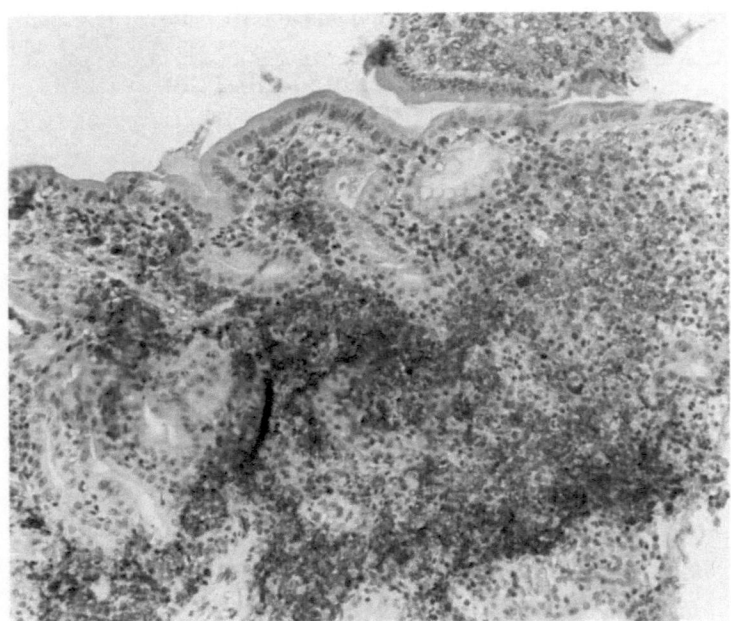

A

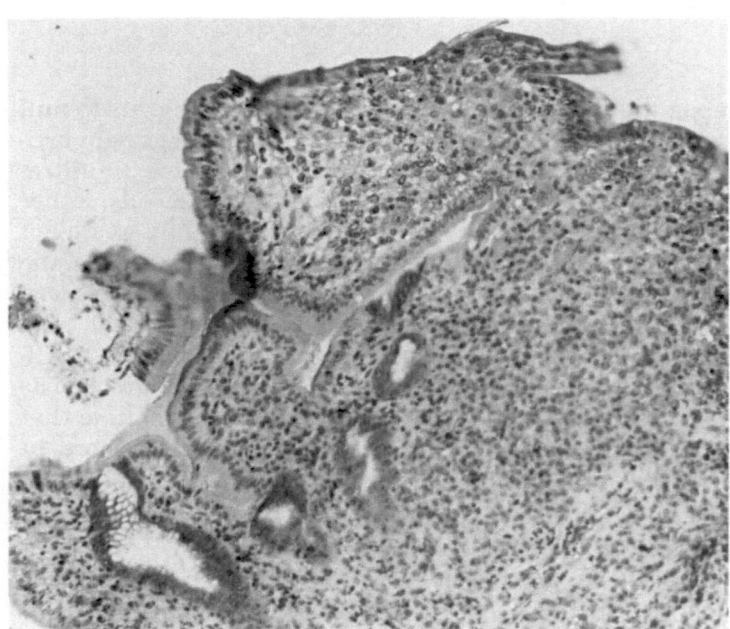

B

Figure 10-12. Immunoperoxidase staining of gastric lymphoma. (Courtesy of Dr. Glezerov.) **A.** Leukocyte common antigen staining is positive. X100, reproduced at 95%. **B.** Epithelial membrane antigen staining is negative in the lymphomatous infiltrate and positive in gastric foveolae. X100, reproduced at 95%.

The major discrepancy in the literature concerns the frequency of true histiocytic lymphoma as indicated by positive staining for lysozyme and α_1-antitrypsin plus polyclonal staining for light chains, presumably due to the phagocytosis by the neoplastic cells. Isaacson and co-workers[29] reported that half of their 66 cases of primary gastrointestinal lymphomas were of true histiocytic origin, including 4 of 7 gastric cases. Seo and co-workers[43] reported that 4 of 18 gastric lymphomas were histiocytic. They further stated that such cases were not separable from other lymphomas on morphologic grounds.

Figure 10-13. Gastric lymphoma. Note the mucosal and submucosal spread. H&E, X4, reproduced at 95%.

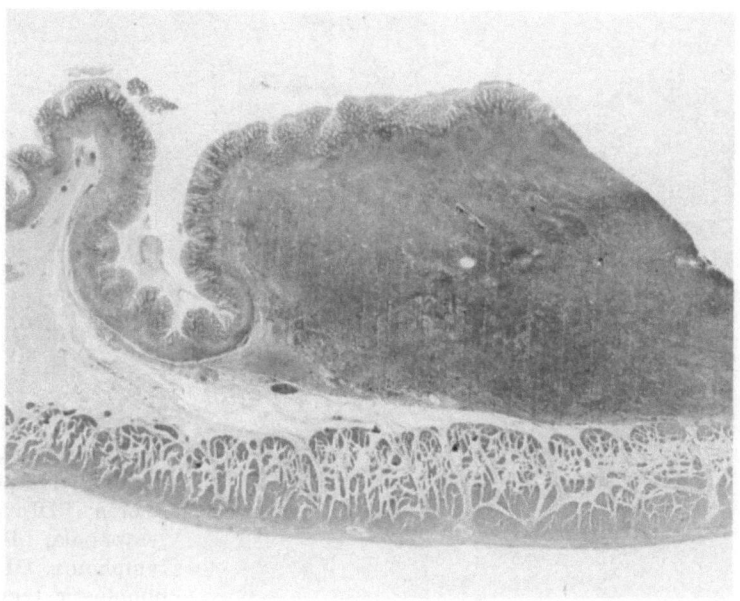

On the other hand, most other series have shown no such cases[27,44] or only an occasional case.[45] The discrepancy is partially explained by overinterpreting stains for histiocytic markers on fixed tissue sections.[44] Infiltration of lymphomas by benign histiocytes, according to Kahn and co-workers,[46] may range from 20 to 50% of the total cell population. They believe that most such cases can be separated from true histiocytic lymphomas by the concentration of such cells in the periphery of the tumor or the production of a checkerboard pattern of such cells positive for histiocyte markers. Utilization of frozen sections allows for more accurate classification.[44]

Gross and Histologic Features of Lymphoma

The gross and histologic features of lymphoma have already been commented on in our discussion of the differentiation of pseudolymphoma and lymphoma. We will only restate here, in outline fashion, that gastric lymphomas tend to be large and may be polypoid, plaque-like, or diffuse (see Figs. 10-3 and 10-4). Fibrosis, if present, is band-like and does not subdivide the tumor into loci of cellularity. Germinal centers are lacking except in the periphery or subtending lymphoma and necrosis, including destruction of muscle, is frequent. The latter is an important consideration, since involvement of the full thickness of the gastric wall may result in perforation, especially after radiation or chemotherapy. Lymphomas tend to infiltrate along the submucosa and the serosa (Figs. 10-13 and 10-14). Direct spread through the serosa into adjacent organs, such as the liver, spleen, and pancreas, is not uncommon.[47] Brooks and Enterline[14] found that in the majority of gastric lymphomas the mitotic rate was considerably in excess of 10 per 10 high-power fields. This finding contrasts with the low mitotic rate in pseudolymphoma. However, well-differentiated and poorly differentiated lymphocytic lymphoma also showed mitotic rates well below this level (Fig. 10-15).

Stage at Presentation

The staging system used in most of the more recently reported series is the modified Ann Arbor Staging Classification.[48] In this classi-

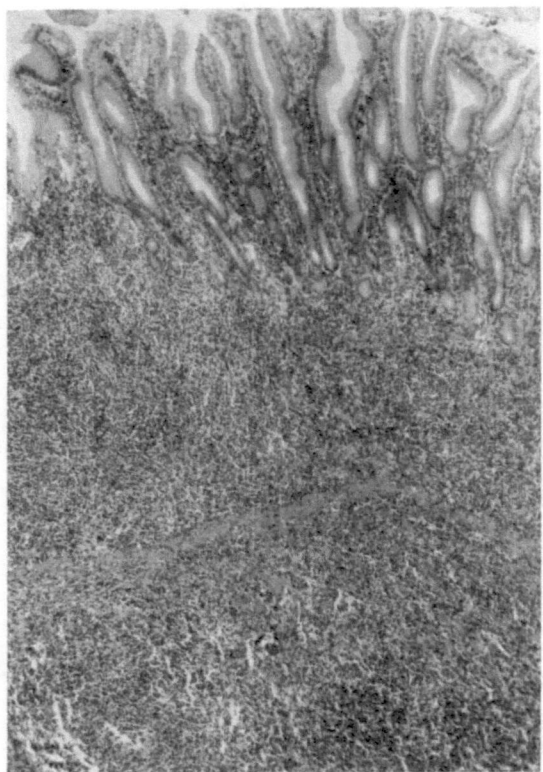

Figure 10-14. Gastric lymphoma. A diffuse lymphocytic infiltrate spreads in the mucosa and submucosa, leaving the muscularis mucosae partially intact. H&E, X40, reproduced at 75%.

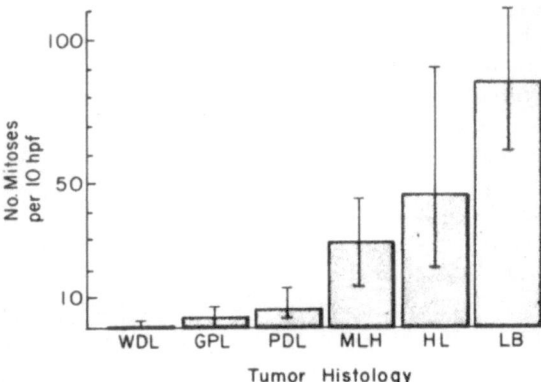

Figure 10-15. Gastric lymphomas: Mitotic index and histologic type. WDL: well differentiated lymphocytic lymphoma; GPL: gastric pseudolymphoma; PDL: poorly differentiated lymphocytic lymphoma; MLH: mixed lymphocytic-histiocytic lymphoma; HL: histiocytic lymphoma; LB: lymphoblastic lymphoma. From Brooks and Enterline,[14] with permission.

fication, as applied to the stomach, Stage I(E) is defined as those lymphomas confined to the stomach without node involvement. Stage II(E) is those with involvement of gastric or other intraabdominal nodes. Stage II is divided into Stage II(E$_1$), those with limited regional node involvement, and Stage II(E$_2$), those with more extensive intraabdominal involvement. Stage III are those cases with involvement above and below the diaphragm, and Stage IV constitutes those with dissemination to the liver, bone marrow, or other distant extranodal sites.

It is possible that focal gastric lymphoma (such as those arising within pseudolymphoma) may remain localized for long periods. However, gastric lymphomas at the time of diagnosis show a marked tendency to spread. In an effort to avoid secondary cases, many series understate or ignore Stages III and IV; thus, figures for later dissemination are difficult to obtain. For Stage IV, Platz[5] quotes figures varying from 12 to 65%. It is clear that lymph nodes, at least the regional gastric nodes, are involved in 50% or more cases in most series (Table 10-7).

The use of tomography for staging has some problems, since regional nodes in gastric lymphoma may be quite large and yet be only hyperplastic.[14,49,50] Tumors whose invasion is restricted to the submucosa most often are Stage I(E) and tend to be less than 7 cm in diameter,[14] but there are sufficient exceptions to render this criterion of little practical value. Stage IV cases may involve the liver, spleen, lung, bone marrow, skin, brain, and, of particular note, Waldeyer's ring,[51] as well as other sites in the gastrointestinal tract. Similarly, Stage I or II cases may disseminate to such sites at a later time.

Survival

The overall survival rate in a recent compilation of the literature[14] averaged out to 53% at

Table 10-7. Distribution of Stage of Gastric Lymphoma at Presentation

Stage	Lim et al[49] (N=50)	Brooks and Enterline[14] (N=58)	Weingard et al[4] (N=76)	Dragosics et al[27] (N=105)
I	58%	34%	38%	20%
II	38%	65%	49%	76%

5 years and 44% at 10 years. When only death from disease is considered, 2-year overall survival rates as high as 78% have been reported.[27] Most patients who die of disease will do so within the first 2 years.[14,27] Spontaneous regression has been observed in rare cases.[52]

It has often been stated that the prognosis from primary gastric lymphoma is better than that for carcinoma. However, when compared stage for stage, this improvement in prognosis is not nearly as apparent[49] (Table 10-8).

Whether, as sometimes thought, gastric lymphoma has a better prognosis than lymphomas in general has been critically analyzed.[5] Platz concluded that the answer is not yet clear.

Prognostic Factors

The factors relating to prognosis that have been analyzed in most series include histologic type, size, depth of penetration, and stage.

Histologic Type and Survival
The influence of histologic type on survival remains unsettled. Most series are relatively small and therefore, when broken down by subtype and compared stage for stage, it is difficult to attain statistically significant results. Also, not all series use the same classification and other factors, such as size and stage, interrelate with type.[51,53] Many authors have concluded that the histologic type is of only minor prognostic significance compared with stage at presentation.[14,27,30,54] However, despite lack of statistical significance, most believe that prognosis is better for nodular as opposed to diffuse lymphoma and for the diffuse small and mixed forms (62 to 73% 5-year survival) as opposed to large cell lymphomas (57% 5-year survival). On the other hand, other authors state that the histologic type is indeed important. For instance, Filippa and co-workers[6] analyzed 60 cases of gastrointestinal primary lymphoma, of which 45 were of gastric origin. In their series (site not specified) patients with low-grade lymphoplasmacytoid tumors did well, with 74% either being alive or dying of other disease without evidence of lymphoma, with a median follow-up of 171 and 147 months, respectively. They also showed a low rate of recurrence and dissemination. In contrast, the other categories did much more poorly, with 60% dying of disease at an average of 7 months and with a high incidence of extraabdominal recurrences. They admit the difficulty of stage-for-stage comparison because of numbers. Dworkin and co-workers[53] also reported a favorable outcome for patients with lymphoplasmacytoid forms. Using various classifications, Dragosics and co-workers[27] reported a distinctly better prognosis at 2 years for those with low- and median-grade malignant

Table 10-8. Comparison by Stage of Survival in Gastric Lymphoma and Gastric Adenocarcinoma*

Stage	Lymphoma (N=50)	Carcinoma (N=1202)
I_A (mucosa)	90%	85%
I_C (serosa)	33%	47%
II_{E1} (adjacent nodes)	33%	21%
II_{E2} (regional nodes)		12%
IV	0%	4%

*Modified from Lim et al.[49]

Table 10-9. Literature Summary, Gastric Lymphomas: Five-Year Survival versus Stage of Disease, All Histologic Types*

Author	Stage I	Stage II
Hoerr et al[56]	10/12 (83%)	2/7 (29%)
Rudders et al[57]	2/2 (100%)	0/1 (0%)
Shani et al[58]	4/4 (100%)	–
Herrmann et al[3]	10/14 (71%)	8/14 (57%)
Brooks and Enterline et al[14]	11/13 (85%)	11/26 (42%)
Total	37/45 (82%)	21/48 (44%)

*Only those articles employing newer classifications of lymphoma.
From Brooks and Enterline,[14] with permission of the publisher.

Table 10-10. Survival Correlated with Serosal Penetration

Author	Serosa Intact	Serosa Penetrated
Shimm et al[54]	91%	32%
Lim et al[49]	82%	24%
Shiu et al[47]	87%	50%

lymphomas (with 48% survival rate) compared to those with high grade malignant lymphomas (with an 18% survival rate). This comparison was without regard to stage, which they considered more important. Shiu and co-workers[47] reported 16 of 26 patients with gastric histiocytic lymphomas to have died of disease as compared with only 1 of 11 with diffuse well-differentiated lymphocytic tumors. Their unusually high percentage of the latter group (22% in their series) is out of line with other series and raises some questions. Finally, in an immunologically focused study, Seo and co-workers[43] reported a 5-year survival rate of 86% for those cases showing globulin-positive B-cell markers as opposed to only 26% for the nonreactive group. There were no survivors in the four cases considered to be truly histiocytic. Similar results are also reported by Saraga and co-workers,[18] although their cases were not site specified. Accumulation of more information is clearly needed.

Stage and Survival

The stage at presentation is agreed by all to be a very important prognostic indicator. Platz[5] in his review, indicates survival rates of 60 to 88% for Stage I(E) as opposed to 21 to 55% for Stage II(E). Involvement of lymph nodes cuts survival roughly in half[14] (Table 10-9). Involvement of nonadjacent abdominal

nodes further reduces survival.[6,27] There are too few Stage III and IV cases for analysis in most reports; however, Rosenfelt and Rosenberg[55] report a 27% survival rate for patients with gastrointestinal diffuse histiocytic lymphoma (DHL) Grade III and IV, site not specified.

Depth of Penetration and Survival

Lymphomas confined to the submucosa have a distinctly favorable prognosis.[5,14] Cases in which the serosa is penetrated, on the other hand, have a much worse survival rate than those in which the serosa is intact (Table 10-10). Direct involvement of adjacent organs and perforation are also ominous signs.[31]

Size and Survival

Survival is inversely proportional to size. Brooks and Enterline[14] reported better survival of patients with tumors measuring less than 7 cm, and Saraga et al[18] made similar observations with a cut-off point at 5 cm. Hande and co-workers[59] reported complete remission for only 1 of 13 cases with tumors larger than 10 cm.

Summary of Prognostic Factors

These various prognostic factors are to some extent interrelated, and their assessment permits a reasonably clear prognosis. Thus, Shimm and co-workers[54] noted that all of six patients with Stage I tumors, confined to the submucosa and with uninvolved serosal margins, were free of tumor with a mean follow-up of 5 years. By multivariate analysis the most important prognostic factor is extragastric spread of lymphoma, either into adjacent organs or abdominal lymph nodes.[31] DNA aneuploidy, demonstrable by flow cytometry in 50% of gastric lymphomas, correlates with a poor prognosis but also with extragastric spread.

Relation of Lymphoma to Adenocarcinoma

There are rare reports of adenocarcinoma as a complication of gastric lymphoma. In general, these have followed partial gastrectomy for lymphoma by many years and may be coincidental or, perhaps, related to factors associated with gastrectomy.[58]

Plasmacytoma and Plasma Cell Granuloma of the Stomach

Extramedullary plasmacytomas may be defined as true localized extraosseus neoplasms of plasma cells that can be proved to be monoclonal for Ig subclasses and for kappa or lambda light chains. The bulk of such tumors occur in the upper respiratory passages. Plasmacytomas primary to the stomach form only 3 to 5% of the total of such cases.[60,61] Henry and Farrer-Brown[62] considered 30% of their gastric lymphoid neoplasms to be plasmacytomas. They included all tumors with morphologic evidence of IgG (except "secretory" plasma cell tumors) under the heading of plasmacytomas. This would include cases of small cell lymphomas with some plasmacytomas. This would include cases of small cell lymphomas with some plasmacytoid differentiation (i.e., lymphocytic immunocytoma), which are not considered plasmacytomas by most authors. The majority would restrict the term plasmacytoma to purely plasmacytic neoplasms.[63] As so defined, they are rare tumors of the stomach with less than 100 acceptable cases reported to date. In most instances, the lack of bone marrow involvement (at presentation) and of abnormal serum globulins easily differentiates these cases from myeloma. In most instances

there is no problem in distinguishing these purely plasmacytic lesions from chronic inflammation. However, three cases composed almost exclusively of plasma cells and presenting as localized gastric masses have been reported under the term "plasma cell granuloma." The histology of these cases was that of completely mature plasma cells, without mitoses, which were arranged in streams and associated with a fibrotic reaction.[64-66] In the two cases in which immunologic techniques were applied, the lesions proved to be polyclonal for both globulins and light chains.

Scott and co-workers[67] reviewed 66 cases of gastric plasmacytoma and reported occurrence over a wide age range (27 to 87 years, mean 52 years) and with male to female predominance of 3 to 2. Serum proteins were usually normal, but Bence Jones protein has been reported with recurrence or dissemination. The plasma cells are usually fairly mature, though with varying degrees of atypia and mitotic figures. In those cases in which immunocytochemistry was tested, most have shown IgG or IgA, although IgM has also been reported.[61] Follow-up has often been sketchy; however, Scott and co-workers state that in their review of 66 patients 30 were dead within 2 years. The high death rate suggests that some patients, in reality, may have had immunoblastic lymphomas. At the same time, a few cases of very long-term survival were noted. In his general discussion of extramedullary plasmacytomas, Wiltshaw[60] stresses that when dissemination does occur in extramedullary plasmacytomas, as a rule it does not mimic that seen in myeloma but involves lung, lymph nodes, skin, and liver; if bone is involved it often is only one or several areas, and not necessarily in hematopoetic areas of bone.

An interesting case was reported by Ferrer-Roca[68] in which the plasma cells were markedly distorted by needle-shaped cytoplasmic crystals.

The lack of initial serum abnormalities has been commented on by many authors and various opinions have been expressed, such as that the tumors are too small, the cells form but do not secrete globulin, or globulins are secreted by too few of the cells. Preud Homme and Galien[63] favor rapid degradation of the globulins as the most reasonable explanation.

Leukemia

Leukemic infiltrates commonly involve the gastrointestinal tract, at least late in the disease. The incidence of such involvement at autopsy has varied from 23 to 63% of cases.[69,70] The stomach is less commonly involved than the intestinal tract. In the stomach such infiltrates are usually submucosal and may present as diffuse rugal thickening, localized multiple plaques, or nodular or polypoid masses. The localized plaque, usually ulcerated, is said to be the most common gastric presentation.[70] Associated massive bleeding may occur either as a result of such ulcerated infiltrates or due to associated peptic ulceration.

Less well known is the occurrence of granulocytic sarcomas (chloromas), which have been reported in the stomach although they are more common elsewhere. Most coexist with developed granulocytic leukemia, but rarely they may precede overt leukemia. The diagnosis is readily established by the positivity of such cells for napthol AS-D chloracetate. Chloromas may be confused with lymphoma unless the diagnosis is considered.[71]

An isolated case of gastric involvement with Richter's syndrome (i.e., chronic lymphocytic leukemia complicated by diffuse large cell lymphoma) of the stomach has been described. Both cell types stained for IgG lambda.[72]

References

1. McNeer G, Berg JW: Clinical behavior and management of primary malignant lymphoma of the stomach. Surgery 1959;46:829–840.

2. Ehrlich AN, Stalder G, Geller W, et al: Gastrointestinal manifestations of lymphoma. Gastroenterology 1968;54:1115–1121.

3. Herrmann R, Panahon AM, Barcos MP, et al: Gastrointestinal involvement in non-Hodgkin's lymphoma. Cancer 1980;46:215–222.

4. Weingrad DN, DeCosse JJ, Sherlock P, et al: Primary gastrointestinal lymphoma: A 30-year review. Cancer 1982;49:1258–1265.

5. Platz CE: Lymphoid proliferations of the stomach, in Appelman HD (ed): Pathology of the Esophagus, Stomach, and Duodenum. New York: Churchill Livingstone, 1984, chap 8.

6. Filippa DA, Lieberman PH, Weingrad DN, et al: Primary lymphomas of the gastrointestinal tract: Analysis of prognostic factors with emphasis on histologic type. Am J Surg Pathol 1983;7:363–371.

7. Young JL, Percy CL, Asire AJ: Surveillance, epidemiology and end results: Incidence and mortality data 1972–1977. National Cancer Institute Monograph no. 57. Washington, DC: U.S. Government Printing Office, 1981.

8. Fu Y, Perzin KH: Lymphosarcoma of the small intestine. Cancer 1972;29:645–659.

9. Brooks JJ, Enterline HT: Gastric pseudolymphoma: Its three subtypes and relations to lymphoma. Cancer 1983;51:476–486.

10. Smith J, Helwig EB: Malignant lymphoma of the stomach (abstract). Am J Pathol 1958; 34:553.

11. Helwig EB: Diseases of the alimentary tract. 12th Annual Seminar of the Indiana Association of Pathologists, 1960 (unpublished).

12. Jacobs DS: Primary gastric malignant lymphoma and pseudolymphoma of the stomach. Am J Clin Pathol 1963;40:379–394.

13. Ranchod H, Lewin KJ, Dorfman RF: Lymphoid hyperplasia of the gastrointestinal tract: A study of 26 cases and review of the literature. Am J Surg Pathol 1978;2:383–400.

14. Brooks JJ, Enterline HT: Primary gastric lymphomas: A clinicopathologic study of 58 cases with long term followup and literature review. Cancer 1983;51:701–711.

15. Tokunaga O, Watanabe T, Movinatsu M: Pseudolymphoma of the stomach. A clinicopathologic study of 15 cases. Cancer 1987;59:1320–1327.

16. Ioachim HL: Lymph Node Biopsy. Philadelphia: JB Lippincott, 1982, chap 21.

17. Toth J, Ronay P: Gastric pseudolymphomas resembling angioproliferative lymph node hyperplasia. Oncology 1974;30:244–253.

18. Saraga P, Hurlimann J, Ozello L: Lymphomas and pseudolymphomas of the alimentary tract, an immunohistochemical study with clinicopathologic correlations. Hum Pathol 1981;12: 713–723.

19. Hyjek E, Kelenyi G: Pseudolymphoma of the stomach–a lesion characterized by progressively transformed germinal centers. Histopathology 1982;6:61–68.

20. Platz CE: Extranodal lymphomas and pseudolymphomas. Presented at Tutorial on Neoplastic Hematopathology, Chicago, September 1972.

21. Eimoto T, Futami K, Naito H, et al: Gastric pseudolymphoma with monotypic cytoplasmic immunoglobulin. Cancer 1985;55:788–793.

22. Burke JS, Sheibani K, Nathwani BN, et al: Monoclonal small (well-differentiated) lymphocytic proliferations of the gastrointestinal tract resembling lymphoid hyperplasia: A neoplasm of uncertain malignant potential. Hum Pathol 1987;18:1238–1245.

23. Levy N, Nelson J, Meyer P, et al: Reactive lymphoid hyperplasia with single class (monoclonal) surface immunoglobulin. Am J Clin Pathol 1983;80:300–308.

24. Galton DAG, Catovsky D, Wiltshaw E: Clinical spectrum of lymphoproliferative diseases. Cancer 1978;42:901–909.

25. Murayama H, Kikuchi M, Eimoto T, et al: Early lymphoma coexisting with reactive lymphoid hyperplasia of the stomach. Acta Pathol Jpn 1984;34:679–684.

26. Wolf JA, Spjut HJ: Focal lymphoid hyperplasia of the stomach preceding gastric lymphoma. Cancer 1981;48:2518–2523.

27. Dragosics B, Bauer P, Radaszkiewicz T: Primary gastrointestinal non-Hodgkin's lymphoma. A retrospective clinicopathologic study of 150 cases. Cancer 1985;55:1060–1073.

28. Najem AZ, Porcaro JL, Rush BF: Primary non-Hodgkin's lymphoma of the duodenum. Case report and literature review. Cancer 1984;54: 895–898.

29. Isaacson P, Wright DH, Judd MA, et al: Primary gastrointestinal lymphoma: A classification of 66 cases. Cancer 1979;43:1805–1819.

30. Lewin KJ, Ranchod M, Dorfman RF: Lymphomas of the gastrointestinal tract. Cancer 1978;42:693–707.

31. Joensuu H, Söderström K-O, Klemi P, Ecrola E: Nuclear DNA content and its prognostic value in lymphoma of the stomach. Cancer 1987;60:3042–3048.

32. Cabré-Fiol V, Vilardell F: Progress in the cytologic diagnosis of gastric lymphoma: A report of 32 cases. Cancer 1978;41:1456–1461.

33. Martin SE, Zhang H, Magyarosy E, et al: Immunologic methods in cytology: Definitive diagnosis of non-Hodgkin's lymphomas using immunologic markers for T and B cells. Am J Clin Pathol 1984;82:666–673.

34. Ernst C: Personal communication.

35. Solidoro A, Salazar F, de la Fior J, et al: Endoscopic tissue diagnosis of gastric involvement in the staging of non-Hodgkin's lymphoma. Cancer 1981;48:1053–1057.

36. Isaacson RG, Spencer J: Malignant lymphoma of mucosa-associated lymphoid tissue. Histopathology 1987;11:445–462.

37. Isaacson PG, Spencer J, Finn T: Primary B-cell gastric lymphoma. Hum Pathol 1986;17: 72–82.

38. Berger F, Coiffier B, Bonneville C, et al: Gastrointestinal lymphomas. Immunohistologic study of 23 cases. Am J Clin Pathol 1987;88: 707–712.

39. National Cancer Institute Sponsored Study of Classifications of Non-Hodgkin's Lymphomas: Summary and description of a working formulation for clinical usage. The Non-Hodgkin's Lymphoma Pathologic Classification Project. Cancer 1982;49:2112–2135.

40. Warnke RA, Rouse RV: Limitations encountered in the application of tissue section immunodiagnosis to the study of lymphomas and related disorders. Hum Pathol 1985;16:326–331.

41. Dean PJ, Moinuddin SM, Emerson LD: Application of anti-leukocyte common antigen and anti-cytokeratin antibodies to the biopsy diagnosis of gastric large cell lymphoma. Hum Pathol 1987;18:918–923.

42. Riddell RH, Lewin KJ: Surgical pathology of the gastrointestinal tract: Diagnostic problems and evolving concepts. IAP Short Course no. 14, 1985.

43. Seo IS, Binkley WB, Warner TFCS, et al: A combined morphologic and immunologic approach to the diagnosis of gastrointestinal lymphomas. 1. Malignant lymphoma of the stomach (a clinicopathologic study of 22 cases). Cancer 1982;49:493–501.

44. Grody WW, Weiss LM, Warnke RA, et al: Gastrointestinal lymphomas. Immunohistochemical studies on the cell origin. Am J Surg Pathol 1985;9:328–337.

45. Vimadalal SD, Said JW, Voyles H III: Gastric

lymphoreticular neoplasms: An immunologic study of 36 cases. Am J Clin Pathol 1983;80: 792–798.

46. Kahn LB, Mir R, Selzer G: True histiocytic lymphoma of the gut. Gastroenterologic Pathology Club Scientific Session, March 11, 1984.

47. Shiu MH, Karas M, Nisce L, et al: Management of primary gastric lymphoma. Ann Surg 1982;195:196–202.

48. Musshoff K: Klinische Stadieneinteilung der nicht-Hodgkin Lymphome. Strahlentherapie 1977;153:218–221.

49. Lim FE, Hartman AS, Tan EGC, et al: Factors in the prognosis of gastric lymphoma. Cancer 1977;39:1715–1720.

50. Berg JW: Primary lymphoma of the human gastrointestinal tract. Natl Cancer Inst Monog 1969:32(hematopoeitic neoplasms):211–220.

51. Saul SH, Kapadia SB: Primary lymphoma of Waldeyer's ring. Clinicopathologic study of 68 cases. Cancer 1985;56:157–166.

52. Strauchen JA, Moran C, Goldsmith M, et al: Spontaneous regression of gastric lymphoma. Cancer 1987;60:1872–1975.

53. Dworkin B, Lightdale CJ, Weingrad DN, et al: Primary gastric lymphoma: A review of 50 cases. Dig Dis Sci 1982;27:987–992.

54. Shimm DS, Dosoretz DE, Anderson T, et al: Primary gastric lymphoma: An analysis with emphasis on prognostic factors and radiation therapy. Cancer 1983;82:2044–2048.

55. Rosenfelt F, Rosenberg SA: Diffuse histiocytic lymphoma presenting with gastrointestinal tract lesions. Cancer 1980;45:2188–2193.

56. Hoerr S, McCormack L, Hertzer N: Prognosis in gastric lymphoma. Arch Surg 1973;107: 155–158.

57. Rudders R, Ross M, DeLellis R: Primary extranodal lymphoma. Cancer 1978;42:406–416.

58. Shani A, Schott AJ, Weiland LH: Primary gastric lymphoma followed by gastric adenocarcinoma. Cancer 1978;42:2039–2044.

59. Hande KR, Fisher RI, DeVita VT, et al: Diffuse histiocytic lymphoma involving the gastrointestinal tract. Cancer 1978;41:1984–1989.

60. Wiltshaw E: The natural history of extramedullary plasmacytoma and its relation to solitary myeloma of bone and myelomatosis. Medicine 1976;55:217–238.

61. Funakoshi N, Kanoh T, Kobayashi Y, et al: IgM producing gastric plasmacytoma. Cancer 1984;54:638–643.

62. Henry K, Farrer-Brown G: Primary lymphomas of the gastrointestinal tract. I. Plasma cell tumors. Histopathology 1977;1:53–76.

63. Preud Homme JL, Galien A: Extramedullary plasmacytoma with gastric and lymph node involvement. Cancer 1980;46:1753–1762.

64. Soga J, Saito K, Suzuki N, et al: Plasma cell granuloma of the stomach. A report of a case and review of the literature. Cancer 1970;25: 618–625.

65. Isaacson P, Buchanan R, Mepham B: Plasma cell granuloma of the stomach. Hum Pathol 1978;9:355–363.

66. Domenichini E, Martiarena HM, Rubio HH: Gastric plasma cell granuloma. Report of a case. Endoscopy 1982;14:148–150.

67. Scott FET, Dupont PA, Webb J: Plasmacytoma of the stomach. Diagnosis with the aid of the immunoperoxidase technique. Cancer 1978; 41:675–681.

68. Ferrer-Roca O: Primary plasmacytoma with massive intracytoplasmic crystalline inclusions—a case report. Cancer 1982;50:755–758.

69. Everett CR, Haggard ME, Levin WC: Extensive leukemic infiltration of the gastrointestinal tract during apparent remission in acute leukemia. Blood 1963;22:92–99.

70. Cornes JS, Jones TG: Leukaemic lesions of the gastrointestinal tract. J Clin Pathol 1962;15: 3051–313.

71. Brugo EA, Marshall RB, Riberi AM, et al: Preleukemic granulocytic sarcomas of the gastrointestinal tract. Am J Clin Pathol 1977;68: 616–620.

72. Brousse N, Solal-Celighy P, Herrera A, et al: Gastrointestinal Richter's syndrome. Hum Pathol 1985;16:854–855.

CHAPTER 11

Gastric Smooth Muscle, Nerve Sheath, and Related Tumors

Smooth Muscle Tumors

Small gastric smooth muscle tumors are common in adults at autopsy. Meissner in 1944[1] observed them in almost 50% of such cases by careful manual examination of the stomach wall. More recently, microleiomyomas of 5 mm or less diameter were detected in 16.4% of resected stomachs, mostly in the upper half.[2] Thus, the larger leiomyomatous tumors of the stomach must, in current parlance, be suspected of possessing increased receptor activity for certain undefined growth factors. Platelet-derived growth factor (PDGF), a smooth muscle growth stimulant, might be involved.[3] Estrogens, of course, stimulate uterine leiomyoma growth, which ceases in their absence, but estrogens do not appear to affect similar gastric tumors that are equally common in men and women. Clinically, gastric smooth muscle tumors, benign or malignant, are asymptomatic when small unless they ulcerate and bleed. Larger solid intramural stomach tumors are spheroidal and may bulge into the lumen, stretch the serosa, or both. The classic radiologic and endoscopic appearance of gastric leiomyoma or leiomyosarcoma is a protrusive hemispherical mass in the fundus or body of the stomach, which stretches the mucosa and has an apical central volcano-like cratered ulcer that bleeds.

Weight loss, upper abdominal pain, and an epigastric mass are less common presentations. Obstruction may develop if the tumor is antral, a more common site for bizarre leiomyomas (leiomyoblastomas). Endoscopic biopsies may be insufficiently deep to identify viable tumor tissue. Frozen-section and gross pathologic diagnoses are generally not totally reliable in discriminating between a benign gastric leiomyoma and a sarcoma.

Unlike uterine leiomyomas, which have been reported to be monoclonal,[4] gastric smooth muscle tumors may represent either hyperplasias or genuine neoplasms. Modern investigative methods have evidently not yet been applied to determine their clonality. Also, in both these sites and elsewhere in soft tissues, either the arterial or venous smooth muscle or the visceral muscularis propria of diverse sites may develop tumors.[5] In the stomach, the muscularis mucosae is not considered a tumor source, but any of the three coats of gastric muscularis propria may be involved.

A caveat discovered by ultrastructural and immunohistochemical studies is that all spindle-celled gastric tumors are not leiomyomas. The controversy of nerve sheath versus smooth muscle origin is an old one,[6] now sometimes resolved by finding immunohistologic markers of Schwann cells in occasional gastric neurilemomas or neurofibromas, as considered further below.

Leiomyoma

The typical, clinically evident tumor, said to constitute up to 10% of gastric resections for tumor,[7] is bulky and protrudes as a smooth

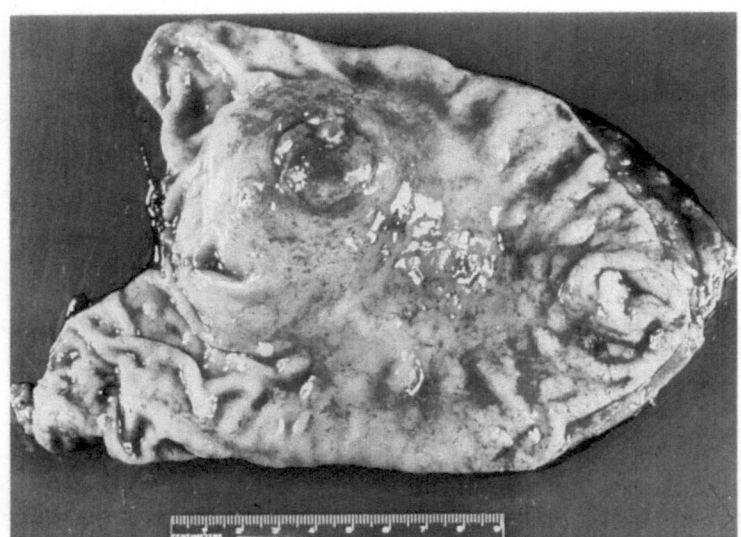

Figure 11-1.A. Leiomyoma of the gastric fundus. The tumor is spheroidal, with a round apical ulceration. **B.** This gastric leiomyoma, 4.5 cm in diameter, has a typical 1.2-cm mucosal ulcer crater.

A

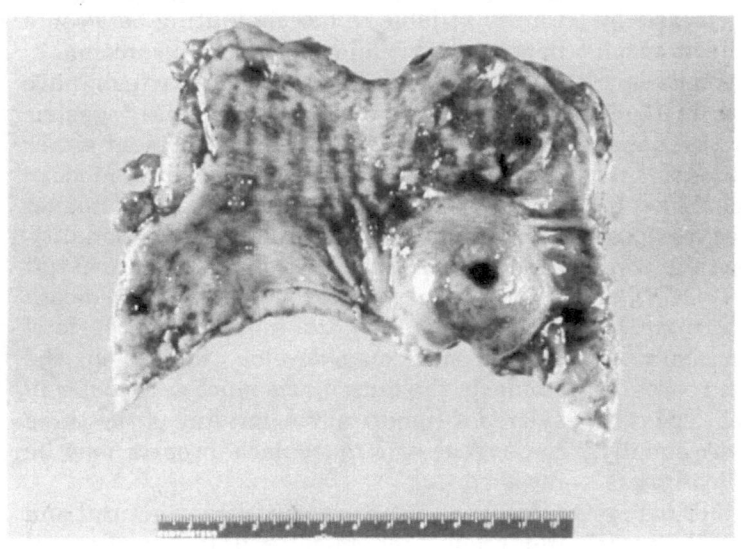

B

mass into the gastric lumen, with an apical, 0.5- to 2.5-cm, ulcerated mucosal crater that bleeds (Fig. 11-1). On cutting it, the mass has a whorled, solid, pinkish gray surface comparable with that of the ordinary uterine fibroid. There are typically dull glassy regions of hyaline degeneration and cystic foci with clear fluid contents. Necrosis in these benign tumors typically is rather limited, in contrast to the more massive necrosis and hemorrhage found in gastric sarcomas. Red degeneration is practically unknown.

Some gastric leiomyomas protrude endogastrically so that on x-ray examination, they appear polypoid. Others are pedunculated subserosal tumors with only a plaque-like base involving the peripheral gastric muscularis propria. Occasional leiomyomas are composed of multiple, closely adjacent, lobulated masses (Fig. 11-2). A few stomach leiomyomas are calcified[8] or subtotally necrotic (Fig. 11-3).

Microscopically, four different growth patterns characterize gastric leiomyomas: 1)

Figure 11-2A & B. Adjacent gastric leiomyomas both protrude into the stomach lumen, with central hemorrhagic ulcerations showing rolled margins. On section, the smaller ordinary leiomyoma is pale and dense, while the larger bizarre leiomyoma is hemorrhagic and soft.

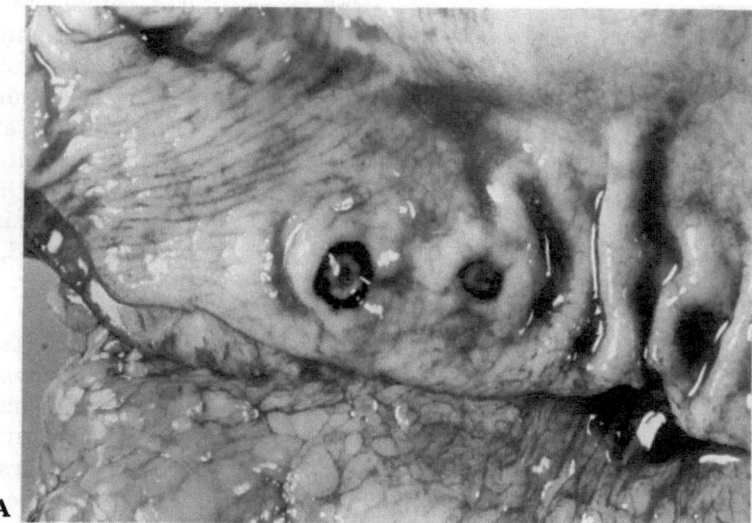

A

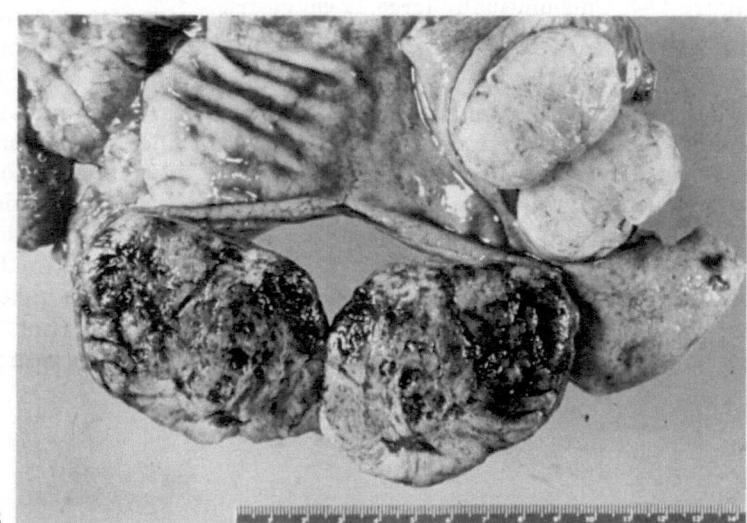

B

ordinary smooth muscle tumors, 2) cellular leiomyomas, 3) epitheloid (bizarre) leiomyomas (leiomyomblastomas), and 4) atypical leiomyomas.

Ordinary Smooth Muscle Tumors
Quite like the uterine fibroid, there are interlacing herringbone patterns of spindle cells, with elongated cigar-shaped uniform nuclei, sometimes perinuclear vacuoles, and reasonably abundant acidophil cytoplasm classically with longitudinal myofibrils (Fig. 11-4).[9] Compared with the adjacent unin-

volved muscularis, the tumor growth pattern is irregular and lacks the smooth undulating fasciculations of normal muscularis propria. Notable palisading of smooth muscle nuclei aligned like canoes is sometimes overt and sometimes focal or absent.[10] Since Antoni type A bodies of schwannomas are indistinguishable on routine examination, nuclear palisading is not diagnostically decisive. Hyaline, ischemic, vacuolar, and cystic degeneration are likely to be present except in the smallest leiomyomas. Fibroblastic interstitial overgrowth is prominent in

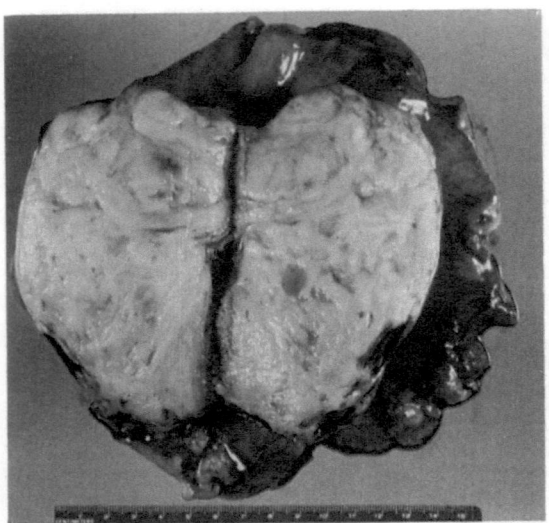

Figure 11-3. This unusually large 12-cm gastric leiomyoma has a tan reticulated appearance.

larger gastric leiomyomas. Mitoses are not found. The tumor margins are reasonably clear-cut, since the surrounding muscle and other tissues are compressed peripherally (Fig. 11-5).

Cellular Leiomyomas
As in comparable uterine tumors, many nuclei are compressed close together, with less cytoplasm, less hyalinization than in ordinary leiomyomas, and sometimes with focal necroses and hemorrhages. Mitoses are relatively easier to find (Fig. 11-6), but most of Appelman and Helwig's[11] 49 cases had less than 1 mitosis in 50 high power (X430) fields (HPF). One tumor with 5 mitoses /50 HPF metastasized, but three cellular leiomyomas with 8, 10, and 11 mitoses /50 HPF did not.[11]

Epithelioid (Bizarre) Leiomyomas (Leiomyoblastomas)
Some consternation may afflict the pathologist who examines frozen sections of what grossly appears to be a gastric leiomyoma. The histologic picture is that of closely packed round or polygonal clear cells with central uniform nuclei (Fig. 11-7). Possibilities of histiocytomas, xanthomas, histiocytosis, hairy cell leukemia, or clear cell renal carcinoma pass through the observer's mind. Then a memory of Stout's[12] term "leiomyoblastoma" resolves the dilemma. Although Evans[13] regarded the term as undesirable, it is very useful in teaching pathology residents and in the practical differential diagnoses of gastric surgical specimens or biopsies that otherwise may temporarily represent rather sinister mysteries.

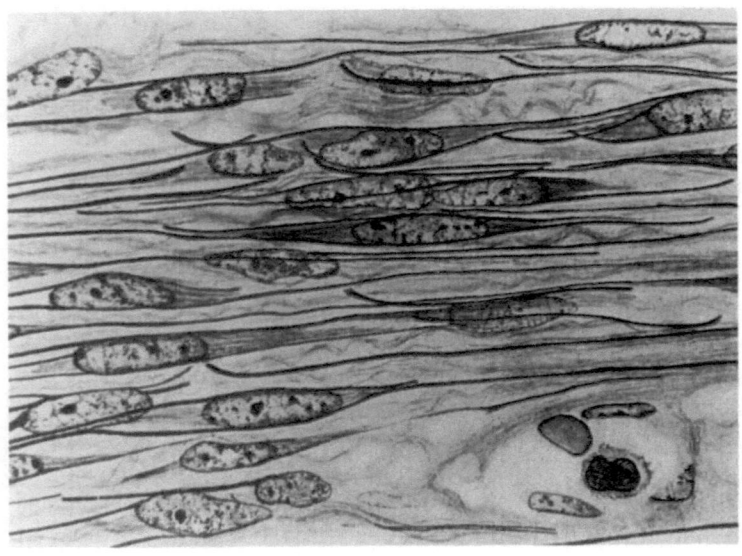

Figure 11-4. Drawing from Mallory[9] demonstrating cytoplasmic details with longitudinal myofibrils and local nuclear palisading in leiomyoma. Reproduced with permission of W.B. Saunders Co.

Leiomyoblastomas vary in size from 5 mm to 20 cm.[14] Characteristically, they are antral,[15] whereas other leiomyomas more often involve the gastric body or fundus. Grossly, these tumors resemble ordinary smooth muscle tumors, but microscopically their growth is infiltrative. The histologic peculiarity of small- or medium-sized cells with rounded or polygonal shapes, central rather bland nuclei, and clear perinuclear cytoplasm gives the tumor its name.[12,15-17] Also, mitotic counting does not provide clear evidence of metastatic potential, nor indeed does the tumor size.[18,19] The great majority are clinically benign, and in larger series, the incidence of malignancy in gastric leiomyoblastomas has been estimated as 1 to 12%.[15,19] However, among 49 so-called gastric "stromal" tumors, Appelman[20] reported that epithelioid leiomyosarcomas were the most common entity, more than twice as common as the benign analog.

Atypical Leiomyomas

Grossly and microscopically these intramural gastric tumors are unlike either classic uterine fibroid-type leiomyomas or clearly malignant smooth muscle neoplasms.[21] They tend to be irregularly nodular, partly lobulated, and to bulge unevenly either into the

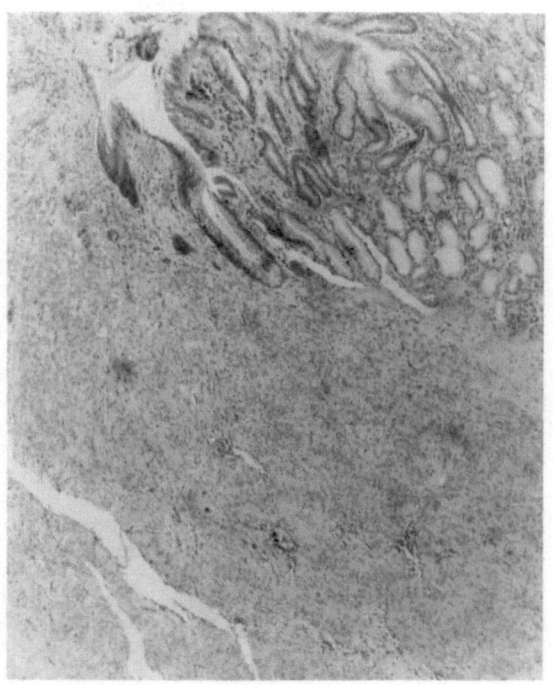

Figure 11-5. An intramural gastric leiomyoma has compressed the overlying submucosa and mucosa. HPS, X16, reproduced at 60%.

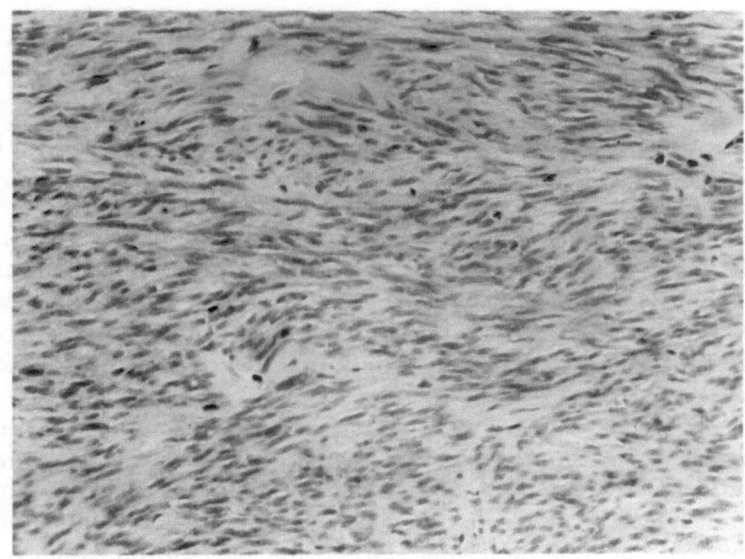

Figure 11-6. Closely packed, uniform spindle cells are present in a cellular gastric leiomyoma. HPS, X100, reproduced at 65%.

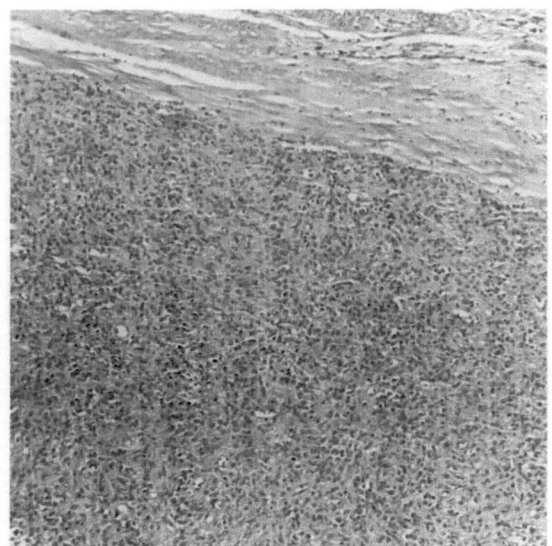

Figure 11-7.A. The distinct margin, cellularity, and peculiar epithelioid pattern of a gastric leiomyoblastoma are demonstrated. HPS, X40, reproduced at 65%. **B.** At higher magnification, the rather pale uniform nuclei and abundant pale or clear cytoplasm characterize leiomyoblastoma of the stomach. Mitosis is evident. HPS, X100, reproduced at 65%.

A

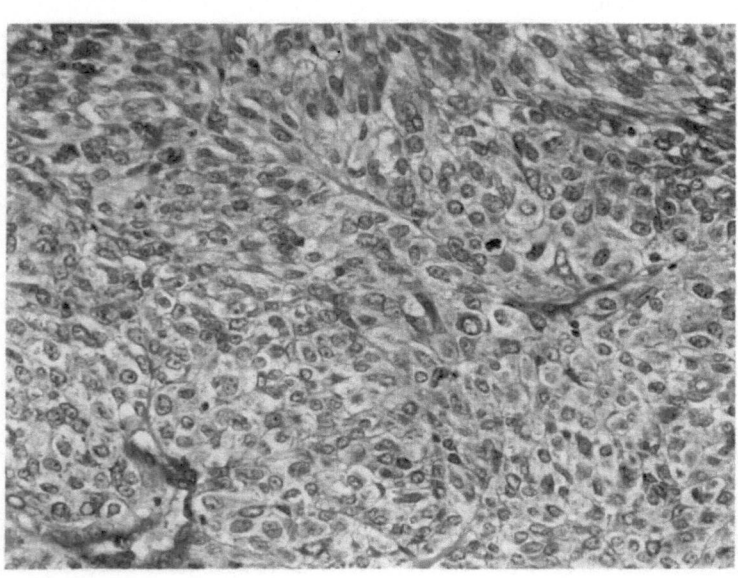

B

stomach or beneath the serosa. Some are dumbell-shaped (Fig. 11-8). Cut surfaces are tan and somewhat smooth without either the whorled, watered, silk whitish areas typical of fibroid tumors or the slick fish-flesh appearance of sarcomas.

Microscopically, atypical gastric leiomyomas are irregular in growth pattern and cytology. Various layers of spindle or partly rounded cells meet at angles. Nuclei vary two-fold in size, and some larger nuclear shapes are oval. Localized or diffuse nuclear hyperchromatism is found (Fig. 11-9). Mitoses are few or restricted to a few regions. Peripheral tumor may protrude tongue-like into the surrounding muscularis or connective tissue. No clear-cut adjacent tissue or vascular invasion is found. The histopathology is not identifiable as either that of a benign or malignant neoplasm. It is not a question of bizarre leiomyoma (leiomyoblastoma).

Several problems are present: 1) A better grasp of the malignant potential is obtained if both the gross and microscopic observations are carefully made. 2) Sampling of the tumor for microscopy may initially be inadequate or misleading. Further sections may clarify the problem. For example, there may be only peculiar clusters of syncytial multinucleated cells (Fig. 11-10). These changes, found also in some uterine fibroids, appear regressive rather than cancerous. 3) Mitotic counting alone cannot be relied on to give a clear prognostic indication unless there are many mitoses spread throughout the tumor.[22] Likewise, histochemistry, immunostaining, and ultrastructure do not solve the diagnostic difficulty. 4) Atypical leiomyomas, as Ewing[23] noted, may be neither clearly benign nor malignant, but in the process of becoming malignant. Consultation cases of atypical leiomyomas, while not infrequently diagnosed initially as leiomyosarcoma, have generally had a benign clinical outlook.

Leiomyosarcoma

Some gastric wall tumors are grossly clear cancers since they are large, lobulated, and irregular soft masses with invasive margins,

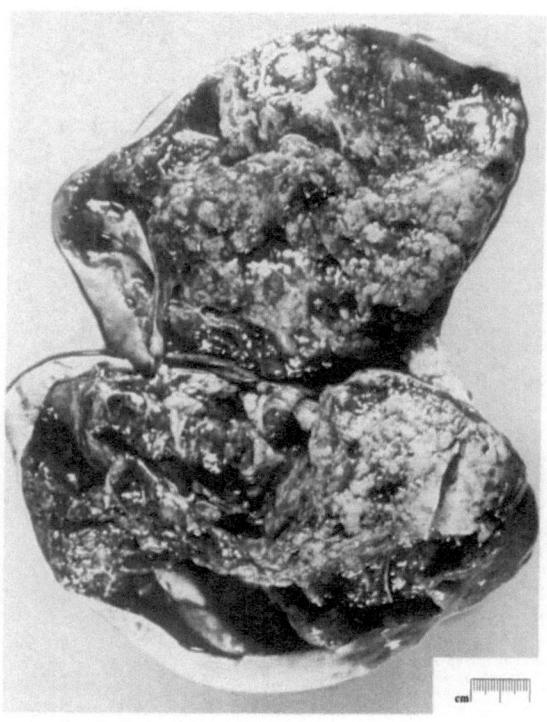

Figure 11-8. A 25-cm atypical gastric leiomyoma was grossly encapsulated, degenerated, and focally necrotic.

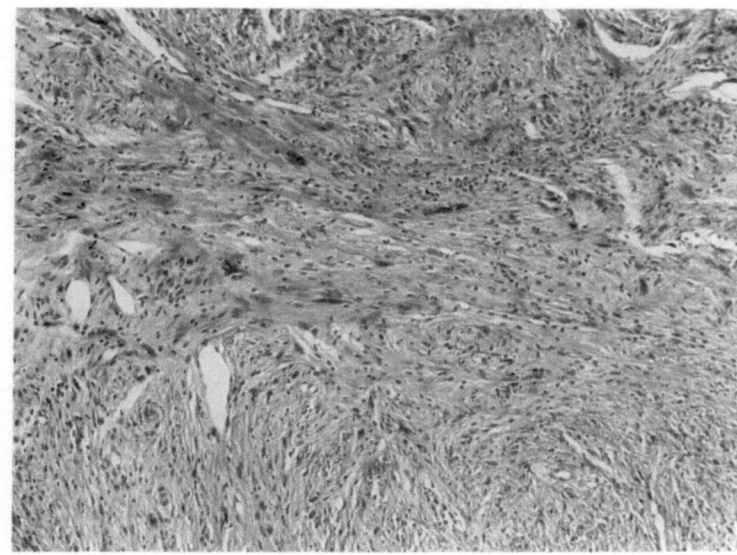

Figure 11-9. Irregularly arranged spindle and oval cells and focal enlargement of heavily or poorly stained nuclei are found in atypical leiomyomas. HPS, X40, reproduced at 65%.

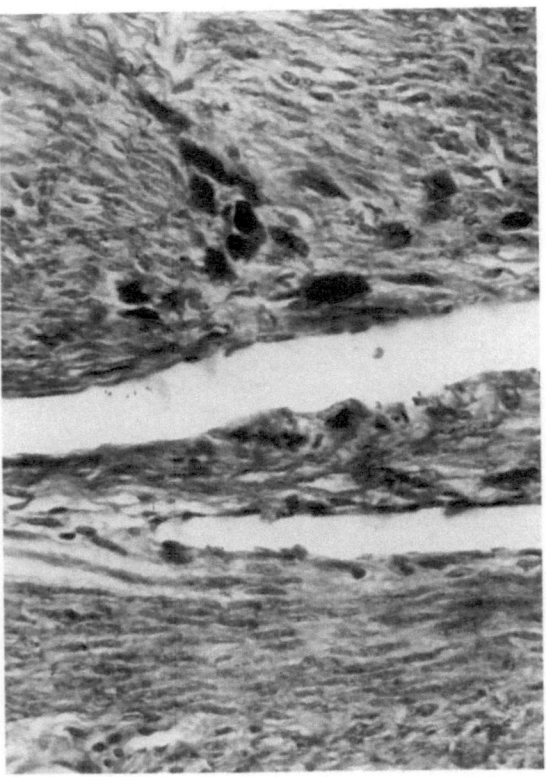

Figure 11-10. Heavily stained syncytial giant nuclei are degenerative and do not by themselves indicate leiomyosarcoma. HPS, X100, reproduced at 90%.

mucosal penetration, notable necrosis, and the slick raw fish-flesh cut surface appearance typical of diverse sarcomas (Fig. 11-11). The posterior gastric wall is involved twice as often as the anterior wall. Most are intramural, with half protruding into the peritoneum and one-third protruding into the gastric lumen. In 70%, the mucosa is ulcerated.[24] Before microscopic examination, the main problem is how to classify the obviously malignant tumor.[25]

Other gastric leiomyosarcomas are merely partly or wholly softer than expected and have the relatively yellow tan color common in cellular neoplasms. These tumors may be of any size, but the larger they are, the greater the suspicion of lethal cancer (Figs. 11-12 and 11-13).[24,26] In a report of 30 gastric leiomyosarcomas and a review of metastases in 161 collected cases, among various gross and microscopic attributes, the potential of metastasis was most closely correlated with tumor size.[27] A high risk of metastasis has been predicted in tumors 6 cm or more in diameter, with mitoses easily found.[20]. However, even a gastric leiomyosarcoma 1 cm in diameter proved fatal.[13]

Finally, gastric leiomyosarcoma may simply be a fibroid tumor mass of any size that on microscopic examination proves unexpect-

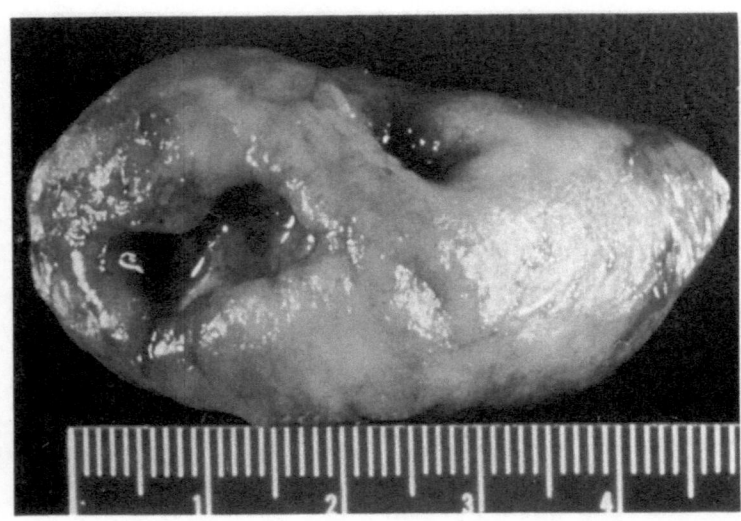

Figure 11-11. An ulcerated 5.5-cm gastric smooth muscle tumor has the typical smooth, slick sarcomatous surface.

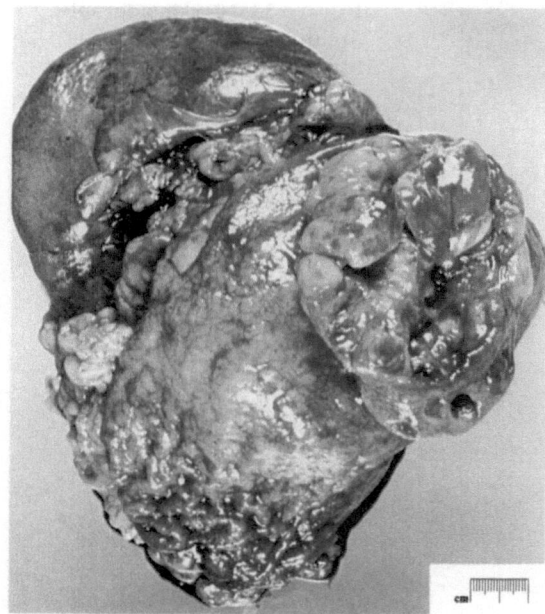

Figure 11-12. A large leiomyosarcoma of the stomach, 13 cm in diameter, is not grossly distinguishable from a leiomyoma.

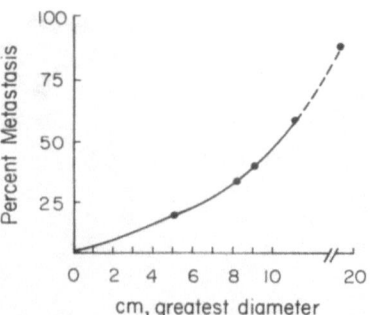

Figure 11-13. Graphic relationship between the size of gastric leiomyosarcoma and the percent with metastasis, derived from Appelman and Helwig,[24] Shiu and co-workers,[26] Berg and McNeer,[32] and Appelman.[34]

edly anaplastic, invasive, or both. The age range of patients is reported to be 12 to 75 years (mean of 50 years) with two-thirds of patients aged 40 to 80 years.[24] The natural history of gastric leiomyomas and leiomyosarcomas is practically unknown. Before symptoms develop, a tumor of considerable size may have formed, which is of indeterminate duration. Once identified, the tumor is promptly excised surgically. One woman had a "benign gastric tumor"[28] found at cholecystectomy 14 years before a leiomyosarcoma was diagnosed.* About all that is currently known is that human gastric leiomyosarcoma is polyclonal.[29] The tumor volume-doubling time of various cancers has a mean value of 58 days, and diverse sar-

comas have a significantly shorter volume-doubling time than do carcinomas.[30]

Microscopically, gastric leiomyosarcomas are conveniently subdivided by degrees or grades of smooth muscle differentiation:

Undifferentiated or Pleomorphic Leiomyosarcoma

No question usually exists that the tumor is a sarcoma, but the problem is its accurate classification. A wild tangle of spindle, rounded, and oval cells is observed without an organoid pattern and with numerous normal and abnormal mitoses.[24,27] Bizarre tumor giant cells are present. The margins of tumor invade adjacent structures and blood vessels and reach the mucosal and serosal surfaces (Fig. 11-14).

The concept of gastric stromal sarcoma or undifferentiated mesenchymal cell sarcoma with focal smooth muscle differentiation has been advanced to explain some undifferentiated and poorly differentiated gastric leiomyosarcomas.[26,31] Stroma means the supporting or matrix tissue of an organ, such as the connective tissue and vessels, as distinguished from the functioning parenchymal tissue. Leiomyomatous neoplasms are consequently not accurately designated as stromal. The theory of stem cell origin of diverse epithelial, soft tissue, hematopoietic,

---

*Dr. Robert E. Scully kindly provided the tumor diameter (9 cm). Based on the average volume-doubling times of sarcomas, the preclinical latent growth period is estimated at about 3 years and 3 months (range 2.1 to 11 years and 8 months).

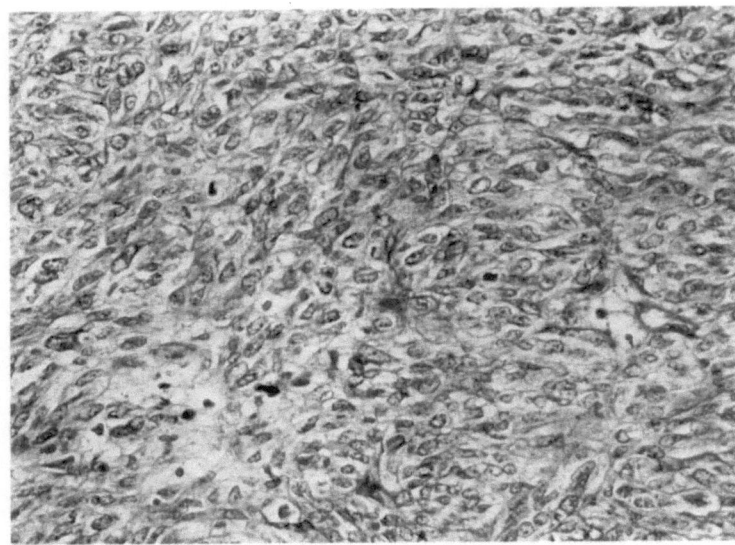

Figure 11-14. Considerable architectural and cytologic atypism and nuclear pleomorphism characterize undifferentiated leiomyosarcoma. HPS, X100, reproduced at 65%.

and connective tissue neoplasms is familiar, but here it is more a handicap than an aid to precise tumor classification. Prognostic evaluations at present are, indeed, based partly on the reliable histopathologic identification of tumor type, besides grading and staging.[14,24,27,32-34]

The prognosis of undifferentiated or pleomorphic leiomyosarcoma, as expected, is the worst of any gastric smooth muscle tumor.[24,27,32]

Poorly Differentiated Leiomyosarcoma
A grossly suspicious or overtly sarcomatous mass proves microscopically to be very cellular, with over 400 nuclei per high power (X400) field (HPF) at 6-micra thickness (Fig. 11-15).[35] Slide thickness is germane, because the now vanished entity "leiomyosarcoma, clinically benign" was based on the hypercellularity of celloidin plastic-embedded sections 30-micra thick. The crowded hyperchromatic nuclei are oval or blunt-ended, they vary slightly to notably in size, and mitoses are abundant. Mitotic counts of 2 to 5 per 10 HPF (10 to 25/50 HPF) in different parts of such tumors have been regarded by Stout[22] and other investigators[13,27,32-34] as a very important criterion of a definitely malig-

nant smooth muscle tumor. In 1920, Evans[36] listed the criteria of leiomyosarcoma as:

1. increased size of tumor cells,
2. enlarged nuclei of irregular sizes and shapes,
3. unequally stained and hyperchromatic nuclei,
4. collagenous stromal fibers absent between tumor cells,
5. thin or absent vessel walls,
6. large (meaning abnormal) mitoses, and
7. mitotic counts between 5.5 and 30 per 10 HPF (or 28 to 150/50 HPF).

Evans[36] emphasized a composite of characteristics supported the diagnosis of leiomyosarcoma. He also included other criteria: shorter and plumper tumor cells, rounded and vesicular nuclei, lack of cell differentiation, and tumor giant cells with hyperchromatic nuclei. Evans[36] counted mitoses in 100 oil immersion fields and calculated 2200 to 12,000 mitoses per mm³. Benign smooth muscle tumors had 1 or 2 mitoses per mm³.

Stout and his co-workers[10,12,22] have counted mitoses in 50 high-power fields (HPF), either at X200 or X400 to help identify various sarcomas, particularly leiomyosarcoma. This

Figure 11-15. Hypercellularity, elongated pointed, or blunt-end nuclei and mitoses are evident in poorly differentiated gastric leiomyosarcoma. HPS, X100, reproduced at 65%.

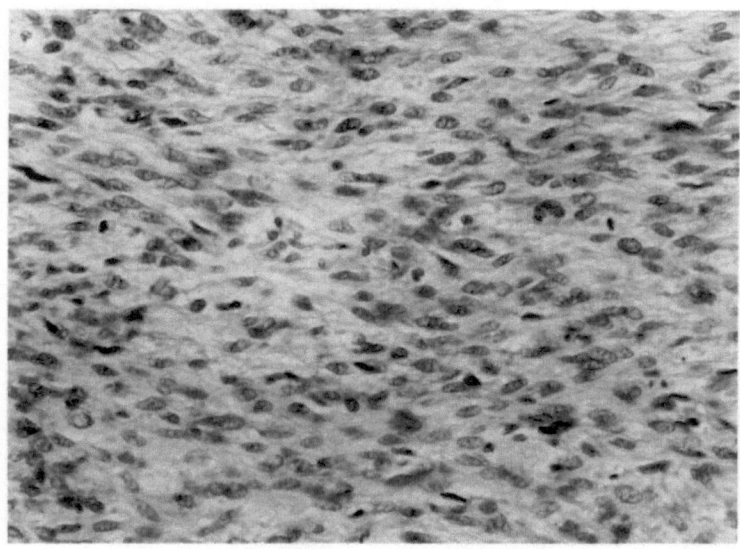

criterion of cancer is discussed further later in this chapter.

Small Cell Leiomyosarcoma

Small cell leiomyosarcoma is a separate histopathologic subcategory of poorly differentiated leiomyosarcoma.[24] The crowded nuclei are half the usual size, elongated, hyperchromatic, and separated by scanty cytoplasm. Appleman and Helwig[24] termed this as "epithelioid leiomyosarcoma" because the nuclei were angulated and the cells were clustered or formed tight perivascular whorls or balls of small spindle-shaped cells. It is not difficult to distinguish this tumor type from small cell (oat cell) carcinoma of the stomach, lung, or elsewhere. Small cell leiomyosarcoma also differs from malignant leiomyoblastoma, which is a separate clinicopathologic entity to be described subsequently.

Leiomyosarcoma with Heterotopic Elements

Leiomyosarcomas with heterotopic elements occur as tumors that contain isolated islands of ossification, cartilaginous, angiomatous, hemangiopericytomatous, or liposarcomatous differentiation.[22,32] Under Stout's teaching that three or more types of differentiation other than fibroblastic are required to des-

ignate a sarcoma as malignant mesenchymoma,[10] such limited heterologous foci are ordinarily appended as a note to the main diagnosis of leiomyosarcoma. The clinical importance of such foci is unknown.

Malignant Leiomyoblastoma

Generally, leiomyoblastomas are regarded as low-grade sarcomas,[12,15,16,19] although some are highly malignant.[19,27] Judged by more recent large series,[15,19] approximately 1 to 2% metastasized. Stout's original 69 cases included two (3%) with metastases to liver or lymph nodes.[12] Neither grossly nor microscopically is the diagnosis of malignancy made easily unless metastasis is evident. Foci of high mitotic counts (e.g., 13 and 19 mitoses /50 HPF) were found in the two original tumors that metastasized, but other regions had only 2 mitoses/50 HPF.[12] Conversely, at least five other leiomyoblastomas with abundant mitoses did not recur, which was also confirmed at autopsy in some cases (Fig. 11-16).

Appleman and Helwig[24] considered small cell leiomyosarcomas of the stomach to represent malignant leiomyoblastomas. Of their cases, 63% metastasized, usually within 2 years. Others have noted an alveolar arrange-

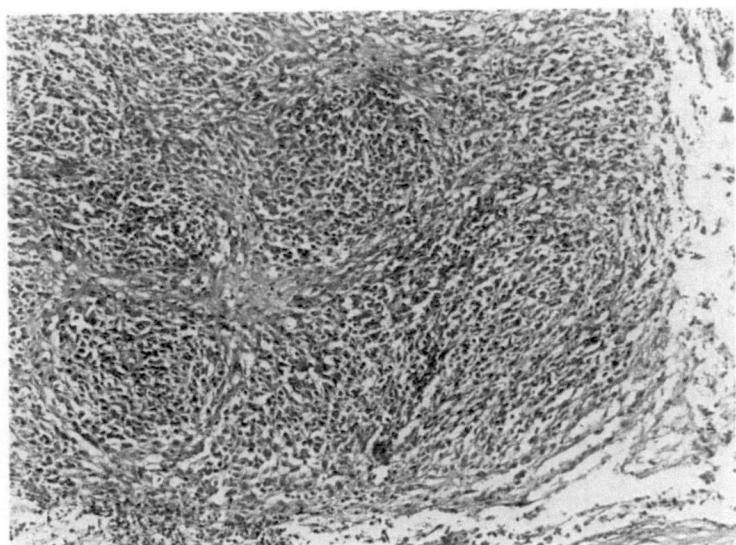

Figure 11-16. An atypical but clinically benign gastric leiomyoblastoma has a loosely arranged multinodular growth pattern without clearcut invasion. The cells have small nuclei and abundant clear cytoplasm. H&E, X40, reproduced at 65%.

ment of malignant leiomyoblastoma cells.[17] Unless gross or microscopic invasion is found, criteria to identify leiomyoblastoma as malignant are not definitive, and the biological course is decisive.

Well Differentiated Leiomyosarcoma

Most authors[13,24-26,36] have concluded that the three grades of undifferentiated, poorly differentiated, and well differentiated smooth muscle sarcomas are enough to be distinguished. Thus, moderately differentiated leiomyosarcoma is believed to be a dispensable grade.

Well differentiated leiomyosarcomas are a source of disagreement and controversy. Usually, the gross tumor appears fibroid, rubbery, or slightly softer and more tan or yellow in places than does the familiar uterine leiomyoma. If it is a consultation case, the gross appearance is either not provided or not carefully described.

Microscopically, the growth is clearly smooth muscle, interspersed with collagenous stromal fibroblasts and small blood vessels. The margins are pushing and not overtly invasive. Hyaline degeneration is found, but usually there are no particular necrotizing or hemorrhagic alterations. The tumor cells are somewhat enlarged and double-sized polypoid nuclei are easily found (Fig. 11-17).

Mitoses are reported to distinguish between atypical leiomyoma and well differentiated leiomyosarcoma. Evans[36] reported that none of 72 suspicious but clinically benign smooth muscle tumors had more than between 2 and 5 mitoses per 10 HPF (10 to 25/50 HPF) (800 to 2000 per mm³), and quoted Ewing that "sarcomatous tendencies or precancerous changes do not constitute real sarcoma or cancer." Berg and McNeer[32] found that a high mitotic rate (not quantified) throughout a tumor was predictive of death from leiomyosarcoma. As noted before, Stout[22] believed that 2 to 5 mitoses per 10 HPF (10 to 25/50 HPF) *in different parts* of a leiomyomatous tumor were persuasive of malignancy. Appleman and Helwig[11] observed one metastasizing smooth muscle tumor that had only 1 mitosis per 10 HPF (5/50 HPF), while the subsequent metastatic liver leiomyosarcoma had 4.8 per 10 HPF (24/50 HPF). In their 44 overt gastric sarcomas, the mitotic counts were usually more than 4 per 10 HPF (>20/50 HPF).[24] Ranchod and Kempson[33] described 54 gastric smooth muscle tumors

Figure 11-17. Well differentiated leiomyosarcoma of the stomach is composed of laminated atypical but clearly recognizable smooth muscle cells with enlarged, hyperchromatic, and variable-sized nuclei. HPS, X100, reproduced at 65%.

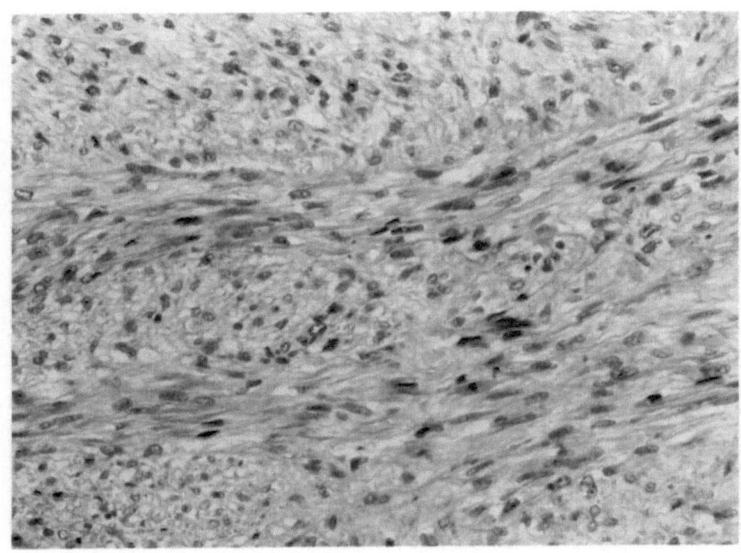

among 100 gastrointestinal cases they analyzed; all tumors with 5 or more mitoses per 10 HPF ($\geq$ 25/50 HPF) behaved aggressively. However, approximately 40% of the leiomyosarcomas they reported had fewer mitoses. Shiu and co-workers[26] found that seven of nine cases of gastric myosarcoma survived 5 years if there were 9 or fewer mitoses per 10 HPF ($\leq$ 45/50 HPF), but only one of five survived if there were more mitoses. Mazur and Clark[25] reported from 2 to more than 10 mitoses per HPF (10 to 50/50 HPF) in the seven leiomyosarcomas they studied, and 3 of their 21 benign tumors had 2 mitoses per 10 HPF (10/50 HPF). Appleman[34] recently concluded that metastases were likely if mitoses exceeded 2 per 10 HPF (> 10/50 HPF), which he reported is about one-third of the number of mitoses found in typical uterine leiomyosarcomas.

One woman with gastric angiomatous leiomyosarcoma survived 45 years after an 11-cm mass was resected from the lesser curvature at age 10 years.[37] At autopsy, the liver metastasis had an undifferentiated mesenchymal sarcomatous appearance.

Counting mitoses in a few fields of limited amounts of blocked gastric smooth muscle tumors is not recommended as a sound independent method to discriminate between typical leiomyoma and genuine leiomyosarcoma or for judging prognosis. Between laboratories and observers, there are widely differing methods, magnifications, and definitions of mitosis.[38] A panel of two or three pathologists is preferable to count mitoses, and four or more tissue blocks are desirable. Some observers count as mitoses small dark blue blobs that others may regard as pyknotic neuclei or lymphocyte emperipolesis. Mitotic spindles are less subject to argument. As Evans[36] observed, abnormal mitoses are worth emphasis, since they are indirect indicators of both abundant cell divisions and aneuploidy.

When making a decision of benign versus malignant tumor, one must consider all available gross and microscopic pathologic features of gastric smooth muscle tumors. Mitotic counts by themselves are a quick-fix approach with wide variables and an uncertain usefulness. For interest, the comparability of reported mitotic counts in distinguishing benign from malignant smooth muscle tumors in other organs are included (Fig. 11-18).[10,13,21,22,33-36,38-48]

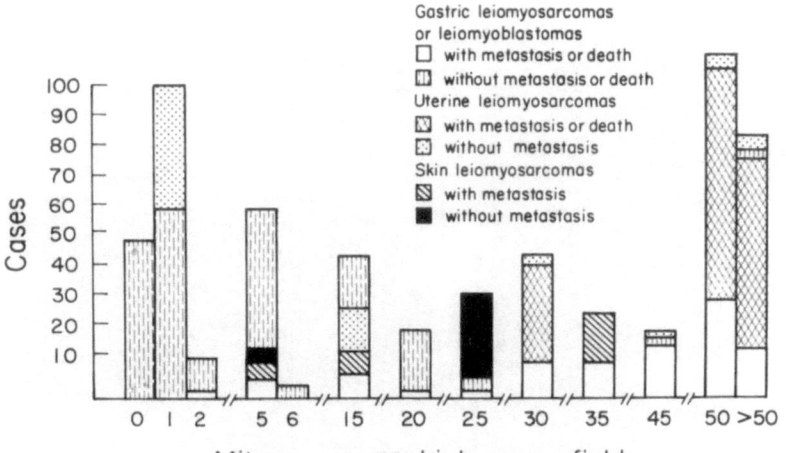

Figure 11-18. Mitotic counts of leiomyosarcomas of the stomach, uterus, and skin correlated with the presence or absence of metastasis or death from cancer.

Nerve Sheath Tumors

Gastric neurilemomas or schwannomas and neurofibromas exist, but their identification is difficult[25,49,50] and requires immunohistochemical and/or electron microscopic study (see below).[51-55] Most reports suggest that perhaps 1 in 50 to 100 gastric intramural solid tumors is of the nerve sheath type.[34] Even in von Recklinghausen's neurofibromatosis, a gastrointestinal nodule may be a leiomyoma.[56] A unique, slightly pigmented, gastric antral, 5-cm melanotic schwannoma with a 19-cm extragastric mass showed no recurrence at autopsy.[57] Ming[58] reported not finding a single neurogenic stomach tumor at his hospital, and cited from the literature that 3% of benign gastric tumors are of nerve sheath origin. A few individual cases were reported 40 years ago,[55,59] and others have recently been described accompanying neurofibromatosis.[60,61]

Grossly, the uncommon gastric nerve sheath tumor appears indistinguishable from leiomyoma, and origin from a peripheral nerve has not been discovered (Fig. 11-19). Microscopically, nuclear palisading of Antoni type A bodies may be regarded as diagnostic, but this pattern, as already noted, is equally characteristic of leiomyomas or

leiomyosarcomas (Fig. 11-20). Toker's[62] "porpoises in the waves" ripple pattern of neurofibroma has not been found. At present, ultrastructural features such as the complex interdigitated cell processes and the basal laminae that separate the individual cells of neurilemomas[63-66] plus immunohistochemical demonstration of S-100 protein[67,68] and glial fibrillary acidic protein (GFAP)[69] may be needed for proof. Mazur and Clark[25] concluded that one small benign gastric tumor (1.5 cm in diameter) was a schwannoma based on these special studies, and that nine other cases (either benign or malignant) had some attributes of perineurial mesenchymal cells. Although the most common differential diagnosis of a gastric leiomyoma or leiomyosarcoma is with a benign or malignant nerve sheath tumor, it has rarely proved to be the latter. Malignant gastric schwannoma, pheochromocytoma, and intracerebral sarcomas occurred together in two men with neurofibromatosis.[60,61]

Myenteric Schwannoma

Myenteric schwannoma is ordinarily a small subserosal nodule found incidentally on the stomach surface. A myenteric nerve enters the tumor, which lies at the interface

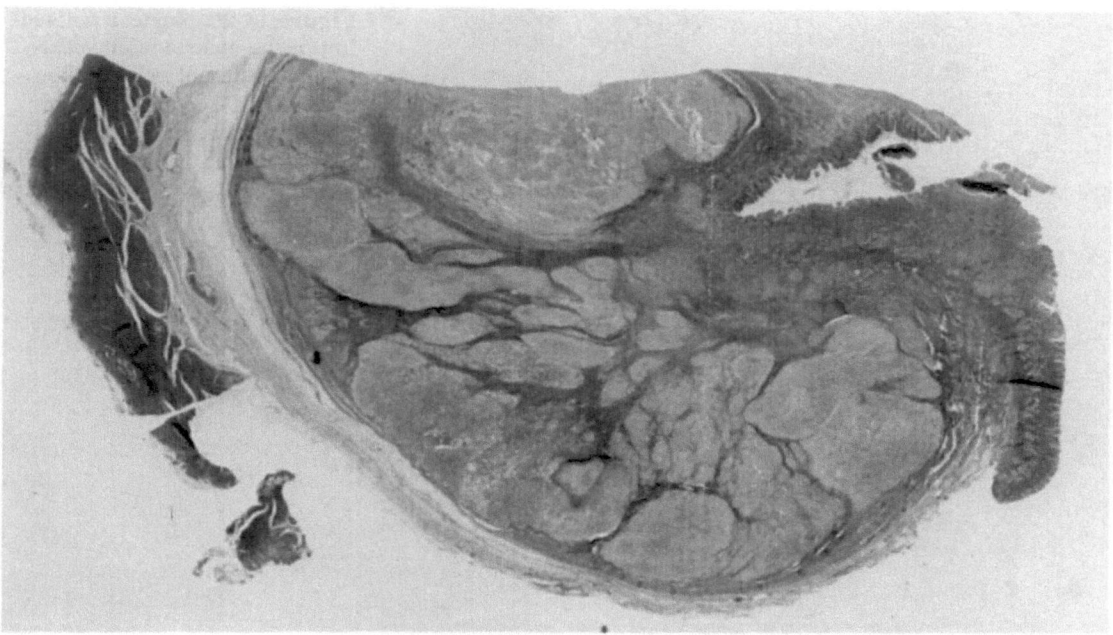

Figure 11-19. Low-power view of a nerve sheath and ganglion cell tumor of the stomach wall, sparing the mucosa at the upper right and stretching the muscularis propria at the left. H&E, X6.5, reproduced at 90%.

of the external muscularis propria and sub-serosal connective tissue. The ultrastructure is that of Schwann cells, with collections of basement membrane or collagenous material.[20]

Gastric Gangliocytic Paraganglioma

While not apparently reported in the literature gastric gangliocytic paraganglioma does exist. Figure 11-21 represents an example from Johns Hopkins Hospital, originally diagnosed as a ganglioneuromatous hamartoma. Best known in the duodenum, the tumor is a distinctive neoplastic or hyperplastic growth.[70] It is characterized by neuroectodermal ganglion cells, neuroectodermal Schwann cells, and endodermal epithelial cells of the ventral pancreatic primordium.[70] Approximately 38 duodenal and 2 jejunal cases of this benign paragangliomatous growth have been reported. Some accompany neurofibromatosis.[71]

Gut Autonomic Nerve (GAN) Tumor

A newly described entity, gastrointestinal or gut autonomic nerve tumor, has been reported.[72,73] One ileal wall and mesenteric GAN sarcoma metastasized to the liver. The gastric GAN tumors, 4 to 8 cm in diameter, remained localized. Grossly and by light microscopy, the appearance is indistinguishable from the ordinary spindle cell leiomyoma. There were less than 3 mitoses per 10 HPF, and staining for S-100 protein was negative. By electron microscopy, long interwoven cytoplasmic filaments, abundant cytoplasm, and free or membrane-bound ribosomes are found. No basal lamina or cytoplasmic filaments are evident. Axons with synaptic densities are present. Dense core granules are

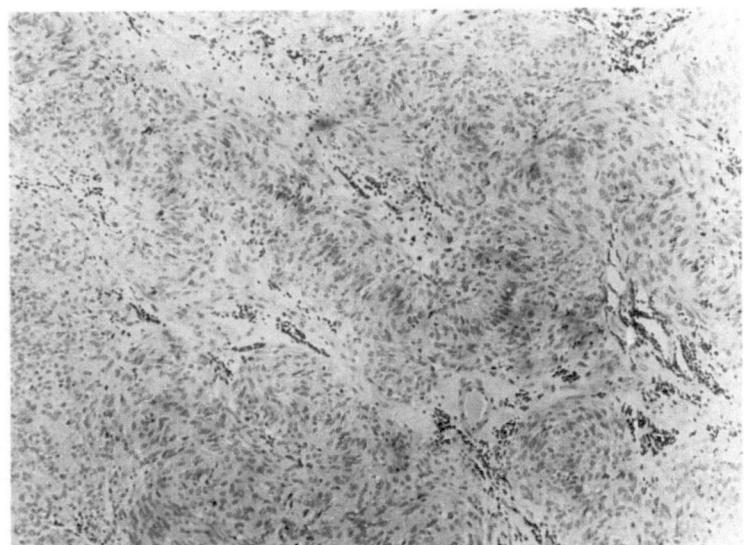

Figure 11-20. Nuclear palisading in the gastric leiomyosarcoma should not be mistaken for Antoni A bodies found in schwannomas. HPS, X40, reproduced at 65%.

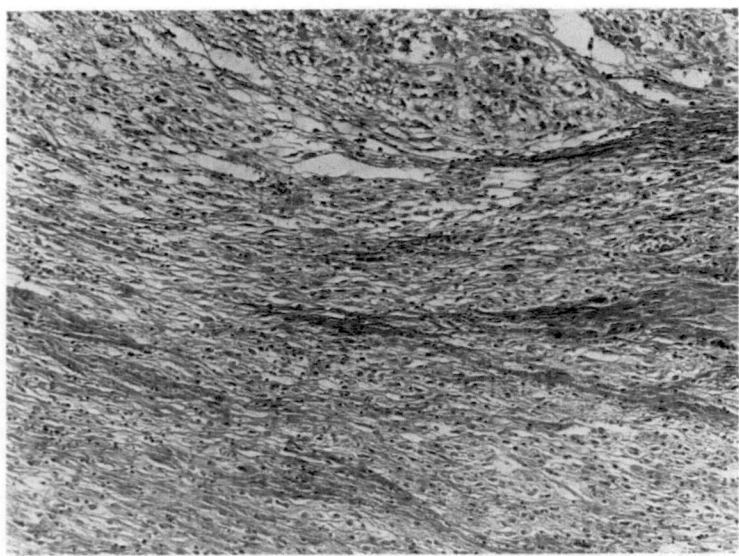

Figure 11-21. Microscopic appearance of the gastric gangliocytic paraganalioma also shown in Figure 11-19. Much of the mass is composed of loosely arranged nerve sheath and Schwann cells. Foci of distorted but differentiated nerve ganglion cells are scattered through the tumor. No invasion or apparent malignant change was found. H&E, X40, reproduced at 65%.

identified here as well as in the Golgi apparatus and, in particular, just beneath the plasma membrane. Empty smooth vesicles occur adjacent to the Golgi apparatus and in axons.[72]

Whether GAN tumors are larger examples of myenteric schwannoma[20] is uncertain. One case also had a retroperitoneal paraganglioma, and thus possessed two-thirds of the attributes of Carney's triad (gastric stromal tumor, extra-adrenal paraganglioma, pulmonary chondromal).[74] This suggests that ultrastructural analysis of Carney's gastric tumor might result in reclassifying some as nerve sheath neoplasms.

Figure 11-22. Gastric osteosarcoma with a polymorphous pattern of atypical polygonal and spindle cells, with intercellular deposits of osteoid and bone. Masson trichrome stain, X40, reproduced at 65%.

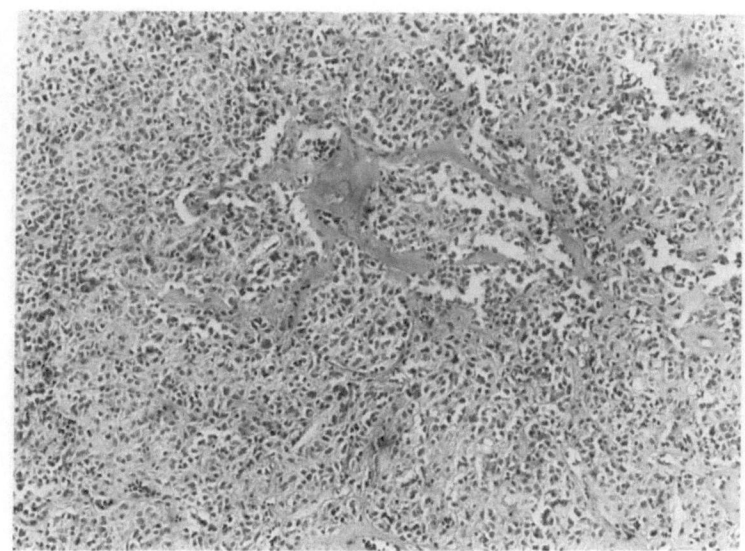

Miscellaneous Solid Intramural Gastric Tumors

Other partly or wholly spindle cell tumors of the gastric wall are considered below.

Fibrosarcoma

A few primary or metastatic sarcomas of fibroblastic type are known, but scarcely any have been reported in 25 years. Osteosarcoma with fibrosarcomatous regions occurs as a rare primary gastric tumor (Fig. 11-22).

Malignant Fibrous Histiocytoma

Two cases of primary gastric malignant fibrous histiocytoma were reported by 1988.[75] Such tumors need to be distinguished from secondary spread of malignant fibrous histiocytomas arising elsewhere, as well as from pleomorphic leiomyosarcoma.

Glomus Tumor

About 70 gastric tumors, mostly pyloric, greater curvature, intramural, 1.5 to 2.5 cm stenosing nodules, have been collected with or without obstruction or ulceration.[76-77] Microscopically, the glomus tumors are benign vascular masses with prominent pericytes and glomus cell groups, but sometimes lack smooth muscle (Fig. 11-23).[76] Endocrine granules (100 to 500 μm in size), a few cilia, zonulae adherentes, long intercellular junctions, and thin cytoplasmic filaments have been described by electron microscopy.[77-78]

Granular Cell Tumor

Twenty cases have been reported, frequently in black people.[79] Twelve were submucosal, three intramural, and two subserosal. Apparently all were benign and relatively small (e.g., 1 cm in diameter). Similar skin and vulvar tumors have been present without neurofibromatosis.[80] Microscopically, rounded, rather bland cells had abundant granular acidophilic cytoplasm (Fig. 11-24). There was S-100 protein immunoreactivity, and ultrastructurally the tumor cell clusters had enveloping basal laminae and adjacent neuraxons. As elsewhere, these granular cell tumors were considered to be likely of schwannian origin.[79,80]

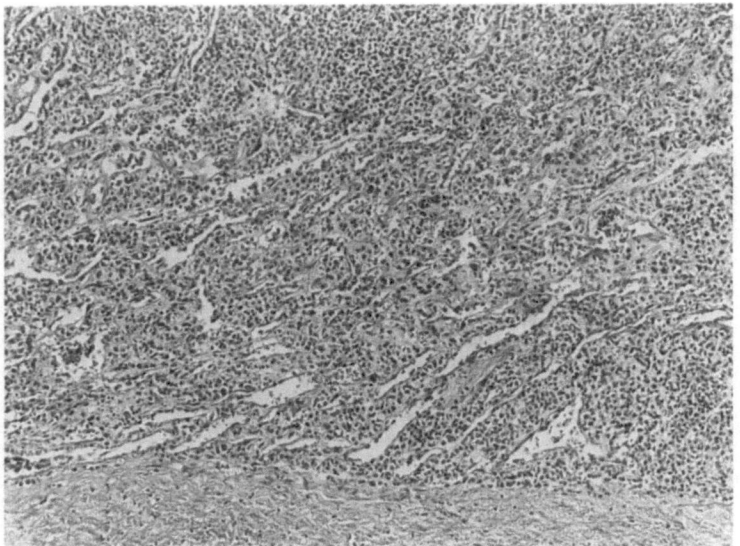

Figure 11-23. The sinusoidal vascular structure and perivascular groups of small regular cells characterize this glomus cell tumor of the stomach. The margin is sharp, an indication of benignancy. H&E, X40, reproduced at 65%.

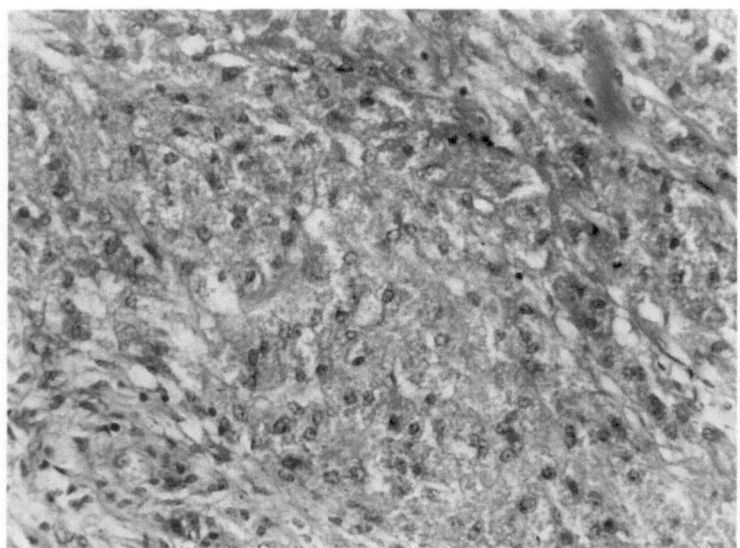

Figure 11-24. Polygonal cells with abundant cytoplasmic granularity and rather small nuclei characterize granular cell tumors of the stomach and elsewhere. H&E, X100, reproduced at 65%.

Hemangiopericytoma

Stout,[22] who introduced the term, considered that some tumors so classified shaded off into leiomyosarcomas. This was before the myofibroblast became a recognized cell type. Among his original approximately 200 cases, 7 involved the gastrointestinal tract.[81] One available gastric case is demonstrated in

Figure 11-25 and 11-26. Overall, about 50% are malignant, but the histopathology of the original tumor gives no clear prognostic information, so that a long follow-up is necessary.[82] Electron microscopy is now considered the most effective way of confirming the diagnosis; there are concentrically arranged cell whorls invested partly or completely by basal membrane laminar material. Prominent

Figure 11-25. A gastric hemangiopericytoma, confirmed by Dr. A.P. Stout, who introduced the term, formed a soft brown spongy encapsulated mass 8 cm in diameter.

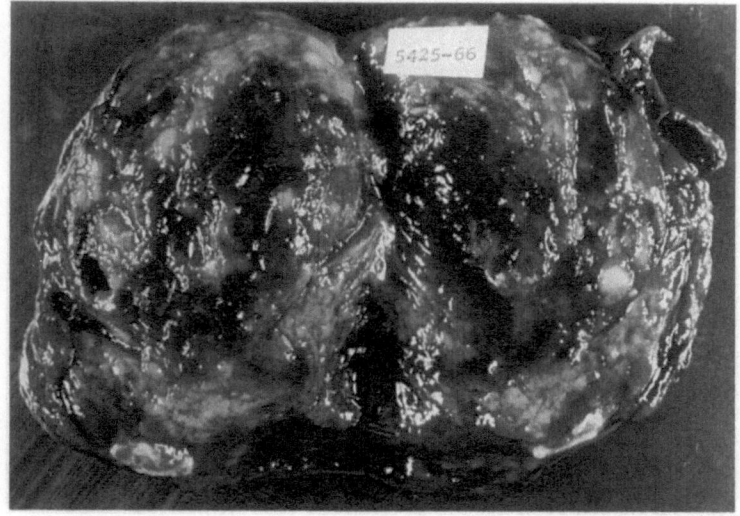

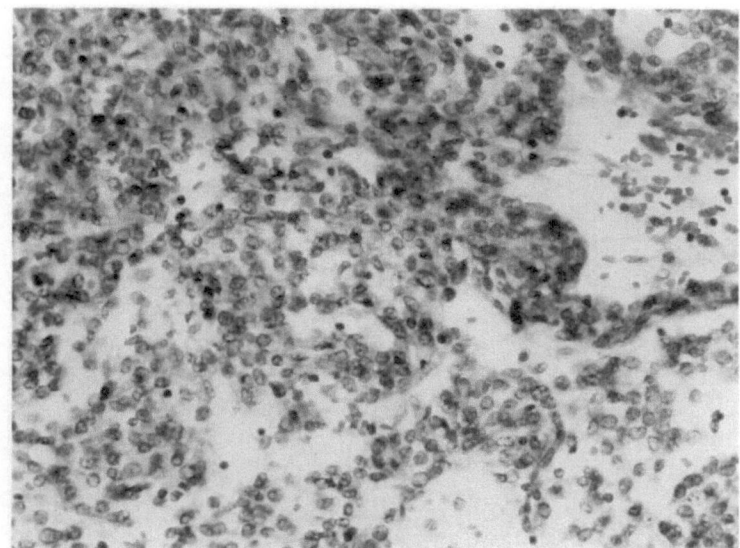

Figure 11-26. Small oval or carrot-shaped cells form a lacy or compact perivascular growth pattern around capillary vessels in hemagiopericytoma. H&E, X100, reproduced at 65%.

myogenic type cytoplasmic filaments, dense bodies, interdigitated cytoplasmic vacuoles, and pinocytotic vesicles are also found. Basal lamina separates the pericytes from vascular endothelium.[83]

Kaposi's Sarcoma

Visceral involvement without skin lesions has been reported for many years prior to AIDS.[84] A rare case presented with a primary gastric lesion.[85] Not only patients with AIDS[86,87] but also immunosuppressed recipients of kidney transplants[88] have had visceral Kaposi's sarcoma involving the stomach. Polypoid or flat hemorrhagic lesions, single or multiple, can be seen (Fig. 11-27). In disseminated Kaposi's sarcoma, a thick plaque of intramural tumor may grossly resemble linitis plastica (Fig. 11-28).

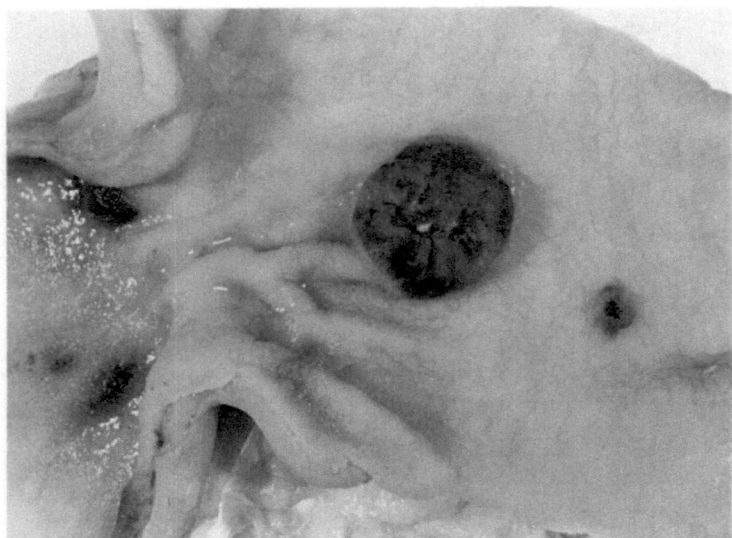

Figure 11-27. A case complicating AIDS with gastrointestinal dissemination of Kaposi's sarcoma had gastric plaques and a polypoid nodule of hemorrhagic appearance.

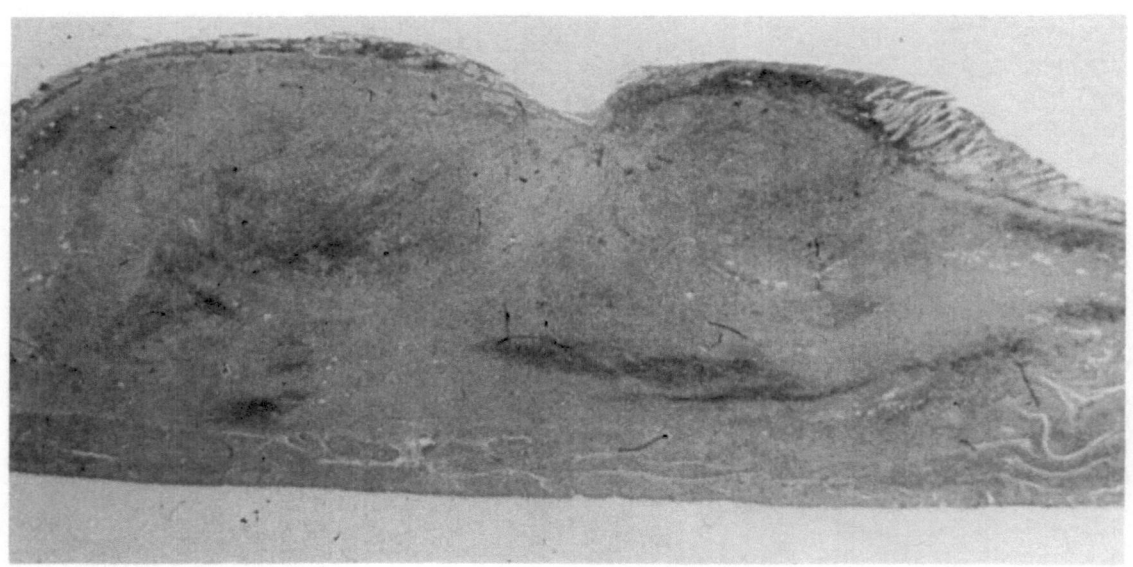

Figure 11-28. Kaposi's sarcoma primarily occupies the submucosa, but may penetrate and ulcerate the mucosa. H&E, X16, reproduced at 90%.

Figure 11-29. Kaposi's sarcoma grows as compact spindle cells, with intercellular erythrocytes leaked from vascular slits, both features of diagnostic value. HPS, X100, reproduced at 65%.

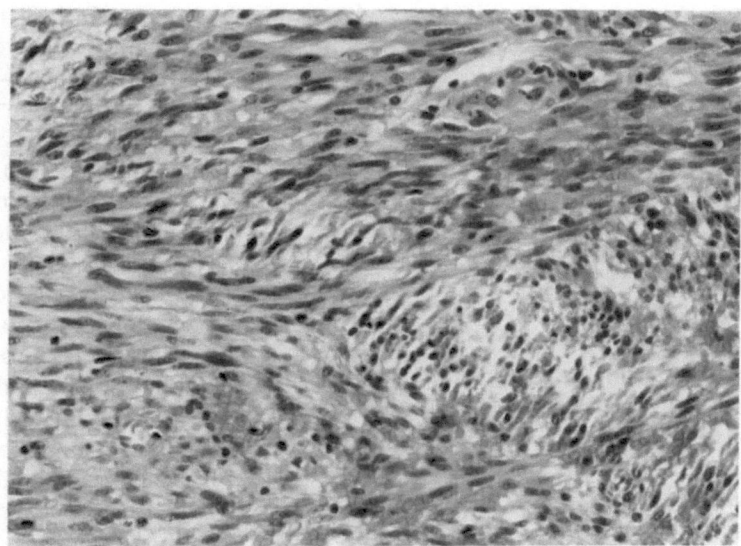

Microscopically, Kaposi's sarcoma grows in the submucosa as plump spindle cells with characteristic vascular slits, erythrocytic leakage, and hemosiderin pigment deposits between the sarcoma cells (Fig. 11-29). In most cases in this laboratory, factor VIII immunostaining has been positive. Electron microscopy demonstrates erythrocytes between adjacent sarcoma cells.

Mesenchyoma

No benign or malignant gastric tumor entity has received this diagnosis. If one accepts the concept that gastric leiomyomas and sarcomas develop from mesenchymal (stromal) stem cells that differentiate partly as smooth muscle and partly as Schwann cells or perineural fibroblasts, mesenchymoma would then apply to a neoplasm with all three specialized cell types intermingled.[10,89] Tissue culture, immunostaining, and electron microscopy are needed to support a multidifferentiated mesenchymal histogenesis.

Paraganglioma

Two examples of nonfunctioning gastric carotid body type paraganglioma have been reported.[90] One was a 5-cm, prepyloric, lesser curvature mass with a 1.5-cm ulcer. It was slightly chromaffin. The description, gross drawing, and photomicrographs suggest that it was actually a leiomyoblastoma.[90] Note also gangliocytic paraganglioma, as described above.[70,71]

Rhabdomyosarcoma

No case has been reported in the stomach, including either pleomorphic or alveolar rhabdomyosarcoma.[91]

Teratoma

The stomach is the rarest of all possible sites in which teratomas can occur, and only 51 such cases were reported until 1981.[92] All had a benign course. Infants and children are affected mostly, particularly males less than one year of age. The greater curvature is the most common location. As elsewhere, gastric teratomas may be solid or cystic and contain tissue from more than one germ cell layer. They are frequently calcified. Congenital anomalies are associated in 10 to 15%.

Gastroscopic Biopsies and Surgical Samples

Endoscopic tissue specimens are often inadequate to evaluate submucosal or intramural stomach lesions. Sometimes overt sarcoma or a considerably degenerated benign leiomyoma is recognized. Ulcerated leiomyomas, leiomyoblastomas, or leiomyosarcomas are accessible to gastroscopic biopsies. However, as discussed, since some specimens may require special studies including immunohistochemistry, electron microscopy, or both to reach a diagnosis, too much should not be made of minute tissue fragments.[7] Nonetheless, the diagnosis has been made by percutaneous needle biopsy.[93]

Immunopathology and Electron Microscopy

Pathology practice in classifying gastric intramural tumors usually involves only light microscopy and special stains such as Masson's trichrome, reticulin, PAS, and Grimelius. Exigencies of time, availability, expertise, and economics usually limit employment of the newer techniques to research, unless the neoplasm is quite unusual by light microscopy.

Special immunohistologic studies of intermediate fibers such as vimentin and desmin showed they were markers for leiomyosarcoma as well as rhabdomyosarcoma, while gastric leiomyomas were desmin-positive but vimentin-negative.[94] Myosin is not regarded as a useful marker to identify poorly differentiated leiomyosarcoma. A more recent report emphasizes that 46 Bouin-fixed gastric smooth muscle tumors were all vimentin-positive and S-100 protein-negative. Desmin was positive in 17 of 37 gastric leiomyomas (46%) and 6 of 9 leiomyosarcomas (67%), with fewer reactive cells in the malignant tumors.[95] Using other fixation and immunostaining methods, 12 gastric stromal tumors

were found to be vimentin- and actin-positive, but desmin-negative, without differences between benign and malignant tumors.[96] Nerve sheath tumors are S-100 protein-positive,[67,68] while neuron-specific enolase (NSE) and glial fibrillary acidic protein (GFAP) may sometimes be useful.[57,69] Grimelius and chromogranin positivity is expected in paragangliomas.

Electron microscopy has shown that some leiomyomas, leiomyoblastomas, and leiomyosarcomas possess attributes of smooth muscle cells, including interdigitated cytoplasmic processes, plasma membrane-associated dense patches, incomplete basement membranes, junctional complexes, random filaments lacking periodicity, cytoplasmic dense bodies, pinocytotic vesicles, clustered mitochondria, and rare cilia (Fig. 11-30).[34,97] The perinuclear clear vacuoles of normal smooth muscle cells and of leiomyomas are evident ultrastructurally and are not artifacts.[98]

However, Weiss and Mackay[31] observed smooth muscle features in only 5 of 20 leiomyosarcomas, 10 each of spindle cell and epithelioid cell type. Dedifferentiation was evident, but the leiomyoblastomas were considered to originate from smooth muscle. Tumors lacking attributes of smooth muscle were divided into poorly differentiated and mesenchymal subtypes. Mazur and Clark,[25] as discussed previously, found cytoplasmic myofibrils with myofilament densities in only 2 of 28 gastric tumors previously diagnosed as leiomyomas or leiomyosarcomas; 8 were positive for S-100 protein, and 9 showed neither feature. Possible origin of such neoplasms from mesenchymal stem cells or the myenteric nervous system was discussed.

Schwannomas are positive with S-100 protein immunostaining, while perineurial cells and tumors are negative.[65,67] If ganglion and epithelioid cells are also present, anti-NSE and anti-neurofilament staining of these elements is positive.[99,100] However, in one report, only two-thirds of malignant schwannomas stained for S-100 protein.[100] Two malignant melanocytic epithelioid schwannomas were

Figure 11-30. Electron micrography demonstrates gastric leiomyoma cells that contain abundant cytoplasmic organelles. Myofibrils and long tight junctions with myofibrillar attachments are shown in the inset. X10,000, X65,000, reproduced at 50%. (Courtesy of Scott Weaver, Lenox Hill Hospital.)

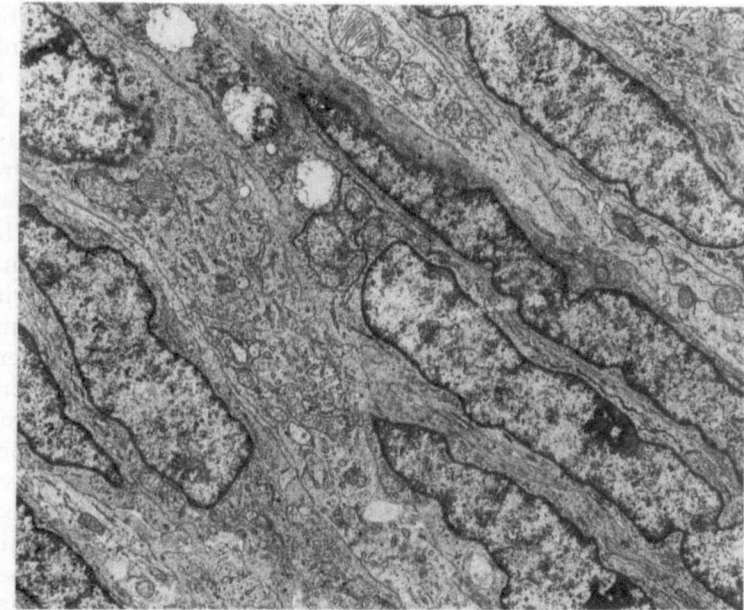

A

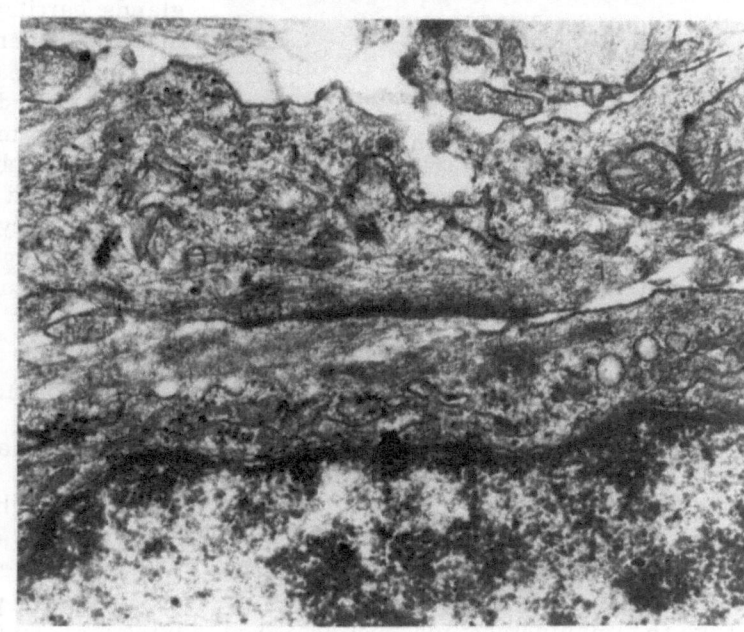

B

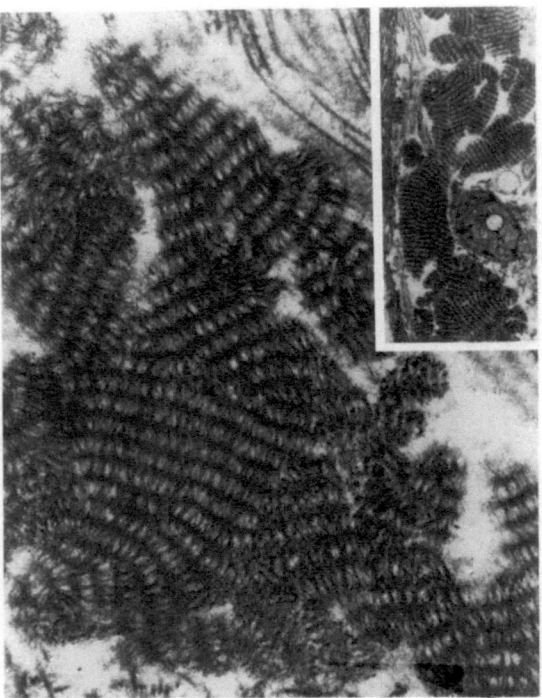

Figure 11-31. Schwannomas may sometimes be identified in part by their characteristic long-spaced collagen. From Ghadially.[123] Reproduced with permission of the author and Butterworths.

S-100 protein-positive, and one stained focally for GFAP.[57,100] S-100 immunoreactivity may also be found in some (5%) gastric stromal tumors classified as smooth muscle tumors by light microscopy.[101] Another group[69] found that most schwannomas and four of eight neurofibromas were GFAP-positive. Desmin is not found in nerve sheath tumors. Vimentin is present in Schwann cells, but because it is seen in more than 10 other cell types, this is not diagnostically valuable.[102]

Like the immunoreactives just described, the ultrastructural features of nerve sheath tumors are controversial. Schwannomas with Antoni A bodies have cells with long and complexly entangled processes, spiral cytoplasmic myelinoid wraps around collagen fibrils, as well as pseudomesaxons or straight processes.[64,65] If present, long-spaced collagen characterizes schwannomas (Fig. 11-31).

Reduplicated basal laminae, basement membrane material, and collagen are present.[64] Granular cell tumors also have basal laminae and some angulate lysosomes.[77] Intermediate filaments and primitive cell junctions are evident. One gastric schwannoma (2.5 cm in diameter) had numerous notched or needle-shaped crystals with 7.8 µm periodicity.[103]

Neurofibromas ultrastructurally recapitulate endoneurial and perineurial cells, which lack basal laminae and rough endoplasmic reticulum. Nerve remnants are found.[63,65,66] Malignant peripheral nerve sheath tumors may be heterogeneous and difficult to classify by electron microscopy.[63,104] Some constituent cells have Schwann cell-like processes. Remnants of basal lamina remain. Cell junctions are primitive, and some ultrastructural attributes resemble malignant fibrous histiocytomas. Rarely, there are heterologous glands, cartilage, bone, or rhabdomyosarcomatous elements present. Neurofibrosarcomas may have elongated plaque junctions of closely apposed cells. Ordinary fibrosarcoma by electron microscopy may demonstrate some myofibroblasts with subplasmalemmal myofibrils and anchoring fibrils. Other cells contain intracytoplasmic collagen fibrils. As in many malignant tumors, the nuclei have complex irregular outlines.

Tumor Syndromes

Neurofibromatosis

Von Recklinghausen's disease, as already noted, may be associated with typical gastric leiomyomas.[56,60,105] More frequently (e.g., 12% of 219 affected patients) there are gastric and intestinal, single or multiple neurofibromas, or less commonly neurofibrosarcomas,[106] or malignant schwannoma.[50,60,61] These tumors may be incidental findings at autopsy, or may lead to gastrointestinal obstruction, bleeding, perforation, or a palpable abdominal mass. It is notable that neurofibromatosis tumors are polyclonal, indicating multiple cell origin.[107]

Postirradiation neurilemomas and neuro-fibrosarcomas are believed to be radiation-induced, with a mean latent period of 14 to 15.6 years, and in about half the cases of malignancy, there were stigmata of neuro-fibromatosis.[108-110] Fibroblasts from individuals with von Recklinghausen's disease also are experimentally susceptible to Kirsten murine sarcoma viral neoplastic transformation.[111]

Carney's Triad[112]

Approximately 20 cases have presented with the combination of multiple gastric leiomyo-blastomas or gastric leiomyosarcoma, extra-adrenal paraganglioma, and pulmonary hamartomatous chondroma.[113-115] Eighteen were females aged 9 to 24 years and two were males (one was 21 years old).[111] The malignant gastric leiomyoblastomas metastasized. Nine ultrastructural attributes of smooth muscle cells were observed.[118] The paragan-gliomas included carotid body tumors, right-sided pheochromocytoma, glomus jugulare tumor, aortopulmonary paraganglioma, and two malignant mediastinal paragangli-omas—the last in females aged 15 and 18 years. However, overall survival data were favorable. Of note is the recent description of a gastric autonomic nerve (GAN) tumor in Carney's triad.[73]

Hypoglycemia

Bulky solid retroperitoneal, pleural, or abdominal tumors are sometimes associated with hypoglycemia, which is relieved by debulking operations. Leiomyosarcomas, mostly weighing 1 to 9 kg, including gastric primary tumors, have been implicated.[116-118]

Pseudotumors

Certain gastric conditions of unknown or inflammatory nature may occasion uncertainty if only small endoscopic biopsies are available.

Plasma Cell Granuloma

This lesion is rare in the stomach. A gray, white, gummy tissue mass up to 10 cm in diameter may obstruct the cardia. Microscopically, there were transmural proliferations of fibroblasts and prominent mature plasma cells in hyalinized collagenous stroma, forming an inflammatory pseudotumor.[119] Recently, Spencer[120] reviewed pulmonary plasma cell granulomas and concluded that they shared features of fibrous histiocytomas, either benign or occasionally malignant. The same may apply to the stomach.

Chemotherapy-Induced Atypia

Antimetabolic chemotherapeutic treatment for lymphnodal lymphomas or bone marrow leukemias not involving the gastrointestinal tract may be associated with suspiciously atypical reactive cells proliferating in the beds of gastric peptic ulcers. Atypical spindle cell plaques have close-packed disproportionately large nuclei and nucleoli. Immunostaining and electron microscopy demonstrate the multiple connective tissue cell types and capillaries of atypical granulation tissue. Conservatism is advisable to avoid a mistaken diagnosis of gastric leiomyosarcoma or Kaposi's sarcoma that is not supported by other clinical or endoscopic observations.

Malakoplakia

Gastric malakoplakia with granular acidophilic mononuclear cell infiltrates may rarely form a tumor encircling the stomach.[121] Electron microscopy revealed Michaelis-Gutman bodies and plasmacytoid cells containing unusual crystalloids in the dilated rough endoplasmic reticulum cisternae.

Inflammatory Fibroid Polyps

Gastric inflammatory fibroid polyps were once thought to have a neuromatous spindle cell structure,[122] although this claim is now largely discredited. As discussed previously discriminating between inflammatory and neoplastic gastric spindle cell proliferations is made more difficult or impossible if only minute endoscopic biopsy specimens are available.

References

1. Meissner WA: Leiomyoma of the stomach. Arch Pathol 1944;38:207–209.
2. Yamada Y, Kato Y, Yanagisawa A, et al: Microleiomyomas of the human stomach. Hum Pathol 1988;19:569–572.
3. Antoniades HN: Platelet-derived growth factor and malignant transformation. Biochem Pharmacol 1984;33:2823–2828.
4. Linder D, Gartler SM: Glucose 6-phosphate dehydrogenase mosaicism: Utilization as a cell marker in the study of leiomyomas. Science 1965;150:67–69.
5. Duhig JT, Ayer JP: Vascular leiomyoma. AMA Arch Pathol 1959;68:424–430.
6. Foot NC: Pathology in Surgery. Philadelphia: JB Lippincott, 1945, pp 224–226.
7. Rotterdam H, Sommers SC. In: Biopsy Diagnosis of the Digestive Tract. New York: Raven Press, 1981:111.
8. Garbarini J, Price HP: Calcified leiomyoma of the stomach. N Engl J Med 1950;243:406–407.
9. Mallory FB: The Principles of Pathologic Histology. Philadelphia: WB Saunders, 1914:305 (Fig. 216).
10. Lattes R: Tumors of the Soft Tissues. AFIP Atlas of Tumor Pathology, 2nd Ser, Fasc 1 Revised, Washington DC, 1982:160.
11. Appelman H, Helwig EB: Cellular leiomyomas of the stomach in 49 patients. Arch Pathol Lab Med 1977;101:373–377.
12. Stout AP: Bizarre smooth muscle tumors of the stomach. Cancer 1962;15:400–409.
13. Evans HL: Smooth muscle tumors of the gastrointestinal tract. Cancer 1985;56:2242–2250.
14. Nanni G, Zaatar E, Bergamini C, et al: Unusual presentation of a giant leiomyoblastoma of the stomach. NY State J Med 1986;86:316–319.
15. Abramson DJ: Leiomyoblastomas of the stomach. Surg Gynecol Obstet 1973;136:118–125.
16. Cornog JL Jr: Gastric leiomyoblastoma. Cancer 1974;34:711–719.
17. Frimodt-Møller PC, Klunder K, Svanholm H: Benign and malignant epithelioid leiomyoma (leiomyoblastoma) of the stomach. Acta Chir Scand 1979;145:257–261.
18. Smithwick W III, Biesecker JL, Leand PM: Leiomyoblastoma: Behavior and prognosis. Cancer 1969;24:996–1003.
19. Appelman HD, Helwig EB: Gastric epithelioid leiomyoma and leiomyosarcoma (leiomyoblastoma). Cancer 1976;38:708–728.
20. Appelman HD: Stromal tumors of the esophagus, stomach, and duodenum. In: Appelman HD (ed). Pathology of the Esophagus, Stomach, and Duodenum. New York: Churchill Livingstone, 1984:195–242.
21. Fechner RE: Atypical leiomyomas and synthetic progestin therapy. Am J Clin Pathol 1968;49:697–703.
22. Stout AP: Seminar on tumors of the soft tissues. Am Soc Clin Pathol (Chicago) 1953:34.
23. Ewing J: Neoplastic Diseases. Philadelphia: WB Saunders, 1940:228, 521.
24. Appelman HD, Helwig EB: Sarcomas of the stomach. Am J Clin Pathol 1977;67:2–10.
25. Mazur MT, Clark HB: Gastric stromal tumors. Am J Surg Pathol 1983;7:407–419.
26. Shiu MH, Farr GH, Papachristou, Hajdu SI: Myosarcomas of the stomach. Cancer 1982;49:177–187.
27. Roy M, Sommers SC: Metastatic potential of gastric leiomyosarcoma. Submitted for publication.
28. Cabot case. N Engl J Med 1951;245:30–32.
29. Okabe T, Suzuki A, Hirono M, et al: Establishment of different clonal strains from a human sarcoma of the stomach: Tumorigenic heterogeneity in athymic nude mice. Cancer Res 1983;43:5456–5461.
30. Sommers SC: Growth rates, cell kinetics, and mathematical models of human cancers. Pathobiol Annu 1973;3:309–340.
31. Weiss RA, Mackay B: Malignant smooth muscle tumors of the gastrointestinal tract. Ultra Pathol 1981;2:231–240.
32. Berg J, McNeer G: Leiomyosarcoma of the stomach. Cancer 1960;13:25–33.
33. Ranchod M, Kempson RL: Smooth muscle tumors of the gastrointestinal tract and retroperitoneum. Cancer 1977;39:255–262.
34. Appelman HD: Smooth muscle tumor of the gastrointestinal tract. Am J Surg Pathol 1986;10(Suppl 1):83–99.

35. Roy M, Sommers SC: Unpublished data.
36. Evans N: Malignant myomata and related tumors of uterus. Surg Gynecol Obstet 1920; 30:225–239.
37. Hart GD, Soots ML, Yoshida S: Leiomyosarcoma of the stomach with 45-year survival. Can Med Assoc J 1972;107:1208–1211.
38. Silverberg SG: Reproducibility of the mitosis count in the histologic diagnosis of smooth muscle tumors of the uterus. Hum Pathol 1976;7:451–454.
39. Franklin GO, Antler AS, Thelmo WL, Rosenthal WS: Esophageal Leiomyosarcoma. NY State J Med 1982;82:1100–1103.
40. Starr GF, Dockerty MB: Leiomyomas and leiomyosarcomas of the small intestine. Cancer 1955;8:101–111.
41. McBrien MP, Jarrett PEM: Leiomyosarcoma of the duodenum. Br J Surg 1971;58:685–689.
42. Olurin EO, Solanke TF: Case of leiomyosarcoma of the duodenum and a review of the literature. Gut 1968;9:672–677.
43. Akwari OE, Dozois RR, Weiland LH, Beahrs OH: Leiomyosarcoma of the small and large bowel. Cancer 1978;42:1375–1384.
44. Lane D: Leiomyosarcoma of the rectum. Med J Aust 1969;1:163–164.
45. Hart WR, Billman JK Jr: Reassessment of uterine neoplasms originally diagnosed as leiomyosarcoma. Cancer 1978;41:1902–1910.
46. Shmookler BM, Lauer DH: Retroperitoneal leiomyosarcoma. Am J Surg Pathol 1983; 7:269–280.
47. Conference case: Clinicopathologic Conference. Am J Med 1985;78:1010–1016.
48. Stout AP, Hill WT: Leiomyosarcoma of the superficial soft tissues. Cancer 1958;11: 844–854.
49. Cabot case: N Engl J Med 1946;234:535–537.
50. Croker JR, Greenstein RJ: Malignant schwannoma of the stomach in a patient with von Recklinghausen's disease. Histopathology 1979;3:79–82.
51. Brown EF, Banner BF, Gould VE: Differential diagnosis of gastrointestinal schwannomas and leiomyomas: A detailed histologic study with electron microscopic correlation. Lab Invest 1984;50:7A.
52. Pike A, Appelman HD, Lloyd R: Differentiation of gut stromal tumors: An immunohistochemical study. Lab Invest 1986;54: 50A.
53. Rast ML, Saul SH, Brooks JJ: Immuno-histochemistry of GI stromal tumors. Lab Invest 1986;54:51A.
54. Kido H: Benign nerve sheath tumor of the stomach: A histologic and immunohistochemical analysis of 18 cases. Fukuoka Acta Med 1986;77:253–262.
55. Daimaru Y, Kido H, Hashimoto H, et al: Benign schwannoma of the gastrointestinal tract: A clinicopathologic and immunohistochemical study. Hum Pathol 1988;19:257–264.
56. Devereux RB, Koblenz LW, Cipriano P, Gray GF: Gastrointestinal hemorrhage–an unusual manifestation of neurofibromatosis. Am J Med 1975;58:135–138.
57. Burns DK, Silva FG, Forde KA, Mount PM, Clark HB: Primary melanocytic schwannoma of the stomach. Cancer 1983;52:1432–1441.
58. Ming S-C: Tumors of the Esophagus and Stomach. 2nd series, Fasc 7 AFIP, Washington DC, also 1973:82, 215; also Supplement 1985:S57–58.
59. Cabot case: N Engl J Med 1949;240:347–350.
60. Chatterjee D, Powell A: Mesenchymal tumors of the stomach: Report of cases, review of literature and analysis of leiomyosarcomas. Br J Clin Pract 1982;36:26–33.
61. Petersen JM, Ferguson DR: Gastrointestinal neurofibromatosis. J Clin Gastroenterol 1984;6:529–534.
62. Toker C: Tumors: An atlas of differential diagnosis. Baltimore: University Park Press, 1983:333, 347.
63. Erlandson RA, Woodruff JM: Peripheral nerve sheath tumors. Cancer 1982;49:273–287.
64. Gould VE, Kraft JR: "Case 14." Ultra Pathol 1983;5:359–368.
65. Erlandson R: Course in electron microscopy. Seattle, Department of Pathology, University of Washington School of Medicine, 1984.
66. Woodruff J: Arthur Purdy Stout and the evolution of modern concepts regarding peripheral nerve sheath tumors. Am J Surg Pathol 1986;10(Suppl 1):63–67.
67. Clark HB, Minesky JJ, Agrawal D, et al: Myelin basic protein and P 2 protein are not immunohistochemical markers for Schwann cell neoplasms. Am J Pathol 1985;121:96–101.
68. Cabot case:37-1985. N Engl J Med 1985;313: 680–688.
69. Memoli VA, Brown EF, Gould VE: Glial fibrillary acidic protein (GFAP) immunoreac-

tivity in peripheral nerve sheath tumors. Ultra Pathol 1984;7:269–275.

70. Perrone T, Sibley RK, Rosai J: Duodenal gangliocytic paraganglioma. Am J Surg Pathol 1985;9:31–41.

71. Kheir SM, Halpern NB: Paraganglioma of the duodenum in association with congenital neurofibromatosis. Cancer 1984;53:2491–2496.

72. Walker P, Dvorak AM: Gastrointestinal autonomic nerve (GAN) tumor. Arch Pathol Lab Med 1986;110:309–316.

73. Dvorak AM: Gut autonomic nerve (GAN) tumors. Dig Dis Pathol 1988 (in press).

74. Tortella BJ, Matthews J, Antonioli D, et al: Gastric autonomic nerve (GAN) tumor and paraganglioma in Carney's triad. Ann Surg 1987;205:221–225.

75. Wright JR, Kyriakos M, DeSchryver-Kecskemeti K: Malignant fibrous histiocytoma of the stomach. Arch Pathol Lab Med 1988; 112:251–258.

76. Kay S, Callahan WB Jr, Murray MR, Randall HT, Stout AP: Glomus tumors of the stomach. Cancer 1951;4:726–736.

77. Kim B-H, Rosen Y, Suen KC: Endocrine type granules in cells of glomus tumor of the stomach. Arch Pathol 1975;99:544–547.

78. Almagro UA, Schulte WJ, Norback DH, Turcotte JK: Glomus tumor of the stomach. Am J Clin Pathol 1981;75:415–419.

79. Seo IS, Azzarelli B, Warner TF, et al: Multiple visceral and cutaneous granular cell tumors. Cancer 1984;53:2104–2110.

80. Johnston J, Helwig EB: Granular cell tumors of the gastrointestinal tract and perianal regions. Dig Dis Sci 1981;26:807–816.

81. Stout AP: Tumors featuring pericytes. Lab Invest 1956;5:217–223.

82. Piluk HC, Conn J Jr: Hemangiopericytoma. Am J Surg 1979;1137:413–416.

83. Nunnery EW, Kahn LB, Reddick RL, Lipper S: Ultrastructure of hemangiopericytoma. Cancer 1981;47:906–914.

84. Stats D: Visceral manifestations of Kaposi's sarcoma. J Mt Sinai Hosp 1945/1946;12:971–983.

85. Balthazar EJ, Richman A: Kaposi's sarcoma of the stomach. Am J Gastroenterol 1977;67:375–379.

86. Friedman SL, Wright TL, Altman DF: Gastrointestinal Kaposi's sarcoma in patients with acquired immunodeficiency syndrome. Gastroenterology 1985;89:102–108.

87. Rotterdam H: The pathology of the gastrointestinal tract in AIDS. Dig Dis Pathol 1988 (in press).

88. Stribling J, Weitzner S, Smith GV: Kaposi's sarcoma in renal allograft recipients. Cancer 1978;42:442–446.

89. Stout AP: Recent observations on mesenchymal tumors in adults and children. Can Med Assoc J 1963;88:453–456.

90. Jones CK, McKee FW: Gastric paraganglioma with ulceration. Arch Pathol 1949; 48:570–577.

91. Keyhani A, Booher RJ: Pleomorphic rhabdomyosarcoma. Cancer 1968;22:956–967.

92. Cairo MS, Grosfeld JL, Weetman RM: Gastric teratoma: Unusual cause for bleeding of the upper gastrointestinal tract in the newborn. Pediatrics 1981;67:721–724.

93. Graham SM, Ballantyne GH, Modlin IM: Gastric epithelioid leiomyosarcoma: A curable gastric neoplasm. Am J Gastroenterol 1987;82:82–84.

94. Denk H, Krepter R, Artlieb U, et al: Proteins of intermediate filaments. Am J Pathol 1983;110:193–208.

95. Saul SH, Rast ML, Brooks JJ: The immunohistochemistry of gastrointestinal stromal tumors. Am J Surg Pathol 1987;11:464–473.

96. Pike A, Appelman H, Lloyd R: Immunostaining of gastric stromal tumors (abstract). Lab Invest 1986;54:50A.

97. Knapp RH, Wick MR, Goellnee JR: Leiomyoblastomas and their relationship to other smooth-muscle tumors of the gastrointestinal tract. Am J Surg Pathol 1984;8:449–461.

98. Morales AR, Fine G, Pardo V, Horn RC Jr: The ultrastructure of smooth muscle tumors. Pathol Annu 1975;10:65–92.

99. Natsunou H, Shimoda T, Kakimoto S, et al: Histopathologic and immunohistochemical study of malignant tumors of peripheral nerve sheath (malignant schwannomas). Cancer 1985;56:2269–2279.

100. Daimaru Y, Hashimoto H, Enjoji M: Malignant peripheral nerve-sheath tumors (malignant schwannomas). Am J Surg Pathol 1985;9:434–444.

101. Hjermstad BM, Maj MC, Sobin LH, Helwig EB: Stromal tumors of the gastrointestinal tract: myogenic or neurogenic? Am J Surg Pathol 1987;11:383–386.

102. Miettinen M, Lehto V-P, Virtanen I: Antibodies to intermediate filament proteins in the

diagnosis and classification of human tumors. Ultra Pathol 1984;7:83–107.

103. Marcus PB, Couch WD, Martin JH: Crystals in a gastric schwannoma. Ultra Pathol 1981; 2:139–145.

104. Ducatman BS, Scheithauer BW: Malignant peripheral nerve sheath tumors with divergent differentiation. Cancer 1984;54:1049–1057.

105. Kleitsch WP, Kehne JW, Gutch CF: Gastrointestinal hemorrhage due to neurofibromatoses. JAMA 1951;147:1434–1436.

106. Cameron AJ, Pairolero PC, Stanson AW, Carpenter HA: Abdominal angina and neurofibromatosis. Mayo Clin Proc 1982;57:125–128.

107. Fialkow PJ, Sagebiel RW, Gartler SM, Rimoin DL: Multiple cell origin of hereditary neurofibromas. N Engl J Med 1971;284:298–300.

108. Riccardi VM: von Recklinghausen neurofibromatosis. N Engl J Med 1981;305:1617–1627.

109. Sordillo PP, Helson L, Hajdu SI, et al: Malignant schwannoma—clinical characteristics, survival and response to therapy. Cancer 1981;47:2503–2509.

110. Shore-Freedman E, Abrahams C, Recant W, et al: Neurilemomas and salivary gland tumors of the head and neck following childhood irradiation. Cancer 1983;51:2159–2163.

111. Bidot-Lopez P, Frankel JW: Enhanced viral transformation of skin fibroblasts from neurofibromatosis patients. Ann Clin Lab Sci 1983;13:27–32.

112. Carney JA, Sheps SG, Go VLW: The triad of gastric leiomyosarcoma, functioning extra-adrenal paraganglioma and pulmonary chondroma. N Engl J Med 1977;296:1517–1518, also Carney JA: Cancer 1979;43:374–382.

113. Wick MR, Ruebner BH: Gastric tumors in patients with pulmonary chondroma or extra-adrenal paraganglioma. Arch Pathol Lab Med 1981;105:527–531.

114. Chander S, Oliverio R Jr, Fermon C, Chander P: Triad of neoplasms (paraganglioma, gastric sarcoma, chondroma). NY State J Med 1981;81:392–393.

115. Grace MP, Batist G, Grace WR, Gillooley JF: Aorticopulmonary paraganglioma and gastric leiomyoblastoma in a young woman. Am J Med 1981;70:1288–1292.

116. Silverstein MN, Wakim KG, Bahn RC, Decker RH: Role of tryptophan metabolites in the hypoglycemia associated with neoplasia. Cancer 1966;19:127–133.

117. Carey RW, Pretlow TG, Ezdinli EZ, Holland JF: Studies on the mechanism of hypoglycemia in a patient with massive intraperitoneal leiomyosarcoma. Am J Med 1966;40:458–469.

118. Froesch ER, Zapf J, Widmer U: Letter to editor. N Engl J Med 1982;306:1178.

119. Soga J, Saito K, Suzuki N, Sakai T: Plasma cell granuloma of the stomach. Cancer 1970; 25:618–625.

120. Spencer H: The pulmonary plasma cell/histiocytoma complex. Histopathology 1984;8:903–916.

121. Flint A, Murad TM: Malakoplakia and malakoplakialike lesions of the upper gastrointestinal tract. Ultra Pathol 1984;7:167–176.

122. Goldman RL, Friedman NB: Neurogenic nature of so-called inflammatory fibroid polyps of the stomach. Cancer 1967;20:134–143.

123. Ghadially FN: Diagnostic Ultrastructural Pathology. London: Butterworths, 1984:11 (Fig. 11).

CHAPTER 12

Miscellaneous Gastroduodenal Pathology

Foreign Bodies

Foreign bodies in the stomach and duodenum can be categorized into three types: true foreign bodies (i.e., environmental objects that should normally never be in stomach or duodenum); bezoars, or foreign bodies composed of substances that normally pass through the gastrointestinal tract in small quantities; and bodies that are foreign to the stomach or duodenum, but not to the human body as such.

True Foreign Bodies

The ingestion of true foreign bodies is a common problem in hospital emergency rooms and causes approximately 1500 deaths in the United States every year.[1,2] Most swallowed foreign bodies pass spontaneously, and even among individuals seeking medical help for the problem, only 43% have symptoms, primarily abdominal pain.[3] Most ingestions occur accidentally in children and the elderly.[4] Intentional ingestion is frequent among prisoners and psychiatric patients.[5] The most commonly swallowed foreign bodies are bones, needles, pins, buttons, coins, and razor blades. Less common are wristwatches, thermometers, pens, pencils, spikes, nails, tacks, forks, spoons, broken glass, and toothbrushes.[6,7] The more unusual foreign bodies are found in mental patients. There are rare reports of accidental ingestion of endodontic instruments,[8] dental prostheses,[9] and endotracheal tubes in neonates.[10] Antireflux prostheses implanted at the esophagogastric junction may loosen and become an intragastric foreign object.[11]

In mental patients, multiple objects are frequently observed, either accumulated over time or removed at different intervals. A total of 71 metal objects were present in the stomach of an asymptomatic schizophrenic man. These included a wrench, wire springs, buttons and eyeglasses.[1] Five consecutive endoscopic removals of a paper clip from the duodenum and a key chain, thermometer, two open safety pins, an aluminum ashtray, coat hanger wire, and four thumb tacks from the stomach were described in a chronic alcoholic.[12]

Most foreign bodies, even pointed and sharp objects like open pins or razor blades, travel through the gastrointestinal tract uneventfully.[4] The so-called mural withdrawal reflex relaxes the intestinal wall whenever an object comes into contact with its mucosa. Locations at which this passage is likely to be delayed or blocked are the lower esophageal sphincter, the pylorus, the duodenal curve, and the ligament of Treitz. Whereas the stomach is the site of lodgement more frequently than the duodenum, the latter preferentially harbors stiff, long objects such as wires or an endotracheal tube.[3,8]

Complications include nonpassage, obstruction, bleeding, abscess formation, perforation, and release of toxic substances from ingested batteries or bags of heroine or cocaine.[1] Perforation is said to occur in less than 1% of all ingested foreign bodies, but in up to 35% of sharp and pointed items.[3] Ten percent of intestinal perforations are caused by toothpicks, usually accidentally swallowed by individuals with dentures.[13] In such instances, the site of perforation is most commonly the ileo-cecal region, but stomach and duodenum may perforate as well.[3,14] Duodenal perforation and formation of a duodeno-renal fistula were described in a 2½-year-old child who swallowed a broken hair pin.[14]

Bezoars

Bezoars are various types of concretions found in the stomach and intestines of animals and man. Trichobezoars are composed of hair, phytobezoars of fruit and vegetable fibers, trichophytobezoars of a mixture of the two, lactobezoars of concentrated formula in neonates, and medication bezoars of medications such as antacids or polystyrene sodium sulfonate (Kayexalate).[15-17] Rarely, bezoars form out of tar, shellac, sand, resin, or laundry starch.[18,19]

The origin of the word "bezoar" is not entirely clear. Possible sources are the Arab "bedzehr," the Persian "padzahr," and the Hebrew "beluzaar," all of which translate into "antidote" or "antipoison."[15] The fourth stomach of a Persian wild goat was the alleged site of origin of the first bezoar. For centuries, Arabs, ancient Hindus, and medieval pharmacists believed in the curative value of bezoars, which became an accepted remedy for plague, small pox, and all types of fever. The last prescription containing the mystical "Lapis Bezoar Orientalis" appeared in the *London Pharmacopea* in 1746.[20] The first human bezoar was described in the Western literature in 1779 as an autopsy finding.[21] Extensive and frequently quoted reviews of the subject were published in 1938 and 1939 by DeBakey and Ochsner.[22,23]

Bezoars were found in 6 of 1400 gastroscopies,[24] and approximately 300 cases were recorded in the world literature until 1979.[20] The phytobezoar is more common in a general hospital population, whereas the trichobezoar is more common among children and mental patients. Most bezoars develop as a complication of previous gastric surgery, with an unusually high incidence of 14% reported in postgastrectomy patients.[25] Loss of normal pyloric function, hypoperistalsis, and low gastric acidity are predisposing factors. Diabetic gastroparesis has a similar effect.[26] Cimetadine treatment-associated bezoar formation can be explained on the basis of low acidity.[27] Emotional disturbances are common, especially in patients with trichobezoars.[23,28] Although most bezoars are formed and remain lodged in the stomach, occasional intraduodenal locations may occur.[29]

Phytobezoars are composed of a variety of vegetables and fruits with an unusually high fiber content, such as berries, persimmon, orange or grapefruit pulp, figs, apple skins, string beans, cabbage, potatoe peels,[26] or corn (Fig. 12-1). The bezoar composition will reflect the regional diets (e.g., fibers of unripe persimmon are frequent in patients from the southern United States and Japan, and orange pulp is common in the northern United States).[30]

Trichobezoars are formed from the hair of the patient, other humans, or animals, bristles, raffia, carpet fibers, wool fibers, and doll hair. They are an occupational hazard among brushmakers, blanket weavers, and wool workers.[22,23] More than 90% of patients with trichobezoars are female, usually younger than 30 years of age, with long hair and a history of emotional imbalance.[18] In the early stages, swallowed hair strands get caught in the gastric folds. As they accumulate, peristalsis causes them to be enmeshed and form a ball which, too large to leave the stomach, causes gastric atony and finally outlet obstruction. In order of decreasing frequency, symptoms include abdominal pain, nausea and vomiting, and alteration in bowel habits.[22] A mild hypochromic anemia from mild blood loss and leucocytosis are common laboratory findings.

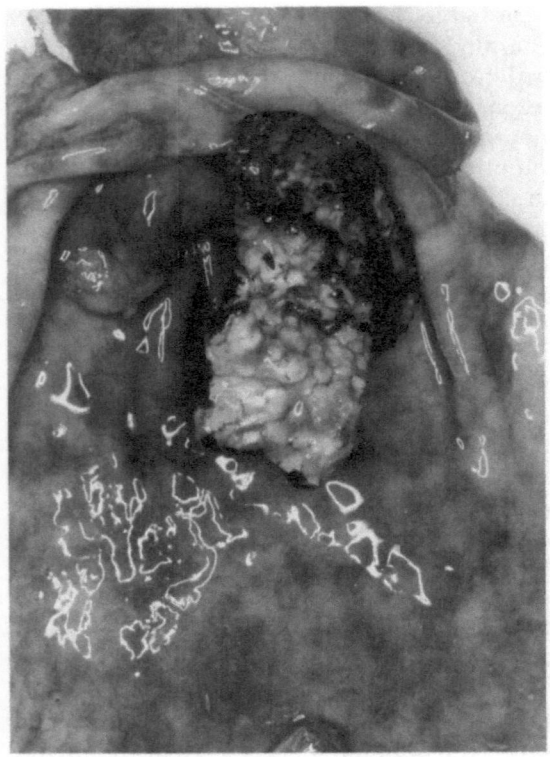

Figure 12-1. Phytobezoar in the stomach of a mental patient.

Trichobezoars may attain considerable size and weight before they become symptomatic. A 1000-g bezoar in a 14-year-old girl extended from the stomach, throughout the small intestine, and into the transverse colon. Such giant trichobezoars are referred to as "Rapunzel syndrome."[18] The patient died as a result of duodenal necrosis. Gastric ulceration, the more common complication, occurs in 10% of cases, 30% of which progress to perforation.[23]

Gallstones

Gallstone perforations into the gastrointestinal tract occur in 5.7% of patients with gallstones.[31] Gallstone ileus develops in 0.3 to 4% of patients, most (80%) of whom have a cholecystoenteric fistula.[32] Of these fistulas, 70% involve the duodenum, 25% the colon, and 5% the stomach. Gallstones with a diameter

larger than 2.5 cm can cause intermittent obstruction, usually ending in irreversible obstruction of the terminal ileum. Gastric outlet obstruction is rare and was first described by Bouveret in 1896.[33] About 170 cases have been reported since. Previously, surgery was considered the only possible treatment, but endoscopic removal of an intragastric gallstone can at times be achieved. Duodenal obstruction by a gallstone primarily affects the bulb.[34]

Depositions

A variety of substances may be deposited in the gastric and duodenal wall, usually as part of a systemic disorder, but occasionally as a localized finding. Deposition of amyloid, pigments (iron among others), calcium, and lipid will be discussed.

Amyloidosis

The gastrointestinal tract may be involved in all types of amyloidosis—primary, secondary, myeloma-associated, familial, and isolated tumor-like. At autopsy, the incidence of amyloid deposits in the different segments of the gastrointestinal tract was reported as 25/57 for the stomach, 31/57 for the small bowel, and 21/57 for the large bowel.[35] In primary amyloidosis, gastrointestinal involvement is found in approximately 70% of cases[36] and in secondary amyloidosis in 55%.[37] Among eight cases of gastric amyloidosis diagnosed by endoscopic biopsy, three were of the primary type, four were myeloma-associated, and one had macroglobulinemia.[38] Immunoglobulin-G (IgG) and IgA myeloma as well as myeloma with Bence-Jones proteinuria showed gastric amyloid. Only rarely is gastric amyloidosis the first manifestation of myeloma.[39] Familial amyloid polyneuropathy, common in Japan and Sweden, produces gastric deposits in many if not all cases. Each of 12 Japanese patients undergoing gastroscopic biopsy[40] and 12 of 43 Swedish patients undergoing radiologic and endoscopic examination[41] had evidence of gastric amyloid. Gastric biopsy may, indeed, prove as reliable as rectal biopsy in detecting gastrointestinal involvement in all types of amyloidosis, as suggested by two studies from Japan.[35,40] Multiple gastric biopsies indicate preferential involvement of the antrum and distal body when deposition is patchy, and involvement of proximal body and fundus when deposition is more diffuse.[38]

Symptoms related to gastric amyloidosis include ulceration, bleeding secondary to vascular amyloid deposits, and reduced motility secondary to intramuscular amyloid.[39-41] Endoscopically, ulcers, hemorrhagic spots, enlarged gastric and duodenal mucosal folds, pseudopolyps, yellow-white nodules, and mucosal friability have been observed.[39,41]

Histologically, amyloid can be seen in blood vessels of all layers of the gastric wall, in the mucosal stroma, and within the muscularis propria.[38] Vascular deposition is most apparent in the submucosa (Fig. 12-2) and is consistently present in all cases of gastric amyloidosis, regardless of type.[42] Deposition in the muscularis mucosae and external layer of the muscularis propria is characteristic of myeloma-associated amyloid (AL), whereas deposition in the lamina propria is more common in secondary amyloidosis (AA). Of practical interest is the finding of more frequent mucosal amyloid deposition in the stomach than in the rectum in the AL type, suggesting that gastric biopsy may be of greater diagnostic value than the customary rectal biopsy in cases of myeloma.[42] Positive identification of amyloid requires staining with Congo red and proof of green-orange dichroism under polarized light or electron microscopic demonstration of the typical nonbranching 60- to 85-Å fibrils.[43]

Isolated tumor-like amyloidosis of the stomach is a rare condition, and only 11 cases were found in reviews of the recent Western literature.[43-46] Such amyloidomas may present as large ulcerated masses up to 14 cm in diameter[46] or as diffuse gastric wall thickening,[43] mimicking carcinoma. Localized amyloid deposits are mainly submucosal, but extend into the mucosa and muscularis pro-

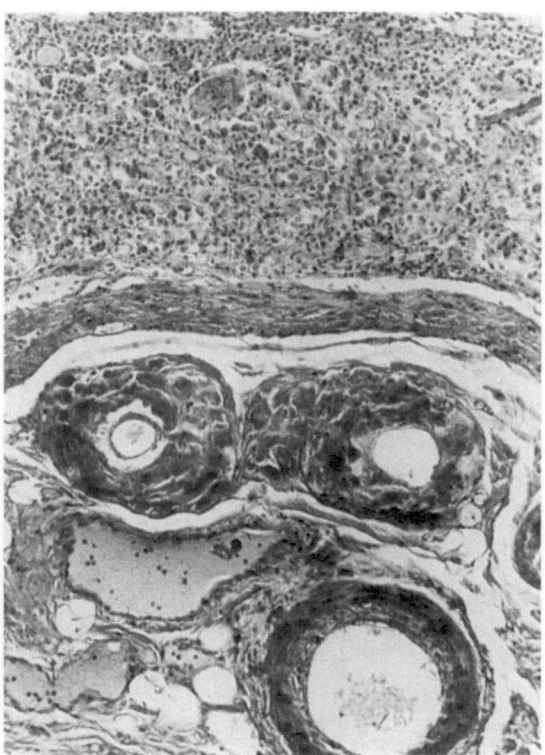

Figure 12-2. Amyloidosis of the stomach. Submucosal vessels are stiff and their walls markedly thickened due to medial deposits of amyloid. Hematoxylin-Phloxine-Saffranin, X100, reproduced at 65%.

pria for short distances. Blood vessels and regional lymph nodes may also be involved.[44] A marked lymphocytic or plasma cell infiltrate accompanies some amyloidomas. Myofibroblasts containing fibrils ultrastructurally identical to amyloid fibrils were demonstrated in one case, suggesting that myofibroblasts play a role in the formation of local amyloid.[43]

Pigment Deposition

Pigment deposition in the stomach and duodenum is rare. Four pigments may be found: melanin, pseudomelanin, hemosiderin, and lipofuscin.

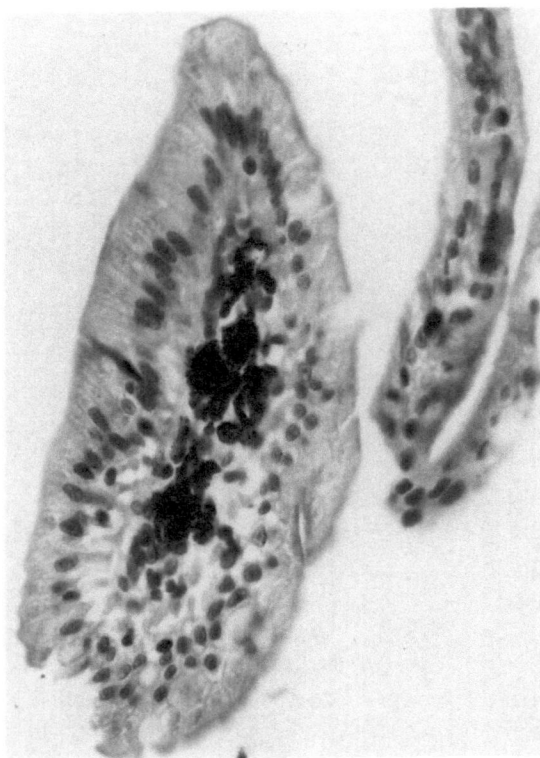

Figure 12-3. Pseudomelanosis duodeni. The tips of villi contain coarse dark pigment granules within macrophages. H&E, X400, reproduced at 65%.

Melanosis (i.e., deposition of true melanin), in our experience, occurs only in association with metastatic malignant melanoma. Melanin pigment, formed and released by tumor cells, is ingested by melanophages in the adjacent normal tissue and produces true melanosis. Reticular pigmentation of gastric and duodenal mucosa has been described in von Recklinghausen's disease.[47] Although not analyzed, such pigmentation most likely is due to melanin deposition.

Pseudomelanosis duodeni is characterized by deposition of a melanin-like pigment that is brown or brown-black on hematoxylin-eosin stain, stains positive with Fontana, but in contrast to true melanin, is periodic acid-Schiff (PAS)-positive and acid-fast. Lack of fluorescence and lack of staining with oil-red O excludes lipofuscin.[48] Pseudomelanosis duodeni was first described as melanosis duodeni in the English literature in 1976,[49] and only six further cases were reported as of 1985.[50] Most affected patients were female, 60 to 70 years old, and had other gastroduodenal pathology such as ulcers, polyps, or gastritis. Many were hypertensive and were receiving multiple oral antihypertensive agents, suggesting that the combined effects of gastrointestinal hemorrhage and certain oral medications may play an etiologic role. Significantly, there is no association with laxative abuse and melanosis coli.

Endoscopically, the duodenal mucosa of the first and second portions appears peppered. Pigment is deposited primarily in the tips of duodenal villi, within macrophages of the lamina propria, and only rarely extracellularly (Fig. 12-3). Ultrastructurally, pigment granules are of markedly variable shape and size, membrane-bound, and apparently within lysosomes. Coating of granules with fine electron-dense material, observed in one case 17 months after the initial diagnosis, coincides with a change from iron-negative to iron-positive staining and most likely reflects pigment degredation.[50] This change in histochemical staining property with aging explains the variability of staining results with Prussian blue reported in the literature. Electron-probe x-ray analysis in one case demonstrated the pigment to be essentially ferrous sulfide.[51] In spite of its iron content, it would be inappropriate to designate the lesion "hemosiderosis," since hemosiderin is hydrated iron oxide. Pseudomelanosis may disappear spontaneously after the accompanying disorder has been corrected.[52]

Hemosiderosis of the duodenum has been described in a patient taking oral ferrous sulfate.[53] Considering the frequency of such medication and the rarity of the lesion , an etiologic link seems doubtful. The pigment, in contrast to the pseudomelanin just described, was Fontana- and PAS-negative and resistant to melanin bleach.

Hemochromatosis, especially in its advanced stage, may be associated with diffuse hemosiderin deposition in the gastric and duodenal mucosa. Endoscopic biopsies have demonstrated iron pigment in the basal glands of the body and antrum of the stomach, particularly in parietal and chief cells (Fig. 12-4), as well as in crypt epithelium and Brunner's glands in the duodenum in 6 of 13 patients with hemochromatosis.[54] Iron was also demonstrated in the lamina propria, but in fewer patients. There was no correlation with serum ferritin levels. Since a similar pattern of iron deposition can be found in alcoholics, the diagnostic value of upper gastrointestinal biopsy in primary hemochromatosis is limited.[54]

Intestinal lipofuscinosis (the "brown bowel syndrome") is characterized by brown pigmentation, usually visible grossly, of the small intestine and sometimes part of the stomach.[54] Lipofuscin pigment is deposited in the cytoplasm of smooth muscle cells, especially in the muscularis propria, but also in the muscularis mucosae and the media of blood vessels. The condition is associated with malabsorption of fat and vitamin E deficiency.[55] In spite of its striking gross and microscopic appearance, there seems to be no functional impairment of the muscle.

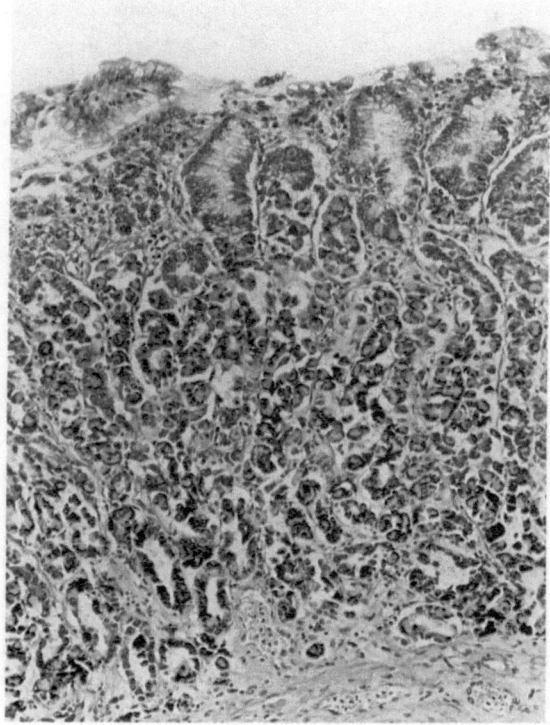

Figure 12-4. Hemochromatosis of the stomach. Chief and parietal cells of the fundus contain abundant iron pigment. Foveolar mucous cells are spared. Prussian blue, X100, reproduced at 65%.

Calcification

Deposition of calcium in any tissue occurs either as local dystrophic calcification or as part of a more generalized process as metastatic calcification. In the latter form, calcium deposits occur most frequently in the lungs, kidneys, and stomach because of local tissue alkalosis at these sites.[56] Most gastric calcifications are of the metastatic type and have been described in patients with renal failure,[57,58] after renal transplantation,[59] in myeloma,[60] and in a patient with diffuse interstitial pulmonary calcification.[56]

Autopsy studies of patients with renal failure cite an unusually high (50 to 60%) incidence of accompanying gastric calcification.[57,58] Among renal transplant patients, the incidence was 20%.[59] Calcium deposits may be reabsorbed when renal function improves and secondary hyperparathyroidism disappears. The fundic mucosa is affected more often than any other part, again as a result of the more pronounced tissue alkalosis at this site. Calcium deposits have been identified in the lamina propria and muscularis mucosae, within the cytoplasm of smooth muscle cells, as well as in the form of large extracellular deposits.[56] If calcifications reach a sufficient size, they may be recognized endoscopically as white, 1 to 2 mm diameter, nodules and can even be detected on bone scans.[60]

Gastric Xanthoma

Deposition of lipid in histiocytes of the gastric mucosa was first described as "lipid islands" in the medical literature in 1929.[61]

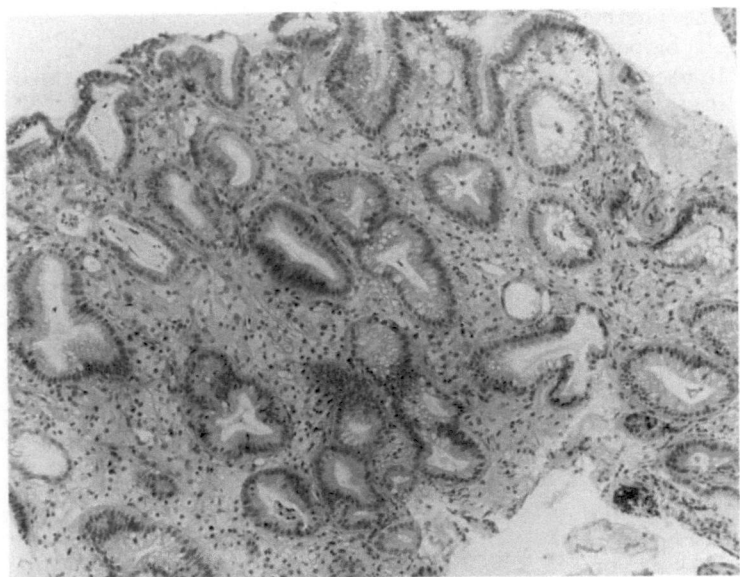

Figure 12-5. Gastric xanthoma. Clusters of foamy histiocytes are seen between intestinalized gastric glands. Hematoxylin-Phloxin-Saffranin. X100, reproduced at 65%.

The increased use of endoscopy has led to a renewed interest in this rather frequent and innocuous lesion , which has been variously reported as "xanthomatosis,"[62] "xanthelasma,"[63] "gastric lipid island,"[64,65] and "xanthoma."[66,67] The latter term is the most recent, and most commonly used. It is certainly preferable to "xanthelasma," which to date has been reserved for lesions of the eyelids. Nonetheless, "xanthoma" is a misnomer since it denotes a neoplastic lesion, which lipid deposition in the gastric mucosa certainly is not.

The incidence of gastric xanthomas at autopsy was reported to be as high as 53% by the discoverers of the lesion[61] and, more recently, as approximately 4% at endoscopy.[62] In gastrectomy patients, the incidence increases to 18%[64] and reaches 60% after 10 to 23 years of age.[65] Although there was no consistent clinical correlation among the 267 cases recorded from the literature in 1982, prolonged inflammation and biliary reflux seem to be the main etiologic factors. The frequent association with intestinal metaplasia is of particular interest because of the known potential of this type of mucosa to absorb fat.[68] There is no correlation with hyperlipidemia. There was associated cholesterolosis of the gallbladder in 5 of 7 cases.[63]

Gastric xanthomas vary in size from 1 to 10 mm in diameter, are usually multiple, and occur most frequently along the lesser curvature of the fundus and prepyloric region.[65,66] Endoscopically, they appear as yellow-white, slightly raised plaques and rarely as nodules. Histologically, there are lipid-laden histiocytes in the lamina propria, displacing gastric glands and foveolae (Fig. 12-5) and occasionally extending into the submucosa.[66] Spontaneous disappearance has been demonstrated.

The importance of the lesion lies in its possible (and actually reported[66]) confusion with the diffuse type of gastric carcinoma. Endoscopists are urged to submit fresh biopsies to allow for lipid staining. In fixed specimens, negative stains for mucin and the lack of significant cytologic atypia help to differentiate xanthoma cells from carcinoma cells.

Emphysema

Intramural gas collections occur in all parts of the gastrointestinal tract, but the stomach is the least often reported site.[69,70] Three pathogenetically different forms are generally distinguished: 1) Emphysematous gastritis, as discussed in Chapter 4 on gastritis, is a form of phlegmonous gastritis caused by gas-forming bacteria. The course is fulminant and patients are toxic and mortality is 60–80%.[69] 2) Pneumatosis of stomach and duodenum is related to idiopathic pneumatosis intestinalis and occurs in patients with asthma and cystic fibrosis.[70] Spontaneous rupture of a subpleural emphysematous bulla releases air into the paraesophageal area, where it gradually dissects downward into the gastric submucosa and subserosa. Patients are generally asymptomatic, and the condition has little clinical significance. 3) Gastric emphysema can be subdivided into the more common traumatic type and the less common obstructive type.[69] Some investigators include pneumatosis in the pulmonary type.[69] Gastric emphysema is usually related to intragastric instrumentation and mucosal trauma that allows air to enter the deeper layers of the gastric wall. In the obstructive type, increased intraluminal gastric pressure due to either severe vomiting, gastroscopic insufflation of air, gastric outlet obstruction, or proximal small bowel obstruction causes a mucosal tear. Air accumulates primarily in the loose submucosa and subserosa, but may extend into gastric ligaments and omentum. Rupture of subserosal or omental vesicles may cause pneumoperitoneum.

Acute Gastric Dilatation

Acute gastric dilatation implies rapid enlargement of the stomach in the absence of actual organic obstruction. The condition is most commonly associated with a surgical procedure that required general anesthesia, but has also been seen after trauma, in bulbar poliomyelitis, typhoid fever, arteriosclerotic heart disease, pneumonia, tuberculosis, debilitating chronic disease, parturition, overeating,[71,72] excessive bicarbonate ingestion, volvulus, malrotation, diabetes mellitus, hypokalemia, anorexia nervosa,[73] and after fundoplication.[74] Acute gastric dilatation has been recognized since the early 19th century under a number of different names that illustrate the variety of associated conditions as well as the suspected pathogenetic mechanisms. These names include acute gastroduodenal atony, gastroenteroplegia, acute paresis of the stomach, acute postoperative dilatation of the stomach, acute gastromesenteric ileus, acute arteriomesenteric compression, cast syndrome,[71] and gas-bloating syndrome.[74] The initial causal event is thought to be a reflex disturbance of the extrinsic gastric innervation, rendering the stomach atonic. Dilatation is then produced by swallowed air and gastric and duodenal secretions. In some patients, especially in thin individuals and those with spinal deformities, mechanical obstruction of the third portion of the duodenum by the superior mesenteric artery may be an additional causal factor.[71] Hypokalemia is a predisposing factor.[75] Dilatation may involve the duodenum to the level of the ligament of Treitz, especially in emaciated patients.[73]

Complications include perforation and infarction (Fig. 12-6). Overdistention of the fundus may lead to occlusion of the cardia, and acute angulation of the antrum will prevent passage of gastric contents through the pylorus. Perforation is unlikely to occur unless the amount of intragastric fluid exceeds 4 liters.[76] In one case in which the amount was actually measured, the stomach contained 8 liters when it ruptured.[73] Most such perforations occur along the lesser curvature near the cardia.[77] Infarction ensues when intragastric pressure exceeds gastric venous pressure.[73] Gastric infarction due to arterial insufficiency has not been recorded. The extensive collateral circulation prevents such an event.[73]

Duodenal Dilatation

Duodenal dilatation without associated intrinsic or extrinsic obstructing lesion is

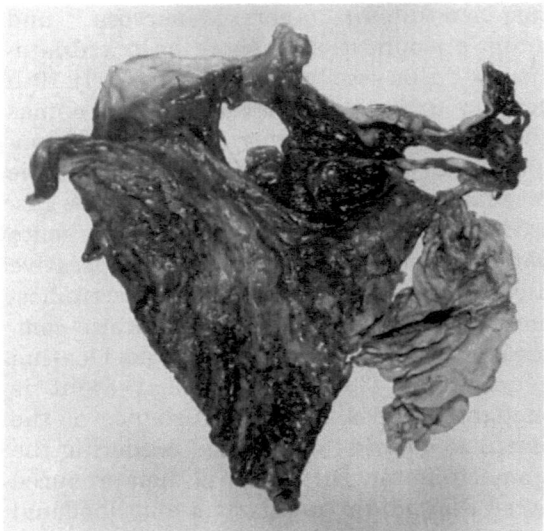

Figure 12-6. Infarction and perforation of stomach. Partial resection.

caused by compression of the fourth portion of the duodenum by the root of the mesentery.[78] The condition was first described by von Rokitansky[79] in 1861, but studied in greater detail by Wilkie[80] in 1921 and, therefore, is sometimes referred to as "Wilkie's syndrome."[81] Other names used in the literature are superior mesenteric artery syndrome, arteriomesenteric duodenal compression syndrome, chronic duodenal ileus, and cast syndrome.[82] Approximately 320 cases were reported as of 1982.[81,82]

Knowledge of the specific topography of the region is necessary for an understanding of the pathogenesis of duodenal dilatation. The transverse or ascending portion of the duodenum, as it crosses the spine, is normally fixed in a space, bounded posteriorly by the spine and aorta, and anteriorly by the mesentery containing the superior mesenteric vessels and nerves. Any condition that impinges on this space will produce distal duodenal compression and proximal duodenal dilatation. It has been pointed out that the extrinsic pressure sufficient to cause anteroposterior compression at this site is minimal, in contrast

to other segments of the small and large intestine where much greater pressures are required for the same effect.[83] A variety of congenital and acquired conditions contribute to produce distal duodenal compression. Short length and high attachment of the ligament of Treitz, high position of the third and fourth portions of the duodenum, and a narrow angle between the aorta and the superior mesenteric artery (15° or less instead of the usual 45 to 60°) are predisposing factors.[78,81] Severe weight loss reduces the amount of supportive tissue in the mesentery and exposes the duodenum to the pressures of surrounding structures. Rapid growth in adolescence may change previously normal anatomic relationships. Severe lumbar lordosis narrows the space between the aorta and the mesenteric root. It is because of positional changes of the lumbar spine that patients with body casts, spinal deformities, extensive burns, and others in long-term nursing care in a supine position may develop duodenal compression.

Symptoms of obstruction, such as vomiting and epigastric pain, are intermittent and characteristically can be relieved by adopting a knee-chest, all-fours, or recumbant position. The diagnosis is best made by simultaneous superior mesenteric artery angiography and hypotonic duodenography.[81] The duodenum up to the level of the mesenteric artery, and occasionally the stomach are dilated and the duodenal wall may be hypertrophied. Treatment consists of removal of any predisposing factor if possible, or of duodenojejunostomy and dextroposition of the duodenojejunal junction.[78]

Spontaneous Gastric Rupture

Gastric rupture may be spontaneous or traumatic. The latter will be discussed under the heading of "Gastroduodenal Injuries." Spontaneous rupture is seen in the newborn and the adult and differs in pathogenesis and pathology in these two populations. Therefore, it will be discussed separately.

Spontaneous Gastric Rupture in the Newborn

Only 1 of 2900 live births at Howard University in Washington D.C. was complicated by spontaneous gastric rupture within the first week of life.[83] The majority of such neonates are premature and suffer from asphyxia or hypoxia at birth.[83,84] A history of vigorous respiratory resuscitative measures, tube feeding, and increased intragastric pressure due to distal obstruction is often present.[83] The cause of rupture is not entirely clear. Focal congenital absence of the muscularis propria was first suggested by Herbut in 1943,[85] but was not found in many subsequently reported cases. Experimentally induced rupture of autopsy specimens of normal neonatal stomachs disclosed separation and retraction of the muscle with increased intragastric pressure, finally resulting in mechanical disruption and perforation.[84]The theory of mechanical disruption as the cause of neonatal gastric rupture is further supported by the identical pathologic characteristics of experimentally induced and spontaneously occurring tears. The tears are linear, 0.5- to 7-cm long, primarily located along the larger curvature near the cardia, and consistently more extensive on the serosal side than in the mucosa.[84]

The specific location, which differs from that in adult gastric rupture, can be explained in several ways. First, the gastric muscle layer is thinnest at the cardia and fundus. Second, the body of the stomach experiences the greatest tension when intragastric pressure increases. Third, and most importantly, the circular muscle layer of the newborn normally contains gaps, mostly in the fundus near the greater curvature, and more commonly in premature than term infants.[84]

Neonatal spontaneous gastric rupture used to have a 100% mortality rate. With improved neonatal medical care, however, the rate is now reduced to 25%.[83]

Spontaneous Gastric Rupture in the Adult

Most of these cases are preceded by acute gastric dilatation, and the predisposing factors have been discussed previously. There are rare reports of postemetic rupture of a herniated cardia[86,87] and gastric rupture following cardiopulmonary resuscitation, in some cases associated with inadvertent esophageal intubation.[88] Gastric dilatation following abnormally large meals accounts for half of all cases of adult gastric rupture.[74] Sixty-seven percent of patients are female.

Adult gastric rupture occurs mostly in the fundus, but in contrast to neonatal rupture, the lesser rather than the greater curvature is involved.[77] Ischemic necrosis, either surrounding the area of rupture or more widespread, has been observed in some cases[74,77] and may precede rupture. Adult gastric rupture is rare, and only 73 cases were found in the literature in 1982.[72]

Gastroduodenal Injuries

Injuries can be classified according to type into penetrating and blunt injuries, and according to extent into 1) hematomas, 2) perforations (i.e, defects involving less than 20% of the lumenal circumference), 3) lacerations (i.e., defects that involve between 20 and 70% of the lumenal circumference), and 4) disruptions (i.e., defects that involve more than 70% of the lumenal circumference).[89] In the following discussion, the term "rupture" is used to include the latter three types of injury.

Blunt injuries to the abdomen are usually the result of motor vehicle accidents in which the steering wheel is pressed against the epigastrium.[88] Penetrating injuries are primarily gunshot and stab wounds. In older publications, blunt trauma was far more frequent than penetrating wounds,[71] but more recent data show the reverse.[89]

Traumatic Gastric Rupture

Blunt abdominal trauma causes rupture of hollow gastrointestinal organs in 11 to 18% of cases.[90] The stomach is the site of rupture in only 0.9 to 1.7% of these, and no more than approximately 100 cases were recorded in the literature as of 1979.[91] Motor vehicle accidents, especially when seat belts were not used (but occasionally with seat belt use), are the major cause, followed by falls, physical violence, and occasionally cardiopulmonary resuscitation.[91,92] Rare causes include injury by a nasogastric suction tube[93] and barotrauma.[94] Most patients are male and most had a large meal prior to gastric rupture. Other serious injuries are present in 77%, most commonly splenic rupture.[92]

Symptoms of peritoneal irritation, such as abdominal pain, tenderness, and rigidity, usually occur immediately after the initiating event. However, delayed rupture up to 17 days after blunt injury has been reported.[95]

Two major mechanisms determine the site of rupture. First, the crushing force is greatest over the vertebral bodies. Second, shearing forces are greatest where mobile parts meet fixed parts.[95] The lesser curvature of the stomach is the most frequent site of traumatic rupture because of its fixed character and its position anterior to the vertebral bodies. The antrum is endangered because of its intermediate position between the mobile body and fundus and the fixed pylorus.[91] The anterior wall is more often affected than the posterior wall.[90,92] Tears tend to be larger on the serosal side than in the mucosa because the initial disruption, even in blunt trauma, is in the seromuscular coat and the mucosa is disrupted only secondarily.[91,95]

Intramural Hematoma

Intramural hematoma affects almost exclusively the duodenum and only rarely the stomach.[96] Nearly 200 cases had been described by 1980.[97] Trauma is the commonest cause, although bleeding disorders, ruptured aneurysms, and acute pancreatitis are some-

times implicated. Sixty percent of duodenal intramural hematomas occur in children, and in most of these cases, injury is due to bicycle accidents in which the duodenum becomes compressed between the handlebar and the lumbar spine.[98] Car accidents account for most adult cases. Endoscopic retrograde cholangiopancreaticography (ERCP) is complicated by duodenal hematoma in 0.2% of cases, and 17 such instances were recorded in 1982.[99] Most of the affected patients had acute pancreatitis, rendering the duodenal mucosa friable.

Vomiting due to obstruction usually occurs only 2 days after the insult, when the hematoma increases in size because of the hyperosmotic action of the liquefying clot. Gastric dilatation and swollen duodenal folds are seen on x-ray study. A palpable mass develops in 50% of cases.

Hematomas most commonly involve the second portion of the duodenum, but may extend along its entire length. Mucosal tears can sometimes be demonstrated. The serosa usually remains intact unless the hematoma extends into the jejunum, where perforation is more likely to occur, than in the duodenum.[97]

Complications include mucosal infarction, late strictures, and other deformities. Surgical evacuation is necessary only for large lesions. Smaller hematomas resolve spontaneously.

Duodenal Rupture

Because of its protected location, the duodenum is infrequently the site of trauma. Duodenum and pancreas account for only 1 to 2% of major abdominal trauma,[100] and the duodenum is affected in only 10% of gastrointestinal tract injuries.[101] Penetrating injuries are more than three times as common as blunt injuries.[88,102] Most patients have associated lesions in liver, colon, pancreas, stomach, or small intestine, and it is these lesions that usually determine the clinical presentation and outcome. Duodenal injury is isolated in only 5% of patients.[102] The second portion of the duodenum is the most frequent site affected, followed, in order to decreasing frequency, by the third, fourth, and first portions. Injuries to the first and second portions carry the greatest morbidity and mortality because of associated trauma to the ampulla and pancreas.

Blunt trauma to the duodenum, like that to the stomach, is most commonly associated with steering wheel injury during a motor vehicle accident.[88] Eighty-one percent of blunt duodenal injuries are ruptures and of these, 59% are perforations or lacerations and 22% are pancreatico-duodenal disruptions. Tears are most often transverse and rarely longitudinal.[103] Mortality rates vary from less than 1% for injuries to the third and fourth portions to 13% for injuries to the second portion.[102] Besides by anatomic location, mortality is greatly influenced by the time interval between injury and surgical intervention. Complications include fistulas, obstruction, and sepsis.

Gastroduodenal Lesions in Systemic Diseases and Diseases of Adjacent Organs

Chronic Renal Failure

Patients with chronic renal failure develop functional and histologic changes of the stomach and duodenum. Hypochlorhydria and chronic superficial or chronic atrophic gastritis are found in approximately 50% of patients.[104] Acid secretion improves with hemodialysis and appears to be dependent on the level of nitrous metabolic products. Histologically, uremic gastritis differs from nonspecific chronic gastritis. There is a predominance of lymphocytes in the mucosal infiltrate, whereas plasma cells are relatively scarce. Among lymphocytes, the ratio of T to B cells is 10 to 1 as compared with 3 to 1 in nonspecific chronic gastritis. Dystrophic and degenerative changes in the superficial epithelium are pronounced.

Nodular duodenitis occurs in 34% of patients with renal failure and presents radiologically and endoscopically with multiple, 2.5- to 7-mm diameter mucosal nodules that are found primarily in the bulb and first portion, but sometimes throughout the full duodenal length.[105,106] Biopsies of such nodules have shown villous blunting and thickening due to fibrosis, lymphoid aggregates, and a chronic inflammatory infiltrate. Erosions may be present on the tip of villi. Besides these nodular lesions, there are diffuse duodenal mucosal changes. The length of villi and crypts is reduced and, ultrastructurally, microvilli are shortened, irregularly distributed, and have been described as "moth-eaten and grainy."[107] These changes may be responsible for reduced calcium reabsorption since both histologic changes and calcium absorption improved with Vitamin D_3-$[1,25(OH)_2D_3]$ therapy.

Diabetes Mellitus

Diabetic gastroparesis (i.e., gastric atony and delayed emptying) is observed mostly in patients with long-standing, insulin-dependent diabetes mellitus,[108] but occasionally is also seen in those receiving oral medications.[109] Almost all have peripheral and autonomic neuropathy. The condition may be asymptomatic or cause (sometimes intractable) nausea and vomiting and abdominal pain; occasionally it will worsen diabetic control as a result of irregular food absorption.[110] Diabetic gastroparesis is thought to be due to vagal nerve damage occurring as part of a more generalized autonomic neuropathy. The stomach is elongated and contains solid residue. The duodenal bulb is dilated, but the remainder of the duodenum is normal in configuration.[109] Histologic studies of autopsy specimens have shown severe loss of myelinated axons and a marked excess of collagen in the vagus nerve.[110] Smooth muscle cells showed hyaline degeneration. Celiac and sympathetic ganglia were inflamed and neurons were vacuolized.

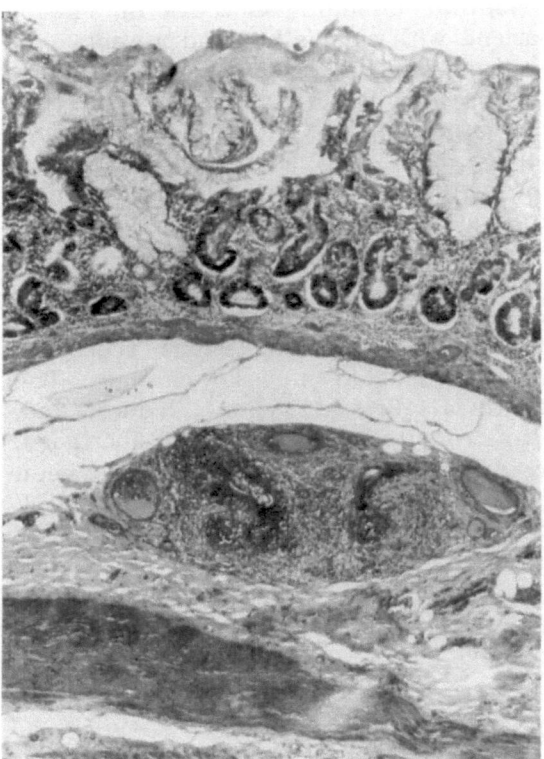

Figure 12-7. Polyarteritis nodosa of the stomach. Submucosal arteries show fibrinoid necrosis and exudative inflammation. Veins are spared. The gastric mucosa shows intestinal metaplasia. Hematoxylin-Phloxine-Saffranin, X50, reproduced at 65%.

Chagas Disease

Chagas disease (also called American trypanosomiasis) is characterized by destruction of intramural neurons in the entire gastrointestinal tract. As a consequence, the stomach is distended, and impaired accommodation to distention produces rapid gastric emptying.[111] The vagus nerve remains intact.

Polyarteritis Nodosa

Virtually any organ may be affected, and the stomach and duodenum are no exception. We have seen marked involvement of gastric submucosal arteries at autopsy (Fig. 12-7). During life, polyarteritis nodosa has been incidentally found in tissues from the cervix, bladder, vas deferens, gallbladder, and bowel, and recently in a gastric polypectomy specimen.[112]

von Willebrand's Disease

Von Willebrand's disease is a coagulation disorder in which a polymeric molecule of the factor VIII antigen, mediating adhesion of circulating platelets to vascular endothelium, is either missing, in the familial form, or inactivated by circulating antibody in the acquired form.[113] Ten cases of gastrointestinal angiodysplasia complicating von Willebrand's disease were reported between 1978 and 1984.[113] Among these, five showed involvement of stomach and/or duodenum. Dilated, ectatic submucosal blood vessels are prone to rupture and bleeding. Immunohistochemical staining for factor VIII antigen was decreased in areas of ectasia, but positive in normal vessels of the adjacent muscularis propria.

Ehlers-Danlos Syndrome

Ligamentous laxity, characteristic of this syndrome, affects not only joints, but also visceral ligaments. Laxity of gastric ligaments and kyphoscoliosis were thought to be causative factors in a case of organo-axial torsion of the stomach in a 63-year-old woman previously diagnosed as Ehlers-Danlos syndrome.[114]

Chediak-Higashi Syndrome

This autosomal-recessive disorder occurs in man and a variety of animals and is characterized by oculocutaneous pigmentary dilution, enhanced susceptibility to viral and bacterial infections, and a high frequency of lymphoma resulting in early death. Leukocytes contain large inclusions, probably derived from lysosomes. Gastric chief and parietal cells in mice were shown to contain similar inclusions, originating from zymogen granules and Golgi apparatus.[115]

von Recklinghausen's Disease

Although gastrointestinal involvement in neurofibromatosis is common (up to 25%[116]) isolated gastric or duodenal involvement is rare.[117] Reticular brown pigmentation of gastric and duodenal mucosa[47] as well as a variety of solid tumors, including neurofibromas, schwannomas, neurofibrosarcomas, ganglioneurofibromas, and leiomyomas, have been described.[118] Rare stromal tumors with minimal smooth muscle differentiation recognizable only ultrastructurally may also be found.[118] These tumors are usually multiple and occur in all sizes. The myenteric plexus, rather than the submucosal plexus, is the most common site of origin. Polypoid and finger-shaped lesions have been seen endoscopically. Once detected, tumors should be excised since they are prone to bleeding (40%)—at times life-threatening—and to malignant degeneration (15%).[118]

Behçet's Disease

Since Behçet[119] described the triple-symptom complex of oral and genital ulceration and ocular inflammation in 1937, the disease named after him has come to include manifestations in a variety of other organs such as muscle, joints, kidney, heart, blood vessels, peripheral and central nervous system, pancreas, and the gastrointestinal tract.[120] Intestinal involvement occurs in about 10% of cases, and presents most commonly as localized ulceration of the ileocecal region. Among 136 cases with intestinal ulcers, only 3 had ulcers in stomach or duodenum.[121] Ulcers may be multiple and, in one case, were associated with pyloric stenosis due to edema and hypertrophy of the pylorus resembling congenital hypertrophic pyloric stenosis.[120]

Ulcers in Behçet's disease are usually undermining, penetrating, and prone to perforation. There is marked edema around the ulcer crater. Behçet's disease is rare in the United States, and most publications on the subject are from Japan and Europe.

Celiac Disease and Dermatitis Herpetiformis

It is beyond the scope of this book to discuss in detail the duodenal pathology of diffuse small intestinal diseases such as celiac disease. Suffice it to say that endoscopic duodenal biopsy in patients with celiac disease has demonstrated mucosal lesions with the same accuracy as upper jejunal capsule biopsy.[122] The larger size of suction-capsule jejunal biopsies, however, allows for better orientation and a greater mucosal area to be examined, and is generally preferred by pathologists. Enterochromaffin cells containing 5-hydroxytryptamine are increased in the duodenal mucosa.[123] The increase specifically affects somatostatin, gastric inhibitory peptide (GIP), cholecystokinin (CCK), and glucagon cells. Secretin cells, in contrast, are reduced in number.[124] This altered cell pattern is not a simple reflection of altered mucosal architecture. Although the increase in somatostatin and GIP cells, both normally predominant in the crypts, can be interpreted as a simple sequela of crypt hyperplasia, and the reduction of secretin cells, normally predominant in the villi, as a sequela of villous atrophy, the increase in CCK cells that are evenly distributed in crypts and villi rebukes such an interpretation. The cause and significance of these endocrine cell changes are therefore still elusive.

Enteropathy associated with dermatitis herpetiformis is histologically identical to that of celiac disease, but the changes tend to be less severe and more patchy in distribution.[125] Consequently, duodenal lesions may be present in the absence of demonstrable jejunal involvement and vice versa. In 8 of 48 patients undergoing multiple duodenal and jejunal biopsies, 17% had duodenal lesions only and 4% had jejunal lesions only.

Pancreatitis

Duodenal ulcer is significantly related to exocrine pancreatic insufficiency and was found in 21% of patients with chronic relapsing pancreatitis.[126]

Duodenal obstruction developed in 13% of patients with chronic pancreatitis[127] and in 1% of patients with acute or acute relapsing pancreatitis.[128] Obstruction is the result of the spread of inflammation into the duodenal wall, at times associated with an intramural hematoma, compression by an indurated mesenteric root, or a pancreatic pseudocyst.[127-129] Some patients develop biliary and duodenal obstruction simulating carcinoma.[127] Endoscopically, thickened and fixed mucosal folds are seen in the duodenal sweep. Histologically, there are edema, inflammation, muscle destruction, and fibrosis. Mural inflammation may extend into the distal stomach. Surgical intervention was necessary in some of the reported cases. Duodenitis without obstruction is common in pancreatitis and was discovered radiologically in 25% of cases.[128] Isolated duodenitis (i.e., not associated with gastritis) is particularly frequent in alcoholic pancreatitis and appears to be related to pancreatitis per se and not alcohol consumption, which is associated with gastritis and goblet cell hyperplasia and gastric metaplasia of the duodenal mucosa.[126]

Retroperitoneal Fibrosis

Extension of retroperitoneal fibrosis into the duodenal area was documented in 7 of the approximately 500 cases published as of 1981.[130,131] The third and fourth portions of the duodenum are narrowed and encased by fibrous tissue, whereas the proximal portion is dilated. Symptoms of obstruction are usually preceded by other manifestations of retroperitoneal fibrosis, usually hydronephrosis, but in one case were the first sign of the disease.[130]

Umbilical Hernia

Umbilical hernias usually contain mobile abdominal structures such as omentum, small intestine, or transverse colon. The rare instance of duodenal obstruction due to strangulation of the pylorus and supraampullary portion of the duodenum was reported in 1981.[132] Gastroptosis was apparently a predisposing factor.

Aortoduodenal Fistula

This complication occurs in up to 4% of aortic aneurysm repairs and may develop anytime between a few days or 14 years after surgery.[133] Although aortic fistulas occur at other sites, the duodenum is the site of perforation in the majority of aortoenteric fistulae.[133,134] Possible mechanisms of development are deterioration of a homograft, usually within a mean interval of 2 years, breakdown of the aortoprosthetic anastomotic suture line (usually proximal and within a mean interval of 3 years), and formation of a false aneurysm proximal to the anastomosis. Graft infection, severe atherosclerosis of the anastomosed aortic segment, and failure to interpose omentum or other tissues between the duodenum and graft have been cited as predisposing factors. Bleeding, the presenting sign in all patients, may be massive and lethal, but in approximately half of the cases is less dramatic and intermittent, allowing sufficient time for diagnostic procedures, primarily endoscopy.[129,130] Endoscopic diagnostic accuracy has been reported between 58 and 100%.[134]

The distal duodenum, especially the medial posterior wall, is the most common site of perforation. Endoscopic visualization of the graft is diagnostic, but active hemorrhage, adherent blood clot at the above mentioned site, or the presence of an extramural pulsating mass is highly suggestive. Early diagnosis is essential since salvage rates with surgery performed prior to massive bleeding are 40 to 85% and mortality without surgery is 100%.

Duodenal Erosion of Mesocaval Shunt

Mesocaval shunt operation using a Dacron interposition graft is widely used in the management of portal hypertension. During the procedure, the second and third portions of the duodenum are mobilized, the graft is interposed between the superior mesenteric vein and the inferior vena cava, and the graft is closely applied to the duodenal wall.[135,136] Erosion of the duodenal wall is secondary to pressure and not necessarily associated with rupture or thrombosis of the graft. The exposed graft, however, may become infected and be the source of septicemia.

Postsplenectomy Gastric Deformity

During splenectomy, the short gastric vessels between the spleen and the greater curvature of the stomach are ligated and cut. Ligating several vessels together, rather than each one separately, may cause infolding of the gastric wall and formation of a submucosal polypoid mass that may be mistaken for tumor, radiologically and endoscopically.[137] Biopsy reveals normal mucosa. At surgery, dense adhesions and occasionally foreign body granulomas are found.

Iatrogenic Gastroduodenal Lesions

Iatrogenic lesions occur as a result of treatment by a physician or surgeon and may be related to a diagnostic procedure, medicinal agents, or therapeutic maneuvers. Some of these, such as aspirin-related gastritis, erosions and ulcers, and endoscopy-induced lacerations, perforations, and hematomas, have already been discussed in previous chapters.

Drug-Related Gastroduodenal Injury

Drug-related gastrointestinal injury is common and accounts for an estimated one-third of adverse drug reactions among hospitalized patients.[138] One of every three gastric ulcers is said to be drug-related.[139] The most commonly implicated agents are aspirin, nonsteroidal antiinflammatory drugs (NSAIDS), potassium chloride (KCl), and iron tablets. Although NSAID-induced damage is generally milder than that caused by aspirin, rare NSAID-induced ulcers may perforate and give rise to a gastrocolic fistula.[140]

Potassium chloride preparations available at present include a wax matrix, slow-release tablet and a microencapsulated preparation. The previously used enteric-coated tablet was withdrawn from the market in 1965 because of severe gastrointestinal toxicity.[141] Controlled endoscopic studies of the two newer preparations showed significantly less injuries with the microencapsulated form.[141] Endoscopically, hyperemia, edema, erosions, or ulcerations were seen in the gastric antrum or gastroesophageal junction in all patients taking wax matrix KCl, regardless of whether there were symptoms, but in only one of six taking the microencapsulated preparation. All patients also took a gastrointestinal transit-delaying anticholinergic agent.

Corticosteroid-related gastrointestinal injury has been the subject of many publications yielding conflicting results.[138] A recent endoscopic study found gastroduodenal lesions in 44% of 25 patients with various disorders. Gastric erosions were most common, followed by duodenal and combined gastroduodenal erosions.[142] One patient developed a gastric ulcer. Injury does not appear to be dose-related, but tends to be more severe in patients with rheumatic diseases than in those with inflammatory bowel disease or skin disorders.[138]

Hepatic arterial infusion of 5-fluoro-2'-deoxuridine (5FUDR), most commonly performed as treatment for liver metastases of a colonic adenocarcinoma, causes severe dyspepsia in 50% of patients, many of whom are found to have erosive gastritis, gastric and duodenal ulcers, and/or gastroduodenitis.[138] Inadvertent infusion of 5FUDR into the gastroduodenal and right gastric arteries may cause necrosis of the gastric wall. Gastric ulcers become clinically apparent 10 to 45 days after therapy and characteristically show severe cytologic mucosal atypia that may be mistaken for carcinoma in situ.[143,144] Certain histologic features, however, are distinctive and aid in the differential diagnosis, namely, the mucosal architecture remains preserved; atypia is accentuated in the basal gastric glands; atypia is more bizarre than that of carcinoma cells but cell enlargement tends to be greater, thus preserving a low nucleo-cytoplasmic ratio; the cytoplasm is eosinophilic and vacuolated; mitotic figures are usually rare or absent, but at times are numerous and bizarre[144]; atypia affects epithelial cells as well as fibroblasts and endothelial cells; and intestinal metaplasia is usually absent.[143] Duodenal mucosal necrosis and crypt cell atypia have also been described after chemotherapy for lymphoblastic lymphoma.[145]

Anticoagulant therapy, especially with warfarin, may cause gastrointestinal hemorrhage and intramural hematomas. The latter are most commonly found in the duodenum, the fixed position of which predisposes the submucosal vessels to tear with intraabdominal pressure changes.[138]

Therapeutic transcatheter arterial embolization for hemorrhage from gastric or duodenal ulcers may, on rare occasions, be complicated by duodenal infarction, gastric infarction, superficial duodenal necrosis, and necrosis of gallbladder, liver, and spleen.[146] Spontaneous duodenal infarction is extremely rare because of the dual vascular supply from both the celiac axis and the superior mesenteric artery. In most of the above cases, the circulation had been compromised by previous surgery or severe atherosclerosis.

Radiation Damage

Radiation injury to the stomach is infrequent because of the protective thick muscular layer and the relatively radioresistant gastric neck glands.[147] In acute radiation injury which occurs within 2 weeks after radiotherapy, chief and and parietal cells are damaged first and the surface epithelium later. Pits become elongated. The connective tissue in mucosa and submucosa shows characteristic changes including edema, congestion, swelling of collagen bundles, and fibrin exudation. Intermediate radiation injury occurs in the subsequent months, and results in endothelial swelling and fibrinoid necrosis of blood vessels. Progressive hyalinization in the late stage leads to ischemic degeneration and necrosis. These are rarely seen in the modern era of radiotherapy, but were described in the older literature as primarily affecting the posterior wall and antrum.[148]

The small intestine is the most radiosensitive segment of the gastrointestinal tract and escapes damage mostly as a result of its great mobility. The duodenum has a particularly low tolerance to radiation because of its fixed position. At 4500 rads, there is a 1 to 5% risk of ulceration, perforation, fibrosis, and obstruction. At 6000 rads, the risk increases to 25 to 50%.[147] Chronic injury resulting in stenosis may develop as late as 19 years after completion of radiotherapy.[149]

References

1. Slovis CM: Massive foreign object ingestion. Ann Emerg Med 1982;11:433–435.
2. Devanesan J, Pisani A, Sharma P, et al: Metallic foreign bodies in the stomach. Arch Surg 1977;112(5):664–665.
3. Vizcarrondo FJ, Brady PG, Nord HJ: Foreign bodies of the upper gastrointestinal tract. Gastrointest Endosc 1983;29:208–210.
4. McCaffery TD, Lilly JD: The management of foreign affairs of the GI tract. Dig Dis 1975;20: 121–126.

5. Griffiths WJ, Bird PC, Zantout I, et al: Fiber-optic endoscopic retrieval of swallowed intragastric foreign objects. OSMA 1979;72:67–71.

6. Eldridge WW: Foreign bodies in the gastrointestinal tract. JAMA 1961;178:665–667.

7. Ertan A, Kedia SM, Agrawal NM, et al: Endoscopic removal of a toothbrush. Gastrointest Endosc 1983;29:144–145.

8. Govila CP: Accidental swallowing of an endodontic instrument. Oral Surg 1979;48:269–270.

9. Raff LJ: Fatal ingestion of a radiolucent dental prosthesis. South Med J 1981;74(7):900–901.

10. Mack JW Jr: Swallowed endotracheal tube: A neonatal emergency. Case report. Milit Med 1981;146(5):354–355.

11. Haney PJ, Gunadi IK, Arnold J, et al: Spontaneous penetration of an antireflux prosthesis into the stomach. Gastrointest Radiol 1983;8:303–305.

12. Solammadevi SV, Hundley RF: Removal of multiple foreign objects from the stomach. Gastrointest Endosc 1983;29:64.

13. Wiest JW, Follette DM, Traverso LW: Toothpick perforation of the duodenum. West J Med 1980;132:157–159.

14. Pickard LR, Tepas JJ, Agarwal BL, et al: Duodeno-renal fistula: An uncommon complication of an ingested foreign body. J Ped Surg 1980;15:337–338.

15. Stahlgren LH, Clearfield HR: Trauma, bezoars, and other foreign bodies in the stomach. In: Berk E (ed). Bockus: Gastroenterology, 4th Ed, Vol 2. Philadelphia: WB Saunders, 1985:1381–1388.

16. Menke JA, Stallworth RE, Binstadt DH, et al: Medication bezoar in a neonate. Am J Dis Child 1982;136:72–73.

17. Rosenburg HK: Antacid bezoar in a premature infant. Clin Pediatr 1982;8:503–504.

18. Deslypere JP, Praet M, Verdonk G: An unusual case of the trichobezoar: The Rapunzel syndrome. Am J Gastroenterol 1982;77:467–470.

19. Brown CH, Schneider RW: Large gastric bezoar; report of case treated medically. Cleve Clin Quart 1951;18:203–206.

20. Grant JA, Murray WR, Patel AR: Giant trichobezoar—an unusual case. Scot Med J 1979;24:83–86.

21. Baudamant WW: Mémoire sur des cheveux trouvés dans l'estomac et dans les intestins grêles. L Med Chir Pharm 1779;52:507–514.

22. DeBakey M, Ochsner A: Bezoars and concretions. Surgery 1938;4:934–963.

23. DeBakey M, Ochsner A: Bezoars and concretions. Surgery 1939;4:132–160.

24. Kadian RS, Rose JF, Mann NS: Gastric bezoars—spontaneous resolution. Am J Gastroenterol 1978;80:70–80.

25. Goldstein HM, Cohen LE, Hagen HO, et al: Gastric bezoars: A frequent complication in the postoperative ulcer patient. Radiology 1973;107:341–344.

26. Rider JR, Foresti-Lorenti RF, Garrido J, et al: Gastric bezoars: Treatment and prevention. Am J Gastroenterol 1984;79:357–359.

27. Trent WN Jr: Phytobezoar formation: A new complication of cimetadin therapy. Ann Intern Med 1981;95:70.

28. Lameron AJ: Trichobezoar: Two case reports—a new physical sign. Am J Gastroenterol 1984;79:354–356.

29. Madura MJ, Naughton, Craig RM: Duodenal bezoar: A case report and review of the literature. Gastrointest Endosc 1982;28:26–28.

30. Case records of the Massachusetts General Hospital; Case 22-1978. N Engl J Med 1978;291:1301–1308.

31. Kommerell B: Klinik und Therapie der Gallenerkrankungen. Boecker IV: Gallenblase-Pankreas. Stuttgart: Thieme, 1975.

32. Peters H, Schubert HJ: Gallensteinileus. Münch Med Wschr 1976;118:1521–1524.

33. Bedogni G, Contini S, Meinero M, et al: Pyloroduodenal obstruction due to a biliary stone (Bouveret's syndrome) managed by endoscopic extraction. Gastrointest Endosc 1985;31:36–38.

34. Weingart J, Wilhelm A, Ottenjann R: Obstruction of the duodenal bulb caused by gallstone perforation. Endoscopy 1979;3:190–192.

35. Nakagawa S, Kobori M, Sato K: A report of 57 cases of amyloidosis in Japan. J Jpn Soc Intern Med 1966;54:59–68.

36. Symmers WSC: Primary amyloidosis, a review. J Clin Pathol 1956;9:187–211.

37. Dahlin DC: Secondary amyloidosis. Ann Intern Med 1949;31:105–119.

38. Ohno F, Numata Y, Yamano T, et al: Gastroscopic biopsy of the stomach for the diag-

nosis of amyloidosis. Gastroenterologia Jpn 1982;17:415–421.

39. Coughlin GP, Reiner RG, Grant AK: Endoscopic diagnosis of amyloidosis. Gastrointest Endosc 1980;26:154–155.

40. Makishita H, Manome T, Tsukada N, et al: Biopsy and study of gastric mucosa in familial amyloid polyneuropathy–with special reference to diagnosis. Clin Neurol 1981; 21:201–208.

41. Steen LE, Oberg L: Familial amyloidosis with polyneuropathy: Roentgenological and gastroscopic appearance of gastrointestinal involvement. Am J Gastroenterol 1983;78: 417–420.

42. Yamada M, Hatakeyama S, Tsukagoshi H: Gastrointestinal amyloid deposition in AL (primary or myeloma-associated) and AA (secondary) amyloidosis: Diagnositic value of gastric biopsy. Hum Pathol 1985;16:1206–1211.

43. Balázs M: Amyloidosis of the stomach. Report of a case with ultrastructure. Virchows Arch (Pathol Anat) 1981;391:227–240.

44. Dastur KJ, Ward JF: Amyloidoma of the stomach. Gastrointest Radiol 1980;5:17–20.

45. Giarelli L, Melato M, Manconi R, et al: Amiloidosi isolata dello stomaco: Carratteristiche istochimiche e suo inquadramento. Pathologica 1980;72:113–118.

46. Levenson OS: Isolated tumor-like amyloidosis of the stomach. Arkh Patol 1979;41(9): 50–52.

47. Rutgeerts P, Hendrickx H, Geboes K, et al: Involvement of the upper digestive tract by systemic neurofibromatosis. Gastrointest Endosc 1981;27:22–25.

48. Cowen ML, Humphries TJ: Pseudomelanosis of the duodenum. Gastrointest Endosc 1980; 26:107–108.

49. Bisordi WM, Kleinman MS: Melanosis duodeni. Gastrointest Endosc 1976;23:37–38.

50. Yamase H, Norris M, Gillies C: Pseudomelanosis duodeni: A clinicopathologic entity. Gastrointest Endosc 1985;31:83–86.

51. Pounder DJ: The pigment of duodenal melanosis is ferrous sulfide. Gastrointest Endosc 1983;29:257.

52. Sharp JR, Insalaco SJ, Johnson LF: "Melanosis" of the duodenum associated with a gastric ulcer and folic acid deficiency. Gastroenterology 1980;78:366–369.

53. Steckman M, Bozymski EM: Hemosiderosis of the duodenum. Gastrointest Endosc 1983; 29:326–327.

54. Conte P, Vello P, Brunelli L, et al: Stainable iron in gastric and duodenal mucosa of primary hemochromatosis patients and alcoholics. Am J Gastroenterol 1987;82:237–238.

55. Bauman MB, DiMase JD, Oski F, et al: Brown bowel and skeletal myopathy associated with Vitamin E depletion in pancreatic insufficiency. Gastroenterology 1968;54:93–100.

56. Ou Tim L, Hurwitz S, Tuch P: The endoscopic diagnosis of gastric calcification. J Clin Gastroenterol 1982;4:213–215.

57. Conger JD, Hammond WS, Alfrey AC, et al: Pulmonary calcification in chronic dialysis patients. Ann Intern Med 1975;83:330–336.

58. Kuzela DC, Huffer WE, Conger JD, et al: Soft tissue calcification in chronic dialysis patients. Am J Pathol 1977;86:403–424.

59. Franzin G, Musola R, Mencarelli R: Changes in the mucosa of the stomach and duodenum during immunosuppressive therapy after renal transplantation. Histopathology 1982; 6:439–449.

60. Valdez VA, Jacobstein JG, Permutter S, et al: Metastatic calcification in the lung and stomach demonstrated on bone scan in multiple myeloma. Clin Nucl Med 1979;4:120–121.

61. Feyrter F: Herdförmige Lipoidablagerungen in der Schleimhaut des Magens. Virchows Arch (Pathol Anat) 1929;273:736–741.

62. Mizuoka S: Clinical and endoscopic studies on xanthomatosis of the stomach. Bull Osaka Med Soc 1969;15:46–60.

63. Kimura K, Hiramoto T, Buncher CR: Gastric xanthelasma. Arch Pathol 1969;87: 110–117.

64. Terruzzi V, Minoli G, Butti G, et al: Gastric lipid islands in the gastric stump and in non-operated stomach. Endoscopy 1980;12:58–62.

65. Domellöf L, Eriksson S, Helander HF, et al: Lipid islands in the gastric mucosa after resection for benign ulcer disease. Gastroenterology 1977;73:462–468.

66. Drude RB, Balart LA, Herrington JP, et al: Gastric xanthoma: Histologic similarity to signet ring cell carinoma. J Clin Gastroenterol 1982;4:217–221.

67. Kunze KC, Baum RA, Nasrallah SM: Gastric xanthoma. Gastrointest Endosc 1987;33: 114–115.

68. Rubin W, Ross LL, Jeffries GH, et al: Some physiologic properties of the heterotopic intestinal epithelium. Its role in transporting lipid into the gastric mucosa. Lab Invest 1967;16:813–827.

69. Kussin SZ, Henry C, Navarro C, et al: Gas within the wall of the stomach. Report of a case and review of the literature. Dig Dis Sci 1982;27:949–954.

70. Kowal LE, Glick SN, Teplick SK: Gastric emphysema resembling pneumoperitoneum: Presentation of a case with a review of the literature. Am J Gastroenterol 1982;77:667–670.

71. Clearfield HR, Stahlgren LH: Acute dilatation, volvulus, and torsion of the stomach. In: Berk E (ed). Bockus: Gastroenterology, 4th Ed, Vol 2. Philadelphia: WB Saunders, 1985:1381–1388.

72. Graham WD: Spontaneous rupture of the stomach in the adult. J Roy Coll Surg Edinburgh 1982;27:368–369.

73. Saul SH, Dekker A, Watson CG: Acute gastric dilatation with infarction and perforation. Report of fatal outcome in patient with anorexia nervosa. Gut 1981;22:978–983.

74. Merrill JR: Gastric necrosis and perforation after fundoplication. South Med J 1981;74:1543–1545.

75. Starr KW: Acute postoperative dilatation of the stomach. Ann Roy Coll Surg 1953;12:71–76.

76. Kerstein MD, Goldberg B, Panter B, et al: Gastric infarction. Gastroenterology 1974;67:1238–1239.

77. Tortorelli AF, Crowley JR: Spontaneous rupture of the stomach: Report of a case. J Oral Surg 1981;39:609–612.

78. Haas PA, Akhtar J, Kobylak L: Compression of the duodenum by the root of mesentery. Henry Ford Hosp Med J 1982;30:85–89.

79. von Rokitansky C: Lehrbuch der Pathologischen Anatomie, 1st Ed. Vienna: Braumüller, 1861:187.

80. Wilkie DPO: Chronic duodenal ileus. Br J Surg 1921;9:204–214.

81. Lundell L, Thulin A: Wilkie's syndrome—a rarity? Br J Surg 1980;67:604–606.

82. Sapkas G, O'Brien JP: Vascular compression of the duodenum (cast syndrome) associated with the treatment of spinal deformities. Arch Orthop Traumat Surg 1981;98:7–11.

83. Rosser SB, Clark CH, Elechi EN: Spontaneous neonatal gastric perforation. J Ped Surg 1982;17:390–394.

84. Holgersen LO: The etiology of spontaneous gastric perforation of the newborn: A reevaluation. J Ped Surg 1981;16:508–613.

85. Herbut PA: Congenital defect in the musculature of the stomach with rupture in a newborn. Arch Pathol 1943;36:91–94.

86. Gapp GA, James AC, Iwen GW, et al: Postemetic rupture of herniated cardia of the stomach. JAMA 1982;247:811.

87. Gallivan GJ: Postemetic rupture of herniated cardia of the stomach. JAMA 1982;247:3186–3187.

88. Mills SA, Paulson D, Scott SM, et al: Tension pneumoperitoneum and gastric rupture following cardiopulmonary resuscitation. Ann Emerg Med 1983;12:94–98.

89. Flint LM, McCoy M, Richardson JD, et al: Duodenal injury. Analysis of common misconceptions in diagnosis and treatment. Ann Surg 1981;19:697–701.

90. Yajko RD, Seydel F, Trimble C: Rupture of the stomach from a blunt abdominal trauma. J Trauma 1975;15:177–183.

91. Richardson G, Schiller WR, Shuck J: Gastric rupture from blunt trauma. Rocky Mt Med J 1979;76:309–310.

92. Semel L, Frittelli G: Gastric rupture from blunt abdominal trauma. NY State J Med 1981;81:938–939.

93. Ghahremani GG, Turner MN, Port RB: Iatrogenic intubation injuries of the upper gastrointestinal tract in adults. Gastrointest Radiol 1980;5:1–10.

94. Cramer FS, Heimbach RD: Stomach rupture as a result of gastrointestinal barotrauma in a scuba diver. J Trauma 1982;22:238–240.

95. Lloyd RG: Delayed rupture of stomach after blunt abdominal trauma. Br Med J 1982;285:176.

96. Melato M, Falconier G, Manconi R, Bucconi S: Intramural hematoma and hemoperitoneum occurring in a patient affected by idiopathic myelofibrosis. Hum Pathol 1980;11:301–302.

97. Vellacott KD: Intramural haematoma of the duodenum. Br J Surg 1980;67:36–38.

98. Moore SN, Erlandson ME: Intramural haematoma of the duodenum. Ann Surg 1963;157:798–809.

99. Patel R, Shaps J: Intramural duodenal

hematoma–a complication of ERCP. Gastrointest Endosc 1982;28:218–219.

100. Proctor HJ, Peacock JB: Pancreatic and duodenal injuries: Morbidity and mortality of surgical management. South Med J 1979; 72:1535–1536.

101. Oglesby JE, Smith DE, Mahoney WD, et al: Complete duodenal transection in blunt trauma. Am J Surg 1968;116:914–916.

102. Snyder WH, Weigelt JA, Watkins WL, et al: The surgical management of duodenal trauma. Arch Surg 1980;115:422–429.

103. Gifford RR Sr, Hymes AC: Duodenal rupture after blunt abdominal trauma. Minn Med 1980;63:83–85.

104. Ryabov SI, Ryss ES, Prochukanov RA, et al: Present-day concepts on gastric pathology on patients with chronic renal failure. Int Urol Nephrol 1980;12:189–197.

105. Zukerman GR, Mills DBA, Koehler RE, et al: Nodular duodenitis. Pathologic and clinical characteristics in patients with end-stage renal disease. Dig Dis Sci 1983;28:1018–1023.

106. Mangla JC, Pereira M, Bhargava A: Nodular duodenitis in chronic maintenance hemodialysis patients. Gastrointest Endosc 1985;31: 318–323.

107. Goldstein DA, Horowitz RE, Petit S, et al: The duodenal mucosa in patients with renal failure: Response to 1,25(OH)$_2$D$_3$. Kidney Int 1981;19:324–331.

108. Rock E, Malmud L, Fisher RS: Motor disorders of the stomach. Med Clin North Am 1981;65:1269–1284.

109. Gramm HF, Renter K, Costello P: The radiologic manifestations of diabetic gastric neuropathy and its differential diagnosis. Gastrointest Radiol 1978;3:151–155.

110. Muls EE, Lamberigts GF: Uncontrolled diabetes mellitus due to gastroparesis diabeticorum: Treatment with metoclopramide. Postgrad Med J 1981;57:185–188.

111. Oliveira RB, Troncon LEA, Meneghelli UG, et al: Impaired gastric accommodation to distension and rapid gastric emptying in patients with Chagas' disease. Dig Dis Sci 1980;25:790–794.

112. Mulshine P, Calabrese L, Krakauer RS: Polyarteritis nodosa diagnosed by endoscopic polypectomy. Arthritis Rheum 1980;23:257–258.

113. Duray PH, Marcal JM, LiVolsi V, et al: Gastrointestinal angiodysplasia: A possible component of von Willebrand's disease. Hum Pathol 1984;15:539–544.

114. Padke JG: Ehlers-Danlos syndrome with surgical repair of eventration of diaphragm and torsion of stomach. J Roy Soc Med 1979;72: 781–783.

115. Sato A, Spicer SS: An ultrastructural and cytochemical investigation of the development of inclusions in gastric chief cells and parietal cells of mice with the Chediak-Higashi syndrome. Lab Invest 1981;44:288–295.

116. Davis GB, Berk RN: Intestinal neurofibromas in von Recklinghausen's disease. Am J Gastroenterol 1973;60:410–414.

117. Hoare AM, Elkington SG: Gastric lesions in generalized neurofibromatosis. Br J Surg 1976;63:499–451.

118. Schaldenbrand JD, Appelman HD: Solitary solid stromal gastrointestinal tumors in von Recklinghausen's disease with minimal smooth muscle differentiation. Hum Pathol 1984;15:229–232.

119. Behçet H: Über rezidivierende, aphtöse, durch Virus verursachte Geschwüre am Mund, am Auge, und den Genitalien. Dermatol Wochenschr 1937;105:1152–1157.

120. Satake K, Yada K, Ikehara T, et al: Pyloric stenosis: An unusual complication of Behçet's disease. Am J Gastroenterol 1986;81:816–818.

121. Kasahara Y, Tanaka S, Nishino M, et al: Intestinal involvement in Behçet's disease: Review of 136 surgical cases in the Japanese literature. Dis Colon Rectum 1981;24:103–106.

122. Holdstock G, Eade OE, Isaacson P, et al: Endoscopic duodenal biopsies in coeliac disease and duodenitis. Scand J Gastroenterol 1979;14:717–720.

123. Sjölund K, Alumets J, Berg N-O, et al: Enteropathy of coeliac disease in adults: Increased number of enterochromaffin cells in the duodenal mucosa. Gut 1982;23:42–48.

124. Sjölund K, Alumets J, Berg N-O, et al: Duodenal endocrine cells in adult coeliac disease. Gut 1979;20:547–552.

125. Gillberg R, Kastrup W, Mobacken H, et al: Endoscopic duodenal biopsy compared with biopsy with the Watson capsule from the upper jejunum in patients with dermatitis herpetiformis. Scand J Gastroenterol 1982; 17:305–308.

126. Piubello W, Vantini I, Scuro LA, et al: Gas-

tric secretion, gastroduodenal histological changes, and serum gastrin in chronic alcoholic pancreatitis. Am J Gastroenterol 1982; 77:105–110.

127. Kozarek RA, Sanowski RA: Duodenal and common bile duct obstruction in pancreatitis simulating carcinoma. J Clin Gastroenterol 1981;3:53–59.

128. Bradley EL, Clements JL: Idiopathic duodenal obstruction. An unappreciated complication of pancreatitis. Ann Surg 1981;193: 638–648.

129. Makrauer FL, Antonioli DA, Banks PA: Duodenal stenosis in chronic pancreatitis. Dig Dis Sci 1982;27:525–531.

130. Violon D, Potvliege R: Retroperitoneal fibrosis involving the duodenum. Fortschr Röntgenstr 1981;134:93–94.

131. Siegel GJ, Hall JM, Welling RE: Idiopathic retroperitoneal fibrosis with functional duodenal obstruction. South Med J 1980;73: 946–948.

132. Bjorgsvik D, Baardsen A: Umbilical hernia with duodenal obstruction. Acta Chir Scand 1981;147:295.

133. Brand EJ, Sivak MV, Sullivan BH: Aortoduodenal fistula. Endoscopic diagnosis. Dig Dis Sci 1979;24:940–944.

134. Champion MC, Sullivan SN, Watson WC: Aortoduodenal fistula: Endoscopic diagnosis. Dig Dis Sci 1980;25:811.

135. Wexler RM, Falchuk KR, Horst DA, et al: Duodenal erosion of a mesocaval graft: An unusual complication of mesocaval shunt interposition surgery. Gastroenterology 1980;79:729–730.

136. Osborne DR, Hobbs KEF: Dacron graft erosion of the duodenum: A complication of interposition mesocaval shunt operations. Br J Surg 1981;68:483–484.

137. Ansel HJ, Wasserman NF: Postsplenectomy gastric deformity. Am J Radiol 1982;139: 99–101.

138. Lewis JH: Gastrointestinal injury due to medicinal agents. Am J Gastroenterol 1986; 81:819–833.

139. Kumar GK, Razzaque MA, Naiou VG, et al: Gastrocolic fistula in benign peptic ulcer disease. Ann Surg 1976;18:236–240.

140. Faurel JP, Delas N, Saigot T, et al: Fistule gastro-colique secondaire a un ulcere medicamenteux. Med Chir Dig 1981;10:621–622.

141. Barkin JS, Harary AM, Shamblen CE, et al: Potassium chloride and gastrointestinal injury. Ann Intern Med 1983;98:261–262.

142. Okada M, Fuchigami T, Iida M, et al: Adrenocorticosteroid therapy and gastroduodenal lesions. Gastrointest Endosc 1985;31:188–190.

143. Petras RE, Hart WR, Bukowski RM: Gastric epithelial atypia with hepatic arterial infusion chemotherapy. Its distinction from early gastric carcinoma. Cancer 1985;56: 745–750.

144. Jewell LD, Fields AL, Murray CJW, et al: Erosive gastroduodenitis with marked epithelial atypia after hepatic arterial infusion chemotherapy. Am J Gastroenterol 1985;80:421–424.

145. Lubitz L, Ekert H: Reversible changes in duodenal mucosa associated with intensive chemotherapy followed by autologous marrow rescue. Lancet 1979;2:532–533.

146. Shapiro N, Brandt L, Sprayregan S, et al: Duodenal infarction after therapeutic gelfoam embolization of a bleeding duodenal ulcer. Gastroenterology 1981;80:176–180.

147. Roswit B, Malsky SJ, Reid CB: Severe radiation injuries of the stomach, small intestine, colon, and rectum. Am J Roentgenol Radiol Ther Nucl Med 1972;114:460–475.

148. Warren S, Friedman NB: Pathology and pathologic diagnosis of radiation lesions in the gastrointestinal tract. Am J Pathol 1942;18:499–507.

Index

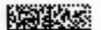